ORTHOPAEDIC CARE
of the
MATURE ATHLETE

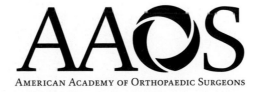

AMERICAN ACADEMY OF ORTHOPAEDIC SURGEONS

ORTHOPAEDIC CARE
of the
MATURE ATHLETE

Andrew L. Chen, MD, MS
Editor

Nicholas A. DiNubile, MD
Richard J. Hawkins, MD
John M. Tokish, MD
Section Editors

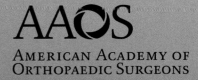

AAOS
AMERICAN ACADEMY OF
ORTHOPAEDIC SURGEONS

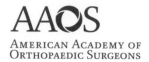

AMERICAN ACADEMY OF
ORTHOPAEDIC SURGEONS

The material presented in *Orthopaedic Care of the Mature Athlete* has been made available by the American Academy of Orthopaedic Surgeons for educational purposes only. This material is not intended to present the only, or necessarily best, methods or procedures for the medical situations discussed, but rather is intended to represent an approach, view, statement, or opinion of the author(s) or producer(s), which may be helpful to others who face similar situations.

Some drugs or medical devices demonstrated in Academy courses or described in Academy print or electronic publications have not been cleared by the Food and Drug Administration (FDA) or have been cleared for specific uses only. The FDA has stated that it is the responsibility of the physician to determine the FDA clearance status of each drug or device he or she wishes to use in clinical practice.

Furthermore, any statements about commercial products are solely the opinion(s) of the author(s) and do not represent an Academy endorsement or evaluation of these products. These statements may not be used in advertising or for any commercial purpose.

Published 2011 by the
American Academy of Orthopaedic Surgeons
6300 North River Road
Rosemont, IL 60018

Copyright 2011
by the American Academy of Orthopaedic Surgeons

ISBN 978-0-89203-633-2

Printed in the USA

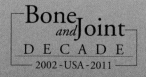

Acknowledgments

Contributors

Joshua Baumfeld, MD
Department of Orthopaedic Surgery
Lahey Clinic
Burlington, Massachusetts

Rob Bell, MD
Chief, Shoulder Section
Department of Orthopaedics
Crystal Clinic Orthopaedic Center
Akron, Ohio

Karen K. Briggs, MPH
Director of Clinical Research
Steadman Philippon Research Institute
Vail, Colorado

Andrew L. Chen, MD, MS
Head Team Physician
United States Ski Jumping
The Alpine Clinic
Franconia, New Hampshire

J.C. Clark, MD
Fellow
Orthopaedic Surgery and Sports Medicine
Steadman-Hawkins Clinic of the Carolinas
Greenville, South Carolina

Alexis Colvin, MD
Assistant Professor
Department of Orthopaedic Surgery
Mount Sinai School of Medicine
New York, New York

Christopher B. Dewing, MD
Lieutenant Commander, United States Navy
Staff Physician
Department of Orthopedic Surgery
Naval Medical Center
San Diego, California

Nicholas A. DiNubile, MD
Clinical Assistant Professor
Department of Orthopaedic Surgery
Hospital of the University of Pennsylvania
Philadelphia, Pennsylvania

Rafael F. Escamilla, PhD, PT, CSCS, FACSM
Professor
Department of Physical Therapy
California State University
Sacramento, California
Results Physical Therapy and Training Center
Sacramento, California
Andrews-Paulos Research and Education Institute
Gulf Breeze, Florida

Evan L. Flatow, MD
Lasker Professor and Chairman
Department of Orthopaedic Surgery
Mount Sinai School of Medicine
New York, New York

Brett Franklin, MD
Sportsmed Orthopaedic Surgery and Spine Center
Huntsville, Alabama

Lawrence W. Gaul, MD
Cardiologist
USSA Nordic Ski Team Physician
Departments of Sport and General Cardiology
Vail Valley Medical Center
Vail, Colorado

Alan M.J. Getgood, MD, FRCS (Tr & Orth)
Clinical Fellow
Fowler Kennedy Sport Medicine Clinic
London, Ontario, Canada

J. Robert Giffin, MD, FRCSC
Associate Professor
Department of Orthopaedic Surgery
Fowler Kennedy Sport Medicine Clinic
University of Western Ontario
London, Ontario, Canada

Laura Dunn Goldberg, MD
Clinical Staff
Department of Orthopedics
Cleveland Clinic Foundation
Lorain, Ohio

Victor M. Goldberg, MD
Professor
Department of Orthopaedic Surgery
University Hospitals Case Medical Center
Cleveland, Ohio

Andreas H. Gomoll, MD
Assistant Professor of Orthopaedic Surgery
Cartilage Repair Center
Brigham & Women's Hospital
Boston, Massachusetts

William Hallier, MD
Orthopaedic Surgery Resident
Department of Orthopaedic Surgery
Wilford Hall Medical Center
San Antonio, Texas

Richard J. Hawkins, MD
Orthopaedic Surgeon
Steadman Hawkins Clinic of the Carolinas
Greenville Hospital System University Medical Center
Greenville, South Carolina

William L. Healy, MD
Chairman
Department of Orthopaedic Surgery
Lahey Clinic
Burlington, Massachusetts

**Todd R. Hooks, PT, SCS, ATC, MOMT,
   MTC, CSCS**
Facility Director
Champion Sports Medicine
Tuscaloosa, Alabama

Atul F. Kamath, MD
Clinical Instructor
Department of Orthopaedic Surgery
University of Pennsylvania
Philadelphia, Pennsylvania

Michael J. Kissenberth, MD
Assistant Professor of Clinical Orthopaedic Surgery
University of South Carolina School of Medicine
Steadman Hawkins Clinic of the Carolinas
Greenville Hospital System
Greenville, South Carolina

Ky Kobayashi, MD
Chief of Hand Surgery
Assistant Professor of Surgery
Uniformed Services University of the Health Sciences
Department of Orthopaedic Surgery
United States Air Force Academy
Colorado Springs, Colorado

Matthew J. Kraay, MS, MD
Kingsbury G. Heiple and Fred A. Lennon Professor of
   Orthopaedics
Department of Orthopaedic Surgery
University Hospitals Case Medical Center
Case Western Reserve University
Cleveland, Ohio

David M. Lutton, MD
Attending Surgeon
Washington Circle Orthopaedics Associates
Washington, DC

Leonard C. Macrina, MSPT, SCS, CSCS
Sports Certified Physical Therapist
Certified Strength and Conditioning Specialist
Champion Sports Medicine
Birmingham, Alabama

Ryan Miyamoto, MD
Attending Surgeon
Fair Oaks Orthopaedics
Fairfax, Virginia

Daniel Fulham O'Neill, MD, EdD
Surgeon
Department of Orthopaedics and Sports Medicine
The Alpine Clinic
Plymouth, New Hampshire

Bradford Parsons, MD
Assistant Professor
Department of Orthopaedic Surgery
Mount Sinai School of Medicine
New York, New York

Brett C. Perricelli, MD
Resident Physician
Department of Orthopaedics
University of Pittsburgh
Pittsburgh, Pennsylvania

Marc J. Philippon, MD
Head of Hip Research
Associate Clinical Professor
Department of Surgery
Faculty of Health Sciences
McMaster University
Hamilton, Ontario, Canada
Steadman Philippon Research Institute
Vail, Colorado

Gita Pillai, MD
Chief Resident
Department of Orthopaedic Surgery
Mount Sinai School of Medicine
New York, New York

Ben C. Robinson, MD
Chief Resident
Department of Orthopaedics
Wilford Hall Medical Center
Lackland Air Force Base, Texas

William G. Rodkey, DVM
Diplomate, American College of Veterinary Surgeons
Chief Scientific Officer
Steadman Philippon Research Institute
Vail, Colorado

Brian J. Sennett, MD
Chief of Sports Medicine
Department of Orthopaedic Surgery
Penn Sports Medicine
University of Pennsylvania
Philadelphia, Pennsylvania

Frederick S. Song, MD
Attending Orthopaedic Surgeon
Princeton Orthopaedic Associates
Princeton, New Jersey

Bruno Goncalves Schröder e Souza, MD
Visiting Scholar in Hip Arthroscopy and Biomechanics
Department of Clinical Research
Steadman Hawkins Research Foundation
Vail, Colorado

J. Richard Steadman, MD
Founder and Chairman
Department of Clinical Research
The Steadman Philippon Research Institute
Vail, Colorado

Gregory Stranges, MD
Assistant Professor
Department of Surgery
University of Manitoba
Winnipeg, Manitoba, Canada

Brett A. Sweitzer, MD
Attending Sports Medicine and Shoulder
*   Reconstruction Surgeon*
Department of Orthopaedic Surgery
Albert Einstein Healthcare Network
Philadelphia, Pennsylvania

Michael Thompson, MD
Department of Orthopaedic Surgery
Lahey Clinic
Burlington, Massachusetts

John M. Tokish, MD
Staff Orthopedic Surgeon
Luke Air Force Base
Peoria, Arizona

Eeric Truumees, MD
Attending Spine Surgeon
Brackenridge University Hospital
Director of Spinal Research
Seton Spine and Scoliosis Center
Austin, Texas

Kevin Wilk, PT, DPT
Associate Clinical Director
Champion Sports Medicine
Birmingham, Alabama

Vonda J. Wright, MD
Assistant Professor
Department of Orthopaedic Surgery
University of Pittsburgh Medical Center
Pittsburgh, Pennsylvania

Douglas J. Wyland, MD
Department of Sports Medicine
Steadman Hawkins Clinic of the Carolinas
Greenville Hospital System
Greenville, South Carolina

Foreword

Musculoskeletal ailments have surpassed the common cold as the number one reason for physician visits in the United States. According to the American Academy of Orthopaedic Surgeons (AAOS), approximately 14% of US healthcare dollars are spent on muscle, bone, and joint problems, which amounts to a staggering 4.6% of the gross national product! Although several factors are responsible for this exponential increase in musculoskeletal problems, a clear driving element is the aging population—especially the aging baby boomers.

In the past 100 years, human life expectancy has nearly doubled. In general, people are living longer and looking better than prior generations, but their musculoskeletal frames are failing. This constitutes what Wharton professor Jeremy Siegel calls "the granddaddy of all demographic shifts," a demographic shift that has occurred in a relatively short period of time and will have dramatic economic, social, and health consequences. From an orthopaedic perspective, a mismatch exists between longevity and durability. Evolution certainly does not act fast enough to close that gap anytime soon, so musculoskeletal issues will remain a dominant factor in the healthcare equation. This scenario, in which people seemingly have outlived the warranty on their frames, has created significant challenges.

One of the keys to optimal aging is exercise. Being fit and being active is the closest thing available to the legendary Fountain of Youth. The baby boomers have embraced this concept and were the first generation in which large numbers of individuals have stayed active on aging musculoskeletal frames. Unfortunately, their frames have not always been cooperative, resulting in an explosion of "boomeritis." *Boomeritis* is a term I coined to describe the many musculoskeletal ailments and vulnerabilities of the boomer generation, who, with their tendinitis, arthritis, and bursitis and their "fix-me-itis" mindset have become frequent flyers in many orthopaedic and sports medicine practices.

The good news is that many things can be done to keep individuals active and pain free as they age, including those who wish to compete at high levels in a variety of sports. In fact, a great deal has been learned from the mature athlete in terms of the potential of the human body, as well as its limitations. In many ways, these active, fit, determined individuals have pushed physicians, researchers, and other healthcare providers to innovate in terms of both nonsurgical and surgical solutions.

This first-of-its-kind book, *Orthopaedic Care of the Mature Athlete,* has emerged from an outstanding AAOS conference titled "Boomeritis: Care of the Mature Athlete." I have had the pleasure and honor to be part of the distinguished faculty of this annual comprehensive conference, driven by the leadership and vision of Dr. Richard Hawkins, and originally inspired by a wonderful article, "Orthopaedic Care of the Aging Athlete" by Dr. Andrew Chen. The "Boomeritis" conference has brought together experts in a wide range of both nonsurgical and surgical specialties relating not only to the mature athlete, but also to anyone striving to "extend the warranty" on their frame. *Orthopaedic Care of the Mature Athlete* will prove invaluable to practitioners who treat and advise these individuals.

Dr. Ernst Wynder, one of the fathers of preventive medicine, once said that "it should be the function of medicine to have people die young as late as possible." A healthy frame, or musculoskeletal system, is a critical factor in achieving this goal of healthy, functional aging. *Orthopaedic Care of the Mature Athlete* provides the necessary tools and cutting-edge information for physicians and other healthcare professionals to help active individuals of all ages, especially the mature athlete, age successfully, living both longer and stronger, with an "extended warranty" on their frames.

Nicholas A. DiNubile, MD

Preface

With the aging of the baby boomer population, mature athletes represent the fastest growing sector of the athletic population. Recent media attention has brought issues relevant to the aging athlete to the forefront, and orthopaedic clinicians should be aware of the issues that these athletes face when attempting to return to sport in the presence of musculoskeletal issues. The same "can do" attitude of the baby boomers that contributed to the explosive industrial and financial growth of the United States in the late 20th century also drives the mature athlete to excel in avocation and sport, often in the presence of known musculoskeletal limitations.

Whereas prior generations have forgone athletic activity with age, whether because of injury, lack of interest, or medical comorbidities, the expectations of the contemporary aging population include maintenance of sports activities well into the sunset years, and many of these athletes participate not only at the recreational but also at the competitive level. Accordingly, injury rates in this rapidly expanding population are on the rise. Moreover, most masters athletes have lifelong histories of training and competition and may continue to apply training practices from their youth to their aging frames, which may increase the risk of injury and functional compromise.

The use of nutritional and anti-aging supplements, ergogenic aids, and hormone replacement therapies by masters athletes has become a multibillion-dollar industry. Unfortunately, much of the hype surrounding the use of such therapies is without a scientific basis and has been driven largely by industry. Even medications used in off-label fashion have by and large not been shown to have health benefits and, ironically, in many cases may be detrimental to overall health and longevity.

Increased recent interest in sport-related injury in mature athletes has resulted in much-needed evidence to guide the clinician in a field that historically has been anecdotally based. Historical recommendations were either predicated on the old adage, "If it hurts, don't do it," and consequent decrease in overall activity, or by extrapolation from the care of younger athletes. Fortunately, in keeping with the expectations of today's mature athletes who wish to return to sport, many clinicians now base treatment paradigms on physiologic rather than chronologic age, a practice supported by an ever-growing base of data. Although practical considerations still limit the orthopaedic surgeon's ability to accrue the highest levels of evidence in many cases (for example, it is not feasible to prospectively randomize patients to either participate or not participate in sports for the rest of their lives after total joint arthroplasty), ample evidence now exists to support the notion that mature athletes may participate in sports even in the presence of orthopaedic injury or arthritis, or after surgery.

Orthopaedic Care of the Mature Athlete features the outstanding contributions of respected leaders in the emerging field of sports medicine as applied to the mature individual. The chapters that review nonsurgical issues feature topics that are frequently discussed in the patient interview but are seldom covered in the orthopaedic literature. The surgical topics that are covered emphasize the mature athlete and provide a comprehensive overview to guide the clinician based on the currently available evidence.

I owe a debt of gratitude to the section editors—Nick, Hawk, and J.T.—for their significant contributions in helping to shape this book. I also would like to thank the authors for contributing their valuable time. In addition, I would like to acknowledge the efforts of Marilyn Fox, PhD, Director of Publications; Laurie Braun, Managing Editor; Michelle Bruno, Publications Assistant; and the production staff at the American Academy of Orthopaedic Surgeons for supporting the development of this book and seeing it to completion. Finally, I applaud the efforts of investigators worldwide who continue to expand the horizon in the nascent field of sports medicine as applied to the mature athlete, and I dedicate this book to them. Without their invaluable contributions, *Orthopaedic Care of the Mature Athlete* would not have been possible.

Andrew L. Chen, MD, MS
Editor

Table of Contents

SECTION 1

OVERVIEW AND BASIC SCIENCE OF CHANGES WITH AGING

Andrew L. Chen, MD, MS
Section Editor

Chapter 1

Overview and Demographics of the Aging Athlete

Andrew L. Chen, MD, MS

Key Points
- The rate of expansion of the aging population of the United States currently far exceeds that of the general population.
- Although aging is inevitable, the anatomic and physiologic changes of aging may be modifiable by regular exercise. The natural history of many disease processes has similarly been shown to be favorably altered by regular exercise.
- Increasingly, older individuals are interested in sports and exercise participation; however, there is a paucity of data to guide recommendations on whether such participation is prudent. This is particularly the case in the setting of injury and/or surgery, such as total joint arthroplasty.
- Treatment must be individualized to the patient, in the context of his or her functional capacity and overall health status.

Introduction

Many individuals maintain high levels of athletic participation into middle age and beyond. The recent emphasis on exercise and fitness in this age group has led to an increased awareness of the anatomic, physiologic, and psychosocial differences between older athletes and their younger counterparts. Age-related structural and biochemical changes occur at the molecular level; these changes ultimately manifest in physiologic alterations that affect every organ system. Although such changes are highly individual, it is becoming increasingly clear that athletic capacity may be maintained well into old age and that many of the "inevitable" physiologic consequences of aging may be mitigated or reversed by regular exercise.

Aging represents a constellation of time-related anatomic, cognitive, and physiologic changes that traditionally had been thought to result in physical decline and a progressive loss of functional capacity and adaptive capability. The rate of aging is highly individual, but the net results of aging are the gradual impairment of organ systems and the depletion of functional reserves that result in an increasing vulnerability to environmental stresses, metabolic disturbances, and disease processes.[1] Recent evidence suggests that functional deterioration and loss of independence are not inevitable consequences of chronologic age, however, and that the so-called effects of aging may be more a result of a long-term sedentary lifestyle.[2,3]

Some authors have suggested a linear decline in the functional reserves of most body systems after the third decade of life,[1] but studies of masters athletes indicate that regular exercise may minimize the effects of aging. Maintenance of an active lifestyle is important for physical and mental well-being, and it may affect longevity.[2] Regular exercise has been shown to reduce premature mortality from cerebrovascular and coronary artery disease, hypertension, and diabetes mellitus[3] and can have profound effects on musculoskeletal function and obesity.

The Aging Population

In Western industrialized countries, the average life expectancy increased from 47 years in 1900 to 78 years in 2007.[4] Increased life expectancy and a post–World War II baby boom in the United States have contributed to a rapidly growing older population; accordingly, the number of individuals older than 85 years grew 232% from 1960 to 1990, compared with a total population growth of 39% during the same period.[5]

The "baby boomer" population is defined as those born between 1946 and 1964. By 2004, all baby boomers were older than 40 years, and half were older than 50 years. In 2008, the first baby boomer was eligible to collect Social Security benefits.[6] In 2008, the US Census Bureau projected that by the year 2025, Americans older than 55 years would represent almost 30% of the population, whereas more than 47% of the population would be older than 40 years.[7] In 2011, the first baby boomers became eligible for Medicare benefits. By 2030, 20% of the population of the United States will be older than 65 years.[8]

Increasingly, older individuals are asking their healthcare providers about the advisability of continued physical activity and sports.[3] Many are encouraged by healthcare providers to participate in regular physical activity to address conditions such as obesity, cardiovascular disease, diabetes mellitus, and chronic illness, but most people engage in physical activity to maintain general health and for enjoyment. The same "can do" attitude of the baby boomer generation that led to the explosive industrial and financial growth of the United States since the early 1970s often pervades the avocational aspects of their lives, resulting in an unwillingness to curtail or cease physical activity just because they are getting older.

A great deal of recent research has focused on aging as it relates to physical activity and sports. In the general population, regular exercise has been shown to be beneficial in addressing obesity, hypertension, coronary artery disease, diabetes mellitus, osteoporosis, and low back pain. It also has been shown to be beneficial for smoking cessation programs.[9] Moreover, regular exercise has been shown to be effective in reducing anxiety and depression and has been independently linked to improved longevity.[10] As a result, more older individuals participate in regular exercise and sports than ever before.

Orthopaedic surgeons often care for athletes and older individuals, but it is the group of *athletically active older individuals* that is the subject of intense interest in the relatively nascent field of the science of sports and aging. For example, certain surgical procedures, such as anterior cruciate ligament reconstruction, that have historically been reserved for younger athletes are now performed in older patients who are active in sports and in whom nonsurgical management has failed. The emphasis has shifted to physiologic rather than chronologic age. Conversely, other surgical procedures, such as total joint arthroplasty, that were designed for older, more sedentary individuals, are increasingly performed in younger patients who have severe, debilitating arthropathy. These patients are of particular interest because our technical ability to perform such procedures has not been correlated with substantial evidence that such practice is advisable or recommended. That is to say, just because it *can* be done, the question remains— *should* it be done? In general, well-controlled, randomized prospective studies with adequate follow-up (ie, level I and II evidence) are lacking, and, despite a recent emphasis on evidence-based medicine, most data regarding a return to sports after joint arthroplasty come from level IV and V studies (see **Sidebar: Levels of Evidence** on page 3). Higher level evidence is likely to remain scarce because practical considerations limit the ability to effectively randomize physical activity after joint arthroplasty (ie, mandating that a patient either perform or avoid physical activity after surgery) for the more than 15 to 20 years needed to evaluate implant longevity.

Despite such limitations, current evidence for participation in sports after arthroplasty is encouraging, and, as prosthetic techniques and technology continue to develop, patient expectations will evolve as well. For example, goals after joint arthroplasty historically centered on pain relief and basic mobility, deformity correction, and return to activities of daily living. Contemporary expectations, however, also include functional independence, social mobility, psychologic well-being, and, increasingly, a return to exercise and sports.[11,12] The growing aging population coupled with performance of joint arthroplasty in an increasingly younger age group have led to projections that these procedures would be performed in sharply increasing numbers. In 2007, it was projected that between 2005 and 2030, total hip and knee arthroplasty procedures would increase by 174% and 673%, respectively, and revision total hip and knee arthroplasty procedures would rise by 137% and 601%, respectively.[13] It was projected that in 2011, more than 50% of total hip replacements would be performed on patients younger than 65 years, and by 2016, more than 50% of total knee arthroplasty procedures would be performed in this age group.[13] By current estimates, the fastest growing group of patients will be those between 45 and 54 years of age; between 2005 and 2030, the prevalence of total knee and hip arthroplasty procedures in this group is projected to increase 17-fold and 6-fold, respectively.[14] This will have dire implications for the practice of orthopaedic medicine, because current estimates predict a shortage of orthopaedic surgeons who perform total joint arthroplasty and, in particular, surgeons who perform complex revision joint arthroplasty.[13,14] Undoubtedly, this also will have profound implications for the already financially burdened payer system in the United States because most patients who currently undergo total joint arthroplasty are older than 65 years of age and thus are covered by Medicare.

Treating the Aging Athlete

In 1996, the American Academy of Orthopaedic Surgeons established the Committee on Aging to address concerns about the orthopaedic care of the older popu-

lation. Since then, geriatric issues have received increased attention at national orthopaedic meetings,[15,16] with an emphasis on injury prevention and physical fitness.[17]

As general orthopaedic practitioners, team physicians, and consultants to sporting events, orthopaedic surgeons often are the first medical professionals to evaluate an athlete in the immediate postinjury period. With the continued growth of the older population and the acceptance of the importance of physical activity for older individuals, it is increasingly important for the orthopaedic surgeon to maintain a working knowledge of the anatomic and physiologic bases of aging and to be able to differentiate these "normal" processes from

---

Levels of Evidence: Investigating the Results of Treatment

Level I
- High-quality randomized controlled trial with statistically significant difference or no statistically significant difference but narrow confidence intervals
- Systematic review of level I randomized controlled trials (and study results were homogeneous)

Level II
- Lesser-quality randomized controlled trial (eg, <80% follow-up, no blinding, or improper randomization)
- Prospective comparative study
- Systematic review of level II studies or level I studies with inconsistent results

Level III
- Case-control study
- Retrospective comparative study
- Systematic review of level III studies

Level IV
- Case series

Level V
- Expert opinion

Adapted with permission from *The Journal of Bone and Joint Surgery*: Instructions to Authors. Updated February 28, 2011.

---

pathologic entities. From a musculoskeletal standpoint, chronic and overuse injuries predominate, reflecting the ultrastructural and compositional changes that result in diminished flexibility and endurance and in degenerative changes. Importantly, many aging individuals have concomitant medical issues that mandate tailoring the physical activity components of the treatment plan to the patient's general health and functional requirements. The return to athletic participation must be individualized, as it may be affected by underlying musculoskeletal conditions such as osteoarthritis or by surgery such as total joint arthroplasty. Treatment must therefore be customized to the specific functional requirements of the patient in the context of his or her general health. The duration of treatment and the patient's ability to physically or mentally comply with a given treatment plan will ultimately affect the success of functional recovery; it is therefore essential that the physician individualize conditioning or rehabilitative regimens based on known physical or cognitive limitations.

References

1. Menard D, Stanish WD: The aging athlete. *Am J Sports Med* 1989;17(2):187-196.

2. Wilmore JH: The aging of bone and muscle. *Clin Sports Med* 1991;10(2):231-244.

3. US Department of Health and Human Services: *Physical Activity and Health: A Report of the Surgeon General*. Atlanta, GA, Centers for Disease Control and Prevention, National Center for Chronic Disease Prevention and Health Promotion, 1996.

4. National Center for Health Statistics: *Health, United States, 2010: With Special Feature on Death and Dying*. Hyattsville, MD, 2011, p 74. http://www.cdc.gov/nchs/data/hus/hus10.pdf#022. Accessed September 9, 2011.

5. US Department of Commerce, Bureau of the Census: *Current Population Reports: Sixty-Five Plus in America*. Washington, DC, US Government Printing Office, 1993.

6. Porucznik MA: How many orthopaedists does it take to...? Is the United States facing a shortage of orthopaedic surgeons? *AAOS Now* 2007;1(7). http://www.aaos.org/news/bulletin/sep07/cover1.asp. Accessed Apr 28, 2010.

7. US Census Bureau, Population Division: *2008 National Population Projections*. Washington, DC, US Census Bureau. Released August 2008. http://www.census.gov/population/www/projections/2008projections.html. Accessed September 9, 2011.

8. US Department of Commerce, Bureau of the Census: *Current Population Reports: Statistical Abstract of the United States: The National Data Book, 1998*. Washington, DC, US Government Printing Office, 1998.

9. Pollock ML, Wilmore MH: *Exercise in Health and Disease: Evaluation and Prescription for Prevention and Rehabilitation*, ed 2. Philadelphia, PA, WB Saunders, 1990, pp 1-2.

10. Barry HC, Eathorne SW: Exercise and aging: Issues for the practitioner. *Med Clin North Am* 1994;78(2):357-376.

11. Laupacis A, Bourne R, Rorabeck C, et al: The effect of elective total hip replacement on health-related quality of life. *J Bone Joint Surg Am* 1993;75(11):1619-1626.

12. Weiss JM, Noble PC, Conditt MA, et al: What functional activities are important to patients with knee replacements? *Clin Orthop Relat Res* 2002(404):172-188.

13. Kurtz S, Ong K, Lau E, Mowat F, Halpern M: Projections of primary and revision hip and knee arthroplasty in the United States from 2005 to 2030. *J Bone Joint Surg Am* 2007;89(4):780-785.

14. Kurtz SM, Lau E, Ong K, Zhao K, Kelly M, Bozic KJ: Future young patient demand for primary and revision joint replacement: National projections from 2010 to 2030. *Clin Orthop Relat Res* 2009;467(10):2606-2612.

15. Buckwalter JA, Heckman JD, Petrie DP; AOA: An AOA critical issue: Aging of the North American population: New challenges for orthopaedics. *J Bone Joint Surg Am* 2003;85-A(4):748-758.

16. Cohen PZ, Strauss E: Symposium: The problematic effects of aging on orthopaedic surgery: An epidemic with major impact. *70th Annual Meeting Proceedings*. Rosemont, IL, American Academy of Orthopaedic Surgeons. New Orleans, LA, February 5-9, 2003, pp 294-296.

17. Kober S: Committee on aging brings awareness to needs of elderly. *Orthopedics Today* 2002;11:32-33.

Chapter 2
Systemic Changes With Aging

Andrew L. Chen, MD, MS

Key Points
- Aging is an individual process that is influenced by a variety of factors.
- Systemic effects of aging:
  Cardiovascular function and work capacity gradually decrease.
  Pulmonary aerobic performance decreases as a function of diminished total lung capacity.
  Renal filtration and urine-concentrating capacity decrease.
  Changes occur in peripheral and central nervous system function that may affect motor control, cognition, and judgment.
  Changes occur in endocrine function that may affect hormonal balance and organ function.
- Many older athletes face psychosocial challenges that affect day-to-day life and sports activities.

Introduction

With the recent emphasis on physical activity in older individuals, it is important for the orthopaedic surgeon to maintain a working knowledge of the anatomic and physiologic changes of normal aging and to be able to differentiate them from pathological entities. These changes may explain why declines in physical performance occur with normal aging, as well as provide some understanding of how physical exercise may mitigate, although not completely abolish, the cumulative effects of aging. This chapter reviews current theories of why aging occurs, as well as systemic changes that may be relevant to the treating orthopaedic surgeon.

Physiologic Effects

The etiology of aging is unknown, but many theories have been advanced (**Table 1**).[1-4] Biologic theories generally postulate that cumulative insults from the environment (ultraviolet light, radiation, etc), metabolic waste, or wear and tear result in progressive injuries to cells that are not adequately repaired by the body. Genetic theories suggest that with successive generations of cell division, the fidelity of transfer of genetic information is compromised (eg, by mutation or shortening of telomeres), which results in gradual degradation of the genetic code. Evolutionary and "aging clock" theories postulate that aging occurs in a predetermined, fatalistic fashion, either based on passing reproductive age

Table 1: Theories of Aging[a]

Biologic Theories

Reproductive-cell cycle theory	Antagonistic pleiotropic cell signaling may be regulated by reproductive hormones in a manner that supports growth and development early in life. After the reproductive stage of life, hormonal patterns then drive cell senescence.
Cumulative damage theory	Aging occurs as a result of accumulation of injuries that are incompletely addressed or healed by the body.
Somatic mutation theory	Accumulated somatic mutations occur with time and may ultimately compromise genetic integrity of somatic cells.
Accumulative waste theory	Metabolic by-products and waste accumulation within cells may interfere with cellular efficiency and metabolic processes, thus leading to aging.
Autoimmune theory	In some individuals, autoantibodies may contribute to cellular death.
Cross-linkage theory	Aging results from accumulation of cross-linked compounds that interfere with normal cell function.
Free radical theory	Free radicals and reactive oxygen compounds may lead to cumulative oxidative stress that may interfere with basic metabolic cellular functions. *Mitohormesis* refers to such damage within mitochondria, which may lead to mitochondrial dysfunction.
Misrepair accumulation theory	At the cellular level, defective structures are incorrectly or incompletely repaired to guarantee the immediate survival of the cell. In this theory, misrepair compromises ultimate longevity for short-term survival. The subsequent cellular damage results in suboptimal cellular function that is recognized as aging.

Genetic Theories

Telomere theory	Telomeres are known to shorten with cell division. By a mechanism that is not fully understood, the shortened telomeres discourage further cell division. This is thought to be important in tissues in which cell replication is important, such as arterial endothelium and marrow tissues.
Genetic error accumulation theory	Imperfect genetic proofreading mechanisms may gradually degrade genetic integrity, particularly with passage to successive generations of cells.

Evolutionary and Aging Clock Theories

Evolutionary theory	Subtle differences in cellular makeup may account for observed differences in organism survival.
Aging clock theory	Aging may occur in a programmed cell-death fashion (apoptosis). This is thought to occur in the central and peripheral nervous systems and may occur in the endocrine system as well, leading to altered hormonal patterns as compared with younger individuals.

Table 1: *(continued)*

Societal Theories

Disengagement theory	This controversial theory suggests that aging individuals progressively disengage from active roles in society. Proponents contend that not only is this normal and appropriate, but this benefits both society and older individuals.
Activity theory	This theory suggests that physical and social activity level is correlated with satisfaction with life. Proponents also suggest that greater social activity earlier in life may be related to satisfaction and well-being in adulthood.
Selectivity theory	Well-being and life satisfaction may be related to disengagement in certain aspects of people's lives, and more activity in others.
Continuity theory	Aging individuals attempt to maintain the same habits, personalities, and lifestyle of their younger years; this enables them to adapt to life changes to maintain their sense of self and well-being, although all these habits and activities may be products of their era rather than a valid, universal theory.

[a]Information adapted from references 1 through 4.

(evolutionary theory) or modulated by neuroendocrine pathways (aging clock theory). Societal theories attempt to correlate aging behavior and well-being with societal norms.[1-4] To a certain extent, scientific evidence for most of these theories can be demonstrated in the laboratory, but no theory sufficiently addresses all aspects of the aging process. Aging is a complex and individual process that is influenced by heredity, ethnicity, environment, diet, physical activity, injury, illness, and culture, among other factors.

Although aging is an individual process, age-related structural and functional changes occur at the molecular level and affect the physiologic performance of virtually every organ system (**Table 2**). Regular physical exercise may affect aging to a variable extent,[5] but changes in physiologic function are well documented and occur in a predictable fashion. At the cellular level, aging results in decreased capacity for division and repair. Intracellular accumulation of lipids and pigments occurs, and cell function becomes gradually impaired. Changes in cell membranes impair the exchange of nutrition, waste, and oxygen and affect cellular metabolism and efficiency. At the tissue level, waste products accumulate, particularly in individuals older than 30 years. Lipofuscin, a fatty brown pigment that is deposited from the breakdown and absorption of damaged erythrocytes, collects in many tissues, particularly myocardium and smooth muscle. Because of its known association with senescence, lipofuscin is also referred to as "the aging pigment."

Molecular and ultrastructural changes in connective tissue result in increased stiffness, decreased elasticity, and increased propensity to degeneration and injury. Diminished chondrocyte population and cellular division result in decreased capacity for repair. The biomaterial changes in connective tissues alter the biomechanical performance of these tissues at the organ level, ultimately affecting clinical function and response to injury. This occurs in virtually all connective tissues and affects organs, blood vessels, neural tissues and joints.

Sarcopenia, or loss of muscle mass, which begins in the late 20s in men and in the 40s in women, results in loss of strength and lean body mass. Although the rate at which such atrophy occurs is genetically related, the rate and extent can be modified to a certain extent by diet and exercise. The muscle fibers themselves demonstrate reduced tone and contractility and, as the atrophic changes occur, muscle mass may be replaced by tough, fibrous, noncontractile tissue. These processes are covered in greater detail in chapter 3.

Aging predictably results in the gradual decline of normal organ function. However, because of functional reserve, until advanced loss of function occurs, most individuals do not notice gradual declines in organ

Table 2: Physiologic Effects of Aging

System	Effects of Aging	Modification With Regular Exercise
Cardiovascular	Decreased maximal heart rate Decreased myocardial contractility Decreased stroke volume Decreased oxygen utilization Atherosclerosis Decreased vascular compliance Diminished microcirculation Decreased vascular tone and baroreceptor function	Increased cardiac output Increased oxygen utilization Diminution of atherosclerotic plaques Enhanced vascular compliance Enhanced microvasculature Enhanced vascular tone
Pulmonary	Decreased elasticity Decreased compliance Weaker respiratory effort Increased pulmonary vascular resistance Altered alveolar gas exchange Decreased total lung capacity, vital capacity, and inspiratory/expiratory airflow Increased residual volume Increased ventilation-perfusion ratio	Improved gas exchange Decreased sense of breathlessness Strengthening of respiratory muscles
Renal	Progressive loss of glomeruli Decreased renal perfusion Decreased glomerular filtration rate Decreased specific gravity of urine	Increased renal blood flow, mainly via increased cardiac output
Neurologic	Impaired hearing, short-term memory, cognition, judgment Decreased coordination, balance, fine-motor skills Increased motor response time Decreased visual-spatial orientation Altered sensation and proprioception Decreased peripheral nerve conduction velocity, amplitude, motor unit recruitment	Improved sport-specific skills Improved coordination, balance Improved visual-spatial orientation
Ophthalmologic	Decreased visual acuity and accommodation Diminished peripheral vision, contract sensitivity Impaired ability to adapt to low-light situations	None

Reproduced from Chen AL, Mears SC, Hawkins RJ: Orthopaedic care of the aging athlete. *J Am Acad Orthop Surg* 2005;13(6):407-416.

performance. For example, the potential cardiac functional capacity of a healthy 20-year-old is 10 times that necessary for sustaining life. After age 30 years, however, this capacity declines by an average of approximately 1% annually. The loss of functional reserve often results in diminished capacity to deal with metabolic stress, such as that introduced by medications, injury or illness, psychologic insults, or changes in physical demand (eg, increased level of physical activity).

Cardiovascular System

Age-associated structural changes within the myocardium result in functional changes that may be clinically relevant. With time, fatty deposits may occur within the myocardium, and the development of fibrous tissue may interrupt the normal conduction pathways that control rhythm. Loss of sinoatrial nodal cells may result in gradual slowing of the heart rate with age. Additionally, cardiac disease may result in arrhythmias. Gradual hypertrophy of the myocardium contributes to overall increase in heart size with age and may disproportionately affect the left ventricle, resulting in decreased left ventricular volume and slower filling time. Lipofuscin deposits are commonly found in the myocardium of older individuals. Cardiac valves may thicken and lose compliance. Heart valve incompetence, which is not uncommon, may result in cardiac murmurs.

An age-associated decline in cardiac output may be attributed to reductions in the maximal heart rate, myocardial contractility, and stroke volume.[6] The consequence of these changes is an age-related drop in the mVO_2 (myocardial oxygen consumption/utilization) beyond age 35 years; by age 60 years, it is only 75% to 80% of that of a 20-year-old.[7] The reduction in physical work capacity associated with aging, as defined by mVO_2, is caused not just by alterations in cardiac physiology but also by the physical deconditioning that occurs with an increasingly sedentary lifestyle.[8] Regular cardiovascular exercise and endurance training have been shown to increase mVO_2 in individuals up to age 70 years.[9] Perhaps of greatest concern to the aging athlete is exercise-induced myocardial injury. Atherosclerosis and decreased cardiac performance increase the risk of acute myocardial events with heavy physical exertion; this risk is compounded in individuals with sedentary lifestyles who begin intensive training regi-

mens abruptly rather than increasing regular exertion gradually.[10]

Alterations in vascular physiology occur with age and are related to changes in vascular compliance, microcirculation, tone, and baroreceptor function. In North America, atherosclerosis is almost universal, with histologically demonstrable atherosclerotic changes present as early as the first decade of life.[11] Independent of disease-related changes to the vasculature, age-associated collagen deposition, cross-linking, and elastocalcinosis occur by age 35 years and result in measurable increases in vessel wall rigidity. Consequent increases in peripheral vascular resistance limit vascular flow and increase blood pressure and thereby necessitate increased cardiac effort to maintain cardiac output.[12] Injection studies have demonstrated that with age, the microvascular supply to major organs and peripheral tissues gradually diminishes, with consequent alterations in metabolic activity and healing.[11] Capillary walls thicken, causing a slight decrease in nutrient, oxygen, and waste exchange. Finally, age-related alterations in vessel wall baroreceptor sensitivity result in aberrant responses in vascular tone, which can contribute to orthostatic hypotension. This may be of clinical consequence in those older individuals with vascular disease who wish to pursue physical activity.

Normal aging results in a reduction in total body water. Accordingly, blood volume decreases. Hematopoiesis slows and hemoglobin and hematocrit levels diminish correspondingly. This further limits the efficient transfer of nutrients, oxygen, carbon dioxide, and waste, and it may contribute to fatigue.

Pulmonary System

The aging process results in numerous pathophysiologic changes that reduce the functional efficiency of the respiratory system. Progressive degeneration of the collagenous and elastic elements of the lung parenchyma result in compromise of the structural integrity (which, in its advanced form, is referred to as senile emphysema) and capacity for elastic recoil.[13] Decreased lung compliance is exacerbated by stiffening of the costovertebral and sternocostal cartilage, weakness of the respiratory and accessory muscles, arthritis, and obesity, which may further restrict pulmonary function. In normal development, new alveoli and corresponding pulmonary microvasculature are formed through the second decade of life, after which the number gradually dwindles.

Age-related reductions in pulmonary microvasculature and number of alveoli result in increased resistance to blood flow; these changes, in conjunction with presumed collagen deposition at the level of the alveolar basement membrane, may limit gas exchange and increase the alveolar-capillary diffusion gradient.[5,8] From a physiologic standpoint, these changes result in decreases in total lung capacity, vital capacity, inspiratory and expiratory air flows, and maximum blood flow, with associated increases in residual volume and ventilation-perfusion ratio.[13] Aerobic performance is thus affected by limitations in oxygen exchange and an increased sense of respiratory effort expended during exercise. Although pulmonary reserve gradually decreases with age, regular exercise in older individuals has been shown to improve pulmonary exchange and decrease breathlessness, probably via strengthening of respiratory muscles.[12]

Renal System

With increasing age, the kidneys experience a progressive loss of mass and number of glomeruli, from an average of 500,000 to 1,000,000 at age 40 years to half this number by the seventh decade of life.[12] Increased vascular rigidity and atherosclerosis contribute to decreased renal blood flow from 670 mL/min in the second decade of life to 350 mL/min by the eighth decade. The glomerular filtration rate decreases 46% in the same time period.[12] These changes may be further exacerbated by coexisting renal disease or nephrotoxic medications. Such medications are of particular concern in the aging individual, because commonly used medications such as nonsteroidal anti-inflammatory drugs (NSAIDs) or angiotensin-converting enzyme (ACE) inhibitors may precipitate acute renal failure. If prolonged use of potentially nephrotoxic agents is anticipated, as in the individual with osteoarthritis managed with ibuprofen, it is important that laboratory blood tests be performed every 3 to 6 months.

The urine-concentrating ability of the kidneys decreases with age. As the specific gravity of urine decreases from an average of 1.032 during youth to 1.024 at age 80, the relative water output is greater, rendering

adequate hydration a challenge; this is exacerbated by insensible losses during exercise as well as alterations in the sensitivity of the thirst mechanism with age.[12,14] Depletion of intravascular volume typically precedes activation of thirst mechanisms. This can affect cardiac output, athletic performance, and cognitive function and result in serious metabolic disturbances in advanced stages of dehydration. It is thus imperative for the older athlete to maintain adequate hydration during periods of exercise; often this requires serial weight monitoring and scheduled rehydration despite a lack of thirst.

Ultrastructural changes to collagen and connective tissues result in a decrease in compliance of the urinary bladder. Moreover, progressive muscle weakness may result in incomplete voiding with urination. Difficulties with urination may also be exacerbated by coexisting prostate disease in males, or pelvic floor incompetence in females.

Neurologic Function

Alterations in central and peripheral nervous function also occur with aging. Progressive central nervous system deterioration can result in impaired hearing, short-term memory, balance, fine motor skills, and cognition.[5,8] Extrapyramidal dysfunction can result in impaired coordination and rapidity of motions and increased motor response time. Vestibular function can be affected by age-related calcification or vascular disease of the inner ear, resulting in impaired balance and spatial orientation. Altered sensation, in particular proprioception, can occur with age and may reflect a combination of central and peripheral dysfunction. Integration of sensory stimuli and coordination of motor responses ("hand-eye coordination") occurs at several levels within the central nervous system and may be affected by numerous factors that commonly affect the elderly, including dementia, cerebrovascular events, decreased cognition, medications, depression, and tumors.[8] Changes in cognition and judgment may be related to the presence of neurofibrillary tangles and senile plaques, which are found in 90% of individuals older than 90 years but are uncommon in those younger than 50 years.[12] Such plaques and tangles may occur as a result of accumulation of metabolic waste or from breakdown of neural tissue. Lipofuscin may accumulate in neural tissue as well.

Age-related peripheral nerve dysfunction can be exacerbated by coexisting disease processes such as diabetes mellitus and may result in decreased conduction velocity, amplitude, and motor unit recruitment, as well as altered motor unit potentials. Even in the absence of known neurologic disease, vibration and position sense at the ankles has been shown to be reduced in 30% to 50% of the elderly population.[15] Although further research is necessary to elucidate the mechanisms by which neurodegenerative processes occur, medical control of identifiable disorders, such as Parkinson disease and diabetes mellitus, may allow for participation in athletic activities.

Vision

Progressive impairment of visual perception typically occurs with age and is commonly associated with decreased visual acuity, accommodation, contrast sensitivity, peripheral vision, and ability to adapt to low-light situations.[16] Other age-related conditions that may result in visual compromise include cataracts, glaucoma, and macular degeneration. Corrective lenses may be beneficial for daily activities, but these are not of great benefit for athletic activities. The bifocal lenses frequently worn by the elderly for presbyopia provide good visual acuity for reading and distant objects but not for vision in the mid-range (<20 m), which is usually important for sporting activities.[8]

Endocrine System

The endocrine system is affected by age. With time, hormone levels gradually decline. This is a normal consequence of aging, although it may be exacerbated by pathologic conditions or surgery, such as oophorectomy or thyroidectomy.

In general, the rate of coronary artery disease in premenopausal women is lower than in age-matched men. After menopause, however, the risk climbs until it is equal to that of age-matched men; in fact, coronary heart disease is the leading cause of mortality in women aged 65 to 74 years and is the second leading cause of death among women aged 45 to 64 years.[17]

Approximately every 25 seconds, an American experiences a cardiac event; about every 60 seconds, one dies

from one.[18] In 2001, the American Heart Association stated that postmenopausal women would benefit from hormone replacement therapy to prevent the increase in risk of coronary artery disease observed after menopause.[19] In 1991, the National Institutes of Health launched the Women's Health Initiative (WHI), a prospective, multicenter observational study of 161,000 healthy, postmenopausal women. The aim of the study was to investigate the risks and benefits of hormone replacement therapy in postmenopausal women. Although the study period was to last until 2005, the estrogen-plus-progestin arm of the study was halted in 2002 and the estrogen-alone arm was halted in 2004 because of the recognition of a statistically significant increase in adverse outcomes. The estrogen-plus-progestin cohort demonstrated a 26% increased risk of breast cancer, a 41% increased risk of cerebrovascular events, a 29% increased risk of myocardial infarction, and a 100% increased risk of deep vein thrombosis and pulmonary embolism, although there were no differences in total number of cancer cases or mortality. The use of estrogen plus progestin also was found to be associated with a 37% reduction in colorectal cancer and 37% fewer hip fractures. The estrogen-alone cohort demonstrated a 39% increased risk of cerebrovascular events, a 37% increase in deep vein thrombosis, and a statistical trend toward an increased risk of pulmonary embolism. Estrogen-alone replacement therapy was not associated with an increased risk of coronary artery disease, colorectal cancer, breast cancer, other cancers, or mortality, and the risk of hip fracture decreased by 39%. The WHI investigators were careful to point out that although the increased risk for various conditions appeared to be alarming, they must be taken in the context of the absolute risk to the individual. For example, in the WHI study, for every 10,000 women who took estrogen plus progestin for 1 year, 8 more cases of breast cancer occurred compared with those who did not take hormone replacement therapy; thus, although this represented a 26% increase in risk, the absolute risk to the individual remained relatively low.[20,21] Recent evidence has shown that the timing of the initiation of hormone replacement therapy may be important. Compared with no use of hormone replacement, continuous estrogen-plus-progestin use was associated with a 2.36-fold risk of developing coronary heart disease for the first 2 years. Initiation of hormone replacement within 10 years after menopause was associated with abatement of the increased risk of coronary heart disease to a 1.29-fold risk for the first 2 years, but by 6 years after initiation of therapy, continuous estrogen-plus-progestin use demonstrated a cardioprotective effect (0.64-fold risk).[22]

Psychosocial Effects of Aging

Despite the fact that many older athletes compete at a high level, they typically face different psychosocial pressures than their younger counterparts. In general, the aging athlete demonstrates a greater than average commitment to sports activity, which frequently necessitates exceptional discipline and motivation to include competitive sports in their lives amid vocational, familial, and social obligations. Some older athletes often fail to derive the excitement, pleasure, and satisfaction that are typically associated with physical exertion because they perceive their training to be another commitment that demands their time, intensity, and concentration. Others view their athletic pursuits as extensions of their vocational lives, in which their athletic performance is motivated purely by their desire to succeed. Unfortunately, these situations frequently lead to errors in training and diminished performance, with an associated increase in susceptibility to injury. Most successful older athletes, however, benefit from lifetimes of athletic experience and possess advanced levels of self-understanding that allow them to maximally benefit from their training while minimizing their risk of injury.[5]

Summary

Current trends suggest that the growth of the aging population will be associated with a greater number of older individuals who participate in athletic pursuits. Accordingly, in addition to addressing any musculoskeletal ailments, it is incumbent upon the treating orthopaedic surgeon to have at least a basic understanding of the so-called normal age-related changes, how they differ from pathologic entities, and how they may affect performance and treatment. Treatment should be individualized in the context of the patient's overall health in order to set realistic goals for functional recovery and successful return to athletics.

References

1. Schulz TJ, Zarse K, Voigt A, Urban N, Birringer M, Ristow M: Glucose restriction extends Caenorhabditis elegans life span by inducing mitochondrial respiration and increasing oxidative stress. *Cell Metab* 2007;6(4): 280-293.

2. Hamilton IS: *The Psychology of Aging: An Introduction.* London, United Kingdom, Jessica Kingsley Publishers, 2006.

3. Willis SL: *Adult Development and Aging.* New York, NY, Harper Collins College Publishers, 1996.

4. Bowling A: *Ageing Well: Quality of Life in Old Age.* London, United Kingdom, McGraw-Hill Open University Press, 2005.

5. Menard D, Stanish WD: The aging athlete. *Am J Sports Med* 1989;17(2):187-196.

6. Ogawa T, Spina RJ, Martin WH III, et al: Effects of aging, sex, and physical training on cardiovascular responses to exercise. *Circulation* 1992;86(2):494-503.

7. Schuman JE: Some changes of aging. *J Otolaryngol* 1986;15(4):211-213.

8. Flanagan SR, Ragnarsson KT, Ross MK, Wong DK: Rehabilitation of the geriatric orthopaedic patient. *Clin Orthop Relat Res* 1995;(316):80-92.

9. Astrand PO: Exercise physiology of the mature athlete, in Sutton JR, Brock RM, eds: *Sports Medicine for the Mature Athlete.* Indianapolis, IN, Benchmark Press Inc, 1986, pp 3-13.

10. Mittleman MA, Maclure M, Tofler GH, et al: Triggering of acute myocardial infarction by heavy physical exertion: Protection against triggering by regular exertion. *N Engl J Med* 1993;329(23): 1677-1683.

11. Goldman R: Speculations on vascular changes with age. *J Am Geriatr Soc* 1970;18:765-779.

12. Siegel AJ, Warhol MJ, Lang G: Muscle injury and repair in ultra-long distance runners, in Sutton JR, Brock RM, eds: *Sports Medicine for the Mature Athlete.* Indianapolis, IN, Benchmark Press Inc, 1986, pp 35-43.

13. Jones NL: The lungs of the masters athlete, in Sutton JR, Brock RM, eds: *Sports Medicine for the Mature Athlete.* Indianapolis, IN, Benchmark Press Inc, 1986, pp 319-328.

14. Maharam LG, Bauman PA, Kalman D, Skolnik H, Perle SM: Masters athletes: Factors affecting performance. *Sports Med* 1999;28(4):273-285.

15. Dorfman LJ, Bosley TM: Age-related changes in peripheral and central nerve conduction in man. *Neurology* 1979;29(1):38-44.

16. Tinetti ME, Speechley M: Prevention of falls among the elderly. *N Engl J Med* 1989;320(16):1055-1059.

17. CDC: *Leading Causes of Death in Females, United States, 2006.* Hyattsville, MD, Department of Health and Human Services. http://www.cdc.gov/women/lcod. Accessed October 12, 2010.

18. Lloyd-Jones D, Adams R, Carnethon M, et al: Heart disease and stroke statistics: 2009 update. A report from the American Heart Association Statistics Committee and Stroke Statistics Subcommittee. *Circulation* 2009;119(3):e21-e181.

19. Mosca L, Collins P, Herrington DM, et al: Hormone replacement therapy and cardiovascular disease: A statement for healthcare professionals from the American Heart Association. *Circulation* 2001;104(4):499-503.

20. Rossouw JE, Anderson GL, Prentice RL, et al: Risks and benefits of estrogen plus progestin in healthy postmenopausal women: Principal results from the Women's Health Initiative randomized controlled trial. *JAMA* 2002;288(3):321-333.

21. Anderson GL, Limacher M, Assaf AR, et al: Effects of conjugated equine estrogen in postmenopausal women with hysterectomy: The Women's Health Initiative randomized controlled trial. *JAMA* 2004;291(14): 1701-1712.

22. Toh S, Hernández-Díaz S, Logan R, Rossouw JE, Hernán MA: Coronary heart disease in postmenopausal recipients of estrogen plus progestin therapy: Does the increased risk ever disappear? A randomized trial. *Ann Intern Med* 2010;152(4):211-217.

Chapter 3

Basic Science of Aging Musculoskeletal Tissues

John M. Tokish, MD

Key Points

- Aging affects diverse biologic systems, but processes are common at all levels that hold the key to healthy longevity.
- In muscle, senile sarcopenia results in a loss of one third of skeletal muscle mass. This loss is multifactorial, including a loss of neural stimulation, decreased nutrition, and loss of trophic hormones.
- Aging collagen demonstrates decreased fibroblast content, altered fibril mechanical properties, and decreased blood supply, resulting in a decrease in healing capacity and structural failure of tendon and meniscus.
- Articular cartilage does not age well. Chondrocytes cease matrix production, and proteoglycan structure changes, resulting in a more rigid construct, which is vulnerable to injury at normal loads.
- Understanding the common pathways of aging offers promise in optimizing longevity. From anti-oxidants, to platelet-rich plasma (PRP), to even simple lifelong exercise, aging can be confronted at the cellular, matrix, and systemic levels.

Introduction

Aging is not a disease. Although musculoskeletal tissues undergo consistent changes with senescence, these changes do not progress uniformly, and intervention may alter this progression.[1] With the aging of the so-called baby boomers (Americans born between 1946 and 1964), the care of the aging musculoskeletal system has received increased emphasis. In 2009, the 76 million baby boomers spent more than $72 billion on products and services to slow the aging process.[2] Unfortunately, much of this money will have been spent on empty promises rather than valid treatment. Successful care of the aging athlete hinges on understanding and manipulating the differences between normal and pathologic aging. This chapter reviews the normal aging process throughout the musculoskeletal system to provide a framework for future strategic application of injury prevention and treatment in seasoned athletes.

Common Denominators of Aging

Aging of the musculoskeletal tissues is a complex process that involves multiple interactions, from the cellular level to the extracellular matrix to each system of the organism. Although these biologic systems are

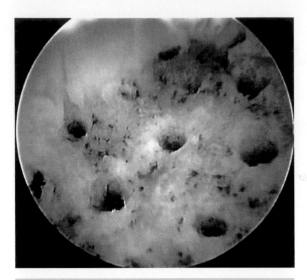

Figure I   Arthroscopic view of a knee that has undergone microfracture. An awl has been used to create holes that penetrate the subchondral bone, allowing pleuripotential cells to repopulate the cartilage defect. These cells have the ability to mature into chondrocytes.

diverse in structure and function, processes that are common at all levels may hold the key to optimizing health across systems in the aging athlete.

At the cellular level, aging can be represented by two main changes. First, differentiated cells have a limited capacity to divide[3,4] or to replicate DNA. Second, these senescent cells lose the ability to synthesize compounds, leading to a decrease in material for use in the extracellular matrix and the compounds that protect the cell itself against stress, injury, or harmful oxidative byproducts. Clinical applications directed toward aging at this level include cartilage restoration procedures such as microfracture or autologous chondrocyte implantation (ACI). In the former, an awl is used to create a vascular channel in the base of a cartilage defect, allowing pleuripotential undifferentiated cells to populate the defect (**Figure 1**). These cells can differentiate into chondrocytes and produce varying quantities of hyaline-like cartilage. In ACI, new chondrocytes are amplified in vitro and then reimplanted, giving the defect a new source of cells to produce hyaline-like cartilage.

Within the extracellular matrix, chemical modifications take place throughout life and older molecules are partially degraded or modified. These molecules can accumulate in the matrix and can affect normal cell processes. Collagen, for example, becomes more soluble as a result of increased cross-linking that may affect its mechanical properties.[1] Accumulation of hyaluronic binding proteins may interfere with normal proteoglycan aggregates[5,6] in articular cartilage. Scavenging or reducing these accumulated cell by-products is one approach to anti-aging. The use of so-called antioxidant vitamins or newer products such as resveratrol supplements may reduce these oxidative byproducts and slow senescence at the cellular and extracellular levels.[7]

At the systemic level, aging is associated with a decrease in trophic hormones such as testosterone and insulin-like growth factor.[8-10] One well-studied example of these changes is in skeletal muscle, where decreases in these hormones directly contribute to senile sarcopenia,[11] an age-related decrease in muscle mass. In bone, osteoporosis, or loss of bone mass with aging, is associated with a decrease in circulating hormones (see chapter 4). These changes form the basis of the multibillion-dollar anti-aging hormone supplementation industry[2,10] discussed in chapter 6.

Another systemic change common in aging tissues is the progressive loss of blood supply to collagenous tissues. This is well demonstrated throughout the musculoskeletal system, from meniscal cartilage to rotator cuff tendons, and may significantly affect the ability of the tissues to respond to injury.

The aging of musculoskeletal tissues follows similar patterns at the cellular, extracellular, and systemic levels. Such patterns are important to recognize in individual tissues if a systemic approach is to be applied to slow or reverse pathologic aging. Reviewing these patterns within individual soft tissues of the musculoskeletal system can provide a framework for understanding the diversity of aging across all soft tissues.

Muscle

Perhaps no tissue is as susceptible to the aging process as muscle. Between the ages of 50 and 80 years, the average man will lose one-third of his muscle mass.[12] The cause of this so-called senile sarcopenia is multifactorial. Disuse atrophy certainly plays a role,[13] but it does not fully

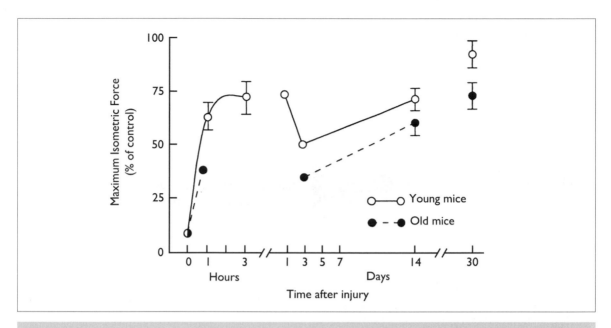

Figure 2   Graph shows maximum isometric force in young and old mice after injury. Both groups show a marked decrease in maximum force after injury, as well as recovery with time, but the same injury caused a more severe decrease in muscle force and slower recovery in the muscles of the older animals. (Reproduced with permission from Buckwalter JA, Woo SL, Goldberg VM, et al: Soft-tissue aging and musculoskeletal function. *J Bone Joint Surg Am* 1993;75[10]:1533-1548.)

explain the phenomenon.[14] With aging comes a loss of motor neurons,[15] which are trophic to the muscle and necessary for its maintenance.

At the cellular level, recent research has highlighted the importance of the satellite cell in muscle regeneration and response to injury.[16] Satellite cells live on the periphery of the myofiber and are normally quiescent. They become activated in response to trauma, however, and direct cellular proliferation and regeneration. In degenerative conditions, aging, and denervated muscle, satellite cell numbers and proliferative capacity significantly decrease.[17] Strategies to stimulate these cells in an aging population are currently being studied in an effort to prevent senile sarcopenia.

In the extracellular matrix, aging muscle is characterized by increased total collagen content, decreased mitochondrial activity, and increased cross-linking in the actin-myosin chains.[18,19] These changes may cause muscle units to become stiffer and therefore more susceptible to injury.[19] To make matters worse, older skeletal muscle is less able to regenerate damaged muscle,[20]

creating a spiral of injury and incomplete recovery that may lead to a significant decrease in mechanical properties in response to injury (**Figure 2**).

At a systemic level, aging affects blood supply to contractile muscle. Recent work has demonstrated that advanced age significantly impairs capillary proliferation, density, and hemodynamics, which may play a role in reduced exercise capacity of aging populations.[21] Decreasing concentrations of sex hormones such as testosterone undoubtedly play a factor[11] in the development of senile sarcopenia as well. Approximately 20% of 60-year-olds and 50% of 80-year-olds exhibit total serum testosterone levels below the normal range for young men.[22] Hormone replacement therapy to restore more normal levels has been shown to increase and maintain muscle mass.[23]

An additional systemic contributor to muscle loss in the aging population is a lack of adequate nutrition. This "anorexia of aging"[15] consists of a decreased protein intake, increased protein catabolism, and a higher requirement for dietary protein. One study investigated

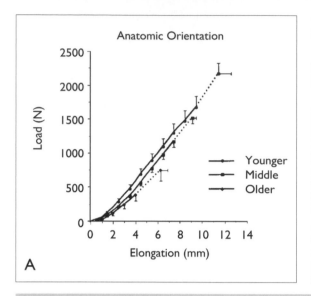

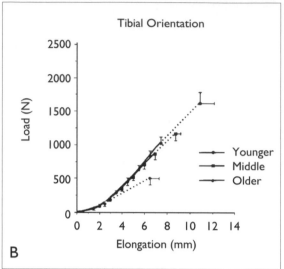

Figure 3   Graphs show the structural properties for anterior cruciate ligament complexes tested at 30° of flexion in the anatomic orientation (**A**) and tibial orientation (**B**) for younger, middle-aged, and older human donors. (Adapted with permission from Woo SLY, Hollis JM, Adams DL, Lyon RM, Takai S: Tensile properties of the human femur-anterior cruciate ligament-tibia complex: The effects of specimen age and orientation. *Am J Sports Med* 1991;19[3]:217-225.)

the relationship between nitrogen balance and protein intake in an older population.[24] At the recommended daily allowance of 0.8 g/kg of body weight per day, participants were found to be in a negative nitrogen balance, and it took nearly double this amount to put them into a positive nitrogen balance. The protein requirements were found to be even higher in older individuals engaged in resistance training. Thus, one simple strategy to combat aging effects on skeletal muscle is to ensure that patients optimize nutrition, a subject covered in greater detail in chapter 5.

Perhaps the best therapy for these changes of aging is simply sustained exercise. Numerous studies have shown that exercise can restore muscle mass and improve strength,[25-27] even in patients as old as 90 years.[28] Aging affects muscle at the cellular level with decreased regeneration, at the matrix level with actin-myosin dysfunction, and at the systemic level with decreased trophic hormone levels. Fortunately, promising therapies exist at each of these levels that may at least flatten the curve of senile sarcopenia.

Tendon and Ligament

The aging of connective tissue also follows predictable patterns at the cellular, extracellular matrix, and systemic levels. The structure of both ligament and tendon changes with aging. In ligaments, the insertion site changes histologically, from resembling articular cartilage to more of a fibrocartilage construct.[29] Aging ligament has fewer fibroblasts and fewer Ruffini mechanoreceptors,[30] which may contribute to a decline in structural properties such as ultimate failure load and mechanical stiffness.[31] One study showed that the ultimate failure load for ligament complexes from older individuals was less than one third that of younger individuals.[32] These changes are nearly universal in aging collagenous tissues[32,33] (**Figures 3** and **4**). Research into modification of the structural properties of injured tendon and ligament is ongoing but remains largely experimental. One available strategy that appears to combat these age-related changes is loading exercise. Woo et al[34] showed that exercise could increase ultimate load, tensile strength, and mechanical stiffness

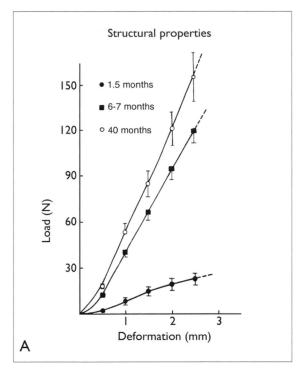

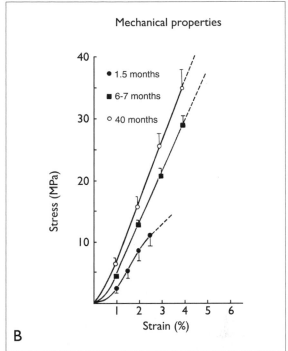

Figure 4   Graphs show the structural (**A**) and mechanical (**B**) properties of the medial collateral ligament complex for three different age groups: 1.5 months (open epiphysis), 6 to 7 months (closed epiphysis), and 40 months (closed epiphysis). (Adapted with permission from Woo SLY, Young EP, Kwan MK: Fundamental studies in knee ligament mechanics, in Daniel D, Akeson WH, O'Connor JJ, eds: *Knee Ligaments: Structure, Function, Injury, and Repair.* New York, NY, Raven Press, 1990, pp 115-134.)

in ligamentous tissues. Although ligament injury itself is not generally considered to be a big problem in the boomer population, these structural changes may affect the joint environment and are perhaps complicit in the progression of osteoarthritis.

Tendon injury, on the other hand, is an epidemic in the boomer athlete. Rotator cuff tendinitis, lateral epicondylitis, and posterior tibialis dysfunction are a few examples that demonstrate the far-reaching impact of pathologic tendon. At the cellular level, aging tendon demonstrates fewer fibroblasts and increased degenerative changes;[35] at the matrix level, it reveals less optimal tendon fibril diameter and Sharpey fiber diameter.[36] These changes, as in ligament, lead to a decline in mechanical properties such as modulus of elasticity and failure load.[37] As with ligament, exercise has been shown to reverse these deleterious effects in tendon.[37,38]

At the systemic level, blood supply to tendon becomes less robust, leading to so-called watershed areas where microtears cannot heal, eventually leading to structural failure. Unlike with ligament, an emerging body of literature describes using biologic supplementation to enhance treatment of these structural failures in tendon. Treatment of tissues with PRP, which attempts to increase cellular and matrix responses in tendon healing by enhancing local growth factor concentrations, is one such emerging technology. Another area of research is the modification of surgical implants, such as the cannulation of suture anchors to allow bleeding from a bony reattachment site to nourish the healing tendon. Other interventions such as collagen scaffolds, growth factor introduction, and mechanical stimulation have all shown promise.

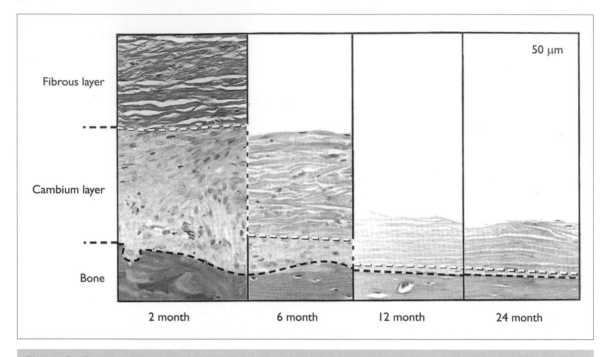

Fibrous layer

Cambium layer

Bone

50 μm

2 month   6 month   12 month   24 month

Figure 5 Composite photomicrograph shows age-related decline in the number of mesenchymal stem cells in rabbit tibia. Note the marked reduction in total cell number in the cambium layer, which contains chondrocyte precursors. (Reproduced from O'Driscoll SW, Saris DB: Articular cartilage repair, in Einhorn TA, O'Keefe RJ, Buckwalter JA, eds: *Orthopaedic Basic Science: Foundations of Clinical Practice*, ed 3. Rosemont, IL, American Academy of Orthopaedic Surgeons, 2007, pp 349-364.)

Articular Cartilage

Articular cartilage does not age gracefully. First, it has a very poor maintenance program. Once skeletal maturity is reached and the tidemark is closed, few, if any, new chondrocytes are produced, and those that remain do not synthesize matrix products well[1,39,40] (**Figure 5**). The cells produce more variable matrix proteoglycans, which may render them less effective in the replacement of degraded macromolecules or in response to injury.[1] Furthermore, because cartilage has no blood supply, no vehicle exists to provide a hematogenous response to injury or degradation. Given this decline in cellular function, there is a corresponding decline in the structure and function of the extracellular matrix. In healthy, younger articular cartilage, large negatively charged proteoglycan molecules attract positively charged hydrogen molecules in water to create the characteristic shock absorption and stress distribution characteristics of cartilage. With age, however, water content decreases, and the concentration of proteoglycan changes with a decrease in chondroitin and an increase in keratan. Hyaluronan, the central core molecule of the proteoglycan aggregate, decreases in size and increases in concentration with age[41] and carries fewer aggrecan complexes with more variability (**Figure 6**). Proteolytic degradation occurs, which breaks down the large proteoglycan aggregates. The smaller fragments can then bind to hyaluronan, which can inhibit the formation of normal proteoglycan structure.[42]

The collagen in articular cartilage is also subject to change with age. Older collagen fibrils have a larger fibril diameter, with greater cross-linking and less flexibility. These changes result in a more rigid construct; combined with a decrease in water content, this construct can limit the normal tissue response to loads, leading to fissure or shear injury.[1] Taken in total, it is easy to see why aging and arthritis are so frequently associated.

Strategies to maintain and restore articular cartilage continue to be investigated. Surgical procedures such as microfracture and ACI seek to increase the number of functioning chondrocytes and therefore the quantity and quality of the extracellular matrix. Nutritional supplements such as glucosamine and chondroitin sulfate are based on the idea of improving biologic levels of proteoglycan substrates, and viscosupplementation injections attempt to locally replenish large hydrophilic molecules directly to the joint.

Meniscus

Meniscal tissue shares many of the aging characteristics of other collagenous tissues. On an ultrastructural level, these changes can range from intrameniscal degeneration to complete structural failure with advancing age. In an often-quoted study, Jerosch et al[43] demonstrated that MRI-diagnosed meniscal tears are evident in 40% of asymptomatic patients older than 50 years. Although these tears in and of themselves are of questionable clinical significance, they certainly change the biomechanical environment and stress distribution in the joint. These changes may contribute to an increase in chondral breakdown and osteoarthritis. Understanding the aging process in the meniscus may lead to advances in delaying or preventing these changes and their potential deleterious effects.

Like other aging tissues, the meniscus demonstrates characteristic changes at the cellular, extracellular matrix, and systemic levels. At the cellular level, there are fewer fibroblasts and decreased production of matrix material for maintenance and injury response. In the extracellular matrix, the meniscal collagen demonstrates increased cross linking and a change in the cross-linking structure.[44] The proteoglycans of the meniscus also change, as they do in articular cartilage, with a characteristic decrease in chondroitin and an increase in keratan concentrations.[45] At a more systemic level, it is well understood that the meniscus undergoes a significant decrease in blood perfusion to its more central portions. This vascular perfusion of the meniscus is 100% at birth, but it gradually retracts to just one third at age 30 years, and to 25% at age 50 years.[46] Thus, the

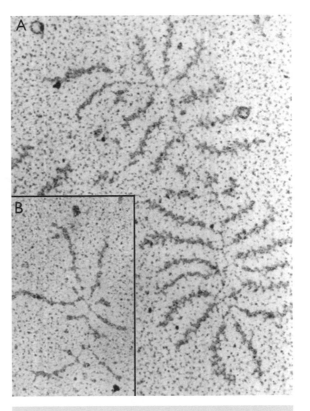

Figure 6 Electron micrographs show proteoglycan aggregates in human articular cartilage. Main image (**A**) shows cartilage from a human newborn; it contains some 30 aggrecan molecules. The inset (**B**) shows skeletally mature human cartilage; it contains 12 aggrecan molecules, which are more variable in length than those in the newborn. (Reproduced with permission from Buckwalter JA, Woo SL, Goldberg VM, et al: Soft-tissue aging and musculoskeletal function. J Bone Joint Surg Am 1993;75[10]:1533-1548.)

more central portions of the meniscus must switch from a hematogenous source of nutrition and reparation to one of diffusion from the synovial fluid.

Preservation or restoration of meniscal function has become more of a focus with improved surgical techniques. More aggressive repair with fibrin blood clots, the use of PRP, and meniscal transplantation are all attempts to restore functional meniscal tissue in compromised knees, and are covered in depth in other chapters.

Summary

As the boomer generation ages, health care will be increasingly focused on age-related pathologies. Treatment of these pathologies will undoubtedly require a multidisciplinary approach; however, the core of this approach should be an increased understanding of the difference between normal and pathologic aging at the basic science level. Research into reversing decreased proliferation at the cellular level, decreased production at the extracellular matrix level, and decreased hematologic and hormonal support at the systemic level will hopefully improve treatment across the entire musculoskeletal system, leading to increased mobility and independence and improved quality of life for millions of patients.

References

1. Buckwalter JA, Woo SL, Goldberg VM, et al: Soft-tissue aging and musculoskeletal function. *J Bone Joint Surg Am* 1993;75(10):1533-1548.

2. Selling the promise of youth. *Business Week.* New York, NY, McGraw-Hill, March 20, 2006.

3. Goldstein S: Replicative senescence: The human fibroblast comes of age. *Science* 1990;249(4973):1129-1133.

4. Stanulis-Praeger BM: Cellular senescence revisited: A review. *Mech Ageing Dev* 1987;38(1):1-48.

5. Buckwalter JA, Rosenberg LC: Electron microscopic studies of cartilage proteoglycans. *Electron Microsc Rev* 1988;1(1):87-112.

6. Buckwalter JA, Kuettner KE, Thonar EJ: Age-related changes in articular cartilage proteoglycans: Electron microscopic studies. *J Orthop Res* 1985;3(3):251-257.

7. Karuppagounder SS, Pinto JT, Xu H, Chen HL, Beal MF, Gibson GE: Dietary supplementation with resveratrol reduces plaque pathology in a transgenic model of Alzheimer's disease. *Neurochem Int* 2009;54(2):111-118.

8. Ferrini RL, Barrett-Connor E: Sex hormones and age: A cross-sectional study of testosterone and estradiol and their bioavailable fractions in community-dwelling men. *Am J Epidemiol* 1998;147(8):750-754.

9. Liu H, Bravata DM, Olkin I, et al: Systematic review: The safety and efficacy of growth hormone in the healthy elderly. *Ann Intern Med* 2007;146(2):104-115.

10. Liu H, Bravata DM, Olkin I, et al: Systematic review: The effects of growth hormone on athletic performance. *Ann Intern Med* 2008;148(10):747-758.

11. Matsumoto AM: Andropause: Clinical implications of the decline in serum testosterone levels with aging in men. *J Gerontol A Biol Sci Med Sci* 2002;57(2):M76-M99.

12. Borst SE: Interventions for sarcopenia and muscle weakness in older people. *Age Ageing* 2004;33(6):548-555.

13. Morley JE: Anorexia, sarcopenia, and aging. *Nutrition* 2001;17(7-8):660-663.

14. Goodpaster BH, Park SW, Harris TB, et al: The loss of skeletal muscle strength, mass, and quality in older adults: The health, aging and body composition study. *J Gerontol A Biol Sci Med Sci* 2006;61(10):1059-1064.

15. Brooks SV, Faulkner JA: Skeletal muscle weakness in old age: Underlying mechanisms. *Med Sci Sports Exerc* 1994;26(4):432-439.

16. Ehrhardt J, Morgan J: Regenerative capacity of skeletal muscle. *Curr Opin Neurol* 2005;18(5):548-553.

17. Jejurikar SS, Kuzon WM Jr : Satellite cell depletion in degenerative skeletal muscle. *Apoptosis* 2003;8(6):573-578.

18. American College of Sports Medicine Position Stand: The recommended quantity and quality of exercise for developing and maintaining cardiorespiratory and muscular fitness, and flexibility in healthy adults. *Med Sci Sports Exerc* 1998;30(6):975-991.

19. Kaplan FS, Hayes WC, Keaveny TM, Boskey AE, Einhorn TA, Iannotti JP: Form and function of bone, in Simon SR, ed: *Orthopaedic Basic Science.* Rosemont, IL, American Academy of Orthopaedic Surgeons, 1994, pp 127-184.

20. Brooks SV, Faulkner JA: Contraction-induced injury: Recovery of skeletal muscles in young and old mice. *Am J Physiol* 1990;258(3 Pt 1):C436-C442.

21. Copp SW, Ferreira LF, Herspring KF, Musch TI, Poole DC: The effects of aging on capillary hemodynamics in contracting rat spinotrapezius muscle. *Microvasc Res* 2009;77(2):113-119.

22. Harman SM, Metter EJ, Tobin JD, Pearson J, Blackman MR, Baltimore Longitudinal Study of Aging: Longitudinal effects of aging on serum total and free testosterone levels in healthy men. *J Clin Endocrinol Metab* 2001;86(2):724-731.

23. Isidori AM, Giannetta E, Greco EA, et al: Effects of testosterone on body composition, bone metabolism and serum lipid profile in middle-aged men: A meta-analysis. *Clin Endocrinol (Oxf)* 2005;63(3):280-293.

24. Campbell WW, Crim MC, Young VR, Evans WJ: Increased energy requirements and changes in body composition with resistance training in older adults. *Am J Clin Nutr* 1994;60(2):167-175.

25. Sullivan DH, Wall PT, Bariola JR, Bopp MM, Frost YM: Progressive resistance muscle strength training of hospitalized frail elderly. *Am J Phys Med Rehabil* 2001;80(7):503-509.

26. Hauer K, Specht N, Schuler M, Bärtsch P, Oster P: Intensive physical training in geriatric patients after severe falls and hip surgery. *Age Ageing* 2002;31(1): 49-57.

27. Frontera WR, Meredith CN, O'Reilly KP, Knuttgen HG, Evans WJ: Strength conditioning in older men: Skeletal muscle hypertrophy and improved function. *J Appl Physiol* 1988;64(3):1038-1044.

28. Fiatarone MA, Marks EC, Ryan ND, Meredith CN, Lipsitz LA, Evans WJ: High-intensity strength training in nonagenarians: Effects on skeletal muscle. *JAMA* 1990;263(22):3029-3034.

29. Wang IE, Mitroo S, Chen FH, Lu HH, Doty SB: Age-dependent changes in matrix composition and organization at the ligament-to-bone insertion. *J Orthop Res* 2006;24(8):1745-1755.

30. Aydoğ ST, Korkusuz P, Doral MN, Tetik O, Demirel HA: Decrease in the numbers of mechanoreceptors in rabbit ACL: The effects of ageing. *Knee Surg Sports Traumatol Arthrosc* 2006;14(4):325-329.

31. Woo SL, Ohland KJ, Weiss JA: Aging and sex-related changes in the biomechanical properties of the rabbit medial collateral ligament. *Mech Ageing Dev* 1990; 56(2):129-142.

32. Woo SL, Hollis JM, Adams DJ, Lyon RM, Takai S: Tensile properties of the human femur-anterior cruciate ligament-tibia complex: The effects of specimen age and orientation. *Am J Sports Med* 1991;19(3):217-225.

33. Woo SL, Kwan MK: Fundamental studies in knee ligament mechanics, in Daniel D, Akeson WH, O'Connor JJ, eds: *Knee Ligaments: Structure, Function, Injury, and Repair*. New York, NY, Raven Press, 1990, pp 115-134.

34. Woo SL, Gomez MA, Woo YK, Akeson WH: Mechanical properties of tendons and ligaments: II. The relationships of immobilization and exercise on tissue remodeling. *Biorheology* 1982;19(3):397-408.

35. Kannus P, Józsa L: Histopathological changes preceding spontaneous rupture of a tendon: A controlled study of 891 patients. *J Bone Joint Surg Am* 1991;73(10):1507-1525.

36. Chen H, Yao XF, Emura S, Shoumura S: Morphological changes of skeletal muscle, tendon and periosteum in the senescence-accelerated mouse (SAMP6): A murine model for senile osteoporosis. *Tissue Cell* 2006;38(5):325-335.

37. Reeves ND: Adaptation of the tendon to mechanical usage. *J Musculoskelet Neuronal Interact* 2006;6(2): 174-180.

38. Langberg H, Ellingsgaard H, Madsen T, et al: Eccentric rehabilitation exercise increases peritendinous type I collagen synthesis in humans with Achilles tendinosis. *Scand J Med Sci Sports* 2007;17(1):61-66.

39. Buckwalter JA, Rosenberg L: Structural changes during development in bovine fetal epiphyseal cartilage. *Coll Relat Res* 1983;3(6):489-504.

40. O'Driscoll SW, Saris DB: Articular cartilage repair, in Einhorn TA, O'Keefe RJ, Buckwalter JA, eds: *Orthopaedic Basic Science: Foundations of Clinical Practice*, ed 3. Rosemont, IL, American Academy of Orthopedic Surgeons, 2007, pp 349-364.

41. Holmes MW, Bayliss MT, Muir H: Hyaluronic acid in human articular cartilage: Age-related changes in content and size. *Biochem J* 1988;250(2):435-441.

42. Roughley PJ, White RJ, Poole AR: Identification of a hyaluronic acid-binding protein that interferes with the preparation of high-buoyant-density proteoglycan aggregates from adult human articular cartilage. *Biochem J* 1985;231(1):129-138.

43. Jerosch J, Castro WH, Assheuer J: Age-related magnetic resonance imaging morphology of the menisci in asymptomatic individuals. *Arch Orthop Trauma Surg* 1996;115(3-4):199-202.

44. Takahashi M, Suzuki M, Kushida K, Hoshino H, Inoue T: The effect of aging and osteoarthritis on the mature and senescent cross-links of collagen in human meniscus. *Arthroscopy* 1998;14(4):366-372.

45. Karube S, Shoji H: Compositional changes of glycosaminoglycans of the human menisci with age and degenerative joint disease. *Nippon Seikeigeka Gakkai Zasshi* 1982;56(1):51-57.

46. Petersen W, Tillmann B: Age-related blood and lymph supply of the knee menisci: A cadaver study. *Acta Orthop Scand* 1995;66(4):308-312.

Chapter 4

Osteoporosis and Osteomalacia

Eeric Truumees, MD

Key Points

- Osteoporosis is the most common metabolic bone disorder. As the population ages, orthopaedic surgeons will encounter bone loss more and more frequently.
- Osteomalacia, which is less common, is frequently misdiagnosed as osteoporosis.
- Bone loss affects not only the types of injuries to which a mature athlete is susceptible, but also the effectiveness of common treatment strategies.
- The orthopaedic surgeon must understand the results of common testing methods, including the dual-energy x-ray absorptiometry (DEXA) scan, and the implications of these measures on bone strength and fixation.
- Newer treatment strategies, including anabolic agents such as teriparatide, may allow patients to rebuild bone, decreasing risk of reinjury or construct failure.

Introduction and Epidemiology

In North America, 35 million people have risk factors for osteoporosis, the most common metabolic bone disorder. That number is expected to triple over the next 3 decades given the aging population. Osteomalacia, the adult form of rickets, on the other hand, is considered a rare disease according to the National Institutes of Health (NIH) Office of Rare Diseases. Since the introduction of vitamin D–fortified milk, its incidence in wealthy, Western nations has dropped to 0.1%. In poorer cultures, including ethnic and cultural subgroups in North America, that rate increases to 15%.[1,2]

Although both osteoporosis and osteomalacia can occur at any age, osteomalacia has a much flatter age distribution curve across the decades than does osteoporosis. Osteomalacia has traditionally been identified in patients with kidney disease or other chronic illness, but its incidence in the active, ambulatory population either is rising or was previously underestimated.[3,4] Often-missed clinical factors include low sun exposure (or sunscreen use) and gastrointestinal disorders such as celiac disease.[5-8] A recent study of Finnish military recruits with stress fractures found a correlation between fractures and low serum vitamin D levels.[4]

Often mistaken for osteoporosis, osteomalacia goes undiagnosed in as many as one third of cases.[9] In one series, 7.7% of patients who were treated for hip fracture and had no clinical features of osteomalacia were found to have classic osteomalacic findings at biopsy.[10] What is emerging, therefore, is a subgroup of osteomalacia patients presenting with isolated injury rather than generalized bone pain.

Not only is the population aging, but they are remaining more active later in life as well. The rate of middle-aged and older women participating in sports has risen in particular.[11] Disordered eating, menstrual dysfunction, and osteoporosis have become known as the "female athlete triad."[12] Generally, this phenomenon refers to younger female patients, but a similar risk is seen in perimenopausal women.

Like hypertension, bone loss is initially clinically silent. With progression, patients may develop a thoracic kyphosis or sustain a low-energy fracture. Older athletes are vulnerable to several bony injuries ranging from stress fractures of the fifth metatarsal to displaced fractures of the femoral neck and dens. Many of these injuries, such as vertebral compression fractures (VCFs), were thought to be benign. Population-wide studies show, however, that mortality rates in patients with VCFs, even those with so-called "subclinical" fractures, exceed those of patients who have never suffered an osteoporotic injury.[13]

Typically, osteoporosis affects trabecular bone first. In the United States, VCFs are the most common osteoporosis-related injury, outnumbering hip and wrist fractures combined, with 700,000 VCFs diagnosed each year. In a population-based European study, VCFs were recorded in 12% of men and women aged 50 to 79 years. The direct medical costs associated with these fractures have been estimated at $13.8 billion annually in the United States alone. By 2030, annual direct costs are projected to exceed $60 billion, or $164 million per day. The indirect costs in lost productivity and human pain and suffering are incalculable.[14]

Osteoporosis and osteomalacia affect the management of mature athletes in several ways. First, bone loss puts the athlete at risk for injuries otherwise seen only after high-energy trauma. Stress fractures are more common in athletes with bone loss.[15] Although much of the skeleton is at risk, lower extremity injuries—of the

sacrum, proximal femur, foot, and tibia—predominate.[16-18] The risk for stress fractures is variable by sport; running is reported in association with many cases. Because older athletes tend to participate in repetitive-stress, endurance-type sports, this is clinically significant.

Second, osteoporosis and osteomalacia can lead to gradual deformity, such as thoracic kyphosis or acetabular protrusio.[19,20] These deformities can cause pain and increase the risk of other injuries. For example, with osteoporotic height loss, patients may report pain caused by the ribs rubbing on the ilium.

Third, bone loss complicates the treatment plan of other orthopaedic interventions. For example, the surgical strategy for stabilization of a long-bone fracture must consider the patient's bone stock and the reliability of fixation.[21-23] When osteoporotic patients are treated nonsurgically, the physician must remember that bracing precipitates further bone loss (ie, "disease" osteopenia) and may thereby increase the risk of other, regional injuries when removed.[24] This may affect surgical measures as well. For instance, the surgeon must consider whether the anticipated fixation will terminate in a region already susceptible to insufficiency fractures. For example, fixation of a hip fracture using a short trochanteric nail that terminates in the subtrochanteric region may increase the risk of subsequent fracture; therefore, use of a longer nail to span this region may be needed. Any clinician treating athletic injuries in the mature patient population must have a solid understanding of the biology and biomechanics of osteoporosis and osteomalacia.[25]

Pathophysiology

Normal bone is a composite of mineral, protein, water, and cells. The exact composition varies by anatomic site, age, diet, and disease. Approximately 70% of the dry weight of bone is in its mineral phase, the largest component of which is hydroxyapatite, $Ca_{10}(PO_4)_6(OH)_2$. The loss of hydroxyapatite weakens the bone's resistance to compressive loading. The bone organic matrix fills in the remaining 30%. Collagen comprises 90% of that matrix. When bone loses organic matrix, it becomes more brittle.[26]

Bone is a dynamic and well-organized tissue that is modulated at both the molecular and organ levels.

Response to strain patterns occurs in the apatite crystal at the molecular level and in the trabecular network at the organ level. Together, the molecular, cellular, and tissue components of bone create a lightweight structure with the tensile strength of cast iron. The loading mechanics of bone depend on the direction of force application. Typically, bone is strongest parallel to the long axis of the collagen molecules and is weakest in torsion or shear.[27]

Mature, lamellar bone is found in two forms: trabecular (spongy or cancellous) and cortical (dense or compact). Trabecular bone, which comprises 20% of total bone mass, is found in long-bone metaphyses and epiphyses as well as in cuboid bones (eg, vertebrae). In these areas, bone composition includes internal beams (trabeculae) that form a three-dimensional branching lattice along mechanical stress lines. This open architecture exhibits eight times the metabolic turnover of cortical bone.

Cortical bone, which comprises 80% of total bone mass, has four times the mass per volume of trabecular bone. Whereas trabecular bone varies by the stress applied, cortical bone maintains a fairly uniform density. The "envelope" of cuboid bones and the diaphysis of long bones are made up of cortical bone.[28]

In osteoporosis, both the crystalline (inorganic) and collagenous (organic) phases of bone are lost. Clinically, osteoporosis may be thought of as a disorder characterized by decreased bone quantity. In osteomalacia, the organic phase of bone remains, but it is inadequately mineralized.[29] It may therefore be considered a disorder characterized by both decreased quantity and quality of bone. The body constantly remodels bone by removing old bone and creating new bone. Osteoporosis stems from disregulation between bone formation and resorption; bone forms more slowly than it is destroyed. In contradistinction, in osteomalacia, normal osteoid production precedes abnormal mineralization of that osteoid. Histopathology typically reveals osteoid "seams," or rims of inadequately mineralized osteoid. In both, overall bone mineral density (BMD) decreases. Over time, unbalanced osteoclast activity disrupts the normal connectivity of bony trabeculae. Bone is thus weakened in both a material and an architectural sense. Several environmental, genetic, and pharmacologic factors may precipitate osteoporosis. Although the etiology is not completely understood, the process is probably multifactorial.[30]

Everyone loses at least 0.5% of their bone mass per year after the age of 35, but not everyone develops osteoporosis. The mechanisms of age-related bone loss are poorly understood but are equivalent in women and men. The two most important determinants for clinical significant loss are peak bone mass and the rate of loss.[31]

Peak bone mass is achieved by the early part of the fourth decade of life. The most effective way to prevent osteoporosis is to increase peak bone mass in pubertal patients. Eating disorders such as anorexia and exercise-induced amenorrhea lead to profound osteoporosis.[32] A lack of weight-bearing exercise and dietary changes may increase the osteoporosis risk in upcoming generations.[33] After bone mass peaks, changes in gonadal hormone levels, such as are experienced at menopause, and several genetic, environmental, and nutritional conditions and chronic disease states modulate the bone loss rate. Estrogen deficiency such as occurs postmenopausally directly accelerates bone loss up to 2% to 3% per year for 10 years.[34]

Osteoporotic patients have traditionally been divided into three categories: type I (postmenopausal), type II (senile), and type III (secondary). Type I obviously affects women more often than men, but hypogonadic men can suffer from this form as well. Most type I patients show signs or symptoms in their 50s and 60s. Trabecular bone fractures (such as commonly occur in the wrist and spine) predominate. Type II osteoporosis arises in men and women equally in their 70s and 80s. More women are affected because more women survive to these ages. With type II osteoporosis, cortical bone is increasingly affected.[35]

Medications and disease states precipitate type III osteoporosis. Elevated endogenous or exogenous cortisol levels are among the most common offenders. Hypercortisolism is deleterious to bone mass because of decreased calcium absorption across the intestinal lumen, increased renal calcium loss, and direct inhibition of bone matrix formation.[36]

Pathomechanics

Osteoporosis and osteomalacia confer several critical mechanical risks. First, weak bone carries a greater risk of fracture. Second, increasing bone loss implies a greater risk of failure with surgical management. Third, bone loss subjects patients to skeletal deformity, such as protrusio acetabuli, kyphosis, and spondylolisthesis.

The distribution of injuries reflects the influence of both mechanical and physiologic factors. A complex interplay among arthrosis, ligament elasticity, muscular changes, and the underlying bone weakness likely occurs. For example, spondyloarthrosis and ligament ossification exert a relative stiffening effect on the midcervical spine (C4 through C7). The upper cervical spine, particularly the atlantoaxial complex, maintains mobility. As a result, older athletes are at increased risk for upper cervical spine injuries, especially through hyperextension mechanisms.[37-40] Lomoschitz et al[41] reviewed 225 cervical spine injuries in patients age 65 years and older, comparing younger (<75 years), more active elderly patients with older (≥75 years) patients. In the younger group, motor vehicle accidents were the main mechanism of injury. In the older group, falls from seated or standing height predominated. In patients older than 75 years, multilevel injuries and fractures at risk for neurologic deterioration were common, occurring in more than 50% of patients.

Because of the altered biomechanics in this patient population, certain injury types occur with greater frequency. Dens fractures, for example, represent 10% of all cervical spine injuries in the general population but are the most common spinal column fracture in patients older than 65 years.[42]

In addition to the sudden displacement or collapse associated with an osteoporotic fracture, osteoporosis also increases the risk for the more gradual loss of alignment and balance associated with spinal deformity and degeneration. For example, loss of bone strength increases the risk of progression of virtually all types of spondylolisthesis—degenerative, isthmic, and iatrogenic.[43] Case reports also describe pars elongation leading to spondylolisthesis in patients with osteoporotic bone.[44] Similarly, the presence of osteoporosis is associated with increased risk of deformity progression with either idiopathic or degenerative scoliosis.[45,46] Given the persistence of osteopenia after treatment of idiopathic scoliosis, even in teenaged girls, the question of its role in scoliosis pathophysiology remains.[47] Some studies suggest that decreased bone mass at the convexity of the curve will foster its propagation.[48]

Finally, ligamentous and muscular factors are underestimated as a cause of deformity. In the spine, several studies have shown progressive kyphosis in osteoporotic patients without significant fracture or bone irregularity. Disk degeneration and spondylotic factors as well as muscular factors have been implicated.[49-51] Other studies have reached similar conclusions in hip fractures and other osteoporotic injuries.[52-54]

Stress fractures occur when repetitive, cyclic loading overwhelms the reparative ability of the bone. Mechanically, one or more of the following factors are present: increased loads are applied; the number or frequency of stress application increases; and the surface area over which load is applied has decreased.[15]

Clinical Presentation and Evaluation

The critical first step in identifying osteoporosis, osteomalacia, or any other bone loss state is to look for it. Despite the mountains of data concerning the frequency of these disorders and their mechanical and prognostic implications, several studies suggest that orthopaedic surgeons do not adequately screen their patients for bone quality.[55-58]

Orthopaedic surgeons are well placed to diagnose bone loss. Often, an athlete's injury pattern is the first indicator of bone mineralization defect.[59,60] Bone loss should be suspected in any at-risk patient or whenever the energy of the insult does not correspond with the severity of the injury (**Table 1**). The possibility of osteoporosis or another abnormal bone state should be considered in any encounter with an older athlete. Understanding a patient's mineralization state is especially important when elective surgery is planned; poor bone stock should not come as an intraoperative surprise. World Health Organization (WHO) criteria for DEXA screening are listed in **Table 2**.[61]

Osteoporosis does not produce symptoms. The first indication is usually a low-energy or fragility fracture. When a patient presents with bone pain, fracture should be considered. Diffuse bone pain is a feature of osteomalacia, mastocytosis, Paget disease, metastatic cancer, multiple myeloma, or lymphoma.[62-65] Similarly, in any patient with a progressive spinal and extremity deformity, underlying bone weakness should be considered among the potential etiologies.

First, the patient's BMD should be determined. BMD is the major determinant of fracture threshold in

Table 1: Risk Factors for Osteoporosis
• Advanced age
• Endocrine abnormalities 　Hypercortisolism 　Hyperthyroidism 　Hyperparathyroidism 　Hypogonadism
• Other diseases 　Tumors 　Chronic disease 　Expression of abnormal collagen or bone 　　matrix genes
• Inactivity or immobilization
• Dietary issues 　Calcium-deficient diet 　Alcoholism 　BMI < 22 kg/m^2
• Smoking

BMI = body mass index.

Table 2: WHO Criteria for DEXA Screening[a]
• All patients 　who have sustained a low-energy fracture 　who have osteopenia on plain radiographs 　with diseases that place them at risk for 　　osteoporosis 　on medications that place them at risk for 　　osteoporosis
• Women who are 　postmenopausal 　older than 65 years 　younger than 65 with one or more risk factors 　　(see Table 1) 　on HRT for prolonged periods 　considering HRT, if BMD will affect decision

BMD = bone mineral density, DEXA = dual-energy x-ray absorptiometry, HRT = hormone replacement therapy, WHO = World Health Organization.
[a]Information adapted from reference 61.

patients with osteoporosis and osteomalacia.[66] Other important factors include cardiovascular status, medications, neuromuscular disorders, body habitus, and falls. Second, in patients with bone loss, osteomalacia, secondary osteoporosis, and the osteopenia of malignancy should be excluded. Third, when osteoporosis is identified, the bone turnover state should be assessed. Orthopaedic surgeons are well positioned to be involved and perhaps should be responsible for the first step. In some settings, referral to an endocrinologist, rheumatologist, or internist may be useful to complete the assessment. Either way, it is incumbent upon the surgeon to ensure that the appropriate workup has been initiated or undertaken.

As a method of assessing bone density, plain radiographs are neither accurate nor precise. A loss of at least 30% of bone mass is necessary to detect osteopenia on radiographs, and technical factors such as exposure of the x-ray may affect recognition of this.[67] On the other hand, radiography can be useful; several classification systems based on plain radiography have been devised to describe trabecular patterns and their impact on bone strength (eg, the Singh index for the proximal femur).[68] Plain radiographs are useful to delineate fracture pattern and severity in injured athletes. Some injury patterns suggest less benign forms of bone loss. For example, in the spine, VCFs of L5 or above T6 are more likely to represent metastatic disease.[69] Similarly, although acetabular injuries occur in postmenopausal osteoporosis, they are more common in osteomalacia.[70]

To assess bone mass and gauge response to treatment, a more accurate method than radiography is needed. Several tools are available, including quantitative CT, quantitative ultrasonography, single x-ray absorptiometry, radiogrammetry,[71-74] and DEXA, which is the current standard because of its accuracy and reproducibility.[75,76]

With DEXA, mineralization status is described by the T-score, which represents the degree to which a patient's BMD deviates from same-sex, young adult bone. A T-score of −1 represents osteopenia and implies 1 SD less bone than in young adults. A BMD below 2.5 SDs (or T-score of −2.5) defines osteoporosis. A T-score less than −2.5 with a history of fragility fractures

Table 3: Comparison of Osteoporosis and Osteomalacia

Factor	Osteoporosis	Osteomalacia
Definition	Bone mass decreased	Bone mass variable
Mineralization	Normal	Mineralization decreased
Age of onset	Generally elderly	Any age
Etiology	Endocrine abnormality	Vitamin D deficiency
	Advanced age	Abnormality of vitamin D pathway
		Idiopathic hypophosphatemia
		Renal tubular acidosis
		Hypophosphatasia
Symptoms	Pain referable to fracture	Generalized bone pain
Signs	Tenderness at fracture	Generalized tenderness
Laboratory findings		
Serum Ca^{2+}	Normal	$\downarrow$ or normal ($\uparrow$ in hypophosphatasia)
Serum phosphate	Normal	$\downarrow$ or normal ($\uparrow$ in renal osteodystrophy)
Alkaline phosphate	Normal	$\uparrow$ (not in hypophosphatasia)
Urinary Ca^{2+}	High or normal	Normal or $\downarrow$ ($\uparrow$ in hypophosphatasia)
Bone biopsy	Normal	Abnormal

meets WHO criteria for severe osteoporosis. Each standard deviation increases fracture risk 1.5 to 3 times.[77,78] For example, a T-score of −1 implies a 30% increased risk of fracture. The Z-score, which is used less frequently, compares the patient's bone with age-matched controls. A Z-score less than −2 should prompt an investigation for neoplasia or osteomalacia.[79]

Although serum calcium and phosphate levels tend to be normal in osteoporosis, these tests are frequently ordered to exclude other causes of bone loss such as osteomalacia, in which these studies are frequently abnormal (**Table 3**). For example, osteomalacia should be suspected when the product of the serum calcium level and the serum phosphate level is less than 25 mg^2/dL^2. Serum alkaline phosphatase levels are elevated and 24-hour urinary calcium excretion may be less than 50 mg.[80] For younger patients and women with a questionable menstrual history, a hormonal profile, including sex hormones (in men, testosterone; in women, testosterone, estrogen, and progesterone), thyroid-stimulating hormone, thyroxine, and parathyroid hormone (PTH) levels, is ordered.[81,82] In patients with unusual fracture patterns or histories suggestive of malignancy or infection, laboratory evaluation may include erythrocyte sedimentation rate, white blood cell count with differential, C-reactive protein level, serum protein electrophoresis (SPEP), urine protein electrophoresis, and prostate antigens (UPEP), such as prostate-specific antigen (PSA).

If serum blood tests alone are insufficient to exclude the diagnosis of osteomalacia, a transiliac bone biopsy or bone marrow aspiration may be indicated. Typically, these procedures are performed in patients younger than 50 years with idiopathic osteopenia, when osteomalacia is highly suspected, or in chronic renal failure patients with skeletal symptoms.[83,84] Two weeks before the biopsy, tetracycline is administered twice each day for 3 days. This dose should be repeated 3 days before biopsy. This tetracycline binds to newly mineralized osteoid and permits the determination of mineralization rates. In osteoporosis, a normal mineralization pattern would be expected as well as two distinct bands of fluorescence, representing the tetracycline labels. With impaired mineralization (ie, osteomalacia), a single band of fluorescence is observed.[85] Although not often necessary, when appropriately indicated, biopsies can have a marked impact on treatment.[84]

Bone biomarker assays are being ordered increasingly for osteoporotic patients. These assays provide information complementary to densitometry. The biomarkers assayed include bone formation markers such as bone-specific alkaline phosphatase (an osteoblast enzyme) and osteocalcin (a bone matrix protein), and bone resorption markers such as urine collagen degradation products (cross-linked telopeptides and pyridinolines). These markers improve future fracture risk prediction and are a sensitive means of monitoring therapy effectiveness.[86]

As with the diagnosis of the bone loss state, identification of insufficiency and stress fractures requires a high index of suspicion and a thorough clinical evaluation. An older athlete presenting with a suspected osteoporotic fracture warrants a careful history to obtain a clear understanding of the mechanism of energy and the energy imparted. Fractures produce focal, intense pain that worsens with loading. These symptoms should be differentiated from muscular pain, which is more typically diffuse and worsens with stretching. The history also should include the time course of the patient's symptoms, as well as a history of the patient's recent athletic endeavors. For example, a change in running distance or surface or issues with shoe wear may suggest a stress injury.

Even osteoporotic fractures should cause mechanical pain. If the pain does not vary in intensity with activity, or if it worsens with recumbency, infection or neoplasm should be considered. Patients with night pain, fevers, chills, unusual weight loss, or bowel or bladder changes require more intense investigation. Relevant past medical history includes previous fractures and prior evaluation and treatment of bone mineralization as well as a history of cancer, tuberculosis, or systemic infection. With axial skeleton injuries in a patient with a history of prior radiation treatments, a more aggressive workup is required.[87]

Physical examination in these patients includes an assessment of concomitant soft-tissue injury. The patient's general condition and sagittal spinal balance should be assessed. Body shape, difficulty breathing, or obesity can affect the efficacy of bracing. Patients with poor bone stock can sustain unstable injuries with few symptoms. In osteoporotic patients sustaining a significant athletic impact, cervical range of motion and tenderness should be assessed.

Similarly, osteoporotic patients may sustain concomitant extremity injuries and thoracolumbar VCFs. Acute VCFs and burst fractures are typically point-tender over the spinous process. The patient should be examined for rib tenderness. A complete neurologic examination should be performed. Although major neurologic deficits are rare (0.05%), many of these patients have spinal stenosis or neuropathy.[88] Sacral insufficiency fractures may cause pain in the tailbone or sacroiliac joint regions. Often this pain will be felt in a band-like distribution across the low back. The Patrick test and other sacroiliac joint–stressing maneuvers will reproduce pain in these patients.

Although most athletic injuries can be treated expectantly before radiographs are ordered, early imaging is beneficial in patients with osteoporosis. With stress fractures, on the other hand, late or repeated plain radiographs may be needed to identify the injury.[15] Bone loss increases the difficulty of identifying subtle fracture lines. In older athletes, interpretation of plain radiographs can be limited by degenerative changes obscuring radiographic landmarks. In axial injuries, plain radiographs should be scrutinized for signs of posterior cortical compromise such as widened pedicles and greater than 50% height loss. End-plate erosions suggest infection or pedicular destruction (eg, the winking owl sign, seen in malignancy).

In patients with symptoms nonresponsive to standard management or in those presenting with red flags, advanced imaging is recommended. With MRI, stress and vertebral fractures are often well delineated on T2-weighted or short tau inversion recovery (STIR) sequences.[89-91] Acute fractures demonstrate decreased signal intensity on T1-weighted images. Both T1 and T2 signal intensity changes normalize over time as the injury heals, although chronic injuries may lead to a fatty marrow, which is seen as increased signal intensity on T1-weighted images. MRI findings such as soft-tissue extension often differentiate neoplasm and infection from osteoporotic injuries.

In patients unable to undergo MRI, CT offers high bone and soft-tissue contrast and clearly delineates cortical compromise. Fracture acuity may be assessed by bone scan.[92-95] Both MRI and CT demonstrate sacral or, more rarely, pubic ramus insufficiency fractures. On a bone scan, these lesions may have the classic "H"

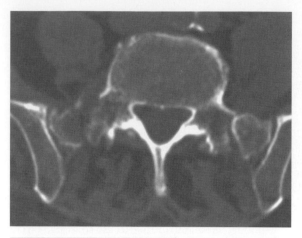

Figure 1   Axial CT demonstrates a bilateral sacral ala fracture in a 64-year-old runner. The patient reported gradually increasing beltline low back and buttock pain that worsened suddenly after a low-energy trip and fall. Subsequently, osteoporosis with a T-score of −2.6 was diagnosed in this otherwise healthy patient.

configuration or may appear as a linear band of increased uptake in the region of the sacral ala[96,97] (**Figure 1**).

Treatment

The treatment of patients with bone loss involves prevention and management of the underlying osteoporosis or osteomalacia as well as management of the presenting athletic injury. Given the frequency and costs of these injuries, the public health implications cannot be ignored. Addressing this problem requires a two-pronged approach. First, orthopaedic surgeons and other health care professionals who treat aging athletes must understand their critical role in screening at-risk patients. Even patients who have been hospitalized for definitive management of an insufficiency fracture sometimes do not receive secondary prevention education for future injuries.[98] Healthcare professionals must do a better job of screening patients for bone loss, and treatment should be initiated or appropriate referral should be made (**Figure 2**).

Second, the population at large, especially men and younger women, must be made more aware of their risk factors.[99] Education, screening, and preventive care can reduce the number of injuries. Leaflets and other edu-

cational materials should be made available in the office setting. Preseason physicals, which have been shown to decrease injury rates in this population, should be recommended, because they are not often mandated prior to participation in the older athletic population as they are in the school-age population.[100]

Once a bone loss state has been identified, its management depends on its cause. When possible, bone-leaching medications should be eliminated and underlying diseases should be managed.[101,102] For example, alternate-day corticosteroid dosing has been shown to decrease bone damage. Calcium, vitamin D, and antiosteoporosis medications are typically added to counter the deleterious effects.[36] Modifying patient activities and addressing the risk of falls are strategies that have been shown to decrease the risk of osteoporosis-related injuries.[103] Some physicians recommend tai chi, for example, which is a low-impact exercise that may improve the patient's balance.

Appropriate treatment should begin *before* the first fracture; it includes supplemental calcium, physiologic vitamin D, and weight-bearing exercise. These measures decrease bone resorption and improve osteoid mineralization, but they do not increase total bone mass. Individuals taking calcium supplementation have one fourth the risk of hip fractures compared with those with low calcium intake. Excessive calcium intake, however, may be harmful.

In perimenopausal women, estrogen supplementation may be helpful to address osteoporosis. Estrogen receptors have been identified in bone-forming cells. Estrogen acts to block the action of PTH on osteoblasts and marrow stromal cells. Estrogen supplementation decreases bone loss by acting to counter the effect of unopposed PTH activity. Without estrogen, osteoblasts and marrow stromal cells secrete increased levels of interleukin-6, which stimulates the osteoclasts to resorb bone. Estrogen does not appreciably alter bone formation rates; therefore, the primary effect of estrogen therapy lies in the maintenance of bone mass. Additionally, women on estrogen have been shown to experience fewer fractures. Recent studies continue to debate the increased coronary artery disease, stroke, pulmonary embolus, and cancer rates reported in the Women's Health Initiative Study.[104,105] These potential untoward side effects have focused attention on selective es-

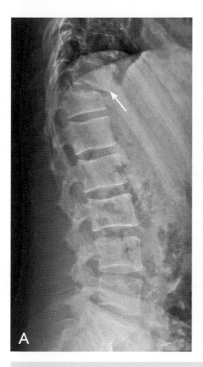
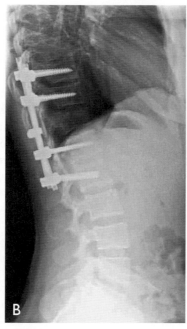
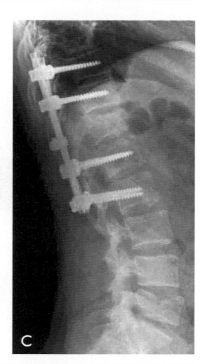

Figure 2   Lateral radiographs of the lower spine of a 38-year-old woman, an active athlete who injured her back while playing rugby. **A,** Preoperative view demonstrates a T11-T12 thoracolumbar fracture-dislocation (arrow). **B,** Radiograph obtained after treatment with a posterior open reduction and internal fixation. At the time, osteoporosis was suspected, and a workup was recommended. Calcium and vitamin D supplementation were prescribed, but unfortunately no DEXA scan was obtained and no additional anti-osteoporosis treatment was undertaken. Two years later, the patient returned, reporting a sudden onset of midline low back pain after weight lifting. An acute L5 compression fracture was found (**C**). The patient improved with bracing and activity restriction. At this point, osteoporosis with a T-score of −3.2 was diagnosed and bisphosphonate therapy was added.

trogen receptor modulators such as raloxifene. These agents appear to have bone-preserving effects similar to estrogen without the cancer and coronary complications.[106,107]

Calcitonin, administered either via subcutaneous injection or nasal spray, decreases osteoclastic bone resorption. Over the short term, calcitonin enhances bone formation, leading to a slight net bone accretion. Over long-term treatment, however, osteoblastic activity slows, and bone mass stabilizes.[108,109]

Traditionally, aggressive pharmacologic management was indicated in patients who had either sustained an insufficiency fracture or had femoral T-scores less than −2.5. More recently, however, several risk-benefit studies have suggested that early, aggressive interven-tion is warranted, especially in younger and more active osteopenic patients.[110-112] Although bisphosphonates have been shown to increase the risk of osteosarcoma, mandibular osteonecrosis, and subtrochanteric fractures, their impact on lifetime fracture risk is thought to justify early implementation.[113] Early treatment is further supported by the idea that, once lost, trabecular connectivity cannot be restored with any later pharmacologic interventions.

The bisphosphonates have dramatic effects in suppressing bone resorption and in preventing fractures of the hip and vertebral bodies.[114-116] These agents act in two ways to inhibit bone resorption. First, they directly stabilize the bone crystal, making it more resistant to osteoclastic bone resorption. Second, they directly inhibit the activity of the osteoclast. Thus, bisphosphonates may help preserve bone architecture as well as overall density. These agents are now available in forms that are administered weekly, monthly, or yearly to facilitate compliance without increased toxicity.

Parodoxically, *intermittent* PTH administration leads to early dramatic increases in bone mass, especially in trabecular areas.[117,118] Daily subcutaneous injections of teriparatide (recombinant PTH) have been shown to lead to clinically relevant improvements in bone mass in as little as 6 months;[119-121] however, the long-term safety and efficacy of these protocols continues to be investigated.

Ultimately, for patients with severe osteoporosis, combination therapies, including those that combine an anabolic agent with an antiresorptive agent (eg, teriparatide plus estrogen), along with calcium and vitamin D supplementation, may prove optimal.[122] Regardless of the regimen selected, appropriate BMD improvements should be assessed with routine DEXA follow-up. Lack of improvement may indicate the presence of osteomalacia or other bone destructive processes or may indicate that a more aggressive treatment regimen is required. For patients on oral agents, compliance should be verified.[123]

When an acute osteoporotic injury occurs, goals of management include decreased pain, early mobilization, and preservation of alignment. Cessation of the precipitating activity is critical, followed by nonsurgical or surgical treatment as indicated.[15] With nonsurgical treatment, pain medications and bracing should be provided as appropriate during the initial, painful interval. Limited activity and, often, bed rest are advised or self-imposed. In the osteoporotic population, however, such bed rest is associated with an additional 4% loss of BMD. Therefore, "active rest," which includes daily, protected weight-bearing activity, is recommended.[124]

Most acute bone pain resulting from an osteoporotic spine fracture lasts 4 to 6 weeks. Narcotic pain medications may be continued until the patient can bear weight comfortably. In older athletes, however, narcotics may cause as many functional problems as the underlying fracture. Adequate fluids and stool softeners may obviate the severe constipation occasionally reported. Nasal calcitonin and bisphosphonates, which are useful in the treatment of osteoporosis, also may be effective in decreasing fracture-related pain.[125]

Several issues complicate bracing programs in older athletes.[24,126] First, the patient's body habitus must be braceable. In patients with preexisting deformity or a short, obese trunk or extremity, brace effectiveness is significantly reduced. Second, many older athletes suffer from decreased range of motion in other joints (eg, the shoulders), which can render donning and doffing of the brace difficult. Compliance, always a problem with bracing regimes, decreases markedly with awkward devices.

The most common osteoporotic spine injuries are between T7 and L2. For these injuries, a limited-contact orthosis such as a tripad Jewett extension brace or Cash brace is easy to fit and wear. Low lumbar injuries (L2 to L4) may benefit from a chair-back brace.[126,127] Rigid collars may be helpful in cervical spine injuries. The short neck and thoracic kyphosis seen in osteoporotic patients often challenges proper fitting. Often, a semicustomized Marlin collar fits best. Upper cervical injuries require more rigid braces, and occasionally a halo-type brace. Cervicothoracic injuries may do well in cervical collars with thoracic extensions. Although thoracolumbosacral orthoses (TLSOs) with thigh cuffs are available to stabilize lower lumbar (below L4), lumbosacral, and sacroiliac injuries, these rigid braces are extremely difficult to don and limit function markedly. As with most injuries requiring rigid bracing like a TLSO, a spine surgery consultation is appropriate in these settings.

Because bracing exacerbates bone loss, once the injury has healed, the athlete should be weaned gradually from the brace.[24] During this interval, physical therapy should be considered to assist the patient in regaining normal gait, core strength, and range of motion. Each osteoporotic patient should receive home strengthening instruction. Over the long term, a combination of weight-bearing, aerobic, and local and core-strengthening exercise should be strived for.

Osteoporotic or osteomalacic patients must consider the additional risks of implant and bone failure relative to the intended benefits of any proposed surgery. For some problems otherwise routinely treated surgically, the risk-benefit ratio may favor nonsurgical management. In patients with nonurgent problems, consideration should be given to treating the underlying osteoporosis before recommending surgery, as improvement of BMD may ultimately improve the chance of surgical success. This should include consideration of the injury's impact on the patient's functional status relative to the months that bone rebuilding requires.

If the decision is made to proceed with surgery, several considerations may improve outcomes (**Table 4**). Iatrogenic destabilization should be minimized whenever possible. Even when implants are used to restabilize the bone or joint, the "race" between fixation failure and bone healing is compromised by less rigid initial fixation. Larger or longer implants with more points of fixation may improve construct integrity, as may achievement of multiplanar stability.[21-23] That is, if a buttress plate is applied, an adequate load-bearing column must be available for it to buttress. Cancellous voids should be packed with graft or extender materials to decrease cantilever forces on the implants. Alternatively, a dynamic or collapsing implant that allows gradual settling into more stable configurations (eg, a sliding hip screw) may be used. Intramedullary implants have been shown to be more load-sharing than load-bearing and may decrease bending moments that affect implant construct failure.

Meticulous soft-tissue handling and careful preservation of the local blood supply accelerate healing. In high-risk cases, bone grafting or use of bone morphogenetic protein should be considered. In many of these patients, postoperative casting or bracing is recommended as a "belt and suspenders" approach. Particularly in the early postoperative period, the local muscular stabilizers, which may also be healing from injury or surgical trauma, are not protecting the region. Immobilization in these patients may result in additional regional osteopenia.

VCFs are the most common osteoporotic fracture in the older athlete. VCFs were previously thought to be benign, self-limited injuries with few, if any, significant long-term sequelae. This conception arose from the fact that nearly two thirds of VCFs are never reported by patients to their physicians. In addition, in many of the cases brought to medical attention, the symptoms respond rapidly to simple nonsurgical treatment. Based on recent population-wide studies, however, it is becoming increasingly evident that any VCF can have significant functional and physiologic effects, such as acute and chronic pain, recurrent fracture, kyphotic deformity, gastrointestinal dysfunction, pulmonary

Table 4: Methods to Improve Fixation in Patients With Osteoporosis
1. Minimize removal of normal bone where possible
2. Improve bone anchorage Longer screws with maximum diameter More anchor points Augment anchor points with PMMA
3. Axial bone to decrease bending forces Spine: anterior column stabilization with bone, cage, or PMMA Metaphyseal areas: Tightly pack cancellous voids with graft Dynamic or collapsing implants Diaphyseal areas: Load-sharing implants (rod versus plate) Axially rigid implants (locking plates)
4. Grafting technique Autograft or BMPs over slower healing agents Meticulous soft-tissue handling
5. Postoperative external bracing
BMPs = bone morphogenetic proteins, PMMA = polymethylmethacrylate.

dysfunction, functional decline, increased hospitalization rates, and, ultimately, increased mortality.[128,129]

Acute VCFs are variably painful. Some patients note only mild and transient symptoms, but others require hospitalization. Although most patients report significant improvement in the first 4 weeks, acute pain can persist for months. After the acute pain subsides, chronic pain disorders may develop. This chronic pain arises from a change in the sagittal balance of the spine. The risk of developing chronic pain increases with the number of VCFs. This pain is intensified with many typical activities of daily living such as standing, sitting, or bending. In many of these patients, standing tolerance decreases.[130]

In patients reporting severe pain and functional limitation nonresponsive to bracing and medications, percutaneous polymethylmethacrylate (PMMA) augmentation of the vertebral body may be considered.[131,132] These percutaneous procedures, including vertebroplasty and kyphoplasty, are often done in the outpatient setting and confer rapid relief and return to function. Complications, while rare, can be devastating, including extravasation of cement into the canal or embolism to the lungs. The most common problems, however, are additional fractures and ongoing muscular or spondylotic pain. Two recent studies in *The New England Journal of Medicine* have questioned the efficacy of vertebroplasty.[133,134] Early criticisms cite bias from the high rates of enrollment refusal, no physical examination data to delineate pre- and posttreatment pain, the chronicity of many of the treated fractures (up to 1 year old), and the very low volumes of PMMA injected.[135] Also, the American Academy of Orthopaedic Surgeons' clinical practice guideline on osteoporotic spinal fractures recommends against vertebroplasty in neurologically intact patients.[136] In my opinion, "the jury is out" at this time. Most patients will benefit from a trial of brace management. On the other hand, for those patients who cannot return to normal function, I believe a vertebroplasty or kyphoplasty should be considered.

Conclusions

Anyone treating older athletes will encounter patients with osteoporosis. Osteomalacia, which is less common, exists on a continuum from simple osteoporosis with low vitamin D levels to a more full-blown condition with diffuse skeletal pain and marked demineralization. Older athletes, especially those from northern states with low levels of sunlight and those with gastrointestinal disorders, will carry a higher risk of osteomalacia.

Providers treating mature athletes must understand osteoporosis and osteomalacia because bone loss affects the types of pathology encountered. From subtle stress fractures to low-energy but possibly devastating dens fractures, a high index of suspicion will lower the rate of missed diagnoses. Furthermore, bone loss affects how even nonosteoporotic musculoskeletal injuries are treated. Awareness of the relative quality of the patient's bone and the proper means of maximizing stability improves outcomes and decreases complications across the spectrum of athletic injuries. For example, the physician who is aware of a patient's bone loss status is more likely to avoid casting an osteoporotic tibia or to take special precautions to prevent plate failure after open reduction and internal fixation of an ankle fracture.

Bone and joint specialists, in an attempt to "own the bone," must understand the quality of the organs they treat. Therefore, consideration of DEXA screening of at-risk patients is of paramount importance. Some may undertake a more complete assessment of bone metabolism and prescribe medications in appropriate cases. At the very least, the patient must receive the proper referral, and appropriate investigations and management must be undertaken. Treatments for bone loss have improved rapidly. But those gains increase the physician's responsibility to ensure patient access to appropriate treatment. In the meantime, vitamin D and calcium intake, along with weight-bearing exercise, should be encouraged.

References

1. Dunnigan MG, Henderson JB, Hole DJ, Barbara Mawer E, Berry JL: Meat consumption reduces the risk of nutritional rickets and osteomalacia. *Br J Nutr* 2005; 94(6):983-991.

2. Prentice A: Vitamin D deficiency: A global perspective. *Nutr Rev* 2008;66(10, Suppl 2)S153-S164.

3. Zuberi LM, Habib A, Haque N, Jabbar A, Vitamin D: Vitamin D deficiency in ambulatory patients. *J Pak Med Assoc* 2008;58(9):482-484.

4. Ruohola JP, Laaksi I, Ylikomi T, et al: Association between serum 25(OH)D concentrations and bone stress fractures in Finnish young men. *J Bone Miner Res* 2006;21(9):1483-1488.

5. Bikle DD: Vitamin D insufficiency/deficiency in gastrointestinal disorders. *J Bone Miner Res* 2007; 22(Suppl 2):V50-V54.

6. Holick MF: High prevalence of vitamin D inadequacy and implications for health. *Mayo Clin Proc* 2006; 81(3):353-373.

7. Lyman D: Undiagnosed vitamin D deficiency in the hospitalized patient. *Am Fam Physician* 2005; 71(2):299-304.

8. Toussaint ND, Elder GJ, Kerr PG: Bisphosphonates in chronic kidney disease: Balancing potential benefits and adverse effects on bone and soft tissue. *Clin J Am Soc Nephrol* 2009;4(1):221-233.

9. Maricic M: Osteomalacia. *Curr Osteoporos Rep* 2008; 6(4):130-133.

10. Riaz S, Alam M, Umer M: Frequency of osteomalacia in elderly patients with hip fractures. *J Pak Med Assoc* 2006;56(6):273-276.

11. Templeton KJ, Hame SL, Hannafin JA, Griffin LY, Tosi LL, Shields NN: Sports injuries in women: Sex- and gender-based differences in etiology and prevention. *Instr Course Lect* 2008;57:539-552.

12. Putukian M: Female athlete triad. *Sports Med Arthrosc* 1995;3(4):295-307.

13. Silverman SL: Quality-of-life issues in osteoporosis. *Curr Rheumatol Rep* 2005;7(1):39-45.

14. Dennison E, Cole Z, Cooper C: Diagnosis and epidemiology of osteoporosis. *Curr Opin Rheumatol* 2005;17(4):456-461.

15. Reeder MT, Dick BH, Atkins JK, Pribis AB, Martinez JM: Stress fractures: Current concepts of diagnosis and treatment. *Sports Med* 1996;22(3):198-212.

16. Pollock N, Hamilton B: Osteoporotic fracture in an elite male Kenyan athlete. *Br J Sports Med* 2008;42(12):1000-1001.

17. Miller C, Major N, Toth A: Pelvic stress injuries in the athlete: Management and prevention. *Sports Med* 2003;33(13):1003-1012.

18. Lee C, Lashari S: Pseudofracture of the neck of femur secondary to osteomalacia. *J Bone Joint Surg Br* 2007;89(7):956-958.

19. Khan MS, Sultan S, Khan A, Younis M: Bilateral protrusion of femoral head into the pelvis in neglected osteomalacia. *J Ayub Med Coll Abbottabad* 2007;19(2):54-55.

20. Cortet B, Houvenagel E, Puisieux F, Roches E, Garnier P, Delcambre B: Spinal curvatures and quality of life in women with vertebral fractures secondary to osteoporosis. *Spine (Phila Pa 1976)* 1999;24(18):1921-1925.

21. Templeman D, Baumgaertner MR, Leighton RK, Lindsey RW, Moed BR: Reducing complications in the surgical treatment of intertrochanteric fractures. *Instr Course Lect* 2005;(54):409-415.

22. Srinivasan K, Agarwal M, Matthews SJ, Giannoudis PV: Fractures of the distal humerus in the elderly: Is internal fixation the treatment of choice? *Clin Orthop Relat Res* 2005;(434):222-230.

23. Ozawa T, Takahashi K, Yamagata M, et al: Insertional torque of the lumbar pedicle screw during surgery. *J Orthop Sci* 2005;10(2):133-136.

24. Hastings MK, Sinacore DR, Fielder FA, Johnson JE: Bone mineral density during total contact cast immobilization for a patient with neuropathic (Charcot) arthropathy. *Phys Ther* 2005;85(3):249-256.

25. Cook SD, Barbera J, Rubi M, Salkeld SL, Whitecloud TS III: Lumbosacral fixation using expandable pedicle screws: An alternative in reoperation and osteoporosis. *Spine J* 2001;1(2):109-114.

26. Shea JE, Miller SC: Skeletal function and structure: Implications for tissue-targeted therapeutics. *Adv Drug Deliv Rev* 2005;57(7):945-957.

27. Zhilkin BA, Doktorov AA, Denisov-Nikol'skii YI: Structure of human vertebral lamellar bone in age-associated involution and osteoporosis. *Bull Exp Biol Med* 2003;135(4):405-408.

28. Gasser JA, Ingold P, Grosios K, Laib A, Hämmerle S, Koller B: Noninvasive monitoring of changes in structural cancellous bone parameters with a novel prototype micro-CT. *J Bone Miner Metab* 2005;23(Suppl):90-96.

29. Mankin HJ, Mankin CJ: Metabolic bone disease: A review and update. *Instr Course Lect* 2008;57:575-593.

30. Zmuda JM, Sheu YT, Moffett SP: Genetic epidemiology of osteoporosis: Past, present, and future. *Curr Osteoporos Rep* 2005;3(3):111-115.

31. Tracy JK, Meyer WA, Flores RH, Wilson PD, Hochberg MC: Racial differences in rate of decline in bone mass in older men: The Baltimore men's osteoporosis study. *J Bone Miner Res* 2005;20(7):1228-1234.

32. Gordon CM, Nelson LM: Amenorrhea and bone health in adolescents and young women. *Curr Opin Obstet Gynecol* 2003;15(5):377-384.

33. Fritton JC, Myers ER, Wright TM, van der Meulen MC: Loading induces site-specific increases in mineral content assessed by microcomputed tomography of the mouse tibia. *Bone* 2005;36(6):1030-1038.

34. Pouillès JM, Trémollieres FA, Ribot C: Osteoporosis in otherwise healthy perimenopausal and early postmenopausal women: Physical and biochemical characteristics. *Osteoporos Int* 2005;17(2):193-200.

35. Aerssens J, Boonen S, Joly J, Dequeker J: Variations in trabecular bone composition with anatomical site and age: Potential implications for bone quality assessment. *J Endocrinol* 1997;155(3):411-421.

36. Cranney A, Adachi JD: Corticosteroid-induced osteoporosis: A guide to optimum management. *Treat Endocrinol* 2002;1(5):271-279.

37. Andersson S, Rodrigues M, Olerud C: Odontoid fractures: High complication rate associated with anterior screw fixation in the elderly. *Eur Spine J* 2000;9(1):56-59.

38. Ritzel H, Amling M, Pösl M, Hahn M, Delling G: The thickness of human vertebral cortical bone and its changes in aging and osteoporosis: A histomorphometric analysis of the complete spinal column from thirty-seven autopsy specimens. *J Bone Miner Res* 1997;12(1):89-95.

39. Dvorak J, Antinnes JA, Panjabi M, Loustalot D, Bonomo M: Age and gender related normal motion of the cervical spine. *Spine (Phila Pa 1976)* 1992; 17(10, Suppl)S393-S398.

40. Karhu JO, Parkkola RK, Koskinen SK: Evaluation of flexion/extension of the upper cervical spine in patients with rheumatoid arthritis: An MRI study with a dedicated positioning device compared to conventional radiographs. *Acta Radiol* 2005;46(1):55-66.

41. Lomoschitz FM, Blackmore CC, Mirza SK, Mann FA: Cervical spine injuries in patients 65 years old and older: Epidemiologic analysis regarding the effects of age and injury mechanism on distribution, type, and stability of injuries. *AJR Am J Roentgenol* 2002;178(3): 573-577.

42. Grauer JN, Shafi B, Hilibrand AS, et al: Proposal of a modified, treatment-oriented classification of odontoid fractures. *Spine J* 2005;5(2):123-129.

43. Benoist M: Natural history of the aging spine. *Eur Spine J* 2003;12(Suppl 2):S86-S89.

44. Tabrizi P, Bouchard JA: Osteoporotic spondylolisthesis: A case report. *Spine (Phila Pa 1976)* 2001;26(13): 1482-1485.

45. Jaovisidha S, Kim JK, Sartoris DJ, et al: Scoliosis in elderly and age-related bone loss: A population-based study. *J Clin Densitom* 1998;1(3):227-233.

46. Sarikaya S, Ozdolap S, Açikgöz G, Erdem CZ: Pregnancy-associated osteoporosis with vertebral fractures and scoliosis. *Joint Bone Spine* 2004;71(1): 84-85.

47. Cheng JC, Guo X, Sher AH: Persistent osteopenia in adolescent idiopathic scoliosis: A longitudinal follow up study. *Spine (Phila Pa 1976)* 1999;24(12):1218-1222.

48. Hans D, Biot B, Schott AM, Meunier PJ: No diffuse osteoporosis in lumbar scoliosis but lower femoral bone density on the convexity. *Bone* 1996;18(1):15-17.

49. Mika A, Unnithan VB, Mika P: Differences in thoracic kyphosis and in back muscle strength in women with

bone loss due to osteoporosis. *Spine (Phila Pa 1976)* 2005;30(2):241-246.

50. Sinaki M, Brey RH, Hughes CA, Larson DR, Kaufman KR: Balance disorder and increased risk of falls in osteoporosis and kyphosis: Significance of kyphotic posture and muscle strength. *Osteoporos Int* 2005;16(8): 1004-1010.

51. Schneider DL, von Mühlen D, Barrett-Connor E, Sartoris DJ: Kyphosis does not equal vertebral fractures: The Rancho Bernardo study. *J Rheumatol* 2004;31(4): 747-752.

52. Wehren LE, Magaziner J: Hip fracture: Risk factors and outcomes. *Curr Osteoporos Rep* 2003;1(2):78-85.

53. Robbins JA, Schott AM, Garnero P, Delmas PD, Hans D, Meunier PJ: Risk factors for hip fracture in women with high BMD: EPIDOS study. *Osteoporos Int* 2005; 16(2):149-154.

54. Leveille SG: Musculoskeletal aging. *Curr Opin Rheumatol* 2004;16(2):114-118.

55. Dipaola CP, Bible JE, Biswas D, Dipaola M, Grauer JN, Rechtine GR: Survey of spine surgeons on attitudes regarding osteoporosis and osteomalacia screening and treatment for fractures, fusion surgery, and pseudoarthrosis. *Spine J* 2009;9(7):537-544.

56. Castel H, Bonneh DY, Sherf M, Liel Y: Awareness of osteoporosis and compliance with management guidelines in patients with newly diagnosed low-impact fractures. *Osteoporos Int* 2001;12(7):559-564.

57. Allen RT, Lee YP, Garfin SR: Spine surgeons survey on attitudes regarding osteoporosis and osteomalacia screening and treatment for fractures, fusion surgery, and pseudoarthrosis. *Spine J* 2009;9(7):602-604.

58. Werner P, Vered I: The diagnosis of osteoporosis: Attitudes and knowledge of Israeli physicians. *Aging Clin Exp Res* 2002;14(1):52-59.

59. Licata AA: Stress fractures in young athletic women: Case reports of unsuspected cortisol-induced osteoporosis. *Med Sci Sports Exerc* 1992;24(9):955-957.

60. Wilson JH, Wolman RL: Osteoporosis and fracture complications in an amenorrhoeic athlete. *Br J Rheumatol* 1994;33(5):480-481.

61. Brown JP, Josse RG, Scientific Advisory Council of the Osteoporosis Society of Canada: 2002 clinical practice guidelines for the diagnosis and management of osteoporosis in Canada. *CMAJ* 2002;167(10, Suppl) S1-S34.

62. Coleman RE: Management of bone metastases. *Oncologist* 2000;5(6):463-470.

63. Angastiniotis M, Pavlides N, Aristidou K, et al: Bone pain in thalassaemia: Assessment of DEXA and MRI findings. *J Pediatr Endocrinol Metab* 1998;11(Suppl 3): 779-784.

64. Berenson JR: Bisphosphonates in multiple myeloma. *Cancer* 1997;80(8, Suppl):1661-1667.

65. Singer FR, Minoofar PN: Bisphosphonates in the treatment of disorders of mineral metabolism. *Adv Endocrinol Metab* 1995;6:259-288.

66. Henry MJ, Pasco JA, Seeman E, Nicholson GC, Sanders KM, Kotowicz MA: Fracture thresholds revisited: Geelong Osteoporosis Study. *J Clin Epidemiol* 2002;55(7):642-646.

67. Weber K, Lunt M, Gowin W, et al: Measurement imprecision in vertebral morphometry of spinal radiographs obtained in the European Prospective Osteoporosis Study: Consequences for the identification of prevalent and incident deformities. *Br J Radiol* 1999;72(862):957-966.

68. Masud T, Jawed S, Doyle DV, Spector TD: A population study of the screening potential of assessment of trabecular pattern of the femoral neck (Singh index): The Chingford Study. *Br J Radiol* 1995;68(808):389-393.

69. Lo LD, Schweitzer ME, Juneja V, Shabshin N: Are L5 fractures an indicator of metastasis? *Skeletal Radiol* 2000;29(8):454-458.

70. Schachter AK, Roberts CS, Seligson D: Occult bilateral acetabular fractures associated with high-energy trauma and osteoporosis. *J Orthop Trauma* 2003;17(5): 386-389.

71. Böttcher J, Pfeil A, Heinrich B, et al: Digital radiogrammetry as a new diagnostic tool for estimation of disease-related osteoporosis in rheumatoid arthritis compared with pQCT. *Rheumatol Int* 2005;25(6): 457-464.

72. Sekioka Y, Kushida K, Yamazaki K, Inoue T: Calcaneus bone mineral density using single x-ray absorptiometry in Japanese women. *Calcif Tissue Int* 1999;65(2): 106-111.

73. Hartl F, Tyndall A, Kraenzlin M, et al: Discriminatory ability of quantitative ultrasound parameters and bone mineral density in a population-based sample of postmenopausal women with vertebral fractures: Results of the Basel Osteoporosis Study. *J Bone Miner Res* 2002;17(2):321-330.

74. Ito M, Lang TF, Jergas M, et al: Spinal trabecular bone loss and fracture in American and Japanese women. *Calcif Tissue Int* 1997;61(2):123-128.

75. Orwoll E, Blank JB, Barrett-Connor E, et al: Design and baseline characteristics of the osteoporotic fractures in men (MrOS) study—A large observational study of the determinants of fracture in older men. *Contemp Clin Trials* 2005;26(5):569-585.

76. Greenwald L, Barajas K, White-Greenwald M: Better bone density reporting: T-score report versus fracture risk report with outcome analysis. *Am J Manag Care* 2003;9(10):665-670.

77. Rozkydal Z, Janicek P: The effect of alendronate in the treatment of postmenopausal osteoporosis. *Bratisl Lek Listy* 2003;104(10):309-313.

78. Swezey RL, Draper D, Swezey AM: Bone densitometry: Comparison of dual energy x-ray absorptiometry to radiographic absorptiometry. *J Rheumatol* 1996;23(10): 1734-1738.

79. Thomas E, Richardson JC, Irvine A, Hassell AB, Hay EM: Osteoporosis: What are the implications of DEXA scanning 'high risk' women in primary care? *Fam Pract* 2003;20(3):289-293.

80. Becker C: Clinical evaluation for osteoporosis. *Clin Geriatr Med* 2003;19(2):299-320.

81. Crandall C: Laboratory workup for osteoporosis: Which tests are most cost-effective? *Postgrad Med* 2003;114(3):35-44.

82. Preston DM, Torréns JI, Harding P, Howard RS, Duncan WE, McLeod DG: Androgen deprivation in men with prostate cancer is associated with an increased rate of bone loss. *Prostate Cancer Prostatic Dis* 2002; 5(4):304-310.

83. Ralston SH: Bone densitometry and bone biopsy. *Best Pract Res Clin Rheumatol* 2005;19(3):487-501.

84. Kann PH, Pfützner A, Delling G, Schulz G, Meyer S: Transiliac bone biopsy in osteoporosis: Frequency, indications, consequences and complications. An evaluation of 99 consecutive cases over a period of 14 years. *Clin Rheumatol* 2006;25(1):30-34.

85. Coen G, Ballanti P, Fischer MS, et al: Serum leptin in dialysis renal osteodystrophy. *Am J Kidney Dis* 2003; 42(5):1036-1042.

86. Bauer DC, Sklarin PM, Stone KL, et al: Biochemical markers of bone turnover and prediction of hip bone

loss in older women: The study of osteoporotic fractures. *J Bone Miner Res* 1999;14(8):1404-1410.

87. Henry AP, Lachmann E, Tunkel RS, Nagler W: Pelvic insufficiency fractures after irradiation: Diagnosis, management, and rehabilitation. *Arch Phys Med Rehabil* 1996;77(4):414-416.

88. Nguyen HV, Ludwig S, Gelb D: Osteoporotic vertebral burst fractures with neurologic compromise. *J Spinal Disord Tech* 2003;16(1):10-19.

89. Chan JH, Peh WC, Tsui EY, et al: Acute vertebral body compression fractures: Discrimination between benign and malignant causes using apparent diffusion coefficients. *Br J Radiol* 2002;75(891):207-214.

90. Kanberoglu K, Kantarci F, Cebi D, et al: Magnetic resonance imaging in osteomalacic insufficiency fractures of the pelvis. *Clin Radiol* 2005;60(1):105-111.

91. Grangier C, Garcia J, Howarth NR, May M, Rossier P: Role of MRI in the diagnosis of insufficiency fractures of the sacrum and acetabular roof. *Skeletal Radiol* 1997;26(9):517-524.

92. Kucukalic-Selimovic E, Begic A: Value of bone scintigraphy for detection and ageing of vertebral fractures in patients with severe osteoporosis and correlation between bone scintigraphy and mineral bone density. *Med Arh* 2004;58(6):343-344.

93. Soubrier M, Dubost JJ, Boisgard S, et al: Insufficiency fracture: A survey of 60 cases and review of the literature. *Joint Bone Spine* 2003;70(3):209-218.

94. Marì C, Catafau A, Carriò I: Bone scintigraphy and metabolic disorders. *Q J Nucl Med* 1999;43(3):259-267.

95. Egol KA, Koval KJ, Kummer F, Frankel VH: Stress fractures of the femoral neck. *Clin Orthop Relat Res* 1998;(348):72-78.

96. Schapira D, Militeanu D, Israel O, Scharf Y: Insufficiency fractures of the pubic ramus. *Semin Arthritis Rheum* 1996;25;(6):373-382.

97. McFarland EG, Giangarra C: Sacral stress fractures in athletes. *Clin Orthop Relat Res* 1996;(329):240-243.

98. Murray AW, McQuillan C, Kennon B, Gallacher SJ: Osteoporosis risk assessment and treatment intervention after hip or shoulder fracture: A comparison of two centres in the United Kingdom. *Injury* 2005;36(9):1080-1084.

99. Skolbekken JA, Østerlie W, Forsmo S: Brittle bones, pain and fractures—Lay constructions of osteoporosis among Norwegian women attending the Nord-Trøndelag Health Study (HUNT). *Soc Sci Med* 2008;66(12):2562-2572.

100. Callaghan MJ, Jarvis C: Evaluation of elite British cyclists: The role of the squad medical. *Br J Sports Med* 1996;30(4):349-353.

101. Feldstein AC, Elmer PJ, Nichols GA, Herson M: Practice patterns in patients at risk for glucocorticoid-induced osteoporosis. *Osteoporos Int* 2005;16(12):2168-2174.

102. Misra M, Papakostas GI, Klibanski A: Effects of psychiatric disorders and psychotropic medications on prolactin and bone metabolism. *J Clin Psychiatry* 2004;65(12):1607-1618, quiz 1590, 1760-1761.

103. Stevens JA, Olson S: Reducing falls and resulting hip fractures among older women. *MMWR Recomm Rep* 2000;49(RR-2):3-12.

104. Stevenson JC: Hormone replacement therapy: Review, update, and remaining questions after the Women's Health Initiative Study. *Curr Osteoporos Rep* 2004;2(1):12-16.

105. Ness J, Aronow WS, Newkirk E, McDanel D: Use of hormone replacement therapy by postmenopausal women after publication of the Women's Health Initiative Trial. *J Gerontol A Biol Sci Med Sci* 2005;60(4):460-462.

106. Siris ES, Harris ST, Eastell R, et al: Skeletal effects of raloxifene after 8 years: Results from the continuing outcomes relevant to Evista (CORE) study. *J Bone Miner Res* 2005;20(9):1514-1524.

107. Prestwood KM, Gunness M, Muchmore DB, Lu Y, Wong M, Raisz LG: A comparison of the effects of raloxifene and estrogen on bone in postmenopausal women. *J Clin Endocrinol Metab* 2000;85(6):2197-2202.

108. Hejdova M, Palicka V, Kucera Z, Vlcek J: Effects of alendronate and calcitonin on bone mineral density in postmenopausal osteoporotic women: An observational study. *Pharm World Sci* 2005;27(3):149-153.

109. Cosman F, Lindsay R: Therapeutic potential of parathyroid hormone. *Curr Osteoporos Rep* 2004;2(1):5-11.

110. Simon JA: Does osteopenia warrant treatment? *Menopause* 2005;12(5):639-648.

111. Cranney A, Adachi JD: Benefit-risk assessment of raloxifene in postmenopausal osteoporosis. *Drug Saf* 2005;28(8):721-730.

112. Waldrop J: Early identification and interventions for female athlete triad. *J Pediatr Health Care* 2005;19(4):213-220.

113. Solomon DH, Rekedal L, Cadarette SM: Osteoporosis treatments and adverse events. *Curr Opin Rheumatol* 2009;21(4):363-368.

114. Rackoff PJ, Sebba A: Optimizing administration of bisphosphonates in women with postmenopausal osteoporosis. *Treat Endocrinol* 2005;4(4):245-251.

115. Nancollas GH, Tang R, Phipps RJ, et al: Novel insights into actions of bisphosphonates on bone: Differences in interactions with hydroxyapatite. *Bone* 2006;38(5):617-627.

116. McClung M: Use of highly potent bisphosphonates in the treatment of osteoporosis. *Curr Osteoporos Rep* 2003;1(3):116-122.

117. Quattrocchi E, Kourlas H: Teriparatide: A review. *Clin Ther* 2004;26(6):841-854.

118. Bazaldua OV, Bruder J: Teriparatide (Forteo) for osteoporosis. *Am Fam Physician* 2004;69(8):1983-1984.

119. Prevrhal S, Krege JH, Chen P, Genant H, Black DM: Teriparatide vertebral fracture risk reduction determined by quantitative and qualitative radiographic assessment. *Curr Med Res Opin* 2009;25(4):921-928.

120. Lindsay R, Miller P, Pohl G, Glass EV, Chen P, Krege JH: Relationship between duration of teriparatide therapy and clinical outcomes in postmenopausal women with osteoporosis. *Osteoporos Int* 2009;20(6):943-948.

121. Glover SJ, Eastell R, McCloskey EV, et al: Rapid and robust response of biochemical markers of bone formation to teriparatide therapy. *Bone* 2009;45(6):1053-1058.

122. Bessette L, Jean S, Davison KS, Roy S, Ste-Marie LG, Brown JP: Factors influencing the treatment of osteoporosis following fragility fracture. *Osteoporos Int* 2009; 20(11):1911-1919.

123. Recker RR, Gallagher R, MacCosbe PE: Effect of dosing frequency on bisphosphonate medication adherence in a large longitudinal cohort of women. *Mayo Clin Proc* 2005;80(7):856-861.

124. Uebelhart D, Demiaux-Domenech B, Roth M, Chantraine A: Bone metabolism in spinal cord injured individuals and in others who have prolonged immobilization: A review. *Paraplegia* 1995;33(11):669-673.

125. Peichl P, Marteau R, Griesmacher A, et al: Salmon calcitonin nasal spray treatment for postmenopausal women after hip fracture with total hip arthroplasty. *J Bone Miner Metab* 2005;23(3):243-252.

126. Lin JT, Lane JM: Nonmedical management of osteoporosis. *Curr Opin Rheumatol* 2002;14(4):441-446.

127. Kaplan RS, Sinaki M, Hameister MD: Effect of back supports on back strength in patients with osteoporosis: A pilot study. *Mayo Clin Proc* 1996;71(3):235-241.

128. Kobayashi K, Shimoyama K, Nakamura K, Murata K: Percutaneous vertebroplasty immediately relieves pain of osteoporotic vertebral compression fractures and prevents prolonged immobilization of patients. *Eur Radiol* 2005;15(2):360-367.

129. McKiernan F, Faciszewski T, Jensen R: Quality of life following vertebroplasty. *J Bone Joint Surg Am* 2004;86A(12):2600-2606.

130. Truumees E: Medical consequences of osteoporotic vertebral compression fractures. *Instr Course Lect* 2003;52:551-558.

131. Brunton S, Carmichael B, Gold D, et al: Vertebral compression fractures in primary care: Recommendations from a consensus panel. *J Fam Pract* 2005;54(9):781-788.

132. Truumees E, Hilibrand A, Vaccaro AR: Percutaneous vertebral augmentation. *Spine J* 2004;4(2):218-229.

133. Buchbinder R, Osborne RH, Ebeling PR, et al: A randomized trial of vertebroplasty for painful osteoporotic vertebral fractures. *N Engl J Med* 2009;361(6):557-568.

134. Kallmes DF, Comstock BA, Heagerty PJ, et al: A randomized trial of vertebroplasty for osteoporotic spinal fractures. *N Engl J Med* 2009;361(6):569-579.

135. Aebi M: Vertebroplasty: About sense and nonsense of uncontrolled "controlled randomized prospective trials". *Eur Spine J* 2009;18(9):1247-1248.

136. American Academy of Orthopaedic Surgeons: *Clinical Practice Guideline on the Treatment of Symptomatic Osteoporotic Spinal Compression Fractures*. Rosemont, IL, American Academy of Orthopaedic Surgeons, September 2010. http://www.aaos.org/research/guidelines/SCFguideline.pdf. Accessed March 28, 2011.

Section 2

General Health, Nutrition, and Exercise

Andrew L. Chen, MD, MS
Section Editor

Chapter 5

Nutritional Supplements and NSAIDs

Andrew L. Chen, MD, MS

Key Points

- Patients often use nutritional supplements, over-the-counter nonsteroidal anti-inflammatory drugs (NSAIDs), and alternative medicine before seeking formal medical treatment.
- Active, older individuals often practice dietary restriction as a method for weight control, which may have a negative effect on the nutritional status of the individual. Dietary modifications may be successful in mitigating or reversing the effects of such practices.
- Maintenance of fluid balance can be challenging but is important in the older athlete.
- In active individuals who maintain a balanced diet, micronutrient deficiencies are rare, and supplementation is typically not necessary. Dietary supplementation with vitamins or other nutrients may be necessary in individuals who have nutritionally restrictive diets.
- Glucosamine and/or chondroitin sulfate may be of benefit to patients with osteoarthritis of the knee. Although many studies document improvement in pain and function, there is a lack of definitive evidence to support that these substances are chondroprotective or that they alter the degenerative course of the disease.
- NSAIDs have been shown to be of short-term benefit for the symptomatic treatment of osteoarthritis. Patients should be aware that the use of NSAIDs may negatively affect bone and soft-tissue healing.

Introduction

Complementary and alternative medicine (CAM) has gained enormous popularity in recent years. Because CAM typically involves over-the-counter substances, such as nutritional supplements, which are easy to obtain, the American public often turns to CAM before seeking conventional medical treatment. In 1997, an estimated $27 to $47 billion was spent on CAM; of this, $12 to $20 billion was paid to CAM providers.[1,2] To put this in perspective, these fees were greater than those paid out of pocket for *all* hospitalizations in 1997, and they represent half the amount paid out for *all* out-of-pocket physician services. In 2007, $14.8 billion was spent on "natural" products (ie, nonvitamin, nonmineral products such as fish oil, echinacea, glucosamine, etc) alone, and CAM was an estimated $100 billion industry in 2010.[1-3]

Table 1: Most Common Conditions for Which CAM Is Used

Condition	%[a]
Back pain	16.8
Upper respiratory	9.5
Neck pain	6.6
Joint pain	4.9
Arthritis	4.9
Anxiety/depression	4.5
Upset stomach	3.7
Headache	3.1
Recurrent pain	2.4
Insomnia	2.2

CAM = complementary and alternative medicine.
[a]Percentage of US adult population.
Data from Barnes P, Powell-Griner E, McFann K, Nahin R: *CDC Advance Data Report #343: Complementary and Alternative Medicine Use Among Adults: United States, 2002.* Hyattsville, MD, US Department of Health and Human Services, DHHS Publication No 2004-1250, 2004.

The terms *complementary* and *alternative* should be considered anachronistic, as CAM use is widespread, common, and mainstream. In a Centers for Disease Control (CDC) report, Barnes et al[4] reported that 74.6% of adults in the United States had used CAM at some point and 62.1% had used such methods in 2002 (**Table 1**). CAM use was more common among women (79% versus 62% of men), educated individuals (74% of those with college degrees versus 37% of those with high school diplomas or less), patients who had been hospitalized within the preceding year, and former cigarette smokers.[4]

Increasingly, patients are inquiring about CAM methods, and it is incumbent upon the physician to have knowledge of these treatments to be able to engage the patient in a meaningful, educated discussion. According to the CDC, 83% of patients wished their doctors would include CAM in treatment discussions, 71% of patients who used CAM brought it up in discussion with their doctor, and 68% of patients would prefer not to see a doctor who refused to consider CAM.[4]

Metabolism, Nutrition, and Aging

One major report on masters athletes discussed weight gain (or lack of weight loss) despite a high level of activity and the same nutritional patterns as when the individuals were younger.[5] This has been shown to be secondary to an age-related decline in resting metabolic rate (RMR), which comprises up to 75% of daily energy expenditure and decreases 10% from childhood to adulthood, and another 10% from adulthood to the sixth decade.[6] RMR has been shown to be affected by many factors (**Table 2**), of which lean body mass, stress level, total body weight, and level of aerobic fitness are potentially modifiable by the individual.[7] A strong correlation has been observed between an individual's RMR and physical training[8]—both endurance and resistance—with geometrically increasing effects noted with cross-training that alternates between endurance and resistance training.[9] The highest degree of correlation has been observed between RMR and lean body mass. Webb[7] observed that replacement of metabolically active muscle tissue (ie, lean body mass) with metabolically inert depot fat was directly correlated with decreased RMR.

Aging athletes who wish to lose weight (usually for physical appearance reasons, regardless of level of aerobic fitness), typically run a negative energy balance. The decreased nutritional intake is typically perceived as a "healthy restriction" of intake. A decrease of dietary intake of 500 calories per day will result in a loss of 1 lb per week; however, more severe dietary restriction may have paradoxical effects. A decrease of intake of more than 1,000 calories per day results in muscle catabolism and decreased metabolic efficiency; chronic negative energy balance to this degree has been shown to result in decreased bone mass and an eightfold increase in stress fracture risk.[10] Moreover, this catabolic effect, compounded by caloric restriction and endurance training, results in a decrease in RMR that drives the athlete to further restrict the dietary caloric intake. Wilmore and Costill[11] thus recommended that athletes consume multiple (4 to 6) smaller meals per day to avoid the "feast or famine" effect.

Because many athletes tend to avoid calcium-rich foods such as cheese and ice cream, restrictive diets often are characterized by insufficient intake of dietary calcium. Beshgetoor et al[12] observed that female masters athletes average only 598 mg of dietary calcium per day. Talbott et al[13] demonstrated that calcium restriction for more than 9 weeks resulted in an irreversible reduction in bone mass. Conversely, calcium supplementation (1,500 to 1,800 mg daily) in conjunction with aerobic training has an independent beneficial effect on cortical bone density of the femoral neck in postmenopausal women. Exercise alone has been shown to increase trabecular bone density in the lumbar vertebrae.[14,15]

The 2002 Institute of Medicine (IOM) nutritional guidelines are summarized in **Table 3**.[14] An average aging individual consumes approximately 0.55 to 0.75 gram of protein per kilogram body weight per day (g/kg/d).[16] The 2002 IOM guidelines suggested that this should be increased to 0.8 g/kg/d, and that for athletes, intake should be 1.2 to 1.8 g/kg/d.[14] This level of protein intake is recommended not only to achieve desired anabolic effects but also to address exercise-induced muscle damage and to replace amino acids that are oxidized with exercise.[17] Evans[18] placed older athletes on a regimen of high protein intake (1.6 g/kg/d) and resistance exercise; increases in skeletal muscle mass and strength were observed. Esmarck et al[19] examined the effects of timing of protein supplementation and found that consuming protein less than 2 hours after exercise was most effective for muscle hypertrophy and strength.

Although the recommendations for carbohydrate intake in aging individuals are similar for athletes and for the general population, the tremendous energy expenditure that occurs during endurance sports often requires a high caloric intake (although, as discussed previously, athletes often "starve" themselves relative to the energy they expend). This intake is usually in the form of carbohydrates, which provide a readily usable, readily available energy source.[15] The 2002 IOM rec-

Table 2: Factors That Influence Resting Metabolic Rate

Thyroid hormones

Genetics

Body/environmental temperature

Body surface area

Sex

Age

Lean body mass[a]

Emotional stress level[a]

Total body weight[a]

Level of aerobic fitness[a]

[a]Potentially modifiable by the individual.
Data from Poehlman E, Danforth E Jr: Endurance training increases metabolic rate and norepinephrine appearance rate in older individuals. *Am J Physiol* 1991;261(2 Pt 1):E233-E239 and Toth MJ, Poehlman ET: Resting metabolic rate and cardiovascular disease risk in resistance- and aerobic-trained middle-aged women. *Int J Obes Relat Metab Disord* 1995;19(10):691-698.

Table 3: 2002 Institute of Medicine Nutritional Guidelines

Nutrient	Recommended Intake Level for the General Population	Recommended Intake Level for Athletes
Carbohydrate	45% to 65%	7 to 12 g/kg/d
Protein	10% to 35% or 0.8 g/kg/d	1.2 to 1.8 g/kg/d
Fat	20% to 35%	Not less than 20%

Data from Manore MM: Exercise and the Institute of Medicine recommendations for nutrition. *Curr Sports Med Rep* 2005;4(4):193-198.

ommendations state that athletes should aim for a daily carbohydrate intake of 7 to 12 g/kg.[14] "Empty calories," or those that come from sugars and short-chain carbohydrates, should be kept to a minimum (as with the general population), although endurance athletes often consume "energy" gels, drinks, or candies for a prerace or in-race burst of energy. During training, however, the consumption of high-quality carbohydrates from whole grain sources provides fiber and micronutrients that improve physiologic function and maximize nutritional advantage, thus ultimately facilitating improved exercise performance. "Carb loading," or consumption of high quantities of carbohydrates 24 to 72 hours before a race, is done to maximize glycogen stores within skeletal muscle. Although this is theoretically desirable, from a physiologic standpoint, glycogen storage is determined more by genetic predisposition and training than by short-term loading. Athletes who consume a nutritionally replete diet have not been shown to gain an advantage in endurance sports (in which this practice is typically used) by "carb loading," as oxidative means of energy production are probably more important for long-term energy production than glycolytic pathways.

In general, athletes should consume the same proportion of calories from fat as the general population (20% to 35% of total calories).[15] Although calories from other sources, such as carbohydrates or protein, may be converted to fat, essential neural lipids and lipoproteins, essential fatty acids, and fat-soluble vitamins are found in exogenous sources that cannot be manufactured by the body. No health or performance benefits have been demonstrated for diets in which fewer than 15% of calories are consumed as fat. Restriction of fat to less than 15% has been associated with nutritional deficiencies of fatty acids and vitamins. Most of this intake should be from plant sources to reduce intake of cholesterol, which is derived only from animal sources.

Fluid Balance

Adequate hydration during athletic activity is important to compensate for fluid loss, maintain performance level, lower submaximal exercise heart rate, and help control core body temperature with exertion.[19] For sedentary individuals, the recommended daily intake of water is 2.2 L for women and 3.0 L for men. During exertion, however, each pound of body weight lost acutely is equivalent to 16 ounces of fluid loss. Dehydration has been shown to be especially problematic in masters athletes because of physiologic changes that occur with aging. From infancy to adulthood, total body water decreases by 10% to 20%. Moreover, older athletes have diminished thirst sensation, decreased renal function and urine-concentrating capacity, and greater insensible fluid losses compared with younger individuals.[20,21]

To maintain adequate hydration during exertion, it is now recommended that athletes should consume "generous" amounts of water 24 hours before exertion. Two hours before exertion, 400 to 600 mL (12 to 20 oz) of water should be consumed. During exertion, 150 to 350 mL (6 to 12 oz) of water should be consumed every 15 to 20 minutes.[20] In general, for exertion less than 1 hour, water is sufficient for fluid replacement. For anticipated exertion greater than 1 hour or if the environment is hot and of low humidity, however, sports drinks (4% to 10% carbohydrate solutions) are recommended, as these have been shown to have enhanced absorption and therefore provide superior rehydration, replace electrolytes, prevent hyponatremia, and replace glycogen.[20]

The postexertion rehydration phase is often overlooked by older athletes, particularly those who do not participate in team sports or formal, organized athletic events. Insufficient rehydration after exertion may contribute to delayed-onset muscle soreness, fatigue, and slow recovery. For optimal recovery, it is now recommended that 150% of weight lost acutely during exercise (typically through sweat or urine) should be replaced with fluid.[20]

Caffeine is commonly consumed by athletes in the form of coffee, tea, or soft drinks. It is also present in various commercially available sports and energy beverages. The use of caffeine during physical exertion has not been shown to enhance physical performance indices such as strength, speed, or reaction time; however, it has been shown to increase exercise-to-exhaustion tolerance, improve mood and concentration, and increase motivation.[21] As such, caffeine is now considered an ergogenic aid that is no longer banned by the International Olympic Committee (IOC) or the World Anti-

Doping Agency (WADA). Moreover, in healthy individuals, caffeine has no adverse effects on fluid-electrolyte balance, hyperthermia, or renal function.[21]

Micronutrients and Nutritional Supplements

In the United States, healthy individuals who follow healthy dietary practices rarely have micronutrient deficiencies; however, such deficiencies may be seen in athletes who intentionally restrict caloric intake, those who use severe weight-loss techniques, those who eliminate one or more food groups from their diet, or those who consume high-carbohydrate diets with low micronutrient density. Micronutrient deficiencies of vitamins or minerals have been shown to compromise aerobic capacity, muscle strength, power, and endurance. Athletes who consume an adequate number of calories to maintain body weight from a variety of foods should not require vitamin or mineral supplementation.[22]

The term *nutritional supplement* originally referred to substances that were intended to make up for dietary nutritional deficiencies, including vitamins, minerals, herbs, amino acids, and botanicals. Today, the term also refers to any dietary supplement with reported health benefits, such as creatine. The term *nutraceutical* has gained popularity; the term refers to a nutritional supplement with pharmaceutical-like intentions; that is, a substance that is intended to not only replete nutritional deficiencies but also to augment physical well-being. For example, ingesting supraphysiologic doses of glucosamine sulfate may allow for an increased bioavailability of substrates to support the synthesis of articular cartilage components. Despite the popularity of this over-the-counter nutraceutical, it was not introduced through the rigorous paradigm of the US Food and Drug Administration (FDA) and therefore is not considered a pharmaceutical product.

Because nutritional supplements are not governed as pharmaceuticals by the FDA, they are not held to specific manufacturing standards, they are not guaranteed to meet product potency or purity ratings, they are not required to prove effectiveness of stated health claims, and they are not required to meet safety or efficacy standards before introduction to the market. Many adverse effects and health risks are discovered after the product is used widely, and, in fact, nutritional supplements are generally withdrawn only if serious health problems or death can be directly attributed to product use. Ginko and garlic, for example, are thought to have blood-thinning effects. Although these may contribute to the purported health benefits, in certain clinical circumstances (eg, concomitant use of warfarin, history of bleeding problems, presurgery), they may be considered undesirable and even dangerous (**Table 4**).

Nonetheless, nutritional supplementation is enormously popular, particularly for the treatment of musculoskeletal symptoms. Nutritional products are used by more people in the United States than any other type of complementary medicine except prayer.[4]

A full review of the numerous commercially available nutritional supplements is beyond the scope of this text. The following sections review several of the more popular nutritional supplements used by the older athlete. Although the popular and scientific literature is replete with reports that nutritional supplements are safe and efficacious, controlled studies are lacking, and patients should be counseled to use these products with caution.

Amino Acids

Amino acids are the building blocks of proteins and are commonly ingested as anabolic aids by athletes of all ages. Although amino acids represent a large fraction of the many billions of dollars spent on nutritional supplements, controlled studies have failed to demonstrate that these supplements provide a clear benefit in athletes who ingest a healthy, balanced diet without severely nutritionally restrictive practices.[22,23] Physiologic breakdown of protein consumed in a healthy diet (especially high-protein diets consumed by athletes) results in an abundance of amino acids to support normal metabolic and even anabolic activities of the body. Commercial claims of increased muscle mass and strength, therefore, may be more related to placebo-mediated increases in workout intensity and duration. Moreover, studies that demonstrate the beneficial effects of amino acid supplementation may be confounded by the positive systemic benefits conferred by regular exercise; thus it may be the exercise that accounts for the observed improvements in systemic function.

In addition to the purported anabolic benefits of amino acid supplementation, other health benefits have

Table 4: Potential Adverse or Dangerous Effects of Popular Nutritional Supplements

Supplement	Uses	Known or Probable Issues
Cayenne pepper	Muscle soreness, GI disorder	Skin blistering, mucosal or eye irritation, hyperthermia with anesthesia
Echinacea	Upper respiratory tract infection, urinary tract infection, bronchitis, wounds, burns	Hepatotoxicity, decreased effectiveness of corticosteroids
Ephedra	Weight loss, antitussive bacteriostatic	Cardiac arrhythmia, enhanced sympathomimetic effects with MAO inhibitors, hypertension with oxytocin use
Feverfew	Migraine headaches, antipyretic	Inhibits platelet function, rebound headache, aphthous ulcers, GI irritation
Garlic	Hyperlipidemia, hypertension, antiplatelet, antioxidant, antithrombotic	Enhances warfarin effect, increases surgical bleeding
Ginger	Antiemetic, antispasmotic, anti-inflammatory	Increases surgical bleeding via inhibition of thromboxane synthetase
Ginko	Circulatory stimulant	Enhances anticoagulant effect
Ginseng	Energy enhancer, antioxidant, adaptogenic	Tachycardia, hypertension, mastalgia, mania in patients on phenelzine, decreases warfarin effect, rebound somnolence, edema, hypertonia
Goldenseal	Diuretic, laxative, hemostatic	Overexcretion of free water, hypernatremia, oxytocic, paralysis, rebound edema, rebound hypertension
Kava-kava	Anxiolytic	Potentiates sedative effects, hepatotoxicity, increases suicide risk in patients with depression
Licorice	GI ulcers, cough, bronchitis	Hypokalemia, hypertension, hypernatremia, edema, renal toxicity, hepatotoxicity
Saw palmetto	Prostatic disease, antiandrogenic	Interference with hormone therapy, antiandrogenic effects
St. John's wort	Depression, anxiety	Prolonged anesthetic effect
Valerian root	Sedative/anxiolytic	Prolonged anesthetic and sedative effect
Vitamin E	Antioxidant, cardiac disease, cancer	Increased surgical bleeding
Vitamin K	Nutritional supplement	Inhibits warfarin effect, hypercoagulability

GI = gastrointestinal, MAO = monoamine oxidase.

been reported. Glutamine has been shown to be important for immunomodulation and is preferentially depleted by stress. Supplementation is therefore thought to improve immune function. L-arginine has been shown to physiologically augment postexercise insulin secretion and thereby facilitate muscle recovery. Ingestion of amino acids within 2 hours after exercise was shown to increase glycogen synthesis and storage by 128%.[23] Additonally, L-arginine was found to decrease plasma lactate and ammonia, and glutamine was felt to be cardioprotective for exercise in patients with a history of myocardial infarction; amino acid supplementation was thus felt to favorably alter cardiac and skeletal muscle metabolism. It appears as if amino acid supplementation may be of benefit in the postexercise recovery period, although ingestion of protein in a meal during the recovery phase may have the same effect.[22,23]

Antioxidants

Antioxidants are molecules capable of preventing oxidation in cells. Oxidation reactions can produce free radicals, which start chain reactions that can damage cells. Antioxidants can reduce these chains and prevent this damage. Diseases thought to be associated with oxidative stress include Alzheimer disease and other neurodegenerative diseases, diabetes, rheumatoid arthritis, and heart disease. Common antioxidants include vitamins C and E, glutathione, melatonin, and carotenes. Supplementation with these antioxidants has been attempted to treat chronic diseases such as cancer and heart disease[24-26] but has not yet been shown to be effective. In fact, meta-analyses of studies on the use of high-dose antioxidant therapy for the prevention of cardiovascular disease have shown that treatment with these antioxidants increases mortality.[27,28] The mechanisms of these disease processes are quite complex and multifactorial, however, and antioxidant treatment may yet prove to be an effective tool in disease prevention and treatment. Supraphysiologic supplementation cannot be recommended at this time, however.

Beta Carotene

Beta carotene is thought to boost immunity, prevent cancer and heart disease, and delay the progression of cataracts and macular degeneration.[26] It also may protect against sunburn, aid in depression, and decrease tremors in patients with Parkinson disease. It is used to boost fertility and may have natural anti-inflammatory effects in the treatment of asthma, psoriasis, and arthritis. Beta carotene may be taken as a daily dietary supplement but is also found in sweet potatoes, carrots, cantaloupe, squash, pumpkins, spinach, kale, and collard greens.

Omega-3 Fatty Acids

Omega-3 fatty acids are thought to exert positive effects on cardiovascular disease.[29] They have been shown to decrease the risk and frequency of cardiac arrhythmias and dysrhythmias. Omega-3 fatty acids have been reported to decrease triglyceride and cholesterol levels, increase high-density lipoproteins (HDLs, or "good" cholesterol), decrease low-density lipoproteins (LDLs, or "bad" cholesterol), lower mean blood pressure, and decrease the growth rate of atherosclerotic plaques. They have been shown to reduce the incidence and severity of exercise-induced bronchospasm in elite athletes by decreasing the release of inflammatory mediators, although similar benefits have not been demonstrated in the management of asthma or chronic obstructive pulmonary disease. Omega-3 fatty acids may have additional beneficial effects on brain function and memory. They are naturally found in "fatty" fish such as salmon and halibut, where the highest concentration is in the subcutaneous layer (eat the skin!), and they also occur in high concentrations in algae and krill. Capsules may be taken as a dietary supplement, but some individuals report that ingesting omega-3 fatty acids in this form causes fishy gaseous odors or regurgitation.

Glutathione

Glutathione is an important cellular antioxidant that helps the body eliminate potentially harmful substances. Benefits of glutathione supplementation have been reported for infertility, cancer, and cataracts, and in the chronic management of HIV. Glutathione is typically ingested as a daily dietary supplement.

Coenzyme Q10

Coenzyme Q10 is a nonessential micronutrient, as it is naturally synthesized by the body. It is thought to boost energy level and vitality and also has been shown to protect against free radical damage. Some studies have demonstrated stimulation of immune function. Coenzyme Q10 is typically ingested as a dietary supplement.

Alpha-Lipoic Acid

Alpha-lipoic acid has been shown to neutralize potentially harmful free radical formation. It is also thought to play an important role in the recycling of crucial antioxidants such as vitamin C and glutathione. Alpha-lipoic acid may be of benefit in patients with peripheral neuropathy; age-related decline of cerebral function, such as Alzheimer disease and senile dementia; and cataracts or glaucoma. Alpha-lipoic acid is naturally found in spinach, broccoli, peas, brewer's yeast, brussels sprouts, and organ meats.

Acetyl L-Carnitine

Acetyl L-carnitine is used as a supplement to facilitate fatty acid oxidation and metabolism. As a supplement, it is used principally to increase metabolism of unwanted body fat. In this role, acetyl L-carnitine is thought to augment the transport of fatty acids across the inner mitochondrial membrane such that they may be oxidized and metabolized. Acetyl L-carnitine is naturally found in meats, leafy vegetables, and whole grains.

Vitamin A

Vitamin A is a fat-soluble antioxidant that is important for vision, particularly night vision. It is thought to aid in soft-tissue and bone healing. Vitamin A plays pivotal roles in reproduction and fetal development, particularly that of the limbs. Vitamin A also has been shown to be important in immunity, and it participates in the destruction of bacteria and viruses. Vitamin A is a naturally occurring substance found in liver, sweet potatoes, carrots, milk, eggs, and mozzarella cheese.

Vitamin C

Vitamin C is a water-soluble antioxidant that may protect against the harmful effects of free radicals. It is important to the health of blood vessels and gums, and it has been shown to participate in the development of bones and teeth. As a supplement, its most common use is for the treatment of infections, particularly upper respiratory infections. Linus Pauling popularized the use of megadoses of vitamin C (up to 10,000 mg daily) to prevent and treat the common cold. Vitamin C is naturally found in fruits (particularly those of the citrus variety), vegetables, cereals, beef, poultry, and fish.

Vitamin E

Vitamin E is a powerful fat-soluble antioxidant that is thought to protect against free radical damage and to exert positive effects in the prevention of cancer and heart disease. Vitamin E also may limit free radical damage to the endothelial lining of the vascular system. It is commonly applied topically for wound healing and for various skin conditions and hypertrophic scars. However, there is no good evidence to support the use of vitamin E supplementation for health benefits, nor is there definitive evidence to support adverse effects on health. Vitamin E is naturally found in almonds, wheat germ oil, safflower oil, corn, soybean oil, mangoes, nuts, and broccoli.

Creatine

Creatine is an amino acid derivative found in skeletal and cardiac muscle and in retinal, testicular, and brain tissues. It is important for the production of adenosine triphosphate (ATP) via production of phosphocreatine. Additionally, it is thought to improve skeletal muscle function by increasing the pH buffering capacity of muscle tissue. During high-intensity exercise, such as sprinting, stored phosphocreatine fuels the initial few seconds of energy. Therefore, although creatine use has been credited with increases in strength and muscle mass (improved high-power performance, increased muscle endurance, increased muscle mass due to skeletal muscle fiber hypertrophy), the observed effects are mainly due to increased available energy substrates and capacity for exercise, rather than a true anabolic effect. In a double-blinded prospective randomized controlled trial, Eijnde et al[30] examined 46 male athletes aged 55 to 75 years who were placed on a daily resistance training program for 6 months, with half of the group additionally taking daily creatine supplementation. At 6 months, the creatine group demonstrated higher peak oxygen uptake rate, increased lean body mass, and decreased body fat. However, 1 year after cessation of creatine supplementation (with continued daily exercise), the study group demonstrated no durable positive effects as compared with the control group. The authors concluded that although creatine may have positive effects on lean body mass gain, continued supplementation with exercise is necessary for maintenance of these effects.[30]

The adverse effects of creatine are principally related to fluid imbalance, which may limit the clinical appropriateness of supplementation in an older population. Reported adverse events include intravascular fluid depletion, extracellular fluid retention, dehydration, nausea, increased incidence and frequency of muscle cramps, increased risk of muscle strain, increased risk of heat-related illness, and increased renal stress and damage.[31]

Glucosamine and Chondroitin Sulfate

Glucosamine is thought to be involved with the maintenance and repair of articular cartilage.[32] It has been shown to stimulate the production of synovial fluid, proteoglycans, and glycosaminoglycans, and it has anti-inflammatory effects. As a nutritional supplement, the recommended dose is 1,200 to 2,000 mg daily, although this has been derived empirically rather than experimentally. Because of altered metabolism and clearance in obese patients, patients with gastrointestinal reflux, and patients who use concurrent diuretics, higher doses may be necessary to obtain the same effects in these patients.[33]

Chondroitin sulfate is thought to act via modulation of joint metabolism. In this regard, chondroitin sulfate has been shown to favorably influence the synthesis and metabolism of glycosaminoglycans, increase total proteoglycan production, inhibit collagenolytic activity of chondrocytes, and increase overall production of synovial fluid.[33,34] It also has been shown to have inherent anti-inflammatory properties, and, as with glucosamine, the recommended dosage of 600 to 1,500 mg daily is empirically derived.

Numerous studies have been performed to determine the effects of glucosamine and/or chondroitin sulfate. Although early reports were encouraging, recent studies with less positive results have tempered the initial popularity of these substances as nutritional supplements for the treatment of osteoarthritis (OA). In a 2002 prospective randomized controlled study of 168 patients with mild to moderate knee OA treated with glucosamine sulfate versus placebo, Pavelká et al[35] concluded that treatment with glucosamine sulfate for at least 12 months decreased the incidence of total knee arthroplasty by 73% at 5-year follow-up.[36] Similarly, in a 2005 prospective randomized controlled trial of

300 patients with mild to moderate knee OA treated for 2 years with chondroitin sulfate or placebo, Michel et al[37] found that chondroitin sulfate was chondroprotective and decreased joint space narrowing in a statistically significant fashion. However, Reichenbach et al[38] performed a meta-analysis of 20 trials including 3,846 patients from 1970 to 2006 and concluded that chondroitin sulfate for the treatment of OA had "minimal or non-existent" benefit and therefore discouraged routine use. It has been postulated in the commercial and popular media that variations in product purity, concentration, or content in different commercially available preparations of glucosamine and/or chondroitin sulfate may account for the observed differences in clinical efficacy.

In 2006, the results of the much-anticipated National Institutes of Health Glucosamine Chondroitin Arthritis Intervention Trial (GAIT) were reported.[39] The GAIT study included 16 centers nationwide that participated in a prospective randomized controlled trial that included five treatment arms: (1) glucosamine 1,500 mg/d; (2) chondroitin sulfate 1,200 mg/d; (3) glucosamine 1,500 mg/d/chondroitin sulfate 1,200 mg/d; (4) celecoxib 200 mg/d; and (5) placebo (acetaminophen, up to 4,000 mg/d). Mean patient age was 59 years (minimum 40 years); patients were treated for 24 weeks. Statistically significant pain relief was observed overall in the celecoxib arm versus placebo ($P < 0.05$). Celecoxib demonstrated pain relief in the mild pain subgroup ($P < 0.05$) but not in the moderate-to-severe subgroup. Interestingly, the glucosamine/chondroitin sulfate treatment arm demonstrated efficacy in the moderate-to-severe subgroup ($P < 0.05$) but not in the mild pain subgroup. Neither glucosamine nor chondroitin sulfate was found to be efficacious when used alone.

A follow-up report on the GAIT study in 2008 demonstrated sustained improvement in the moderate-to-severe pain subgroup.[40] Post hoc analysis revealed decreased knee joint inflammation and effusion for the mild pain subgroup taking chondroitin sulfate, and this effect was observed to be larger for patients with milder pain and less radiographic damage at entry into the trial.[40]

To determine if glucosamine and/or chondroitin sulfate has a chondroprotective effect (as demonstrated by joint space narrowing on plain radiographs), Sawitzke et al[41] examined a subset of 581 knees from the original GAIT cohort with Kellgren-Lawrence grade I and II OA. At 2 years after initiation of the study, follow-up radiographs demonstrated an average joint space loss of 0.166 mm in the placebo group and 0.194 mm in the glucosamine and chondroitin sulfate group ($P > 0.05$). The glucosamine-only group demonstrated a mean loss of 0.130 mm, which was not statistically significant but demonstrated a trend toward improvement in this group.[41] This corroborates other reports that have suggested that glucosamine alone may have chondroprotective effects.[35,36,42]

In summary, glucosamine and/or chondroitin sulfate may be beneficial for moderate to severe osteoarthritis of the knee. The clinical benefit of the combination of glucosamine and chondroitin sulfate does not correlate with the possible chondroprotective effects of glucosamine alone, and it may be that chondroitin sulfate has anti-inflammatory and antinociceptive properties that do not translate to chondroprotection. Most reports have documented that it takes at least 1 to 3 months of daily dosing to realize the benefits,[39] but clearly more research is necessary to establish the efficacy of these substances. Moreover, it seems that certain patients respond better to glucosamine and/or chondroitin sulfate than others; further investigation is therefore necessary to identify subsets of patients for whom these supplements may be of particular benefit.

It is important to note that at the time of writing of this chapter, the American Academy of Orthopaedic Surgeons' (AAOS) Clinical Practice Guideline for the treatment of osteoarthritis of the knee stated that "We recommend that glucosamine and/or chondroitin sulfate or hydrochloride not be prescribed for patients with symptomatic OA of the knee."[43] This was based largely on an Agency for Healthcare Research and Quality (AHRQ) report that cited evidence from one randomized controlled trial and six systematic reviews that concluded that "the best available evidence found that glucosamine hydrochloride, chondroitin sulfate, or their combination did not have any clinical benefit in patients with primary OA of the knee."[44] Of the six systematic reviews that were evaluated by the AAOS workgroup, one found no clinical benefit with the use of glucosamine or chondroitin over placebo. Although

the remaining five systematic reviews concluded that glucosamine and/or chondroitin sulfate were superior to placebo, the AAOS workgroup determined that these reviews failed to provide conclusions on the clinical importance of the superiority of glucosamine and/or chondroitin sulfate to placebo. Based on this, it was decided that these substances "not be prescribed for patients with symptomatic OA of the knee." The author agrees that there is a lack of evidence to substantiate the use of glucosamine and/or chondroitin sulfate for the purposes of chondroprotection or to alter the natural course of knee osteoarthritis; however, it is the author's opinion that as an over-the-counter remedy with few, mild untoward effects, symptomatic relief in terms of pain and improved function may be "clinically important" enough to warrant at least inclusion in the discussion of various treatment strategies that the physician has with the patient.

Other Supplements

The scientific and popular literature is replete with reports of other nutritional supplements used for the treatment of musculoskeletal ailments, but, in general, well-designed, well-performed studies are lacking. S-adenosylmethionine (SAMe) has been reported to stimulate repair of proteoglycans and may therefore be helpful in the treatment of OA. Cetyl myristoleate is thought to be a cyclooxygenase (COX) and lipoxygenase pathway inhibitor that may decrease inflammation and pain. Ginger has been reported to inhibit prostaglandin and leukotriene synthesis to decrease the elaboration of downstream inflammatory mediators. Dimethyl sulfoxide (DMSO) is a topical oxygen radical scavenger that additionally may have intrinsic anti-inflammatory effects. Boron has been shown to affect calcium metabolism and may slow age-related loss of bone mineral density. Avocado/soybean unsaponeifiables (ASUs) have been reported to help decrease pain and degeneration associated with OA of the hip. In general, the practitioner should be aware that although commercially available, over-the-counter nutritional supplements for the treatment of musculoskeletal symptoms represent a multibillion-dollar industry, evidence for their effectiveness remains largely unsubstantiated, and less is known about their safety profiles.[45-48]

Nonsteroidal Anti-Inflammatory Drugs

Prostaglandin synthesis is mediated by the COX-1 and COX-2 enzymes. It is important to note that although the COX-1 and COX-2 enzymes are targeted by various anti-inflammatory agents to decrease production of downstream inflammatory mediators (**Figure 1**), prostaglandins are essential for normal physiologic functions. Among the numerous homeostatic functions of prostaglandins, of critical importance is the maintenance of the gastric lining, renal blood flow, and platelet aggregation. Complications of nonselective COX inhibition may therefore include gastric ulceration, renal insufficiency, and prolonged bleeding time. Nonselective nonsteroidal anti-inflammatory drug (NSAID) use in patients older than 60 years has been associated with a four- to fivefold risk of gastrointestinal ulceration, particularly in those with underlying peptic ulcer disease or concurrent corticosteroid use, proteinuria, azotemia, renal failure, or severe gastric bleeding that requires hospitalization.[49,50] Thus, individuals considered to be at high risk for complications include those older than 60 years; those having a history of peptic ulcer disease, concurrent corticosteroid use, or moderate to high ibuprofen dose (>400 mg/dose); and those with anticipated duration of regular NSAID usage for at least 3 months. In these individuals, it is recommended that a COX-2 selective inhibitor be used rather than a nonselective variety, or that misoprostol and/or a proton-pump inhibitor (PPI; eg, lansoprazole or omeprazole) be added to the regimen.[51]

Numerous studies have investigated the efficacy of NSAIDs for the symptomatic treatment of OA. For mild OA, nonselective NSAIDs have been shown to provide the same degree of pain relief as acetaminophen, although the latter does not possess anti-inflammatory properties.[51,52] For moderate to severe OA, COX-2 selective inhibitors have been shown to be superior to nonselective NSAIDs, and both are more effective than acetaminophen.[52] Moreover, in patients with moderate to severe OA, COX-2 selective inhibitors were observed to have a faster onset of action, and, interestingly, the efficacy of the agent in the first 6 days correlated with the efficacy at 6 weeks of therapy. For chronic management of OA, acetaminophen is safer than either traditional or COX-2 selective inhibitors,

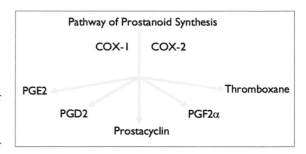

Figure 1   Cyclooxygenase (COX)-mediated synthesis of inflammatory prostaglandins. PGE2 and prostacyclin are major inflammatory vasoactive prostanoids. PGE2 = prostaglandin E2, PGD2 = prostaglandin D2, PGF2α = prostaglandin F2α.

although hepatotoxicity may occur. COX-2 selective inhibitors have been shown to have a lower risk profile than nonselective NSAIDs, which carry risks of severe gastrointestinal complications, renal issues, and bleeding problems. Edema, hypertension, and underlying cardiovascular disease may be an issue with patients who take COX-2 selective inhibitors, and appropriate vigilance and monitoring of patients is essential.[49,50] In 2004, rofecoxib, a COX-2 selective inhibitor that had gained widespread acceptance among physicians and patients for the chronic treatment of OA, was voluntarily withdrawn from the market because of data that associated its use with increased risk of myocardial infarction and cerebrovascular events. Similarly, in 2005, valdecoxib was voluntarily withdrawn from the market due to increased risk of myocardial infarction, stroke, Stevens-Johnson syndrome, and fatal skin reactions. Celecoxib and meloxicam are still widely used for chronic symptomatic management of OA, although once-daily dosing at the lowest effective dose is recommended because of ongoing concerns about COX-2 selective inhibition in patients with underlying cardiac disease or hypertension.

NSAIDs also may negatively affect bone and soft-tissue healing. Glassman et al[53] examined 288 patients who underwent spinal fusion and were assigned to receive either NSAID (ketorolac) or non-NSAID analgesia. Nonunion occurred in 4% of non-NSAID controls and 17% of those who received ketorolac (odds ratio 4:9, $P < 0.05$), with a dose-dependent relationship observed between nonunion rate and keterolac use. Similarly, multiple reports have documented impaired fracture healing (defined as delayed union or nonunion) with concurrent use of COX-2 selective inhibitors in the postfracture or postoperative period[54-62] Cohen et al[63] observed that in rats that went on to heal from rotator cuff repair, those given indomethacin or celecoxib demonstrated lower rates of healing and decreased mechanical integrity compared with non-NSAID–fed controls. It thus appears that not only does NSAID administration after rotator cuff repair affect whether the tendon heals, but it may also result in weaker repairs in those in which healing occurs.[63] Dimmen et al[64] observed similar decreased rates of healing after tendon and cartilage repair. Similar issues with ligament and wound healing have been described.[65] Mounting evidence thus suggests that the clinical effectiveness of COX-2 selective inhibitors in decreasing inflammation may have dire consequences on soft-tissue or osseous healing, particularly if given during the critical 3 weeks following injury or repair. My preference is to discontinue use of these agents, or any systemic NSAID, during the healing period following fracture or soft-tissue repair.

Evidence also suggests that although NSAIDs may be effective in controlling symptoms associated with OA, the natural progression of the disease may be unfavorably altered. In a prospective randomized controlled trial of 2,514 osteoarthritic hips and 874 osteoarthritic knees, Reijman et al[66] randomized patients to either NSAID (diclofenac) or placebo to determine if progression occurred, as defined by increase in Kellgren-Lawrence score or need for total joint arthroplasty. At a mean follow-up of 6.6 years, long-term NSAID use (defined as >180 days) was associated with a 2.4 times higher risk for progression of hip OA (95% confidence interval [CI], 1.0 to 6.2) and a 3.2 times higher risk for progression of knee OA (95% CI, 1.0 to 9.9). It remains uncertain whether the NSAIDs themselves have deleterious effects on joints or whether the pain relief and decrease in inflammation allows for excessive mechanical loading and progression of articular damage.[66]

Recently, there has been renewed interest in the use of topical NSAIDs. Topical NSAIDs are typically applied as a cream, gel, lotion, or ointment but also may be supported on an adhesive medium to be applied as a patch. Numerous products are available over the counter or by prescription, and compounding pharmacies often offer customizable preparations that can include other analgesics, such as menthol or camphor, or even local anesthetics such as lidocaine. Topical diclofenac has been shown to be as effective for pain, stiffness, and function as oral preparations,[67] and it has been shown to be effective in decreasing periarticular and extracapsular pain and inflammation.[68] However, the efficacy of topical NSAID preparations seems to diminish with chronic use. With daily as-needed use of topical diclofenac, symptomatic relief has been shown to be superior to placebo at 2 weeks, but by 4 weeks no benefit over placebo has been shown. Topical NSAIDs may therefore be more appropriate for episodic flare-ups rather than for chronic management.[68,69]

Summary

Throughout history, people have been obsessed with reversing the effects of time on the human body. To this end, complementary and "natural" approaches are frequently used by consumers, and CAM now represents a multibillion-dollar industry. Nutritional supplements may be beneficial for the aging athlete, but well-performed studies are lacking. Glucosamine and/or chondroitin sulfate may be beneficial in certain circumstances, but further investigation is necessary to determine which subsets of patients will best benefit. NSAIDs may be effective for temporizing relief of OA but in general do not favorably alter the natural course of disease.

References

1. National Center for Complementary and Alternative Medicine: *Statistics on Complementary and Alternative Medicine in the United States.* Bethesda, MD, National Institutes of Health. http://nccam.nih.gov/news/camstats. Accessed August 1, 2011.

2. Eisenberg DM, Davis RB, Ettner SL, et al: Trends in alternative medicine use in the United States, 1990-1997: Results of a follow-up national survey. *JAMA* 1998;280(18):1569-1575.

3. Nahin RL, Barnes PM, Stussman BJ, Bloom B: Costs of complementary and alternative medicine (CAM) and frequency of visits to CAM practitioners: United States,

2007. *National Health Statistics Reports*, No. 18. Hyattsville, MD, National Center for Health Statistics, 2009.

4. Barnes P, Powell-Griner E, McFann K, Nahin R: *CDC Advance Data Report #343: Complementary and Alternative Medicine Use Among Adults: United States, 2002.* May 27, 2004.

5. Poehlman ET: A review: Exercise and its influence on resting energy metabolism in man. *Med Sci Sports Exerc* 1989;21(5):515-525.

6. Shephard RJ: Aging and exercise, in Fahey TD, ed: *Encyclopedia of Sports Medicine and Science.* Internet Society for Sport Science, http://sportsci.org, 1998.

7. Webb P: Energy expenditure and fat-free mass in men and women. *Am J Clin Nutr* 1981;34(9):1816-1826.

8. Poehlman ET, Danforth E Jr: Endurance training increases metabolic rate and norepinephrine appearance rate in older individuals. *Am J Physiol* 1991; 261(2 pt 1):E233-E239.

9. Toth MJ, Poehlman ET: Resting metabolic rate and cardiovascular disease risk in resistance- and aerobic-trained middle-aged women. *Int J Obes Relat Metab Disord* 1995;19(10):691-698.

10. Bennell KL, Malcolm SA, Thomas SA, et al: Risk factors for stress fractures in female track-and-field athletes: A retrospective analysis. *Clin J Sport Med* 1995;5(4):229-235.

11. Wilmore JH, Costill DL: Physical energy: Fuel metabolism. *Nutr Rev* 2001;59(1 pt 2):S13-S16.

12. Beshgetoor D, Nichols JF, Rego I: Effect of training mode and calcium intake on bone mineral density in female master cyclist, runners, and non-athletes. *Int J Sport Nutr Exerc Metab* 2000;10(3):290-301.

13. Talbott SM, Rothkopf MM, Shapses SA: Dietary restriction of energy and calcium alters bone turnover and density in younger and older female rats. *J Nutr* 1998;128(3):640-645.

14. Manore MM: Exercise and the Institute of Medicine recommendations for nutrition. *Curr Sports Med Rep* 2005;4(4):193-198.

15. Campbell WW, Geik RA: Nutritional considerations for the older athlete. *Nutrition* 2004;20(7-8):603-608.

16. Munro HN, Suter PM, Russell RM: Nutritional requirements of the elderly. *Annu Rev Nutr* 1987;7: 23-49.

17. American College of Sports Medicine, American Dietetic Association, Dietitians of Canada: Joint Position Statement: Nutrition and athletic performance. American College of Sports Medicine, American Dietetic Association, and Dietitians of Canada. *Med Sci Sports Exerc* 2000;32(12):2130-2145.

18. Evans WJ: Protein nutrition, exercise and aging. *J Am Coll Nutr* 2004;23(6, suppl):601S-609S.

19. Esmarck B, Andersen JL, Olsen S, Richter EA, Mizuno M, Kjaer M: Timing of postexercise protein intake is important for muscle hypertrophy with resistance training in elderly humans. *J Physiol* 2001; 535(pt 1):301-311.

20. Von Duvillard SP, Braun WA, Markofski M, Beneke R, Leithäuser R: Fluids and hydration in prolonged endurance performance. *Nutrition* 2004;20(7-8):651-656.

21. Armstrong LE, Casa DJ, Maresh CM, Ganio MS: Caffeine, fluid-electrolyte balance, temperature regulation, and exercise-heat tolerance. *Exerc Sport Sci Rev* 2007;35(3):135-140.

22. Johnson WA, Landry GL: Nutritional supplements: Fact vs. fiction. *Adolesc Med* 1998;9(3):501-513, vi.

23. Joyner MJ: Glutamine and arginine: Immunonutrients and metabolic modulators? *Exerc Sport Sci Rev* 2005;33(3):105-106.

24. Atalay M, Lappalainen J, Sen CK: Dietary antioxidants for the athlete. *Curr Sports Med Rep* 2006;5(4):182-186.

25. Murphy SP, Subar AF, Block G: Vitamin E intakes and sources in the United States. *Am J Clin Nutr* 1990;52(2):361-367.

26. Stanner SA, Hughes J, Kelly CN, Buttriss J: A review of the epidemiological evidence for the 'antioxidant hypothesis'. *Public Health Nutr* 2004;7(3):407-422.

27. Vivekananthan DP, Penn MS, Sapp SK, Hsu A, Topol EJ: Use of antioxidant vitamins for the prevention of cardiovascular disease: Meta-analysis of randomised trials. *Lancet* 2003;361(9374):2017-2023.

28. Miller ER III, Pastor-Barriuso R, Dalal D, Riemersma RA, Appel LJ, Guallar E: Meta-analysis: high-dosage vitamin E supplementation may increase all-cause mortality. *Ann Intern Med* 2005;142(1):37-46.

29. Simopoulos AP: Omega-3 fatty acids and athletics. *Curr Sports Med Rep* 2007;6(4):230-236.

30. Eijnde BO, Van Leemputte M, Goris M, et al: Effects of creatine supplementation and exercise training on

fitness in men 55-75 yr old. *J Appl Physiol* 2003;95(2):818-828.

31. Chen AL, Mears SC, Hawkins RJ: Orthopaedic care of the aging athlete. *J Am Acad Orthop Surg* 2005;13(6):407-416.

32. Uitterlinden EJ, Jahr H, Koevoet JL, et al: Glucosamine reduces anabolic as well as catabolic processes in bovine chondrocytes cultured in alginate. *Osteoarthritis Cartilage* 2007;15(11):1267-1274.

33. Richy F, Bruyere O, Ethgen O, Cucherat M, Henrotin Y, Reginster JY: Structural and symptomatic efficacy of glucosamine and chondroitin in knee osteoarthritis: A comprehensive meta-analysis. *Arch Intern Med* 2003;163(13):1514-1522.

34. Uitterlinden EJ, Koevoet JL, Verkoelen CF, et al: Glucosamine increases hyaluronic acid production in human osteoarthritic synovium explants. *BMC Musculoskelet Disord* 2008;9:120.

35. Pavelká K, Gatterová J, Olejarová M, Machacek S, Giacovelli G, Rovati LC: Glucosamine sulfate use and delay of progression of knee osteoarthritis: A 3-year, randomized, placebo-controlled, double-blind study. *Arch Intern Med* 2002;162(18):2113-2123.

36. Bruyere O, Pavelka K, Rovati LC, et al: Total joint replacement after glucosamine sulphate treatment in knee osteoarthritis: Results of a mean 8-year observation of patients from two previous 3-year, randomised, placebo-controlled trials. *Osteoarthritis Cartilage* 2008;16(2):254-260.

37. Michel BA, Stucki G, Frey D, et al: Chondroitins 4 and 6 sulfate in osteoarthritis of the knee: A randomized, controlled trial. *Arthritis Rheum* 2005;52(3):779-786.

38. Reichenbach S, Sterchi R, Scherer M, et al: Meta-analysis: Chondroitin for osteoarthritis of the knee or hip. *Ann Intern Med* 2007;146(8):580-590.

39. Clegg DO, Reda DJ, Harris CL, et al: Glucosamine, chondroitin sulfate, and the two in combination for painful knee osteoarthritis. *N Engl J Med* 2006;354(8):795-808.

40. Hochberg MC, Clegg DO: Potential effects of chondroitin sulfate on joint swelling: A GAIT report. *Osteoarthritis Cartilage* 2008;16(suppl 3):S22-S24.

41. Sawitzke AD, Shi H, Finco MF, et al: The effect of glucosamine and/or chondroitin sulfate on the progression of knee osteoarthritis: A report from the glucosamine/chondroitin arthritis intervention trial. *Arthritis Rheum* 2008;58(10):3183-3191.

42. Biggee BA, Blinn CM, McAlindon TE, Nuite M, Silbert JE: Low levels of human serum glucosamine after ingestion of glucosamine sulphate relative to capability for peripheral effectiveness. *Ann Rheum Dis* 2006;65(2):222-226.

43. American Academy of Orthopaedic Surgeons: *AAOS Clinical Practice Guideline: Treatment of Osteoarthritis (OA) of the Knee.* Rosemont, IL, American Academy of Orthopaedic Surgeons, December 2008. http://www.aaos.org/research/guidelines/OAKrecommendations.pdf. Accessed August 1, 2011.

44. Samson DJ, Grant MD, Ratko TA, et al: *Treatment of Primary and Secondary Osteoarthritis of the Knee.* Rockville, MD, Agency for Healthcare Research and Quality, Sep 1, 2007, Report No. 157.

45. Newnham RE: Essentiality of boron for healthy bones and joints. *Environ Health Perspect* 1994;102(suppl 7):83-85.

46. Lequesne M, Maheu E, Cadet C, Dreiser RL: Structural effect of avocado/soybean unsaponifiables on joint space loss in osteoarthritis of the hip. *Arthritis Rheum* 2002;47(1):50-58.

47. Liebman B: Ten myths that can trip you up. *Nutrition Action Healthletter* 2008;3(7).

48. Little CV, Parsons T: Herbal therapy for treating osteoarthritis. *Cochrane Database Syst Rev* 2001;1(1):CD002947.

49. Gabriel SE, Jaakkimainen L, Bombardier C: Risk for serious gastrointestinal complications related to use of nonsteroidal anti-inflammatory drugs: A meta-analysis. *Ann Intern Med* 1991;115(10):787-796.

50. Smalley WE, Ray WA, Daugherty JR, Griffin MR: Nonsteroidal anti-inflammatory drugs and the incidence of hospitalizations for peptic ulcer disease in elderly persons. *Am J Epidemiol* 1995;141(6):539-545.

51. Pincus T, Koch GG, Sokka T, et al: A randomized, double-blind, crossover clinical trial of diclofenac plus misoprostol versus acetaminophen in patients with osteoarthritis of the hip or knee. *Arthritis Rheum* 2001;44(7):1587-1598.

52. Battisti WP, Katz NP, Weaver AL, et al: Pain management in osteoarthritis: A focus on onset of efficacy. A comparison of rofecoxib, celecoxib, acetaminophen, and nabumetone across four clinical trials. *J Pain* 2004;5(9):511-520.

53. Glassman SD, Rose SM, Dimar JR, Puno RM, Campbell MJ, Johnson JR: The effect of postoperative

nonsteroidal anti-inflammatory drug administration on spinal fusion. *Spine (Phila Pa 1976)* 1998;23(7):834-838.

54. Daluiski A, Ramsey KE, Shi Y, et al: Cyclooxygenase-2 inhibitors in human skeletal fracture healing. *Orthopedics* 2006;29(3):259-261.

55. Einhorn TA: Do inhibitors of cyclooxygenase-2 impair bone healing? *J Bone Miner Res* 2002;17(6):977-978.

56. Hochberg MC, Melin JM, Reicin A: Cox-2 inhibitors and fracture healing: An argument against such an effect. *J Bone Miner Res* 2003;18(3):583-587.

57. Simon AM, Manigrasso MB, O'Connor JP: Cyclooxygenase 2 function is essential for bone fracture healing. *J Bone Miner Res* 2002;17(6):963-976.

58. Zhang X, Schwarz EM, Young DA, Puzas JE, Rosier RN, O'Keefe RJ: Cyclooxygenase-2 regulates mesenchymal cell differentiation into the osteoblast lineage and is critically involved in bone repair. *J Clin Invest* 2002;109(11):1405-1415.

59. Goodman S, Ma T, Trindade M, et al: COX-2 selective NSAID decreases bone ingrowth in vivo. *J Orthop Res* 2002;20(6):1164-1169.

60. Kloen P, Doty SB, Gordon E, Rubel IF, Goumans MJ, Helfet DL: Expression and activation of the BMP-signaling components in human fracture nonunions. *J Bone Joint Surg Am* 2002;84-A(11):1909-1918.

61. Gerstenfeld LC, Al-Ghawas M, Alkhiary YM, et al: Selective and nonselective cyclooxygenase-2 inhibitors and experimental fracture-healing: Reversibility of effects after short-term treatment. *J Bone Joint Surg Am* 2007;89(1):114-125.

62. Simon AM, O'Connor JP: Dose and time-dependent effects of cyclooxygenase-2 inhibition on fracture-healing. *J Bone Joint Surg Am* 2007;89(3):500-511.

63. Cohen DB, Kawamura S, Ehteshami JR, Rodeo SA: Indomethacin and celecoxib impair rotator cuff tendon-to-bone healing. *Am J Sports Med* 2006; 34(3):362-369.

64. Dimmen S, Nordsletten L, Madsen JE: Parecoxib and indomethacin delay early fracture healing: A study in rats. *Clin Orthop Relat Res* 2009;467(8):1992-1999.

65. Randelli P, Randelli F, Cabitza P, Vaienti L: The effects of COX-2 anti-inflammatory drugs on soft tissue healing: A review of the literature. *J Biol Regul Homeost Agents* 2010;24(2):107-114.

66. Reijman M, Bierma-Zeinstra SM, Pols HA, Koes BW, Stricker BH, Hazes JM: Is there an association between the use of different types of nonsteroidal anti-inflammatory drugs and radiologic progression of osteoarthritis? The Rotterdam Study. *Arthritis Rheum* 2005;52(10):3137-3142.

67. Banning M: Topical diclofenac: Clinical effectiveness and current uses in osteoarthritis of the knee and soft tissue injuries. *Expert Opin Pharmacother* 2008;9(16):2921-2929.

68. Grace D, Rogers J, Skeith K, Anderson K: Topical diclofenac versus placebo: A double blind, randomized clinical trial in patients with osteoarthritis of the knee. *J Rheumatol* 1999;26(12):2659-2663.

69. Ottillinger B, Gömör B, Michel BA, Pavelka K, Beck W, Elsasser U: Efficacy and safety of eltenac gel in the treatment of knee osteoarthritis. *Osteoarthritis Cartilage* 2001;9(3):273-280.

Chapter 6
Anti-Aging and Ergogenic Aids

John M. Tokish, MD

Key Points

- Great interest exists in the field of anti-aging medicine, which is often driven more by marketing than science.
- Significant scientific work has been done regarding the anti-aging effects of testosterone, human growth hormone, resveratrol, and antioxidant therapy in the prevention of age-related disease.
- Testosterone has potential benefits in the areas of body composition, muscle strength, sexual function, cognition, and prevention of frailty, but much work remains to be done on the logistics of its administration.
- Human growth hormone demonstrates some effect on body composition, but it has no scientific basis as an anti-aging therapy at this time. Significant side effects make this drug a potentially harmful intervention.

Dr. Tokish or an immediate family member serves as a board member, owner, officer, or committee member of the Society of Military Orthopaedic Surgeons and is a member of a speakers' bureau or has made paid presentations on behalf of Arthrex.

Introduction

The search for the "Fountain of Youth" is as active today as it was in 1513, when Juan Ponce de León first explored Florida in search of a cure for aging. But whereas Ponce de León never found the legendary waters, American baby boomers have re-energized this search. In 2006, it was estimated that this segment of the population (born between 1946 and 1964) would number 76 million and would spend more than $72 billion in 2009 alone on products and services to slow the aging process.[1] A large part of this spending is on so-called anti-aging drugs or supplements, designed to either slow the aging process or reverse its effects. Considerable controversy exists, however, as to the safety and efficacy of these drugs and supplements. Many are not controlled by the US Food and Drug Administration, and therefore little oversight is in place to ensure safety and efficacy. Drugs that are controlled are often used off-label, without critical evaluation of indications or results. Nevertheless, a growing body of scientific evidence exists on the efficacy of many of these regimens, and an understanding of that science can help clinicians and consumers separate potential health advances from marketing hype. This chapter reviews several of the products that are at the center of the anti-aging movement, with special attention on the science supporting or refuting their effectiveness as anti-aging treatments.

Testosterone

The performance-enhancing effects and abuses of testosterone in athletic populations have been well publicized since the 1950s, but considerable work also has been done investigating its potential as an anti-aging hormone in older populations. The logic behind this research is relatively simple. Many of the more apparent changes of aging, such as loss of muscle or bone mass, libido, and energy,[2-5] are often the inverse of what is reported in testosterone users. Furthermore, it is well understood that testosterone levels decrease with normal aging.[6-9] Thus it follows that replacing testosterone in an older population may lead to reversal of some of these negative effects.

History

The first reported studies on testosterone were undertaken by Arnold Berthold, who performed a series of experiments on roosters in 1849 while he was curator of the Göttingen Zoo. He castrated the roosters and found that they stopped crowing and fighting, and lost interest in hens. He also found that the combs of these roosters atrophied. The roosters' normal behavior could be restored by reimplantation of the testes into the abdominal wall.[10]

This concept of hormone replacement was further investigated by the French neurologist Dr. Charles Brown-Séquard, who injected testicular extracts into himself to reverse the aging process. He reported in *The Lancet* in 1889 that after treatment, he regained many of his "old powers."[11] Although subsequent studies on his extract showed it to be nearly devoid of androgen, his reported findings led many of the rich elderly of the world to pay large amounts of money for injections of testicular extracts and testicular transplants from human, monkey, and goat sources.[12]

Testosterone was first synthesized in 1935 by Adolf Butenandt and Leopold Ruzicka, earning them the 1939 Nobel Prize in Chemistry. Further studies by Heller and Myers documented the ability to successfully administer synthetic testosterone.[13] Since then, its use to treat various medical conditions has skyrocketed. From athletics for its muscle-building powers, to psychiatry for its antidepressive effects, to urology for its effects on libido, testosterone supplementation has achieved widespread application and increasing accep-

tance. Since 1993, testosterone prescriptions have increased at an annual rate of 25% to 30%, and a 500% increase in overall prescription use has occurred over the last decade.[14] Despite the widespread use of testosterone, much work remains to be done to more clearly define the risks, benefits, and boundaries for its proper application.

Hypogonadism and Testosterone Replacement Therapy

It is well known that testosterone levels in males decrease with age. Approximately 20% of 60-year-olds and 50% of 80-year-olds exhibit total serum testosterone levels below the normal range for young men.[15] Such low levels are commonly associated with erectile dysfunction, loss of libido, muscle weakness, lower bone mass, and frailty.[16]

Defining who is "hypogonadal" and therefore might benefit from testosterone treatment remains somewhat controversial. Total testosterone remains the most common method measured, with some authors suggesting an absolute cutoff value of less than 200 ng/dL, below which an individual should be considered hypogonadal, regardless of age.[17] Others have argued that 300 ng/dL is still within the low range. Because total testosterone includes that which is bound to sex hormone–binding globulin, which is biologically inactive, some have suggested measuring "bioavailable" or "free" testosterone as a more clinically applicable test.[18] Varying assays, diurnal variation, and a wide range of normal values make the diagnosis of hypogonadism difficult to make on the basis of a laboratory value alone. Accordingly, most authors suggest that a low testosterone value plus clinical symptoms such as loss of libido, erectile dysfunction, and a loss of muscle mass or sarcopenia be required for the clinical diagnosis.

Once testosterone replacement therapy has been selected, a variety of regimens should be considered and individualized for a patient. Intramuscular injectible testosterone, such as the enanthate or cypionate varieties, reaches a serum peak value at 24 hours and gradually declines over 2 weeks.[19] This method requires little maintenance, but it results in large fluctuations in serum testosterone levels, leading to mood swings and shifts in sexual function in some men. Transdermal patches can be placed on the scrotum or nongenital

Table 1: Summary of Effects of Testosterone Replacement Therapy[a]

Measurement	Effect	Comment
Total body fat	↓ 1.6 kg (6.2%)	
Lean body mass	↑ 1.6 kg (2.7%)	
Muscle strength	↑ 6%	Seen in dominant muscle groups only
Bone mineral density	↑ 4%	Lumbar spine only
Bone markers	↓ Resorption markers 18%	No effect on bone formation
LDL	No effect	
HDL	↓ 4 to 6%	Predominantly in more hypogonadal subgroups
PSA	↑ 0.6 to 1 ng/dL	Considered clinically insignificant by all authors
Hematocrit	↑ 2% to 5%	
Time to exercise-induced ST-segment depression (measure of cardiac protection)	↑ 22% to 24%	

LDL = low-density lipoprotein ("bad" cholesterol), HDL = high-density lipoprotein ("good" cholesterol), PSA = prostate-specific antigen.
[a]Information adapted from references 16, 22, and 24.

areas and have more favorable pharmacokinetics, with midnormal serum testosterone levels 4 to 8 hours after application and a gradual decrease over 24 hours. These must be changed daily, however, and can be associated with skin irritation.[17] Transdermal testosterone gels have been available in the United States since 2000; these provide a serum testosterone level in the normal range of healthy men. These gels appear to be well tolerated, with tenfold fewer application-site reactions than patch preparations.[20] One potential drawback is transfer of the medication by direct contact. Oral testosterone is perhaps the most problematic delivery method, given low bioavailability and hepatotoxicity due to the first pass effect of the liver. One newer oral formulation that is dissolved in castor oil bypasses the liver via its lymphatic absorption.[21] Other delivery methods, such as sublingual preparations, implantable pellets, and mucoadhesive buccal testosterone, continue to be developed in an effort to provide a stable circulating testosterone level while minimizing adverse side effects.

Scientific Review of the Effects of Testosterone Supplementation

No shortage of data exists on the effects of testosterone replacement in aging men. In fact, several meta-analyses and systematic reviews have been published to evaluate the best data on testosterone supplementation and its effects on body composition,[16,22] muscle strength,[23] bone density,[16,24] sexual function,[25-27] and depression.[28] These findings are summarized in **Table 1**.

Body Composition

Fairly extensive work has been done on the effects of testosterone on the body composition of the aging man. Perhaps the most complete recent review belongs to

Isidori et al,[16] who included 29 randomized clinical trials in a meta-analysis on the topic. Their summary included 1,083 subjects with an average age of 64.5 years and average duration of treatment of 9 months. The studies varied widely in terms of testosterone preparation, drug dosing, protocol design, and gonadal status of enrolled subjects. Treated subjects experienced an average reduction of 1.6 kg of total body fat, which corresponds to a 6.2% decrease of initial body fat. Only one study showed a gain in total fat mass,[29] and only two studies demonstrated a loss of more than 4 kg.[30,31] Active treatment also produced an increase in fat-free mass of 1.6 kg, which corresponds to an increase of 2.7% over initial lean body mass. As noted in the results of fat loss, most studies were homogeneous in their findings, with only two demonstrating a loss of fat-free mass[32,33] and only one showing a gain of more than 6 kg.[34] These findings were in agreement with a separate systematic review of 29 placebo-controlled trials on testosterone supplementation,[22] in which the authors noted a consistent modest increase in lean muscle with a modest fat loss. These authors noted that effects on body composition were more consistently observed in studies with a long duration of supplementation compared with studies in which duration of treatment was 3 months or less.

Muscle Strengthening

The treatment of muscle weakness and age-related sarcopenia with testosterone supplementation is one of the drug's most important applications. Because most falls in the elderly are due to muscle weakness,[14] use of this drug may help prevent falls and the fractures that are associated with them. Muscle strength also is a risk factor for frailty and disability,[35] and supplementation to maintain strength may be effective in facilitating independent living. Several studies have examined the effects of testosterone on muscle strength, with conflicting results. Ottenbacher et al[23] performed the largest meta-analysis on this topic, in 2006. The authors included all randomized clinical trials in refereed English-language journals that provided sufficient statistical information to estimate an effect size. Eleven trials were included, which consisted of 474 men with a mean age of 67 years. Effect sizes were noted to be in the small to medium range, and were larger for measures of lower

extremity muscle strength. Interestingly, effect sizes were larger for administration by injection compared with topical or oral administration. In a separate review of 29 studies on testosterone supplementation, Isidori et al[16] noted that only dominant knee extension and dominant handgrip showed improvement over placebo, and no effect could be detected in the nondominant muscles tested. In the other major review on muscle strength, Gruenewald and Matsumoto[22] found similar modest and conflicting results. These investigators noted that self-assessment of physical functioning at 3 years did not change with testosterone treatment, whereas placebo-treated men demonstrated a significant decline by the end of the study. The greatest effect of testosterone on perception of physical functioning occurred in subjects with the lowest baseline testosterone levels. Taken as a whole, the effect of testosterone supplementation on muscle strength in hypogonadal aging men must be considered modest at best.

Bone Density

At present, no adequately powered interventional trials have evaluated the outcome of testosterone supplementation on fractures. However, several randomized clinical trials on bone density, a critical risk factor for fracture, have been conducted. Tracz et al[24] undertook a meta-analysis of these trials, which included 365 participants. In all of these studies, otherwise healthy older men were treated with either transdermal or injectable testosterone to determine effects on bone. The results demonstrated increases of 4% in both femoral neck and lumbar spine bone mineral density. Studies using transdermal testosterone therapy showed no convincing improvement in bone density, however, whereas studies of injectable testosterone enanthate[36,37] showed an overall 8% increase in lumbar bone mineral density compared with placebo. In summary, the effect of testosterone supplementation on bone mineral density appears to be affected by androgen dose, route of administration, and degree of baseline testosterone deficiency. Several newer studies suggest that the type of testosterone is also crucial in mediating its bone-enhancing effects. Specifically, aromatizability (conversion of androgen to estrogen) appears to be required to affect bone. In a study of minimally aromatizable (nandrolone) versus aromatizable testosterone in equal doses, both augmented muscle strength equivalently, but only the aromatizable form increased lumbar spine bone mineral density.[37] Other studies have demonstrated that aromatizability may mediate up to 70% of testosterone's effect on bone.[38] Thus, although androgen supplementation may play a role in the prevention of fractures, much further study is required to determine optimal type, route of administration, dosing, and duration of treatment of optimal therapeutic use.

Sexual Function

Hypogonadism may be responsible for sexual dysfunction among men due to either primary gonadal failure or pituitary abnormalities. Population-based studies have reported that as many as 50% of aging men report sexual dysfunction.[39,40] Other studies have reported an association between higher testosterone levels and improved self-reported sexual function among elderly men,[41] although these findings are inconsistent across the literature.[26] In 2004, the Endocrine Society commissioned a task force to offer recommendations for the use of testosterone in aging men. As part of that work, a meta-analysis of the effects of testosterone on sexual function was conducted by Boloña et al.[26] This analysis encompassed 17 trials with 862 participants overall, including 11 studies on erectile dysfunction and 10 studies on libido. They found that participants with low testosterone levels showed moderate nonsignificant and inconsistent effects on erectile function but a very large effect on libido stimulation, especially in trials using oral testosterone. It is not surprising that erectile function responded less favorably than did libido, given that participants in these studies were generally older, often with other medical conditions that may have affected the biology of erection. Thus, it appears that testosterone supplementation does not have much of an effect on erectile dysfunction but may stimulate libido quite successfully. This effect on libido has also been demonstrated in women,[42] with transdermal or topical administration being well tolerated. The decision as to whether to use testosterone in the setting of sexual dysfunction should therefore be individualized, with consideration of other aspects of testosterone supplementation and potential side effects.

Cognitive Function

The effects of testosterone on cognitive function remain unclear. Some studies show that supraphysiologic supplementation results in improvement in spatial cognition, spatial and verbal memory, and working memory,[43-45] but another study showed no effect on memory, recall, or verbal fluency.[30] One additional study[46] showed testosterone to be outperformed by placebo with regard to verbal fluency. It should be noted that very few of these studies extended beyond 3 months; therefore, it remains unclear whether longer term testosterone supplementation would have any effect on cognitive function.

Side Effects

As many tissues and organ systems throughout the body are sensitive to testosterone, it follows that supplementation may adversely affect some of these systems. The ideal androgen would be selective, with receptors targeted for positive effects. To this end, selective androgen receptor modulators are being investigated, which may avoid many of the side effects currently associated with testosterone use. Currently, however, no regimen of testosterone replacement therapy is without some risk of side effects.

Dermatologic reactions may include oily skin and acne, and use of the patch can lead to skin irritation severe enough that 10% to 15% of patients cease treatment because of these concerns.[47] Breast enlargement or tenderness is often short-lived and abates with continued treatment. This side effect is commonly reported in younger males who use anabolic steroids but is uncommon at standard dosing levels for hypogonadal males.[17] Erythrocytosis, or elevation of the hematocrit, is actually the most common side effect of testosterone therapy,[14] but typical increases are only in the 3% to 5% range[48,49] and are usually clinically insignificant.

One of the more serious concerns with testosterone supplementation is its potential effect on cardiovascular disease. Studies on common markers such as serum lipoprotein levels have yielded equivocal results. Although high-density lipoproteins (HDLs) have been shown to decrease in young bodybuilders on supraphysiologic testosterone,[50] no such correlation has been found in older populations.[14] In the largest meta-analysis done on cardiovascular effects of testosterone replacement therapy, Haddad et al[51] evaluated 30 trials including 1,642 men. Overall, men with low testosterone levels treated with androgen supplementation experienced inconsequential changes in all lipid fractions, including total cholesterol, HDL, low-density lipoproteins (LDLs), and triglycerides. In other studies on coronary blood flow and coronary artery diameter, testosterone administration has been shown to improve these parameters.[52-54] Thus, the best available data would suggest that testosterone replacement therapy in the aging man may not pose a significant cardiovascular risk.

Benign prostatic hypertrophy (BPH) or prostate cancer is another area of concern with testosterone supplementation. The concern is valid, as the prostate is uniquely responsive to testosterone, and chemical blocking of testosterone is a well-accepted treatment of prostate cancer. Yet, although prostate volume has been reported to increase with testosterone therapy, the increases have been inconsistent and modest without any increase in clinical symptoms of BPH.[18,55] It has been suggested that nonobstructive BPH is not a contraindication to testosterone therapy, although it is not recommended in cases of obstructive BPH.[17] Treatment with testosterone has been associated with minor prostate-specific antigen (PSA) elevation,[56] but general agreement exists that testosterone replacement therapy does not cause prostate cancer.[57] In a recent randomized clinical trial evaluating the effect of testosterone replacement therapy on prostate tissue and biomarkers, Marks et al[58] randomized 44 hypogonadal men to testosterone versus placebo. After 6 months of treatment, testosterone levels were increased to normal, but prostate levels of hormone did not significantly change. In addition, no treatment-related change was observed in prostate histology, tissue biomarkers, or cancer incidence or severity. Treatment-related changes in volume, PSA level, voiding symptoms, and urinary flow were minor. The authors concluded that 6 months of treatment with testosterone normalizes serum androgen levels with little effect on prostate tissue or cellular functions.

In spite of the apparent safety of testosterone replacement therapy regarding the prostate, however, screening is still recommended as follows for all patients:[14]

- PSA testing and digital examination on initial visit and every 3 months thereafter;
- If PSA level is above 4.0 ng/dL, prostate biopsy before beginning testosterone replacement;
- If PSA level rises more than 1.5 ng/dL over 3 to 6 months, repeat test followed by biopsy;
- Contraindicated if there is a history of prostate cancer.

Conclusions

Although increasing evidence exists regarding the benefits of testosterone replacement for aging men, it is estimated that approximately 5,000 to 10,000 men need to be randomized and treated for approximately 5 to 7 years to assess long-term safety and a general recommendation for all men.[59] Until then, the current guidelines are as follows:[14]

- Treatment should be individualized and with informed consent.
- Treatment should be reserved for the symptomatic individual with hypogonadism.
- The benefits and risks should be discussed in detail with the patient.
- Patients should be followed up with PSA testing and hematocrit measures.
- Blood pressure and general heath issues should be addressed.
- Lifestyle modifications, including exercise and weight loss, should be stressed.

Human Growth Hormone

Human growth hormone (hGH) is a peptide hormone secreted by the pituitary gland that stimulates growth and cell production. Deficiencies in growth hormone result in small stature, increased adiposity, and decreased lean body mass, and treatment in children with growth hormone deficiency can be successful.[60] The rationale for its use in anti-aging lies in the age-related decline in activity of the hypothalamic growth hormone–insulin-like growth factor axis, a phenomenon referred to as "somatopause."[61] Pituitary hGH production reaches a peak around the pubertal growth spurt and then declines steadily.[62] After age 40, hGH secretion declines approximately 14% per decade of adult life.[63] Numerous studies show that hGH replacement in young adults with severe deficiency leads to

Table 2: Summary of Effects of hGH Replacement Therapy[a]

Measurement	Effect of hGH supplementation	Comment
Weight	↑ 0.06 kg	Not significant
Fat mass	↓ 2.08 kg	
Lean body mass	↑ 2.1 kg	
VO$_2$ max (exercise capacity)	↑ 0.32 mL/min	Not significant
Bone mineral density	No effect	Not significant
Skin thickness	↑ 0.7 mm	Not significant
LDL	↓ 0.12 mmol/L	Not significant
HDL	↓ 0.01 mmol/L	Not significant
Strength	↓ 0.2 kg	Not significant
Tissue edema	↑ 42%	
Carpal tunnel syndrome	↑ 18%	
Arthralgia	↑ 16%	
New-onset diabetes	↑ 4%	

hGH = human growth hormone, LDL = low-density lipoprotein, HDL = high-density lipoprotein.
[a]Information adapted from references 61, 68, and 69.

improvement in body composition, muscle strength, bone mineral density, physical function, and quality of life.[64-67]

The "birth" of hGH as an anti-aging treatment may have occurred in 1990, when Rudman et al[68] published a report that a short course of hGH therapy could reverse decades of age-related changes in body composition in otherwise healthy elderly men. Since then, the popularity of hGH therapy has experienced exponential growth. Although the exact number of people in the United States on hGH is not known, one study estimated that 30,000 people used the drug for anti-aging purposes in 2004, representing a tenfold increase since the mid-1990s.[69] Annual sales of hGH worldwide now exceed $1.5 billion, and a third of this may be off-label illegal use.[69] The scientific community, however, continues to be reticent to use hGH as a treatment for anti-aging. The American Association of Clinical Endocrinologists has adopted a position statement against its use,[70] and the distribution of hGH for use as an anti-aging therapy in the United States is illegal.[71] Some experts have suggested that the strength-enhancing

properties of hGH among healthy adults have been exaggerated,[72] and others have cited serious health risks and even an association with increased mortality.[73] Thus hGH replacement therapy remains a very controversial topic.

Scientific Review of the Effects of hGH Therapy

Many systematic reviews have been performed on hGH as an ergogenic aid[69] in young athletic populations, as well as in the healthy elderly population.[61] In the first application, 44 studies including 303 participants were reviewed; the second analysis reviewed 31 studies including 220 participants. The results are summarized in **Table 2**.

Body Composition

One of the key outcome measures was the effect of hGH on body composition. Healthy older adults who took hGH experienced no significant weight loss, but they did decrease fat mass by a mean of 2.08 kg and gained 2.13 kg of lean body mass over the treatment period. No association was reported between any body composition outcome and participants who took hGH alone versus those who took it in combination with lifestyle changes, although these findings were largely based on a single trial that specifically addressed this question.[74] Furthermore, no significant differences were reported for outcomes in body composition between those who had more than 26 weeks of therapy versus those who had less than 26 weeks of therapy. In women, hGH treatment did not result in significant changes in body composition, except for a borderline statistically significant decrease in fat mass. No significant differences were found for serum lipid profiles, maximal oxygen consumption rate, bone mineral density, or insulin sensitivity. The authors found little evidence of clinical benefit of hGH therapy in the healthy elderly, and they felt that they could not recommend growth hormone replacement therapy for use in the healthy aging adult.

Effects on Performance

Given the marketing claims of hGH as a performance-enhancing drug, it is surprising how little scientific work has been done on its effect on strength, and the work that has been done does not seem to support the marketing claims. Rubeck et al[75] evaluated all randomized, double-blinded, placebo-controlled trials in the literature on the effects of hGH administration on muscle mass and strength in growth hormone–deficient adults. In their review of 15 trials and 306 patients, muscle volume increased an average of 7%, but no improvement was seen in any measure of muscle strength. Blackman et al[76] performed a randomized clinical trial in healthy elderly men and women on the effects of hormone replacement therapy and hGH in this population. Strength testing was included in this trial. The authors found that the strength of the women did not change in any treatment group, whereas the strength of the men improved marginally (6.8%) when given a combination of testosterone and hGH. No such increase was detected with the administration of hGH alone. In the systematic review by Liu et al[69] of the effect of hGH on athletic performance in a population of healthy 13- to 45-year-olds, hGH supplementation was not found to enhance strength in single-repetition maximal biceps or quadriceps strength, nor did it en-hance maximum strength or muscle circumference throughout the reviewed trials. This lack of any benefit in muscle strength has been confirmed in at least two other trials,[77,78] making the scientific literature to date unanimous on this point.

Side Effects

Numerous side effects have been associated with hGH use, including an approximate 42% increase in soft-tissue edema (with an even higher incidence in women), an 18% increase in carpal tunnel syndrome, a 16% increase in arthralgias, a 6% increase in gynecomastia, and a 4% increase in new-onset diabetes mellitus.[61] Across studies, approximately 27% of patients treated with hGH required a dose decrease.

Conclusions

The best available scientific evidence suggests that supplementation with hGH in the healthy elderly population improves body composition minimally but does not alter clinically relevant outcomes. It should be noted, however, that most studies limited dosing to therapeutic ranges, and it is unknown whether supra-physiologic doses might improve results beyond those reported. Caution should be exercised, however, because even in the doses reported, adverse events were quite common, and dose increases to improve body composition would likely result in even higher adverse events. At this time, hGH supplementation cannot be recommended for use in the healthy elderly population.

Resveratrol

Perhaps the most promising recent supplement with true anti-aging applications is resveratrol, a phytoalexin produced naturally in some plants when under attack by pathogens such as bacteria or fungi.

Scientific Review of the Effects of Resveratrol

Resveratrol garnered international attention after a 2003 study showed that it significantly extended the life span in yeast.[79] Subsequent studies showed up to 33% longer life span in worms,[80] fish, and other species.[81] Baur and Sinclair[82] demonstrated that mice on a high-fat diet supplemented with 22 mg/kg of resveratrol had a 30% lower risk of death than mice on a high-fat diet alone. Gene expression analysis indicated the addition of resveratrol opposed the alteration of 144 out of 155 gene pathways changed by the high-fat diet. Although no study regarding life extension has been done in humans, studies like these make resveratrol a promising treatment for age-related decline.

Mechanism of Action

The mechanism of action of resveratrol is not fully understood, but it appears to mimic several of the biochemical effects of calorie restriction, a well-founded anti-aging regimen. It is suggested that resveratrol acts through activation of the *SIRT1* gene and improves functioning in the mitochondria.[83] This mechanism of action has been implicated not only in life span extension as mentioned above but also in cancer,[84] neurodegenerative diseases,[85] and, more recently, diabetes.[86] Unfortunately, very little work has been done in humans, and extrapolation from animal data would require massive doses. For example, to duplicate the protective effects against high-fat diets seen in mice,[82] a 70-kg person would have to take a daily dose of 1,540 mg of resveratrol. This would be roughly equivalent to 1,500 glasses of red wine, a popular but unconcentrated source of resveratrol. Currently, supplements from the Japanese knotweed are the most common source, and these can be concentrated enough to achieve equivalent doses to the in vitro studies.

Side Effects

Data on the potential side effects of resveratrol supplementation are sparse. One study in healthy volunteers[87] found that a single dose of up to 5 g of resveratrol caused no serious side effects, but this finding is preliminary at best. Another study noted that resveratrol was found to inhibit new blood vessel formation, which suppresses tumors but also inhibits wound healing.[88] Because its mechanism of action is ubiquitous throughout the body, resveratrol may have quite far-reaching effects and requires much further study.

Conclusions

Resveratrol is perhaps the first compound with solid evidence that it slows the actual aging process in lower life-forms. Much further study will be required to see if this is applicable to humans, whether it will confer protection against cancers, or whether it will have detrimental effects in longer term use at therapeutic doses.

Summary

Although the Fountain of Youth remains elusive, scientists are beginning to understand the complex causes of aging. Unfortunately, the marketing of anti-aging products has drastically outpaced the science behind them. Nevertheless, strategies to extend both the length and quality of life receive more scientific attention now than ever before, and progress is being made. All clinicians who treat aging patients should have an open mind for potential anti-aging applications as well as a healthy suspicion for snake oil.

References

1. Selling the promise of youth. *Business Week*. Columbus, OH, McGraw-Hill, 2006.

2. Hughes VA, Frontera WR, Roubenoff R, Evans WJ, Singh MA: Longitudinal changes in body composition in older men and women: Role of body weight change and physical activity. *Am J Clin Nutr* 2002;76(2): 473-481.

3. Liu PY, Pincus SM, Keenan DM, Roelfsema F, Veldhuis JD: Analysis of bidirectional pattern synchrony of concentration-secretion pairs: Implementation in the human testicular and adrenal axes. *Am J Physiol Regul Integr Comp Physiol* 2005;288(2):R440-R446.

4. Nguyen TV, Eisman JA, Kelly PJ, Sambrook PN: Risk factors for osteoporotic fractures in elderly men. *Am J Epidemiol* 1996;144(3):255-263.

5. Santavirta S, Konttinen YT, Heliövaara M, Knekt P, Lüthje P, Aromaa A: Determinants of osteoporotic thoracic vertebral fracture: Screening of 57,000 Finnish women and men. *Acta Orthop Scand* 1992;63(2): 198-202.

6. Ferrini RL, Barrett-Connor E: Sex hormones and age: A cross-sectional study of testosterone and estradiol and their bioavailable fractions in community-dwelling men. *Am J Epidemiol* 1998;147(8):750-754.

7. Gray A, Feldman HA, McKinlay JB, Longcope C: Age, disease, and changing sex hormone levels in middle-aged men: Results of the Massachusetts Male Aging Study. *J Clin Endocrinol Metab* 1991;73(5):1016-1025.

8. Pirke KM, Doerr P: Age related changes in free plasma testosterone, dihydrotestosterone and oestradiol. *Acta Endocrinol (Copenh)* 1975;80(1):171-178.

9. Rubens R, Dhont M, Vermeulen A: Further studies on Leydig cell function in old age. *J Clin Endocrinol Metab* 1974;39(1):40-45.

10. Berthold AA: Transplantation der hoden. *Arch Anat Physiol Wissensch* 1849;16:42-46.

11. Brown-Séquard CE: The effects produced on man by subcutaneous injections of liquid obtained from the testicles of animals. *Lancet* 1889;2:105-107.

12. Morley JE: Hormones and the aging process. *J Am Geriatr Soc* 2003;51(7, Suppl):S333-S337.

13. Heller CG, Myers GB: The male climacteric: Its symptomatology, diagnosis, and treatment. *JAMA* 1944;126:472-477.

14. Tan RS, Culberson JW: An integrative review on current evidence of testosterone replacement therapy for the andropause. *Maturitas* 2003;45(1):15-27.

15. Harman SM, Metter EJ, Tobin JD, Pearson J, Blackman MR, Baltimore Longitudinal Study of Aging: Longitudinal effects of aging on serum total and free testosterone levels in healthy men. *J Clin Endocrinol Metab* 2001;86(2):724-731.

16. Isidori AM, Giannetta E, Greco EA, et al: Effects of testosterone on body composition, bone metabolism and serum lipid profile in middle-aged men: A meta-analysis. *Clin Endocrinol (Oxf)* 2005;63(3):280-293.

17. Wald M, Meacham RB, Ross LS, Niederberger CS: Testosterone replacement therapy for older men. *J Androl* 2006;27(2):126-132.

18. Bhasin S, Bagatell CJ, Bremner WJ, et al: Issues in testosterone replacement in older men. *J Clin Endocrinol Metab* 1998;83(10):3435-3448.

19. Sokol RZ, Palacios A, Campfield LA, Saul C, Swerdloff RS: Comparison of the kinetics of injectable testosterone in eugonadal and hypogonadal men. *Fertil Steril* 1982;37(3):425-430.

20. Bouloux P: Testim 1% testosterone gel for the treatment of male hypogonadism. *Clin Ther* 2005;27(3):286-298.

21. Jockenhövel F: Testosterone therapy—What, when and to whom? *Aging Male* 2004;7(4):319-324.

22. Gruenewald DA, Matsumoto AM: Testosterone supplementation therapy for older men: Potential benefits and risks. *J Am Geriatr Soc* 2003;51(1):101-115.

23. Ottenbacher KJ, Ottenbacher ME, Ottenbacher AJ, Acha AA, Ostir GV: Androgen treatment and muscle strength in elderly men: A meta-analysis. *J Am Geriatr Soc* 2006;54(11):1666-1673.

24. Tracz MJ, Sideras K, Boloña ER, et al: Testosterone use in men and its effects on bone health: A systematic review and meta-analysis of randomized placebo-controlled trials. *J Clin Endocrinol Metab* 2006;91(6):2011-2016.

25. Jain P, Rademaker AW, McVary KT: Testosterone supplementation for erectile dysfunction: Results of a meta-analysis. *J Urol* 2000;164(2):371-375.

26. Boloña ER, Uraga MV, Haddad RM, et al: Testosterone use in men with sexual dysfunction: A systematic review and meta-analysis of randomized placebo-controlled trials. *Mayo Clin Proc* 2007;82(1):20-28.

27. Isidori AM, Giannetta E, Gianfrilli D, et al: Effects of testosterone on sexual function in men: Results of a meta-analysis. *Clin Endocrinol (Oxf)* 2005;63(4):381-394.

28. Zarrouf FA, Artz S, Griffith J, Sirbu C, Kommor M: Testosterone and depression: Systematic review and meta-analysis. *J Psychiatr Pract* 2009;15(4):289-305.

29. Morley JE, Perry HM III, Kaiser FE, et al: Effects of testosterone replacement therapy in old hypogonadal males: A preliminary study. *J Am Geriatr Soc* 1993;41(2):149-152.

30. Sih R, Morley JE, Kaiser FE, Perry HM III, Patrick P, Ross C: Testosterone replacement in older hypogonadal men: A 12-month randomized controlled trial. *J Clin Endocrinol Metab* 1997;82(6):1661-1667.

31. Page ST, Amory JK, Bowman FD, et al: Exogenous testosterone (T) alone or with finasteride increases physical performance, grip strength, and lean body mass in older men with low serum T. *J Clin Endocrinol Metab* 2005;90(3):1502-1510.

32. Boyanov MA, Boneva Z, Christov VG: Testosterone supplementation in men with type 2 diabetes, visceral obesity and partial androgen deficiency. *Aging Male* 2003;6(1):1-7.

33. Clague JE, Wu FC, Horan MA: Difficulties in measuring the effect of testosterone replacement therapy on muscle function in older men. *Int J Androl* 1999;22(4):261-265.

34. Ferrando AA, Sheffield-Moore M, Paddon-Jones D, Wolfe RR, Urban RJ: Differential anabolic effects of testosterone and amino acid feeding in older men. *J Clin Endocrinol Metab* 2003;88(1):358-362.

35. Bhasin S, Tenover JS: Age-associated sarcopenia—Issues in the use of testosterone as an anabolic agent in older men. *J Clin Endocrinol Metab* 1997;82(6):1659-1660.

36. Amory JK, Watts NB, Easley KA, et al: Exogenous testosterone or testosterone with finasteride increases bone mineral density in older men with low serum testosterone. *J Clin Endocrinol Metab* 2004;89(2): 503-510.

37. Crawford BA, Liu PY, Kean MT, Bleasel JF, Handelsman DJ: Randomized placebo-controlled trial of androgen effects on muscle and bone in men requiring long-term systemic glucocorticoid treatment. *J Clin Endocrinol Metab* 2003;88(7):3167-3176.

38. Falahati-Nini A, Riggs BL, Atkinson EJ, O'Fallon WM, Eastell R, Khosla S: Relative contributions of testosterone and estrogen in regulating bone resorption and formation in normal elderly men. *J Clin Invest* 2000;106(12):1553-1560.

39. Bacon CG, Mittleman MA, Kawachi I, Giovannucci E, Glasser DB, Rimm EB: Sexual function in men older than 50 years of age: Results from the health professionals follow-up study. *Ann Intern Med* 2003;139(3):161-168.

40. Feldman HA, Goldstein I, Hatzichristou DG, Krane RJ, McKinlay JB: Impotence and its medical and psychosocial correlates: Results of the Massachusetts Male Aging Study. *J Urol* 1994;151(1):54-61.

41. Tsitouras PD, Martin CE, Harman SM: Relationship of serum testosterone to sexual activity in healthy elderly men. *J Gerontol* 1982;37(3):288-293.

42. Hubayter Z, Simon JA: Testosterone therapy for sexual dysfunction in postmenopausal women. *Climacteric* 2008;11(3):181-191.

43. Cherrier MM, Asthana S, Plymate S, et al: Testosterone supplementation improves spatial and verbal memory in healthy older men. *Neurology* 2001;57(1):80-88.

44. Janowsky JS, Chavez B, Orwoll E: Sex steroids modify working memory. *J Cogn Neurosci* 2000;12(3):407-414.

45. Janowsky JS, Oviatt SK, Orwoll ES: Testosterone influences spatial cognition in older men. *Behav Neurosci* 1994;108(2):325-332.

46. Wolf OT, Preut R, Hellhammer DH, Kudielka BM, Schürmeyer TH, Kirschbaum C: Testosterone and cognition in elderly men: A single testosterone injection blocks the practice effect in verbal fluency, but has no effect on spatial or verbal memory. *Biol Psychiatry* 2000;47(7):650-654.

47. Jordan WP Jr: Allergy and topical irritation associated with transdermal testosterone administration: A comparison of scrotal and nonscrotal transdermal systems. *Am J Contact Dermat* 1997;8(2):108-113.

48. Tenover JS: Effects of testosterone supplementation in the aging male. *J Clin Endocrinol Metab* 1992;75(4): 1092-1098.

49. Wang C, Swerdloff RS, Iranmanesh A, et al: Transdermal testosterone gel improves sexual function, mood, muscle strength, and body composition parameters in hypogonadal men. *J Clin Endocrinol Metab* 2000;85(8):2839-2853.

50. Hurley BF, Seals DR, Hagberg JM, et al: High-density-lipoprotein cholesterol in bodybuilders v powerlifters: Negative effects of androgen use. *JAMA* 1984;252(4): 507-513.

51. Haddad RM, Kennedy CC, Caples SM, et al: Testosterone and cardiovascular risk in men: A systematic review and meta-analysis of randomized placebo-controlled trials. *Mayo Clin Proc* 2007;82(1):29-39.

52. Jaffe MD: Effect of testosterone cypionate on postexercise ST segment depression. *Br Heart J* 1977;39(11):1217-1222.

53. Rosano GM, Leonardo F, Pagnotta P, et al: Acute anti-ischemic effect of testosterone in men with coronary artery disease. *Circulation* 1999;99(13):1666-1670.

54. Webb CM, McNeill JG, Hayward CS, de Zeigler D, Collins P: Effects of testosterone on coronary vasomotor regulation in men with coronary heart disease. *Circulation* 1999;100(16):1690-1696.

55. Meikle AW, Arver S, Dobs AS, et al: Prostate size in hypogonadal men treated with a nonscrotal permeation-enhanced testosterone transdermal system. *Urology* 1997;49(2):191-196.

56. Gerstenbluth RE, Maniam PN, Corty EW, Seftel AD: Prostate-specific antigen changes in hypogonadal men treated with testosterone replacement. *J Androl* 2002;23(6):922-926.

57. Bhasin S, Woodhouse L, Casaburi R, et al: Testosterone dose-response relationships in healthy young men. *Am J Physiol Endocrinol Metab* 2001;281(6):E1172-E1181.

58. Marks LS, Mazer NA, Mostaghel E, et al: Effect of testosterone replacement therapy on prostate tissue in men with late-onset hypogonadism: A randomized controlled trial. *JAMA* 2006;296(19):2351-2361.

59. Bhasin S, Buckwalter JG: Testosterone supplementation in older men: A rational idea whose time has not yet come. *J Androl* 2001;22(5):718-731.

60. Mehta A, Hindmarsh PC: The use of somatropin (recombinant growth hormone) in children of short stature. *Paediatr Drugs* 2002;4(1):37-47.

61. Liu H, Bravata DM, Olkin I, et al: Systematic review: The safety and efficacy of growth hormone in the healthy elderly. *Ann Intern Med* 2007;146(2):104-115.

62. Lamberts SW, van den Beld AW, van der Lely AJ: The endocrinology of aging. *Science* 1997;278(5337): 419-424.

63. Toogood AA: Growth hormone (GH) status and body composition in normal ageing and in elderly adults with GH deficiency. *Horm Res* 2003;60(Suppl 1): 105-111.

64. Carroll PV, Umpleby M, Alexander EL, et al: Recombinant human insulin-like growth factor-I (rhIGF-I) therapy in adults with type 1 diabetes mellitus: Effects on IGFs, IGF-binding proteins, glucose levels and insulin treatment. *Clin Endocrinol (Oxf)* 1998;49(6):739-746.

65. Johannsson G, Grimby G, Sunnerhagen KS, Bengtsson BA: Two years of growth hormone (GH) treatment increase isometric and isokinetic muscle strength in GH-deficient adults. *J Clin Endocrinol Metab* 1997;82(9):2877-2884.

66. Rodríguez-Arnao J, Jabbar A, Fulcher K, Besser GM, Ross RJ: Effects of growth hormone replacement on physical performance and body composition in GH deficient adults. *Clin Endocrinol (Oxf)* 1999;51(1): 53-60.

67. Fernholm R, Bramnert M, Hägg E, et al: Growth hormone replacement therapy improves body composition and increases bone metabolism in elderly patients with pituitary disease. *J Clin Endocrinol Metab* 2000;85(11):4104-4112.

68. Rudman D, Feller AG, Nagraj HS, et al: Effects of human growth hormone in men over 60 years old. *N Engl J Med* 1990;323(1):1-6.

69. Liu H, Bravata DM, Olkin I, et al: Systematic review: The effects of growth hormone on athletic performance. *Ann Intern Med* 2008;148(10):747-758.

70. Gharib H, Cook DM, Saenger PH, et al: American Association of Clinical Endocrinologists medical guidelines for clinical practice for growth hormone use in adults and children—2003 update. *Endocr Pract* 2003;9(1):64-76.

71. Perls TT, Reisman NR, Olshansky SJ: Provision or distribution of growth hormone for "antiaging": Clinical and legal issues. *JAMA* 2005;294(16):2086-2090.

72. Rennie MJ: Claims for the anabolic effects of growth hormone: A case of the emperor's new clothes? *Br J Sports Med* 2003;37(2):100-105.

73. Osterziel KJ, Dietz R, Ranke MB: Increased mortality associated with growth hormone treatment in critically ill adults. *N Engl J Med* 2000;342(2):134-135, author reply 135-136.

74. Hameed M, Lange KH, Andersen JL, et al: The effect of recombinant human growth hormone and resistance training on IGF-I mRNA expression in the muscles of elderly men. *J Physiol* 2004;555(Pt 1):231-240.

75. Rubeck KZ, Bertelsen S, Vestergaard P, Jørgensen JO: Impact of growth hormone (GH) substitution on exercise capacity and muscle strength in GH-deficient adults: A meta-analysis of blinded, placebo-controlled trials. *Clin Endocrinol (Oxf)* 2009;71(6):860-866.

76. Blackman MR, Sorkin JD, Münzer T, et al: Growth hormone and sex steroid administration in healthy aged women and men: A randomized controlled trial. *JAMA* 2002;288(18):2282-2292.

77. Papadakis MA, Grady D, Black D, et al: Growth hormone replacement in healthy older men improves body composition but not functional ability. *Ann Intern Med* 1996;124(8):708-716.

78. Holloway L, Kohlmeier L, Kent K, Marcus R: Skeletal effects of cyclic recombinant human growth hormone and salmon calcitonin in osteopenic postmenopausal women. *J Clin Endocrinol Metab* 1997;82(4):1111-1117.

79. Howitz KT, Bitterman KJ, Cohen HY, et al: Small molecule activators of sirtuins extend Saccharomyces cerevisiae lifespan. *Nature* 2003;425(6954):191-196.

80. Wood JG, Rogina B, Lavu S, et al: Sirtuin activators mimic caloric restriction and delay ageing in metazoans. *Nature* 2004;430(7000):686-689.

81. Valenzano DR, Terzibasi E, Genade T, Cattaneo A, Domenici L, Cellerino A: Resveratrol prolongs lifespan and retards the onset of age-related markers in a short-lived vertebrate. *Curr Biol* 2006;16(3):296-300.

82. Baur JA, Sinclair DA: Therapeutic potential of resveratrol: The in vivo evidence. *Nat Rev Drug Discov* 2006;5(6):493-506.

83. Lagouge M, Argmann C, Gerhart-Hines Z, et al: Resveratrol improves mitochondrial function and protects against metabolic disease by activating SIRT1 and PGC-1alpha. *Cell* 2006;127(6):1109-1122.

84. Cullen JJ, Weydert C, Hinkhouse MM, et al: The role of manganese superoxide dismutase in the growth of pancreatic adenocarcinoma. *Cancer Res* 2003; 63(6):1297-1303.

85. Karuppagounder SS, Pinto JT, Xu H, Chen HL, Beal MF, Gibson GE: Dietary supplementation with resveratrol reduces plaque pathology in a transgenic model of Alzheimer's disease. *Neurochem Int* 2009;54(2):111-118.

86. Palsamy P, Subramanian S: Resveratrol, a natural phytoalexin, normalizes hyperglycemia in streptozotocin-nicotinamide induced experimental diabetic rats. *Biomed Pharmacother* 2008;62(9): 598-605.

87. Boocock DJ, Faust GE, Patel KR, et al: Phase I dose escalation pharmacokinetic study in healthy volunteers of resveratrol, a potential cancer chemopreventive agent. *Cancer Epidemiol Biomarkers Prev* 2007;16(6): 1246-1252.

88. Bråkenhielm E, Cao R, Cao Y: Suppression of angiogenesis, tumor growth, and wound healing by resveratrol, a natural compound in red wine and grapes. *FASEB J* 2001;15(10):1798-1800.

Chapter 7

Corticosteroids and Viscosupplementation for Osteoarthritis

Laura Dunn Goldberg, MD
Victor M. Goldberg, MD

Key Points

- An integrated approach offers the best outcome for osteoarthritis (OA).
- Nonpharmacologic interventions include education, physical/occupational therapy, weight loss, low-impact exercise, quadriceps strengthening, and proprioception training.
- Pharmacologic treatment options include acetaminophen, nonsteroidal anti-inflammatory drugs (NSAIDs), cyclooxygenase-2 (COX-2) inhibitors, opioids, anti-inflammatory creams, and intra-articular corticosteroids.
- Intra-articular corticosteroids are rapidly effective over days, offering short-term benefit (often for acute flares), and may prolong the effect of hyaluronic acid (HA).
- Intra-articular HA injections have a longer onset of action and longer duration of effect; they are best used for chronic pain management.
- Treatment decisions need to be individualized based on patient characteristics and efficacy and tolerability of therapy.
- HA injections may have disease-modifying activity that would expand the therapeutic indications.

Introduction

OA is the most common form of arthritis. It has been estimated that 27 million people in the United States have clinical OA, with 50% of people older than 65 years having OA in at least one joint.[1] OA is second only to ischemic heart disease as a cause of work disability in men older than 50.[2] It is estimated that by 2020, 59.4 million people in the United States will be affected.[2]

OA is a slowly evolving articular disorder characterized by gradual development of joint pain, stiffness, and loss of range of motion. Patients with OA report stiffness or swelling in the morning or after prolonged rest. The pain worsens with activity and weight bearing and improves with rest. OA results from a complex interaction of biomechanical, biochemical, and genetic factors that influence the degradation and repair of cartilage, bone, and synovium with secondary components of inflammation.[3] Several risk factors for the development of OA have been identified, including increased age, obesity, female sex, joint trauma, prolonged occupational or sports stress, joint hypermobility or instability, malalignment, genetic predisposition, and possibly quadriceps weakness.[4] On physical examination, patients may have tenderness to palpation, localized inflammation such as a joint effusion and/or warmth, bony enlargement, crepitus with movement, and limitation of joint motion. Primary or secondary malalignment may be present.

The goals of clinical management of OA are to reduce pain; maintain mobility; minimize disability; and to slow, halt, or reverse disease progression.[5] Treatment requires nonpharmacologic, pharmacologic, and surgical approaches. Patients with OA-related symptoms present to primary care physicians, rheumatologists, and orthopaedic surgeons. Several treatment guidelines exist to guide qualified clinicians, insurance payers, governmental bodies, and healthcare policy makers in caring for these patients.[6-10] **Table 1** summarizes the current guidelines.

Nonpharmacologic Interventions

OA can have a dramatic affect on lifestyle and strongly affect a patient's emotional health. Nonpharmacologic interventions may be used throughout all treatment plans to help patients understand the disease process and the active role they must play in their care. Education of the patient, family, and caregiver as well as social support of the patient enable the patient to better understand and tolerate the symptoms. Several risk factors are modifiable, such as obesity, activity level, and quadriceps strength. Obesity increases the load through the joint and may lead to increased rate of progression. Any weight loss can have an appreciable treatment effect. Aerobic exercise such as biking, walking, or pool exercises of moderate intensity for a minimum of 30 minutes 5 days a week or of vigorous intensity for 20 minutes 3 days a week is recommended for all ages.[11] Such low-impact aerobic exercise helps with weight loss as well as maintaining strength and functional ability. Physical therapy assists with range of motion, muscle strengthening, and maintenance of proprioception, which may be diminished in the arthritic joint. Occupational therapy may be helpful for functional adaptation and maximization of functional capacity. Improving motion, strength, and proprioception offers joint protection and, together with aerobic exercise and weight loss, aids in energy conservation. Assistive devices for mobilization and ambulation such as a walker or cane enable patients to maintain activities, and vocational assistance may delay the need for work disability. The American Academy of Orthopaedic Surgeons (AAOS) guidelines do not support the use of braces and wedged insoles; however, other guidelines suggest that, if tolerated, braces and wedged insoles may alleviate some pressure due to malalignment.[6-8,10]

Pharmacologic Interventions

In the early stages of OA, nonpharmacologic interventions may have dramatic effects, eliminating the need for medications. However, the continuously changing balance of repair and degradation of tissues of the synovial joint often results in recurrent inflammation and/or pain that requires increased intervention. In the increasingly painful joint without evidence of inflammation, acetaminophen (maximum 4 g/d) is universally recommended for mild to moderate pain.[7,8,10,12] In the absence of response or inadequate response to acetaminophen, NSAIDs should be used at the lowest effective dose. In the patient with increased gastrointestinal risk (older than 65 years, history of ulcer or bleeding), COX-2 selective agents or nonselective NSAIDs with a coprescription for a gastroprotective agent such as misoprostol or a proton pump inhibitor (PPI) may be effective.[12] Topical NSAIDs and capsaicin cream can provide effective adjunctive therapy to oral medications. Tramadol (200 to 300 mg divided 4 times per day) is an effective alternative when NSAIDs and acetaminophen fail. Opioid and narcotic analgesics can be considered if the patient has refractory pain despite all nonsurgical treatment modalities or if other treatments are contraindicated.[7,8,10,12]

Intra-articular Injections

Intra-articular injections of corticosteroids have been widely used for more than 50 years in the treatment of knee OA to relieve inflammation and reduce swelling, pain, and disability. Most commonly, intra-articular corticosteroids are used to treat acute flare-ups of pain, as concern regarding the safety of repetitive injections limits their long-term use. The mechanism of action is not fully understood, but some animal research suggests that intra-articular corticosteroids may exert a protec-

Table 1: Guideline Summary for Nonsurgical Treatment of Knee Osteoarthritis[a]

- An integrated approach of nonpharmacologic and pharmacologic treatment modalities offers the best outcome for OA.
- Treatment should be tailored according to:
  - Risk factors (activity level, age, obesity, malalignment or mechanical factors, comorbidity, polypharmacy)
  - Level of pain intensity and disability
  - Signs of inflammation (ie, effusion)
  - Location and degree of structural damage
- Nonpharmacologic interventions include:
  - Patient education and social support
  - Physical therapy (range of motion, quadriceps strengthening, and proprioception training)
  - Occupational therapy (walking aids, insoles, and braces)
  - Weight loss
  - Low-impact exercise
  - Thermal modalities, TENS, and acupuncture may be beneficial
- Pharmacologic treatment options include:
  - Acetaminophen (up to 4 g/d)—initial oral analgesic for mild to moderate pain
  - NSAIDs—lowest effective dose in symptomatic OA;
    - COX-2 inhibitors or add PPI or misoprostol in high-GI-risk patient
  - Topical NSAIDs or capsaicin cream as adjunctive therapy
  - Glucosamine and/or chondroitin sulfate—stop if no effect at 6 months
  - IA corticosteroids are rapidly effective over days, offering short-term benefit (often for acute flares), and may prolong hyaluronan effect
  - Opioid and narcotic analgesics can be used in refractory pain patients where other pharmacologic treatments have failed or are contraindicated. Nonpharmacologic therapies should be continued and surgical treatment should be considered.
- IA hyaluronic acid injections have a longer onset of action and longer duration of effect, best used forchronic pain management.
- Treatment decisions need to be individualized based on patient characteristics as well as the efficacy and tolerability of therapy.

OA = osteoarthritis, TENS = transcutaneous electrical nerve stimulation, NSAIDs = nonsteroidal anti-inflammatory drugs, COX-2 = cyclooxygenase-2, PPI = proton pump inhibitor, GI = gastrointestinal, IA = intra-articular.
[a]Information adapted from references 6 through 10.

tive effect by suppressing destructive circulating cytokines and proteases.[3,13] Chondrocytes in an arthritic knee are deficient in glucocorticoid receptors. The resulting decreased responsiveness to circulating glucocorticoid may increase the degradative effects of circulating cytokines and metalloproteases on cartilage. Further evaluation of the mechanism of action and long-term effects of repetitive use is needed.

The efficacy of intra-articular corticosteroids is well supported in the literature.[14,15] Studies have shown intra-articular corticosteroids to be superior to placebo for pain relief at 1 week, but these effects are not sustained beyond 3 weeks. Functional improvement reported at 1 week after injection was not adequate to find statistically significant or clinically important differences. No statistical difference was detected between

Table 2: Summary of Meta-Analyses of Intra-articular Cortisone Therapy in Knee Osteoarthritis[a]

Authors (Year)	Total No. of Studies	Efficacy Outcome Measures	Key Pooled Results	Conclusions
Arroll and Goodyear-Smith (2004)	10	Symptomatic improvement	RR = 1.66 (95% CI, 1.37 to 2.01)	IA steroids effective <2 weeks
Bellamy et al (2006)	28	WMD in pain on weight bearing vs placebo	1 week (WMD 21.91; 95% CI, −29.93 to −13.89)	IA steroids more effective than placebo at 1 to 3 weeks IA steroids *not* superior to IA HA (similar effects at 1-4 weeks, less sustained duration at 5-13 weeks vs HA)

RR = relative risk, CI = confidence interval, IA = intra-articular, HA = hyaluronic acid, WMD = weighted mean difference.

[a]Information adapted from references 14 and 15.

intra-articular corticosteroids and HA injections at 1 to 4 weeks. Intra-articular corticosteroids were found to be less effective at 5 to 13 weeks than intra-articular HA for one or more of the following variables: Western Ontario and McMaster Universities (WOMAC) OA Index, Lequesne Index, pain, range of motion (flexion), and number of responders. In general, intra-articular corticosteroids and HA injections had similar onset of effect, but HA injections had longer-lasting effects.[3,14,15] **Table 2** summarizes the results of two meta-analyses. In conclusion, intra-articular corticosteroids are effective in short-term symptomatic treatment of knee OA.

Comparisons of different formulations of intra-articular corticosteroids suggest that triamcinolone hexacetonide is superior to betamethasone for pain reduction up to 4 weeks (relative risk [RR], 2.00; 95% confidence interval [CI], 1.10 to 3.63).[6,15] This is thought to be due to the lower solubility of traimcinolone hexacetonide, which may increase the depot effect of the injected steroid. However, the choice of glucocorticoid and the dosage vary widely among studies, from 6.25 to 80 mg prednisone equivalents, with too few head-to-head comparisons to endorse the use of one particular preparation or dose with evidence-based sup-

port.[3,14,16] American College of Rheumatology guidelines from 2000 recommend 40 mg triamcinolone, as some data suggest this dosage may affect length of relief.[8]

Safety of treatment remains a concern. However, no serious adverse events were reported in 28 controlled trials.[15] Potential side effects include joint infection, postinjection flare of pain, synovitis, hemarthrosis, and steroid atrophy. However, concern remains as to whether long-term treatment accelerates destruction of joint and tissue atrophy. One study of repetitive injections of 1 mL of triamcinolone acetonide 40 mg every 3 months for 2 years showed no adverse cartilage effects, and patients had increased range of motion, decreased pain, and decreased stiffness at 1 year.[3] Further studies need to be performed to better evaluate long-term effects of intra-articular corticosteroids.

Current guidelines from the Osteoarthritis Research Society International (OARSI), the AAOS, the American College of Rheumatology, and the Cochrane Systematic Reviews for management of knee OA find intra-articular corticosteroids to be safe and effective for short-term pain relief in symptomatic knee OA and use

Table 3: Potential Disease-Modifying Activities of Hyaluronans[a]

Promotion of Healing and Repair

- Stimulation of chondrocyte growth and metabolism
- Maintenance of chondrocyte vitality (decreased apoptosis)
- Stimulation of synthesis of articular cartilage matrix components (eg, collagen, proteoglycans, endogenous hyaluronans, hyaladherins)

Inhibition of Destruction

- Inhibition of expression and activity of chondrodegradative enzymes (eg, metalloproteinase)
- Inhibition of matrix-destructive inflammatory processes

[a]Information adapted from reference 17.

may be appropriate in conjunction with nonpharmacologic intervention in patients with effusion and/or signs of inflammation. Most experts recommend limited frequency, with repeat injections no more than four times per year.[6-9]

Hyaluronan

Hyaluronan, or hyaluronic acid (HA), is a glycosaminoglycan composed of repeated disaccharide units that form a linear polymer. HA was first proposed for the treatment of arthritis by Balazs in 1942. In the early 1970s, therapeutic studies were begun to test the efficacy of HA on knee OA. The US Food and Drug Administration (FDA) approved the first HA injection in 1998 based on encouraging results with few adverse effects. Early human studies showed improved joint function, which was thought to be due to increased lubrication, but quick degradation and elimination from the joint (48 to 72 hours per labeling studies) suggest alternative biologic mechanisms for efficacy. A growing body of nonclinical evidence exists to show that exogenous hyaluronans have complex effects on joint biochemistry and may have disease-modifying activity in addition to the established symptomatic effects[17] (**Table 3**).

HA is the most abundant glycosaminoglycan in mammalian tissue, with the highest concentration in synovial fluid. HA molecules provide important viscoelasticity and lubricating properties of synovial fluid. In particular, they reduce articular cartilage wear with high shear forces and stabilize the joint at low shear forces. Additionally, HA molecules restrict large plasma protein entry into synovial fluid while facilitating the entry of water and small molecules important for joint nutrition. The synovial fluid in patients with OA has increased levels of proinflammatory cytokines, free radicals, and proteinases, which may lead to production of HA with abnormal molecular weights as well as increased synovial fluid due to inflamed synovial vessels. The abnormal HA coupled with increased fluid lowers the concentration of HA in the synovial fluid and decreases the effects of native HA on joint protection. The goal of an intra-articular HA injection is to restore or supplement HA properties to improve joint function, reduce symptoms, and possibly modify disease activity.[17-20]

Enhancement of synovial fluid with a higher concentration of exogenous HA molecules to between 500 and 4,000 kDa increases synovial fluid viscosity, reduces pain induction, inhibits inflammation, promotes healing and repair, and reduces cartilage deterioration through many potential mechanisms of action. However, smaller HA fragments may be proinflammatory. Increased viscosity restores the shock-absorbing and lubricating ability of synovial fluid.[18-20] The HA-enhanced synovial fluid creates a boundary layer around nociceptors, reducing pain induction via receptor shielding. Inhibition of inflammatory mediators such as cytokines and prostaglandins inhibits cell migration and phagocytosis. The exogenous HAs reduce cartilage deterioration by stimulating cartilage matrix synthesis with chondrocyte growth and collagen biosynthesis.

Table 4: Summary of Product Profiles for FDA-Approved Hyaluronic Acid Therapies

Product (Distributor)	Manufacturing	Active Ingredient	Number of Injections per Course	Molecular Weight (kDa)	Labeling Precaution on Efficacy/Safety
Hyalgan (Sanofi-Aventis, New York, NY)	Naturally derived, purified HA	1% sodium hyaluronate (20 mg)	3 or 5	500-730	No
Synvisc (Genzyme Biosurgery, Philadelphia, PA)	Hylan polymers derived from HA	0.8% sodium hyaluronate derivative (16 mg)	1 (6 mL) or 3 (2 mL)	6,000+ gel	No
Supartz (Smith & Nephew, Tokyo, Japan)	Naturally derived, purified HA	1% sodium hyaluronate (25 mg)	3 or 5	620-1170	Yes
Orthovisc (DePuy Mitek, Raynham, MA)	Fermented, bacteria-derived HA	0.7% sodium hyaluronate (30 mg)	3 or 4	1,100-2,900	Yes
Euflexxa (Ferring, Parsippany, NJ)	Fermented, bacteria-derived HA	1% sodium hyaluronate (20 mg)	3	2,400-3,600	Yes

Product profiles based on package insert of Hyalgan (2001), Synvisc (2006), Synvisc-One (2008), Supartz (2004), Orthovisc (2005), Euflexxa (2005).

FDA = US Food and Drug Administration, HA = hyaluronic acid.

HAs also stimulate endogenous hyaluronate synthesis by synoviocytes through CD44 receptor binding. Inhibition of cartilage degradation is supported through downregulation of matrix metalloproteinases-3 and interleukin-1β expression, increased tissue inhibition of metalloproteinase-1 production, and decreased chondrocyte apoptosis.[17] In summary, current proposed actions include restored shock absorption, reduction of pain transmission, reduction of synovial inflammation, promotion of healing and repair, and reduction of cartilage degradative enzymes.

Five injectable preparations of HA for the knee are currently approved by the FDA: Hyalgan, Synvisc, Supartz, Orthovisc, and Euflexxa. **Table 4** summarizes the product profiles.

The pooled analyses of five meta-analyses of intra-articular HA therapy in knee OA support the efficacy of HA as a class. However, some analyses showed a small effect size.[21-25] These meta-analyses are summarized in **Table 5**. Caution must be exercised in drawing relative conclusions about individual HA preparations, as there are few head-to-head comparisons. The systematic reviews show high variability in outcome measurements, and individual HA preparations had different effect size in various outcome scales. Comparable efficacy of intra-articular HA injections was noted against NSAIDs, and longer term benefits were noted compared to intra-articular corticosteroids.[21] Synvisc-one (Genzyme Biosurgery, Cambridge, MA), a single 6-mL intra-articular injection of hylan G-F 20, was shown to be effective in improving WOMAC A pain scores (−0.15, standard error 0.076, $P = 0.047$) in one randomized, double-blinded, placebo-controlled trial, but this study was not included in the meta-analyses.[26]

Table 5: Summary of Meta-Analyses of Intra-articular Hyaluronic Acid Therapy in Knee Osteoarthritis[a]

Authors (Year)	Total No. of Studies	Efficacy Outcome Measures	Key Pooled Results	Conclusions
Lo et al (2003)	22	Effect size (change from baseline pain vs placebo)	Effect size: 0.32 ($P < 0.001$)	Small treatment effect
Wang et al (2004)	20	Mean difference, ASPID vs placebo	Mean difference for ASPID: 13.4%	Safe and effective
Arrich et al (2005)	22	WMD in pain during/after exercise (VAS) vs control	WMD at 10-14 wks: −4.3 mm ($P = 0.013$) WMD at 22-30 wks: −7.1 mm ($P = 0.013$)	Not effective in measured outcomes
Modawal et al (2005)	11	VAS	WMD at 5-7 wks: 17.6 (95% CI, +7.5, +28.0) WMD at 8-12 wks: 18.1 (95% CI, +6.3, +29.9) WMD at 15-22 wks: 4.4 (95% CI, −15.3, 24.1)	Moderately effective at 5-10 wks, not effective at 15-22 wks
Bellamy et al (2006)	76	WMD in pain on weight bearing vs placebo	% change at 5-13 wks: +26% for pain, +23% for function	Effective treatment of pain, function, patient global assessment, especially at 5-13 wks

ASPID = adjusted sum of pain intensity differences, WMD = weighted mean difference, VAS = visual analog scale, CI = confidence interval.

[a]Information adapted from references 21 through 25.

Most of the current guidelines suggest the use of intra-articular HA for treatment of pain in OA of the knee that has failed to respond adequately to nonpharmacologic therapy and to simple analgesics.[5,6,8,10] Intra-articular HAs are contraindicated if there is known hypersensitivity to HA preparations, if there is a past or present infection, or if there is skin disease in the area of the injection site. HAs are relatively contraindicated in the setting of prior hypersensitivity reaction to HA injection; however, if the patient has previously experienced good relief with HA injections and desires repeat injection, a thorough discussion of the risks and benefits should be undertaken, with an emphasis on the possibility of recurrent reaction. Under these circumstances, it may be reasonable to proceed after a "washout" period of 6 months. The use of an alternative HA preparation should be strongly encouraged. Despite widespread popularity and data to support their use, current AAOS guidelines do not recommend for or against intra-articular HA for knee OA.[7]

The use of a combination injection of HA and a corticosteroid has been advocated by clinicians without any good data to substantiate this approach. A more rational treatment sequence might be to use intra-articular corticosteroid to reduce the inflammatory component of the symptoms, and then, 2 to 3 weeks later, when the joint effusion has subsided, begin the HA injections. Again, no data exist to confirm this treatment protocol.

HA preparations have a favorable safety profile with few serious adverse events. No significant difference was observed in gastrointestinal and cardiovascular events between patients receiving HA and controls, and no drug-drug interactions were reported. More local but fewer systemic adverse events are reported with HA than with NSAIDs.[21,22,25] Pseudoseptic reactions to injections have been reported with hylan G-F 20 derivatives but not with naturally extracted sodium hyaluronates. Symptoms of these pseudoseptic reactions resemble those of a "septic knee" and include severe inflammation with painful effusion generally 24 to 72 hours after injection that often does not resolve within 72 hours without intervention. Prior exposure to HA is often present. Acute management includes rest, cold compresses, analgesics, and NSAIDs. Synovial fluid analysis shows a cellular infiltrate, predominately monocytic, and is negative for crystals or bacteria, distinguishing it from true sepsis or pseudogout. While awaiting cultures, one should consider administering prophylactic oral antibiotics. If the condition deteriorates, intravenous antibiotics may be indicated. Once a septic joint has been ruled out, intra-articular steroids may alleviate severe pain that persists after day 4. If pain persists, the hylan G-F 20 should be discontinued. If the patient benefited from hylan G-F 20 in the past, another HA preparation may be used after initial symptoms resolve. If a chronic granuloma develops, surgical intervention may be required.[27]

HA injections are most commonly used in knee OA, but off-label use of HA injections is being studied, and early results suggest symptomatic efficacy. Qvistgaard et al[28] performed a randomized controlled trial of HA, corticosteroid, and intra-articular injections of isotonic saline in 101 patients with hip OA. Results were significant for improvement of "pain on walking" (effect size 0.6; 95% CI, 0.1 to 1.1; $P = 0.021$) with cortisone and a much smaller clinical effect size of 0.4 (95% CI, –0.1 to 0.9; $P = 0.13$) with HA compared with saline. van den Bekerom et al[29] compared three different HA formulations with 126 total hip arthroplasty candidates, finding significant improvement in visual analog scale and Harris hip scores. After 3 years, 51% of patients still had not undergone total hip arthroplasty. These studies suggest a clinical use for HA in the hip, but indications remain highly individualized given the cost-benefit analysis and slightly increased risk of adverse events with hip injections in general (10% to 30%).[28-30] Studies of other joints suggest clinical use in carpometacarpal joint arthritis,[31,32] chronic shoulder pain from OA, rotator cuff tear and/or adhesive capsulitis,[33] and ankle arthritis.[34] Petralla et al[35] reported on 158 athletes with acute grade 1 or 2 lateral ankle sprains who received periarticular HA or placebo injections within 48 hours. The periarticular HA injections showed significant reduction in visual analog scale pain on weight bearing and walking at 8 days.[35] Huang et al[36] investigated the effects of intra-articular HA injections at 4, 8, and 12 weeks after anterior cruciate ligament reconstruction with a patellar tendon graft; 120 patients were included in the randomized controlled trial. Significant improvement in average Lysholm knee scoring scale was reported in the 8-week intra-articular HA group from 12-week through 1-year follow-up. Future orthopaedic applications may include postarthroscopy therapy, wound healing, and generation of synthetic matrices for use in reconstructive surgery as we learn more about the possible disease-modifying actions of HA, such as stimulation of chondrocyte growth and metabolism, inhibition of chondrodegradation and chondrocyte apoptosis, and suppression of destructive inflammation.[17]

Summary

Nonpharmacologic interventions remain important for the successful management of OA throughout its course. An integrated approach of nonpharmacologic and pharmacologic treatments offers the best outcomes. Pharmacologic treatment options include NSAIDs, COX-2 inhibitors, opioids, anti-inflammatory creams, and intra-articular corticosteroids and HA injections. Intra-articular corticosteroids are rapidly effective over days, offering short-term benefit (often for acute flares), and may prolong the hyaluronan effect. Intra-articular HA injections have a longer onset of action and longer duration of effect and are best used for chronic pain management. Treatment decisions need to be individualized based on patient characteristics and efficacy and tolerability of therapy. Future therapeutic uses for HA may extend to other orthopaedic applications as further investigation into the disease-modifying activity progresses.

References

1. Lawrence RC, Felson DT, Helmick CG, et al: Estimates of the prevalence of arthritis and other rheumatic conditions in the United States: Part II. *Arthritis Rheum* 2008;58(1):26-35.

2. Divine JG, Zazulak BT, Hewett TE: Viscosupplementation for knee osteoarthritis: A systematic review. *Clin Orthop Relat Res* 2007;455: 113-122.

3. Raynauld JP, Buckland-Wright C, Ward R, et al: Safety and efficacy of long-term intraarticular steroid injections in osteoarthritis of the knee: A randomized, double-blind, placebo-controlled trial. *Arthritis Rheum* 2003;48(2):370-377.

4. Kraus VB: Pathogenesis and treatment of osteoarthritis. *Med Clin North Am* 1997;81(1):85-112.

5. Kelly MA, Goldberg VM, Healy WL, Pagnano MW, Hamburger MI: Osteoarthritis and beyond: A consensus on the past, present, and future of hyaluronans in orthopedics. *Orthopedics* 2003;26(10): 1064-1081.

6. Zhang W, Moskowitz RW, Nuki G, et al: OARSI recommendations for the management of hip and knee osteoarthritis, Part II: OARSI evidence-based, expert consensus guidelines. *Osteoarthritis Cartilage* 2008; 16(2):137-162.

7. American Academy of Orthopaedic Surgeons: *Clinical Practice Guideline on Treatment of Osteoarthritis of the Knee (Non-Arthroplasty)*. Rosemont, IL, American Academy of Orthopaedic Surgeons, December 2008. http://www.aaos.org/research/guidelines/OAK guideline.pdf. Accessed March 10, 2011.

8. American College of Rheumatology Subcommittee on Osteoarthritis Guidelines: Recommendations for the medical management of osteoarthritis of the hip and knee: 2000 update. *Arthritis Rheum* 2000;43(9):1905-1915.

9. Zhang W, Doherty M: EULAR recommendations for knee and hip osteoarthritis: A critique of the methodology. *Br J Sports Med* 2006;40(8):664-669.

10. Jordan KM, Arden NK, Doherty M, et al: EULAR Recommendations 2003: An evidence based approach to the management of knee osteoarthritis. Report of a Task Force of the Standing Committee for International Clinical Studies Including Therapeutic Trials (ESCISIT). *Ann Rheum Dis* 2003;62(12):1145-1155.

11. Nelson ME, Rejeski WJ, Blair SN, et al: Physical activity and public health in older adults: Recommendation from the American College of Sports Medicine and the American Heart Association. *Med Sci Sports Exerc* 2007;39(8):1435-1445.

12. Zhang W, Moskowitz RW, Nuki G, et al: OARSI recommendations for the management of hip and knee osteoarthritis, part I: Critical appraisal of existing treatment guidelines and systematic review of current research evidence. *Osteoarthritis Cartilage* 2007;15(9): 981-1000.

13. Young L, Katrib A, Cuello C, et al: Effects of intraarticular glucocorticoids on macrophage infiltration and mediators of joint damage in osteoarthritis synovial membranes: Findings in a double-blind, placebo-controlled study. *Arthritis Rheum* 2001;44(2):343-350.

14. Arroll B, Goodyear-Smith F: Corticosteroid injections for osteoarthritis of the knee: Meta-analysis. *BMJ* 2004;328(7444):869.

15. Bellamy N, Campbell J, Robinson V, Gee T, Bourne R, Wells G: Intraarticular corticosteroid for treatment of osteoarthritis of the knee. *Cochrane Database Syst Rev* 2006;2:CD005328.

16. Smith MD, Wetherall M, Darby T, et al: A randomized placebo-controlled trial of arthroscopic lavage versus lavage plus intra-articular corticosteroids in the management of symptomatic osteoarthritis of the knee. *Rheumatology (Oxford)* 2003;42(12):1477-1485.

17. Goldberg VM, Buckwalter JA: Hyaluronans in the treatment of osteoarthritis of the knee: Evidence for disease-modifying activity. *Osteoarthritis Cartilage* 2005;13(3):216-224.

18. Ghosh P, Guidolin D: Potential mechanism of action of intra-articular hyaluronan therapy in osteoarthritis: Are the effects molecular weight dependent? *Semin Arthritis Rheum* 2002;32(1):10-37.

19. Balazs EA, Watson D, Duff IF, Roseman S: Hyaluronic acid in synovial fluid: I. Molecular parameters of hyaluronic acid in normal and arthritis human fluids. *Arthritis Rheum* 1967;10(4):357-376.

20. Smith MM, Ghosh P: The synthesis of hyaluronic acid by human synovial fibroblasts is influenced by the nature of the hyaluronate in the extracellular environment. *Rheumatol Int* 1987;7(3):113-122.

21. Bellamy N, Campbell J, Robinson V, Gee T, Bourne R, Wells G: Viscosupplementation for the treatment of osteoarthritis of the knee. *Cochrane Database Syst Rev* 2006;2:CD005321.

22. Arrich J, Piribauer F, Mad P, Schmid D, Klaushofer K, Müllner M: Intra-articular hyaluronic acid for the treatment of osteoarthritis of the knee: Systematic review and meta-analysis. *CMAJ* 2005;172(8):1039-1043.

23. Lo GH, LaValley M, McAlindon T, Felson DT: Intra-articular hyaluronic acid in treatment of knee osteoarthritis: A meta-analysis. *JAMA* 2003;290(23):3115-3121.

24. Modawal A, Ferrer M, Choi HK, Castle JA: Hyaluronic acid injections relieve knee pain. *J Fam Pract* 2005;54(9):758-767.

25. Wang CT, Lin J, Chang CJ, Lin YT, Hou SM: Therapeutic effects of hyaluronic acid on osteoarthritis of the knee: A meta-analysis of randomized controlled trials. *J Bone Joint Surg Am* 2004;86(3):538-545.

26. Chevalier X, Jerosch J, Goupille P, et al: Single, intra-articular treatment with 6 ml of hylan G-F 20 in patients with symptomatic primary osteoarthritis of the knee: A randomised, multicentre, double-blind, placebo controlled trial. *Ann Rheum Dis* 2010;69(1):113-119.

27. Goldberg VM, Coutts RD: Pseudoseptic reactions to hylan viscosupplementation: Diagnosis and treatment. *Clin Orthop Relat Res* 2004;419:130-137.

28. Qvistgaard E, Christensen R, Torp-Pedersen S, Bliddal H: Intra-articular treatment of hip osteoarthritis: A randomized trial of hyaluronic acid, corticosteroid, and isotonic saline. *Osteoarthritis Cartilage* 2006;14(2):163-170.

29. van den Bekerom MP, Rys B, Mulier M: Viscosupplementation in the hip: Evaluation of hyaluronic acid formulations. *Arch Orthop Trauma Surg* 2008;128(3):275-280.

30. van den Bekerom MP, Lamme B, Sermon A, Mulier M: What is the evidence for viscosupplementation in the treatment of patients with hip osteoarthritis? Systematic review of the literature. *Arch Orthop Trauma Surg* 2008;128(8):815-823.

31. Roux C, Fontas E, Breuil V, Brocq O, Albert C, Euller-Ziegler L: Injection of intra-articular sodium hyaluronidate (Sinovial) into the carpometacarpal joint of the thumb (CMC1) in osteoarthritis: A prospective evaluation of efficacy. *Joint Bone Spine* 2007;74(4):368-372.

32. Fuchs S, Mönikes R, Wohlmeiner A, Heyse T: Intra-articular hyaluronic acid compared with corticoid injections for the treatment of rhizarthrosis. *Osteoarthritis Cartilage* 2006;14(1):82-88.

33. Blaine T, Moskowitz R, Udell J, et al: Treatment of persistent shoulder pain with sodium hyaluronate: A randomized, controlled trial. A multicenter study. *J Bone Joint Surg Am* 2008;90(5):970-979.

34. Cohen MM, Altman RD, Hollstrom R, Hollstrom C, Sun C, Gipson B: Safety and efficacy of intra-articular sodium hyaluronate (Hyalgan) in a randomized, double-blind study for osteoarthritis of the ankle. *Foot Ankle Int* 2008;29(7):657-663.

35. Petrella RJ, Petrella MJ, Cogliano A: Periarticular hyaluronic acid in acute ankle sprain. *Clin J Sport Med* 2007;17(4):251-257.

36. Huang MH, Yang RC, Chou PH: Preliminary effects of hyaluronic acid on early rehabilitation of patients with isolated anterior cruciate ligament reconstruction. *Clin J Sport Med* 2007;17(4):242-250.

Chapter 8
Tendinopathy and Rehabilitation

Kevin Wilk, PT, DPT
Leonard C. Macrina, MSPT, SCS, CSCS

Key Points

- Tendinopathies are commonly seen in mature athletes.
- Tendon pain is often called tendinitis, whereas careful differential diagnosis often reveals a tendinosis or a degenerative tendon.
- Differential diagnosis is the key to successful rehabilitation and desired outcomes.
- Treatment for a patient with stage 3 tendinopathy is very different from treatment for a patient with tendinitis.
- Tendinopathies respond favorably to a progressive eccentric loading program.

Dr. Wilk or an immediate family member serves as a paid consultant to or is an employee of Empi, Theralase Technologies, and LiteCure Medical and has received nonincome support (such as equipment or services), commercially derived honoraria, or other non–research-related funding (such as paid travel) from Empi, Joint Active Systems, and Biodex. Neither Mr. Macrina nor any immediate family member has received anything of value from or owns stock in a commercial company or institution related directly or indirectly to the subject of this chapter.

Introduction

The rise in competitive sports and the desire to continue to play later in life has led to an increase in overuse injuries. Overuse injuries in the United States are thought to represent 30% to 50% of all sports-related injuries.[1] Rotator cuff tendinitis is one of the most common diagnoses seen, accounting for 2.8 million injuries per year. It is believed that 1% to 2% of the general population has experienced some form of tendon injury of the lateral elbow. A 1987 study[2] showed that 20% of all knee injuries assessed in a sports clinic were diagnosed as patellar tendinopathy. The demands to train longer and compete at a higher level often lead to soft-tissue injuries. Proper recognition and treatment algorithms are necessary to return the athlete to sport as quickly and safely as possible.

Pathology to tendons represents a major problem facing the orthopaedic and sports medicine clinician. During sporting activities, tendons often sustain more than ten times normal body weight; however, the tissue has a relatively slow metabolic rate to maintain healthy tissue. It has been reported that tendon demonstrates only 13% of the oxygen uptake of muscle and requires more than 100 days to synthesize collagen.[3,4] The pain associated with the tendon breakdown often causes tremendous functional limitations that can disable even the well-trained athlete. The specific pathology that causes the debilitating symptoms often influences treatment dramatically. The treating clinician should have a good understanding of the structure and function of the tendon and the best mode of treatment to expedite the patient's return to pain-free function. The goal of this chapter is to provide an overview of the application and the scientific basis

Table 1: Characteristics of Tendinitis Versus Tendinosis

Tendinitis	Tendinosis
Inflammation	Mucoid degeneration
Acute hemorrhage	Sporadic inflammation
Fiber disruption	Fiber disorganization
Neutrophils	Angiofibroblastic hyperplasia

for formulating a rehabilitation program for patients with tendinopathy.

Tendon Anatomy

A tendon is a collection of closely packed collagen fibers that connect muscle to bone and transmit and dissipate the forces created during joint movements. Collagen represents 80% of the dry weight of a tendon; the overall weight of a tendon is 30% collagen, 2% elastin, and 68% water.[5] Other basic elements include ground substance or extracellular matrix, which is a viscous substance with high amounts of proteoglycans. The collagen portion is made up of 97% to 98% type I collagen, with small amounts of other types of collagen. These include type II and type IX collagen in the cartilaginous zones, type III collagen in the reticular fibers of the vascular walls, type IV collagen in the basement membranes of the capillaries, type V collagen in the vascular walls, and type X collagen in the mineralized fibrocartilage near the interface with the bone.[6-8] The low percentage of elastin reflects the limited elasticity of tendon as compared with ligament; however, the tendon's elastic composition assists in its ability to function as a spring. This allows tendons to passively modulate forces during locomotion, providing additional stability with no active work. It also allows tendons to store and recover energy at high efficiency. Collagen provides the tendon with tensile strength, and the ground substance provides structural support.[9-11]

The tendon is covered by the epitenon, which is a fine, loose connective tissue sheath containing the vascular, lymphatic, and nerve supply.[6] The epitenon extends deeper into the tendon as the endotenon. The epitenon is surrounded by paratenon, which is a loose areolar connective tissue consisting mainly of type I and III collagen, elastic fibrils, and synovial cells.[12-14] In certain instances in which high areas of mechanical stress are present, the tendon will be surrounded by a synovial sheath.[6] The synovial sheath functions to reduce the friction forces present as the musculotendinous units contract and pull the tendon within its tunnel.

Acute pain in and around a tendon is often associated with repetitive activities and is termed *tendinitis*. This terminology implies an inflammatory process in which treatment is aimed at controlling inflammation. This tendon pain is often associated with a gradual onset and structural changes of the tendon seen on ultrasonography and MRI.[15,16] Rest, nonsteroidal anti-inflammatory drugs (NSAIDs), and corticosteroid injections often are used in an attempt to relieve the painful symptoms. The problem with this approach is that often little to no inflammation is present by the time the patient presents to the clinician. Traditional modalities aimed at reducing inflammation often are not effective because of the chronicity of the problem and lack of a true inflammatory process.[17-23]

Normal tendon appearance involves collagen fibers organized in a longitudinal pattern with a slightly wave-like presentation.[6,20,24] Because no pathology is present in the normal tendon, fibroblasts and myofibroblasts are not present.[20] The term *tendinopathy* has been used widely in the literature and in many medical diagnoses for patients. This usually denotes a painful condition around or in the tendon arising from overuse. The term *tendinopathy*, as applied today, was first used by Puddu et al[25] in 1976, when they noted that such degeneration was troublesome in athletes and involved a localized, palpable tenderness. Today, *tendinopathy* is used to describe various tendon pathologies, including paratendinitis, tendinitis, and tendinosis, in the absence of biopsy-proven histopathologic evidence[18] (**Table 1**). Histopathologic studies demonstrate degeneration and disorganization of collagen fibers with increased cellularity and tendon thickening.[20,26] Tenocytes are more apparent and abnormal in shape.[20] Often, minimal inflammation is present at the site of the lesion but the tissue demonstrates loss of mechanical properties, cell apoptosis,[27] and increased production of matrix metalloproteinases.[19] The increased cellularity causes fibroblast, chondrocyte, endothelial, osteocyte, and lipocyte infiltration. For example, in symptomatic Achilles tendon pathology, an increase in blood vessels with random orientation, sometimes at right angles to the collagen fibers, is seen. Only with partial rupture of the tendon is an inflammatory lesion or granulation tissue observed.[13,28-32] Nirschl and Ashman[33,34] noted the angiofibroblastic infiltration correlated with the duration of symptoms in cases of lateral epicondylitis. Lian et al[27] performed tissue biopsies of ten patellar tendons with known chronic degeneration. Their results showed an occurrence of nerve ingrowth, substance P nerve fibers, and a decreased occurrence of vascular sympathetic nerve fibers. Therefore, tendinopathy appears to result from an imbalance between the regenerative changes and pathologic responses that result in tendon overuse. The net result from the tissue morphologic changes is tendon mucoid degeneration,[6] weakness, microtearing, pain, and loss of function.

Tendon Response to Exercise

The treatment of tendinopathy is a major challenge for the clinician because knowledge of the exact pathophysiology involved remains incomplete.[35,36] According to a meta-analysis published in 2007,[37] strong evidence to support physical interventions is lacking. This same meta-analysis found a limited level of evidence supporting the role of exercise in reducing pain but suggested that it typically takes approximately 12 weeks of eccentric exercise to accomplish this.[37] Exercise (specifically, eccentric exercise) has been shown to improve outcomes in patients with tendinosis lesions.[37-40] Studies of healthy tendons in animals and humans have shown that collagen turnover, cross-sectional area, and tensile strength of tendons can be improved with exercise.[41-44] Langberg et al[45] demonstrated that physical training increases both synthesis and degradation of collagen but a net collagen synthesis is seen after a long period of training. Langberg et al[46] showed, through microdialysis studies, that 12 weeks of eccentric training significantly increased the propeptide of type I collagen (PICP), a marker for collagen type I synthesis in the area around diseased Achilles tendons in patients with Achilles tendinosis. The collagen degradation marker, carboxyterminal telopeptide of type I collagen (ICTP), did not demonstrate any significant

Table 2: Extrinsic and Intrinsic Factors for Tendon Degeneration

Extrinsic	Intrinsic
Repetitive load	Anatomic
Equipment problems	Aging
Environmental factors	Tissue hypoxia

changes in either the diseased or healthy tissue. This may indicate that the addition of eccentric loading of diseased tendons may lead to an increase in net collagen synthesis. The increase in collagen synthesis was seen only in the injured tendons, which may indicate that chronically injured tendons are the result of chronic mechanical overloading.

Often, the goal of physical rehabilitation is to improve blood flow to the diseased area to aid in tissue healing. The improved blood flow may bring the nutrients needed to initiate and maintain the healing process. Spectroscopy studies have shown increased blood flow to the tendon and peritendinous tissues as activity level increases.[47-50] Positron emission tomography studies have demonstrated an increase in metabolic activity by an increase in glucose uptake within the muscle with activity.[50-52] Therefore, exercises to load the tendon and muscle may aid in improved blood flow, metabolic activity, and tissue healing.

Treatment Principles

Tendinopathy as a result of sports or overuse issues continues to be commonly seen by the sports medicine clinician. A delicate balance exists between tissue strength and the amount of load before the tissue breaks down and becomes injured. If the mechanical loading on a tendon is not matched with the adaptation of new collagen formation, then pathology may result. This overloading exceeds the repair capacity of the tendon tissue.[46] One may consider both the intrinsic and extrinsic factors that contribute to this problem. Extrinsic factors may include repetitive loading of the tendon, equipment issues, and environmental exposures. Intrinsic factors may be anatomic, the age of the patient, and issues with tissue regeneration (**Table 2**). Common diagnoses seen by the orthopaedic clinician may include

Stage	Characteristics
1	Acute, reversible inflammation Involved tissue displays no new angiofibroblastic invasion.
2	Involved tissue may display partial angiofibroblastic invasion. Tissue degeneration has begun. Increased levels of substance P and calcitonin gene-related peptide,[53-55] which may inhibit local growth hormone; increase in protease levels breaks down tissue. Some healing may be present.
3	Extensive angiofibroblastic infiltration usually present

Table 3: Stages of Tendinopathy

lateral epicondylitis (tennis elbow), patellar tendinitis, supraspinatus tendinitis, and Achilles tendinitis. Histologic analysis reveals that in most cases, "-itis" should be replaced with "-osis" or "-opathy."

The recognition and treatment of tendinopathy may be determined by three different distinct stages of the inflammatory process. Each stage often can be delineated by distinct characteristics (**Table 3**). Often, however, there is significant overlap in the characteristics that may confound the best treatment strategy. A good history is critical in determining the best course of rehabilitation.

With stage 1 tendinopathy, the patient reports minor aching after heavy lifting or repetitive activity. Nonsurgical rehabilitation is often successful. The patient is instructed on the use of modalities, including ice and activity modification. Rest, gentle stretching of the agonist and antagonist musculotendinous units, and strengthening exercises are used with good success. Strengthening begins with submaximal, pain-free isometrics to retard muscular atrophy and restore voluntary muscular control while avoiding detrimental forces. Isometrics should be performed at multiple angles throughout the available range of motion (ROM), with particular emphasis on contraction at the end of the currently available ROM. Active ROM activities are permitted when adequate muscular strength has been achieved and symptoms are minimal to absent. NSAIDs are physician-prescribed to decrease the associated pain. The analgesic effects of NSAIDs are often short term (7 to 14 days), so these medications are most effective in patients with a shorter duration of symptoms.

Therapeutic modalities such as massage, cold laser therapy, iontophoresis, ultrasound, nitric oxide, and extracorporeal shock-wave therapy are often used by rehabilitation specialists to decrease inflammation and promote healing. Only very limited evidence exists to support the use of these modalities in isolation. When used in combination with exercise or with other modalities, however, improved tissue quality and outcomes have been reported.[56-74]

In stage 2, the patient often reports pain with activity that remains even after the activity is over. Rest can help alleviate symptoms, but rehabilitation is used to stimulate tendon regeneration and promote healing through gradual strengthening activities. Eccentric-type strengthening is used to synthesize and realign tissue collagen. Many of the modalities mentioned for stage 1 may be used as well.

With stage 3 tendinopathy, the patient reports pain during and after activity and often at rest. This leads to significant functional deficits, including with lifting, reaching, and gripping. Much research has been performed to determine the cause of the pain in tissue with little inflammation. Tissue samples using a microdialysis technique found no prostaglandin E2, which is commonly found in inflammatory tissue. An increase in glutamate production, which is an excitatory neurotransmitter, was noted in higher levels.[75-80]

Rehabilitation for stage 3 tendinopathy includes activities to improve collagen regeneration and alignment. Modalities to promote a warming effect and improve blood flow such as continuous ultrasound, hot packs, and transverse friction massage are often used.

Tendon loading by eccentric exercise and strength training has been shown to improve results in this patient population by increasing collagen synthesis[46] and realigning fiber orientation.[38,81,82] Other modalities, such as cold laser therapy[63-66] and extracorporeal shock-wave therapy,[69-71] have shown promising results as well.

Some emerging treatments have shown promise in treating chronic tendinopathy. The goal of these treatments is to stimulate a regenerative response that has otherwise been difficult to achieve up to this point. Platelet-rich plasma (PRP) is a promising intervention in which a small sample of the patient's own blood is separated out and the platelet-rich layer is injected into the site of injury. One theory of the mechanism of action of PRP is that it delivers supraphysiologic concentrations of humoral mediators and growth factors locally to induce a healing response. Other advantages of PRP are its minimally invasive nature, localized response, and avoidance of inflammatory response. Disadvantages include the cost of treatment; lack of supporting evidence; and staffing time to withdraw the blood, centrifuge it, and reinject it into the site of pathology.

Early research on the clinical application of PRP to promote healing and adaptive responses is promising.[83-92] Mishra and Pavelko[86] showed significant benefits of PRP in patients with chronic lateral epicondylitis. Basic science and controlled studies have yet to provide clear evidence for the efficacy of such a treatment.

Pain stimulation is also used as a treatment for the degenerative tissue before strength training. The primary goal of the pain stimulation is to produce pain at the site of the degenerative tissue. By producing pain, the body will respond by releasing endorphins that will block any pain response felt by the involved tissue. Once a moderate degree of discomfort has been produced by the noxious stimulus, the patient performs eccentric loading exercises specifically designed to progressively load the tendon to produce collagen synthesis and collagen alignment. We have found pain stimulation to be successful in the treatment of patellar and Achilles tendinopathies. The specific parameters are listed in **Table 4**. **Figure 1** illustrates the application and location of the pain stimulation electrodes. The

Table 4: Pain Stimulation Parameters
Frequency: 2,500 Hz
Pulse: 50 pps
Duty cycle: 10 s on and 10 s off
Intensity: to tolerance
Duration: 10-12 min

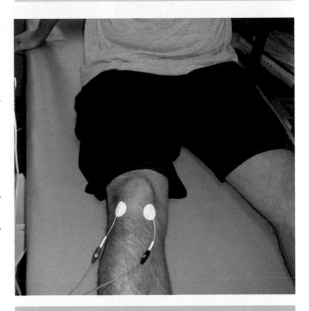

Figure 1 For pain stimulation, electrodes are placed on both sides of the location of tendon pain. Here, electrodes are shown placed on either side of the patella.

patient also may benefit from the use of topical creams to control the symptoms associated with tendinitis and tendinosis.

Strengthening activities are essential to promote a healing response, and they allow the patient to return to pain-free activities. Isometric resistance activities are initiated in a pain-free ROM. Isotonic strengthening exercises are progressed as symptoms allow. For rehabilitation of patellar or Achilles tendinitis, specific closed-kinetic-chain drills designed to dynamically load the lower extremity are recommended. These exercises include front step-downs (**Figure 2**, *A*), lateral step-downs (**Figure 2**, *B*), declining single-leg squats (**Figure 2**, *C*), single-leg leg presses (**Figure 2**, *D*), and single-leg

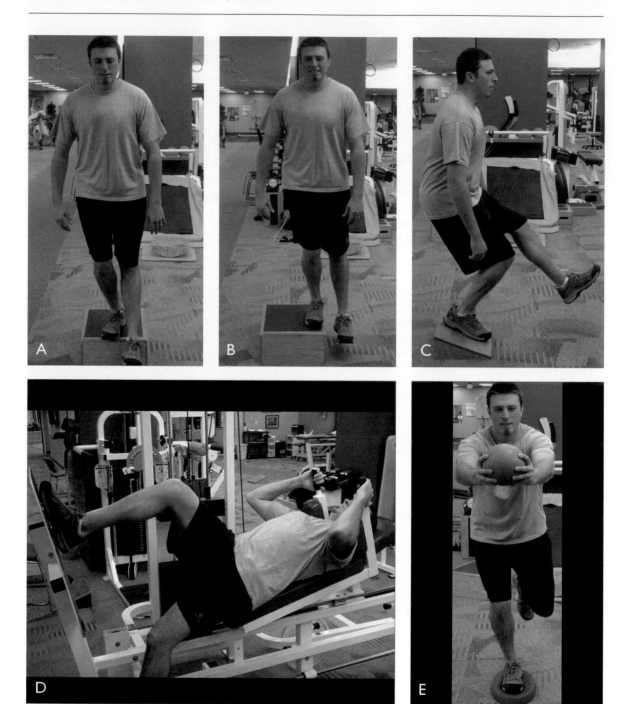

Figure 2 Clinical photographs show eccentric muscle loading. **A,** Single-leg forward step-down performed off an 8-in board. **B,** Lateral step-down off an 8-in board. **C,** Single-leg decline squat. **D,** Single-leg leg press. **E,** Single-leg balance on foam.

balance drills (**Figure 2,** *E*). Plyometric jumping drills also may be performed to facilitate dynamic stabilization and neuromuscular control of the knee joint once pain allows. Plyometric exercises use the muscle's stretch-shortening properties to produce maximal concentric contraction following a rapid eccentric loading of the muscle tissues.[93,94] Plyometric training is used to train the lower extremity to produce and dissipate forces to avoid injury.

Conclusions

Tendinopathy is a common presentation in the athlete and is often difficult to treat. For athletes to return to competition, it is imperative that they regain muscular strength and endurance in the injured extremity. Current rehabilitation programs focus not only on eccentric strengthening exercises but also on modalities used for stimulating the collagen regenerative process. We believe that it is important to use this approach not only for a rehabilitation process, but to also address any possible causes that might predispose the individual to future injury.

References

1. Renström P: Sports traumatology today: A review of common current sports injury problems. *Ann Chir Gynaecol* 1991;80(2):81-93.

2. Kannus P, Aho H, Järvinen M, Niittymäki S: Computerized recording of visits to an outpatient sports clinic. *Am J Sports Med* 1987;15(1):79-85.

3. Vailas AC, Tipton CM, Laughlin HL, Tcheng TK, Matthes RD: Physical activity and hypophysectomy on the aerobic capacity of ligaments and tendons. *J Appl Physiol* 1978;44(4):542-546.

4. Zernicke RF, Garhammer J, Jobe FW: Human patellar-tendon rupture. *J Bone Joint Surg Am* 1977;59(2):179-183.

5. O'Brien M: Functional anatomy and physiology of tendons. *Clin Sports Med* 1992;11(3):505-520.

6. Jozsa L, Kannus P: *Human Tendons: Anatomy, Physiology, and Pathology.* Champaign, IL, Human Kinetics, 1997.

7. Fukuta S, Oyama M, Kavalkovich K, Fu FH, Niyibizi C: Identification of types II, IX and X collagens at the insertion site of the bovine Achilles tendon. *Matrix Biol* 1998;17(1):65-73.

8. Lin TW, Cardenas L, Soslowsky LJ: Biomechanics of tendon injury and repair. *J Biomech* 2004;37(6):865-877.

9. Sharma P, Maffulli N: Biology of tendon injury: Healing, modeling and remodeling. *J Musculoskelet Neuronal Interact* 2006;6(2):181-190.

10. Sharma P, Maffulli N: Tendon injury and tendinopathy: Healing and repair. *J Bone Joint Surg Am* 2005;87(1):187-202.

11. Sharma P, Maffulli N: Basic biology of tendon injury and healing. *Surgeon* 2005;3(5):309-316.

12. Kvist M, Józsa L, Järvinen M, Kvist H: Fine structural alterations in chronic Achilles paratenonitis in athletes. *Pathol Res Pract* 1985;180(4):416-423.

13. Williams JG: Achilles tendon lesions in sport. *Sports Med* 1986;3(2):114-135.

14. Khan KM, Bonar F, Desmond PM, et al: Patellar tendinosis (jumper's knee): Findings at histopathologic examination, US, and MR imaging. *Radiology* 1996;200(3):821-827.

15. Neuhold A, Stiskal M, Kainberger F, Schwaighofer B: Degenerative Achilles tendon disease: Assessment by magnetic resonance and ultrasonography. *Eur J Radiol* 1992;14(3):213-220.

16. Fredberg U, Bolvig L, Pfeiffer-Jensen M, Clemmensen D, Jakobsen BW, Stengaard-Pedersen K: Ultrasonography as a tool for diagnosis, guidance of local steroid injection and, together with pressure algometry, monitoring of the treatment of athletes with chronic jumper's knee and Achilles tendinitis: A randomized, double-blind, placebo-controlled study. *Scand J Rheumatol* 2004;33(2):94-101.

17. Maffulli N, Kahn KM: Clinical nomenclature for tendon injuries. *Med Sci Sports Exerc* 1999;31(2):352-353.

18. Maffulli N, Khan KM, Puddu G: Overuse tendon conditions: Time to change a confusing terminology. *Arthroscopy* 1998;14(8):840-843.

19. Nirschl RP, Pettrone FA: Tennis elbow: The surgical treatment of lateral epicondylitis. *J Bone Joint Surg Am* 1979;61(6A):832-839.

20. Khan KM, Visentini PJ, Kiss ZS, et al: Correlation of ultrasound and magnetic resonance imaging with clinical outcome after patellar tenotomy: Prospective and retrospective studies. *Clin J Sport Med* 1999;9(3):129-137.

21. Ljung BO, Forsgren S, Fridén J: Substance P and calcitonin gene-related peptide expression at the

extensor carpi radialis brevis muscle origin: Implications for the etiology of tennis elbow. *J Orthop Res* 1999;17(4):554-559.

22. Soslowsky LJ, Thomopoulos S, Tun S, et al: Neer Award 1999: Overuse activity injures the supraspinatus tendon in an animal model. A histologic and biomechanical study. *J Shoulder Elbow Surg* 2000;9(2):79-84.

23. Fredberg U: Tendinopathy: Tendinitis or tendinosis? The question is still open. *Scand J Med Sci Sports* 2004;14(4):270-272.

24. Kraushaar BS, Nirschl RP: Tendinosis of the elbow (tennis elbow): Clinical features and findings of histological, immunohistochemical, and electron microscopy studies. *J Bone Joint Surg Am* 1999; 81(2):259-278.

25. Puddu G, Ippolito E, Postacchini F: A classification of Achilles tendon disease. *Am J Sports Med* 1976;4(4): 145-150.

26. Alfredson H, Ohberg L, Forsgren S: Is vasculo-neural ingrowth the cause of pain in chronic Achilles tendinosis? An investigation using ultrasonography and colour Doppler, immunohistochemistry, and diagnostic injections. *Knee Surg Sports Traumatol Arthrosc* 2003;11(5):334-338.

27. Lian O, Scott A, Engebretsen L, Bahr R, Duronio V, Khan K: Excessive apoptosis in patellar tendinopathy in athletes. *Am J Sports Med* 2007;35(4):605-611.

28. Kälebo P, Goksör LA, Swärd L, Peterson L: Soft-tissue radiography, computed tomography, and ultrasonography of partial Achilles tendon ruptures. *Acta Radiol* 1990;31(6):565-570.

29. Merkel KH, Hess H, Kunz M: Insertion tendopathy in athletes: A light microscopic, histochemical and electron microscopic examination. *Pathol Res Pract* 1982;173(3):303-309.

30. Nelen G, Martens M, Burssens A: Surgical treatment of chronic Achilles tendinitis. *Am J Sports Med* 1989;17(6):754-759.

31. Clancy WG Jr, Neidhart D, Brand RL: Achilles tendonitis in runners: A report of five cases. *Am J Sports Med* 1976;4(2):46-57.

32. Fox JM, Blazina ME, Jobe FW, et al: Degeneration and rupture of the Achilles tendon. *Clin Orthop Relat Res* 1975;(107):221-224.

33. Nirschl RP, Ashman ES: Elbow tendinopathy: Tennis elbow. *Clin Sports Med* 2003;22(4):813-836.

34. Nirschl RP, Ashman ES: Tennis elbow tendinosis (epicondylitis). *Instr Course Lect* 2004;53:587-598.

35. Kannus P: Etiology and pathophysiology of chronic tendon disorders in sports. *Scand J Med Sci Sports* 1997;7(2):78-85.

36. Kannus P: Tendons—A source of major concern in competitive and recreational athletes. *Scand J Med Sci Sports* 1997;7(2):53-54.

37. Woodley BL, Newsham-West RJ, Baxter GD: Chronic tendinopathy: Effectiveness of eccentric exercise. *Br J Sports Med* 2007;41(4):188-199.

38. Alfredson H, Pietilä T, Jonsson P, Lorentzon R: Heavy-load eccentric calf muscle training for the treatment of chronic Achilles tendinosis. *Am J Sports Med* 1998;26(3):360-366.

39. Nakamura K, Kitaoka K, Tomita K: Effect of eccentric exercise on the healing process of injured patellar tendon in rats. *J Orthop Sci* 2008;13(4):371-378.

40. Wasielewski NJ, Kotsko KM: Does eccentric exercise reduce pain and improve strength in physically active adults with symptomatic lower extremity tendinosis? A systematic review. *J Athl Train* 2007;42(3):409-421.

41. Rosager S, Aagaard P, Dyhre-Poulsen P, Neergaard K, Kjaer M, Magnusson SP: Load-displacement properties of the human triceps surae aponeurosis and tendon in runners and non-runners. *Scand J Med Sci Sports* 2002;12(2):90-98.

42. Simonsen EB, Klitgaard H, Bojsen-Møller F: The influence of strength training, swim training and ageing on the Achilles tendon and m. soleus of the rat. *J Sports Sci* 1995;13(4):291-295.

43. Tipton CM, Matthes RD, Martin RK: Influence of age and sex on the strength of bone-ligament junctions in knee joints of rats. *J Bone Joint Surg Am* 1978;60(2): 230-234.

44. Tipton CM, Matthes RD, Maynard JA, Carey RA: The influence of physical activity on ligaments and tendons. *Med Sci Sports* 1975;7(3):165-175.

45. Langberg H, Rosendal L, Kjaer M: Training-induced changes in peritendinous type I collagen turnover determined by microdialysis in humans. *J Physiol* 2001;534(pt 1):297-302.

46. Langberg H, Ellingsgaard H, Madsen T, et al: Eccentric rehabilitation exercise increases peritendinous type I collagen synthesis in humans with Achilles tendinosis. *Scand J Med Sci Sports* 2007;17(1):61-66.

47. Langberg H, Bülow J, Kjaer M: Blood flow in the peritendinous space of the human Achilles tendon

during exercise. *Acta Physiol Scand* 1998;163(2): 149-153.

48. Boushel R, Langberg H, Green S, Skovgaard D, Bulow J, Kjaer M: Blood flow and oxygenation in peritendinous tissue and calf muscle during dynamic exercise in humans. *J Physiol* 2000;524(pt 1):305-313.

49. Boushel R, Langberg H, Olesen J, et al: Regional blood flow during exercise in humans measured by near-infrared spectroscopy and indocyanine green. *J Appl Physiol* 2000;89(5):1868-1878.

50. Boushel R, Piantadosi CA: Near-infrared spectroscopy for monitoring muscle oxygenation. *Acta Physiol Scand* 2000;168(4):615-622.

51. Hannukainen J, Kalliokoski KK, Nuutila P, et al: In vivo measurements of glucose uptake in human Achilles tendon during different exercise intensities. *Int J Sports Med* 2005;26(9):727-731.

52. Kalliokoski KK, Knuuti J, Nuutila P: Relationship between muscle blood flow and oxygen uptake during exercise in endurance-trained and untrained men. *J Appl Physiol* 2005;98(1):380-383.

53. Jonhagen S, Ackermann P, Saartok T, Renstrom PA: Calcitonin gene related peptide and neuropeptide Y in skeletal muscle after eccentric exercise: A microdialysis study. *Br J Sports Med* 2006;40(3):264-267.

54. Lian O, Dahl J, Ackermann PW, Frihagen F, Engebretsen L, Bahr R: Pronociceptive and antinociceptive neuromediators in patellar tendinopathy. *Am J Sports Med* 2006;34(11):1801-1808.

55. Ackermann PW, Salo PT, Hart DA: Neuronal pathways in tendon healing. *Front Biosci* 2009;14:5165-5187.

56. Harvey W, Dyson M, Pond JB, Grahame R: The stimulation of protein synthesis in human fibroblasts by therapeutic ultrasound. *Rheumatol Rehabil* 1975;14(4):237.

57. Enwemeka CS: The effects of therapeutic ultrasound on tendon healing: A biomechanical study. *Am J Phys Med Rehabil* 1989;68(6):283-287.

58. Enwemeka CS: Inflammation, cellularity, and fibrillogenesis in regenerating tendon: Implications for tendon rehabilitation. *Phys Ther* 1989;69(10):816-825.

59. Jackson BA, Schwane JA, Starcher BC: Effect of ultrasound therapy on the repair of Achilles tendon injuries in rats. *Med Sci Sports Exerc* 1991;23(2): 171-176.

60. Reddy GK, Gum S, Stehno-Bittel L, Enwemeka CS: Biochemistry and biomechanics of healing tendon: Part II. Effects of combined laser therapy and electrical stimulation. *Med Sci Sports Exerc* 1998;30(6):794-800.

61. Reddy GK, Stehno-Bittel L, Enwemeka CS: Laser photostimulation of collagen production in healing rabbit Achilles tendons. *Lasers Surg Med* 1998;22(5):281-287.

62. Gum SL, Reddy GK, Stehno-Bittel L, Enwemeka CS: Combined ultrasound, electrical stimulation, and laser promote collagen synthesis with moderate changes in tendon biomechanics. *Am J Phys Med Rehabil* 1997;76(4):288-296.

63. Bjordal JM, Lopes-Martins RA, Iversen VV: A randomised, placebo controlled trial of low level laser therapy for activated Achilles tendinitis with microdialysis measurement of peritendinous prostaglandin E2 concentrations. *Br J Sports Med* 2006;40(1):76-80.

64. England S, Farrell AJ, Coppock JS, Struthers G, Bacon PA: Low power laser therapy of shoulder tendonitis. *Scand J Rheumatol* 1989;18(6):427-431.

65. Lam LK, Cheing GL: Effects of 904-nm low-level laser therapy in the management of lateral epicondylitis: A randomized controlled trial. *Photomed Laser Surg* 2007;25(2):65-71.

66. Stergioulas A, Stergioula M, Aarskog R, Lopes-Martins RA, Bjordal JM: Effects of low-level laser therapy and eccentric exercises in the treatment of recreational athletes with chronic Achilles tendinopathy. *Am J Sports Med* 2008;36(5):881-887.

67. Nowicki KD, Hummer CD III, Heidt RS Jr, Colosimo AJ: Effects of iontophoretic versus injection administration of dexamethasone. *Med Sci Sports Exerc* 2002;34(8):1294-1301.

68. Murrell GA, Szabo C, Hannafin JA, et al: Modulation of tendon healing by nitric oxide. *Inflamm Res* 1997; 46(1):19-27.

69. Ko JY, Chen HS, Chen LM: Treatment of lateral epicondylitis of the elbow with shock waves. *Clin Orthop Relat Res* 2001(387):60-67.

70. Wang CJ, Chen HS: Shock wave therapy for patients with lateral epicondylitis of the elbow: A one- to two-year follow-up study. *Am J Sports Med* 2002;30(3): 422-425.

71. Wang CJ, Ko JY, Chen HS: Treatment of calcifying tendinitis of the shoulder with shock wave therapy. *Clin Orthop Relat Res* 2001;387:83-89.

72. Wang L, Qin L, Lu HB, et al: Extracorporeal shock wave therapy in treatment of delayed bone-tendon healing. *Am J Sports Med* 2008;36(2):340-347.

73. Alfredson H: Chronic midportion Achilles tendinopathy: An update on research and treatment. *Clin Sports Med* 2003;22(4):727-741.

74. Paoloni JA, Appleyard RC, Nelson J, Murrell GA: Topical nitric oxide application in the treatment of chronic extensor tendinosis at the elbow: A randomized, double-blinded, placebo-controlled clinical trial. *Am J Sports Med* 2003;31(6):915-920.

75. Alfredson H, Forsgren S, Thorsen K, Fahlström M, Johansson H, Lorentzon R: Glutamate NMDAR1 receptors localised to nerves in human Achilles tendons: Implications for treatment? *Knee Surg Sports Traumatol Arthrosc* 2001;9(2):123-126.

76. Alfredson H, Forsgren S, Thorsen K, Lorentzon R: In vivo microdialysis and immunohistochemical analyses of tendon tissue demonstrated high amounts of free glutamate and glutamate NMDAR1 receptors, but no signs of inflammation, in Jumper's knee. *J Orthop Res* 2001;19(5):881-886.

77. Alfredson H, Ljung BO, Thorsen K, Lorentzon R: In vivo investigation of ECRB tendons with microdialysis technique—No signs of inflammation but high amounts of glutamate in tennis elbow. *Acta Orthop Scand* 2000;71(5):475-479.

78. Alfredson H, Lorentzon R: Intratendinous glutamate levels and eccentric training in chronic Achilles tendinosis: A prospective study using microdialysis technique. *Knee Surg Sports Traumatol Arthrosc* 2003;11(3):196-199.

79. Alfredson H, Lorentzon R: Chronic tendon pain: No signs of chemical inflammation but high concentrations of the neurotransmitter glutamate. Implications for treatment? *Curr Drug Targets* 2002;3(1):43-54.

80. Alfredson H, Thorsen K, Lorentzon R: In situ microdialysis in tendon tissue: High levels of glutamate, but not prostaglandin E2 in chronic Achilles tendon pain. *Knee Surg Sports Traumatol Arthrosc* 1999;7(6):378-381.

81. Shalabi A, Kristoffersen-Wilberg M, Svensson L, Aspelin P, Movin T: Eccentric training of the gastrocnemius-soleus complex in chronic Achilles tendinopathy results in decreased tendon volume and intratendinous signal as evaluated by MRI. *Am J Sports Med* 2004;32(5):1286-1296.

82. Clement DB, Taunton JE, Smart GW: Achilles tendinitis and peritendinitis: Etiology and treatment. *Am J Sports Med* 1984;12(3):179-184.

83. de Mos M, Koevoet W, van Schie HT, et al: In vitro model to study chondrogenic differentiation in tendinopathy. *Am J Sports Med* 2009;37(6):1214-1222.

84. Lyras D, Kazakos K, Verettas D, et al: Immunohistochemical study of angiogenesis after local administration of platelet-rich plasma in a patellar tendon defect. *Int Orthop* 2010;34(1):143-148.

85. Lyras DN, Kazakos K, Verettas D, et al: The effect of platelet-rich plasma gel in the early phase of patellar tendon healing. *Arch Orthop Trauma Surg* 2009;129(11):1577-1582.

86. Mishra A, Pavelko T: Treatment of chronic elbow tendinosis with buffered platelet-rich plasma. *Am J Sports Med* 2006;34(11):1774-1778.

87. Mishra A, Woodall J Jr, Vieira A: Treatment of tendon and muscle using platelet-rich plasma. *Clin Sports Med* 2009;28(1):113-125.

88. Sánchez M, Anitua E, Orive G, Mujika I, Andia I: Platelet-rich therapies in the treatment of orthopaedic sport injuries. *Sports Med* 2009;39(5):345-354.

89. Creaney L, Hamilton B: Growth factor delivery methods in the management of sports injuries: The state of play. *Br J Sports Med* 2008;42(5):314-320.

90. de Mos M, van der Windt AE, Jahr H, et al: Can platelet-rich plasma enhance tendon repair? A cell culture study. *Am J Sports Med* 2008;36(6):1171-1178.

91. Kajikawa Y, Morihara T, Sakamoto H, et al: Platelet-rich plasma enhances the initial mobilization of circulation-derived cells for tendon healing. *J Cell Physiol* 2008;215(3):837-845.

92. Sampson S, Gerhardt M, Mandelbaum B: Platelet rich plasma injection grafts for musculoskeletal injuries: A review. *Curr Rev Musculoskelet Med* 2008;1(3-4):165-174.

93. Wilk KE, Voight ML, Keirns MA, Gambetta V, Andrews JR, Dillman CJ: Stretch-shortening drills for the upper extremities: Theory and clinical application. *J Orthop Sports Phys Ther* 1993;17(5):225-239.

94. Wilk KE, Reinold MM: Plyometric and closed kinetic chain exercise, in Bandy WD, Sanders B, eds: *Therapeutic Exercises: Techniques for Intervention.* Philadelphia, PA, Lippincott, Williams & Wilkins, 2001.

Chapter 9

Exercise and Fitness Considerations

Nicholas A. DiNubile, MD

Dr. DiNubile or an immediate family member is a member of a speakers' bureau or has made paid presentations on behalf of Genzyme and serves as a paid consultant to or is an employee of Genzyme and H-Wave.

Key Points

- Balanced, year-round exercise programs have proven health benefits, especially for the mature athlete.
- Physicians and other healthcare professionals play essential roles in promoting and prescribing exercise, especially for the mature athlete with medical and musculoskeletal issues.
- The ideal exercise prescription is based on the individual's goals, health and/or fitness needs, level of conditioning, and past or present illness or injury.
- Exercise prescriptions must be customized for the large percentage of the population with musculoskeletal ailments. The mature athlete is clearly more vulnerable in this regard.
- A balanced fitness program includes aerobic exercise, strength training, flexibility exercises, and core training. Neuromuscular training is also important to maintain optimal balance and agility.
- Mature athletes often need more recovery time from hard workouts and sports competition than their younger counterparts.

Introduction

In 1513, Juan Ponce de León went in search of the Fountain of Youth. Had he embarked on this journey today, his time would have probably been best spent visiting a local gym or fitness center. Exercise is the closest thing to the Fountain of Youth that exists, even in this modern day and age. Many mature athletes and masters athletes are a testament to this statement. In fact, an active, fit 60-year-old can be in better physiologic shape than a 30-year-old couch potato. Exercise is essential for anyone who wants to prevent or manage a wide variety of diseases and age in a healthful, functional manner. Balanced, year-round exercise programs are especially important for mature athletes, both to help them perform at their optimal level and to prevent the all-too-common musculoskeletal injuries that sideline them. Unfortunately, most active individuals fail to create ideal, balanced exercise programs for themselves. In addition, their routines are often not properly designed to accommodate their musculoskeletal issues or vulnerabilities. Also, far too few physicians promote and prescribe exercise for their patients. Even those who do tend to make a general suggestion to take up exercise, rather than providing a comprehensive, individualized exercise prescription.

According to the 1996 US Surgeon General's report on physical activity and health, less than 30% of physicians in the United States actually discuss exercise with their patients.[1] This is unfortunate, especially in light of the fact that several national surveys that were conducted to determine which factors influence people to become involved in regular exercise programs showed that the most influential factor was their physician's recommendation. Therefore, physicians and other healthcare professionals must assume a leadership role in promoting exercise.

The promotion of exercise as part of health care is not a new concept. Hippocrates, the father of medicine, routinely prescribed exercise for patients with a wide variety of ailments, and scientific data substantiate that Hippocrates was wise to do so. So why don't physicians prescribe exercise more often?

Exercise Is Medicine

In the early 1980s, the journal *The Physician and Sportsmedicine* promoted exercise using the slogan "Exercise Is Medicine." Recently, the American College of Sports Medicine (ACSM) and the American Medical Association (AMA), in cooperation with *The Physician and Sportsmedicine*, launched a national initiative around this concept, with the goal of getting physicians more involved in prescribing exercise for their patients. An ever-growing body of evidence supports the myriad health benefits of exercise. In fact, exercise is a very powerful medicine. Regular exercise is not only essential in achieving optimal health but also is a valuable tool in the prevention and treatment of a wide variety of medical ailments.[2,3] For it to reach full potency, however, exercise must be specific to the individual and must be appropriately applied. In the future, exercise programming must take this specificity into consideration, especially as it relates to the aging population.

Physicians should indeed think of exercise as medicine (*Dorland's Illustrated Medical Dictionary* defines medicine as "any drug or remedy"), and it should be taught as such in every medical school. Few if any medical schools include exercise prescription in the curriculum, so it is no surprise that physicians are not comfortable giving specific exercise advice and direction to their patients. Although the exact relationship between exercise and disease has not been fully defined, data continue to overwhelmingly confirm that enormous benefits result when exercise is used for health promotion and disease prevention and treatment. As with certain medications, exercise not only can be used to prevent and treat many diseases, but regular exercise also results in relatively predictable, specific changes in the human body. These adaptations occur both centrally and peripherally and include structural, hormonal, and biochemical changes. As with medications, a dose-response curve for exercise exists and should be considered when developing safe, sensible, and effective programs. Current scientific work attempts to define optimal dose ranges for a variety of exercise-related effects. It is becoming apparent that the quantity and quality of exercise/activity levels required for certain health-related outcomes may differ from what is needed for fitness benefits or improved performance. Both the acute and longer term beneficial effects of exercise have a half life, with most systemic and structural changes disappearing after just a few months of relative inactivity; thus, for sustained benefit, exercise must be a lifelong habit. Interestingly, exercise also has been linked to allergy (exercise-induced urticaria and exercise-induced anaphylaxis) and addiction (exercise addiction and withdrawal), making the "exercise as medicine" concept even stronger.

The Exercise Prescription

The ideal exercise prescription should include a specific exercise program for the individual based on his or her goals, health and/or fitness needs, level of physical conditioning, and past or present illness or injuries. The prescription should address the frequency, intensity, and duration of exercise, as well as the mode or type. It also should include advice for graduated progression of the activity or activities. Physicians also need to be prepared to modify exercise programs and routines for individuals with certain ailments.[4] This is especially true for those with musculoskeletal conditions such as arthritis, tendinitis, back pain, osteoporosis, and other bone and joint problems that limit the ability to be optimally active.[3,5,6]

Although creating an exercise program can seem complicated, it is usually a simple process. The key is to individualize the program and identify activities the patient will enjoy and hopefully continue for life. Over the years, the ACSM has provided excellent guidelines regarding exercise prescription.[7]

In 1995, the Centers for Disease Control and Prevention (CDC) and the ACSM issued recommendations that "every US adult should accumulate 30 minutes or more of moderate-intensity physical activity on most, preferably all, days of the week."[8] The main goal at that time was to activate the sedentary population. The recommendation was not very specific, nor did it promote comprehensive, balanced exercise routines. Although some progress has been made in getting Americans off the couch, US adults remain far too inactive. In 2005, less than half of US adults met the minimal CDC and ACSM standards regarding physical activity; for those older than 65 years, the percentage was less than 40%.[9] One survey found that less than 25% of adults engage in exercise on a regular basis, and 25% are totally inactive.[1] In 2007, the ACSM and the American Heart Association updated, clarified, and expanded their recommendations.[10] In addition to continuing to promote daily moderate exercise for all Americans, they described the role of vigorous exercise and its benefits to overall health. They added the need for strength training as well as information regarding exercise as it relates to weight control and obesity prevention. They also issued a separate recommendation for Americans older than 65 years and for adults aged 50 to 65 with certain chronic conditions and/or functional limitations.[11] In 2011, the ACSM expanded its adult exercise recommendations to include neuromuscular training to maintain or improve balance, agility, and coordination.[12] The recommendations for older adults with limitations are very similar to those for the general adult population, but they allow for a more gradual progression and include other precautions. For example, supervision is recommended for some individuals when beginning an exercise program. In addition to aerobic exercise and strength training (both of which should be done with less intensity in these particular groups), flexibility exercises are suggested. Also, therapeutic rehabilitation-type exercise routines are encouraged to help treat any specific ailments they might have, or prevent problems from occurring in susceptible individuals with known vulnerabilities. This creates a long-overdue integration of the worlds of fitness training and

rehabilitation. Balance training is suggested for individuals with a history of falls or for those at risk for falls. These recommendations provide a comprehensive, thoughtful approach that is very important in deconditioned adults, the elderly, and those who have had difficulty embarking on a fitness program because of chronic medical conditions.

The Mature Athlete

Mature athletes are in many ways a remarkable group. Although they are typically quite fit and active, they usually can benefit tremendously from solid advice regarding exercise prescription and exercise/activity modification that brings their workouts, and thus their overall fitness, into balance. This will result is less downtime from injuries, an extended "career," and improved performance. Some convincing and a little creativity on the part of the treating physician or healthcare professional may be required, but it is well worth the effort.

Anyone who treats mature athletes on a regular basis will see some common threads. Mature athletes are usually highly motivated and have tremendous focus. Activity and performance are critically important to them, and they will usually continue to push themselves at almost any cost. They tend to be in good shape, but their fitness is not balanced. Because they specialize in one or two activities, their frames develop chronic, often predictable imbalances. They also have a variety of musculoskeletal vulnerabilities from the effects of aging on the musculoskeletal system as well as injuries, both overuse and acute, that they have collected, like trophies, over the years. I have learned a lot from mature athletes. They have inspired me and have also helped change my perspective, and philosophy, on aging.

Program Design
Health Protection, Fitness, and Performance
Exercise prescriptions for adults can have many different forms, with different levels and types of recommendations for different individuals. An active adult or mature athlete cannot be assumed to have an optimal fitness level or even to be fit. Some may have been very fit in the past and count on that prior level of conditioning to get them through. Some engage in old routines that are now known to be suboptimal or even

dangerous at this point in time for them. Some may have missed time from their sport or activity because of injury and now have a misguided desire to make up for lost time. All of these factors need to be considered when assessing a patient's current situation.

When recommending exercise or activity programs for patients, it is generally useful to categorize the individual as either "sedentary" or "active." This has practical applications for program design. Also, the spectrum of activity levels should be considered a continuum, from sedentary, to active (moderate everyday activity), to exercise (planned exercise sessions), to fitness (consistently higher levels of balanced fitness routines). Although there may be some overlap among these levels, it is usually easy to distinguish a couch potato from someone who is active in daily life from someone who exercises regularly and/or has achieved higher levels of physical fitness. If the individual is sedentary, the major emphasis should be simply to activate that person. Discussing the information regarding the many health benefits of moderate activity (ie, avoiding sedentary behavior) should be motivating. Individuals who were once intimidated by vigorous exercise or who stopped because of the level of difficulty of high-intensity exercise programs or because of musculoskeletal ailments can be easily activated by convincing them that even a minor increase in their activity level can produce beneficial results. This increase in activity can be accomplished through exercise sessions or by initiating more active daily routines, such as taking the stairs at work, parking farther away in the parking lot, or walking to the store. Individuals are more likely to make these adjustments if they are reminded on multiple occasions, if they include family or friends in their program, if they keep an activity log, and if positive support and feedback are provided. If physicians can motivate patients to this level, they have done them a tremendous favor. Convincing a patient to take up an appropriate sport or regular activity is another healthy option. For example, tennis is a sport that can be played at almost any age and offers a wide range of documented health benefits, from improved aerobic and anaerobic conditioning to improved bone health, balance, agility, and hand-eye coordination.[13] Also, activities like tai chi and yoga are not only fun but also can help individuals with a variety of medical and orthopaedic issues including arthritis and balance. They also provide stress reduction and improved flexibility, ingredients often lacking in current exercise routines and sport.

I see the activation phase as a hook. Once patients are activated, I have great success moving them along the activity continuum into balanced, specific exercise and fitness programs, in which (in addition to the health protection benefits) the patient can enjoy the benefits of a stronger, more fit, functional body. More comprehensive fitness programs are prescribed for those already involved in exercise programs or those who can be moved further along the fitness continuum. The four basic components of a balanced fitness program are cardiovascular or aerobic exercise, strength training, flexibility exercises, and core training. Because no single sport or exercise routine meets all these needs, cross-training is encouraged. Exercise prescription can be thought of as a puzzle with four large pieces: cardiovascular, strength, flexibility, and core. For a complete picture, individuals should have almost equal amounts of each in a given week. Most individuals, including many athletes, favor one or two over the others and may even ignore some completely. For example, many distance runners have an excellent cardiovascular system and strong calves, but they also have a relatively weak upper body and weak quadriceps, abdominal, and anterior shin muscles, as well as tight low back and hamstrings muscles. Individuals whose workouts are primarily at the gym, where straight-line unidimensional activities prevail, often lack what I call three-dimensional or 3-D fitness, in which agility and balance are consistently called into play.[14] Neuromuscular training will improve balance, proprioception, agility, coordination, and performance, and is included in the most recent ACSM adult exercise recommendations.[12] Given the importance of specificity of exercise in terms of training and remodeling the human frame, all of these considerations are important in program design.

Aerobic Exercise

Aerobic (cardiovascular) exercise strengthens the most important muscle in the body—the heart. Activities that can accomplish this include walking, hiking, cycling, running, stair climbing, aerobic dance, and cross-country skiing. For all intents and purposes, the heart cannot tell the difference as to which activity is being performed. However, aerobic activities that combine the simultaneous use of the upper and lower body (eg, cross-country skiing, water polo, step climbers) provide a more potent stimulus for the cardiovascular system. For a training effect, exercise should be performed within a target heart rate range for at least 30 minutes, three times per week. Gradually increasing the intensity and duration will increase the training effect. Formulas are available for determining target heart rate; it should be noted that recent studies suggest that the standard formula used for many years to determine ideal target heart rate range may not be appropriate or accurate for most women. Perceived exertion scales also can be used. Aerobic exercise improves cardiac function and, because of its metabolic effect with increased caloric consumption, is important in weight control and fat loss. Although the heart cannot feel the difference between different cardiovascular options, the frame certainly can, especially in the mature athlete with certain degenerative or arthritic conditions. For example, individuals with hip or knee arthritis should choose lower impact activities. Water is a terrific environment for individuals with arthritis or for those sidelined with certain injuries such as stress fractures. Individuals with low back problems should avoid rowing ergometers.

Aerobic fitness declines with age. After the age of 30, the average person will experience a decline in aerobic fitness of approximately 1% per year. A 3-month moderate-intensity aerobic training program can regain 15% to 20%. Continued aerobic training is essential for maintaining aerobic fitness, or reversing losses, with age. Some deterioration in cardiopulmonary performance is inevitable because of reduction in maximal heart rate, myocardial contractility, and stroke volume, as well as lowered lung compliance and thoracic cage elasticity. Despite these limitations, as noted previously, an exercising, fit 60-year-old can be in better physiologic shape than a 30-year-old couch potato. Masters athletes are a testament to the ability to maintain high levels of cardiovascular fitness with age, keeping significant declines at bay.

To improve aerobic and anaerobic fitness, interval training should be incorporated into the fitness program. This is accomplished by adding short bursts of higher intensity training. For example, on a treadmill, brisk walking can be interspersed with 30- to 60-second intervals of jogging. On a stationary bike, the pedaling resistance can be increased (as if a steep hill were being climbed) for similar short time periods. Interval training can be incorporated into virtually any aerobic-type activity. These intervals not only increase the anaerobic threshold but also enhance both strength and endurance in the muscles activated.

Strength Training

Exercise for muscular strength and endurance involves the use of resistance exercise to build muscle tone and strength.[3] This can be accomplished with free weights and/or machines. Functional strength training can also be done with elastic bands or a stability ball. Progressively overloading muscle tissue increases strength. This structural response affects not only muscle but also bone and surrounding ligaments and tendons. Strength training programs should be done two or three times per week, with at least one rest day between strength workouts. The athlete should include all major muscle groups of the upper and lower extremities as well as the torso (low back, pelvis, and abdomen). Movements should be slow and controlled to avoid sudden forceful contractions with resultant unnecessary high forces across muscles, tendons, and joints. This is especially important in the mature athlete, whose musculoskeletal frame is more vulnerable to injury for a variety of reasons.[4] Sometimes daily workouts with more sets, lower resistance, and higher numbers of repetitions are necessary for certain muscle groups. This is true when there are weak or painful areas from prior injury or chronic musculoskeletal conditions. Rehabilitation principles are combined with exercise prescription either indefinitely or until the issue is resolved.

Intensity of effort and proper progression appear to be more important than the number of sets of strength exercises. Usually, 12 to 15 repetitions per set, done to momentary muscular failure, are ideal. Movements should be through the full range of motion and should focus on both the concentric (positive) lifting phase as well as the eccentric (negative) lowering phase; otherwise, imbalances can occur in the strength curve that is developed. Eccentric training has also been shown to be extremely effective for many insertional tendinopathies such as tennis elbow, golfer's elbow, jumper's knee, and Achilles tendinitis, all of which are encountered quite commonly in the mature athlete.

Strength training is finally receiving the recognition it has long deserved. Once used only by football players and other select athletes, its indications have broadened significantly. Strength training is equally important for men and women. It has a vital role in strengthening bone tissue and thus is useful in osteoporosis prevention and treatment. Also, age is no barrier.

Muscle mass peaks around the age of 30 and then declines 10% to 15% per decade of life, especially between 50 and 70 years of age. This loss is particularly evident in individuals not involved in strength training. Losses can approach 30% per decade after age 70. Strength can be built and/or maintained at any age, but it does become more challenging with advancing age, especially after the fifth decade, in part secondary to loss of muscle fibers as well as neural and hormonal factors. Testosterone levels decline in men, with resultant loss of muscle tissue. Nutritional factors also play a role; protein needs increase with age because protein is less optimally absorbed. Also, mature athletes may be challenged by chronic muscle or tendon issues that make more intense routines impossible.

The greatest potential benefits of strength training may be for the elderly. Studies have documented improved strength and function in the elderly, even in frail nursing home residents age 90 and older.[15] Understanding this effect is important for efforts to maintain functional independence in an aging population. Many of the physiologic changes attributed to aging are in large part due to inactivity rather than aging, with resultant muscle loss (sarcopenia) being a major factor in functional decline. These changes are preventable and reversible to a large degree. If exercise is indeed the fountain of youth, then strength training is the main secret ingredient.

Strength training has additional benefits. It is helpful in injury prevention, especially in athletes. Also, increasing lean body tissue (muscle) helps in weight and fat control. Muscle is a highly active tissue from a metabolic standpoint. The amount of muscle on a person's frame is a key driver of basal metabolic rate and the amount of calories burned on a day-to-day basis. Sarcopenia, or loss of muscle tissue with aging, is thought to be one of the key reasons for gradual weight gain in middle age. Strength training, in conjunction with aerobic exercise and dietary modifications, should be an integral part of any weight control or reduction program.

Flexibility

Stretching improves muscle and joint flexibility, which becomes more and more important as patients age. Stretching reduces the likelihood of muscle strain and injury. It helps prevent muscle soreness associated with exercise or activity, and it helps maintain mobility and function in arthritic joints when used in conjunction with range-of-motion exercises and strengthening. Unfortunately, for most people, stretching is the most neglected area of the exercise routine.

The major muscle groups of the upper and lower extremities should be stretched. Typical adult problem areas include the anterior shoulder, low back, hamstrings, and calves. Warming up and stretching are different. Ideally, one should warm up before stretching. Warm-up involves a brief cardiovascular activity such as jogging in place, jumping jacks, or stationary cycling—anything that makes the person "loosen up" and break a light sweat. This allows muscles and tendons to behave more elastically, because of temperature-dependent viscoelastic properties, enhancing the stretch and decreasing the likelihood of straining that might occur when a cold muscle is stretched. Gentle stretching can also be done on a cold muscle, but care must be taken to not bounce or overstretch. When stretching, individuals are instructed to use a slow, static-type stretch with no bouncy or ballistic movements. The stretch should be held for 15 to 20 seconds. No added benefit has been observed with stretching more than 30 seconds. A slight pulling sensation should be felt, but not pain. The patient should repeat the stretch several times and try to improve gradually with each session. Stretching can safely be done every day. Yoga is a terrific activity for enhancing overall flexibility.

Dynamic stretching routines also can be used. These involve more ballistic, bouncing movements and represent a more advanced technique better used before participation in sports. It is essential to warm up first and even do some gentle static stretching before embarking on the dynamic routines. Some authors have reported that static stretching might not lessen the risk of injury and may also lead to decreased performance in athletes in certain events (eg, sprinting), but I am not convinced of this (especially for the mature athlete), as many of these studies were done on younger, healthier athletes, whose musculoskeletal systems are much less vulnerable to injury or strain. In mature athletes with less muscle and tendon elasticity, many of whom have prior injuries, I believe that the importance of warm-up and stretching (especially static stretching on a daily basis) cannot be overstated. If a dynamic routine is used, it must follow a warm-up and should be incorporated gradually and cautiously.

Core Training

A strong core (torso) is the foundation for the balanced and optimal use of all the body's musculature, head to toe. Ballet dancers, boxers, expert golfers, baseball sluggers, and practitioners of martial arts have long known that real power comes from the core of the body. To properly train the core, the athlete needs to work a variety of muscle groups, including the abdominal region (front upper and lower and obliques), the low back or spinal extensors, and muscles within the pelvic area. Especially important is the deeper abdominal muscle, the transverse abdominus (transversus abdominis). A Swiss ball, or stability ball, is ideal for building a strong, solid core. Other methods include the use of machines at the gym and floor exercises such as crunches, the Superman exercises, the plank, and the side plank. Pilates classes and certain yoga routines are also effective. A strong core will not only improve athletic performance but will also protect against a variety of injuries and musculoskeletal ailments such as low back pain, patellar pain syndrome, and anterior cruciate ligament tears. Core training should be done 2 or 3 times per week.

Exercise Precautions and Modifications

Certain individuals require medical clearance and/or exercise testing before initiating an exercise program. The ACSM has issued excellent guidelines for this.[7] Variables for clinicians to consider include the presence of risk factors or known disease, the intended level of activity, and the age and sex of the individual. Most healthy, previously sedentary people can safely start a moderate activity program, such as walking, without medical clearance. For the increasingly large segment of the population with musculoskeletal conditions, modified programs will be needed that combine orthopaedic rehabilitation concepts with traditional exercise. This concept of modified exercise programs will become increasingly important as the population ages. This is especially true of the baby boomer population. The importance of exercise modification was documented at the Cooper Clinic, where more than 30% of adults involved in a very conservative, medically supervised exercise program dropped out because of a musculoskeletal injury.[16] I believe that this fallout is both predictable and unnecessary. Exercise-related musculoskeletal issues are very preventable. In my experience, approximately 80% of adults will need some modification of their routines because of musculoskeletal ailments or vulnerabilities. For example, rotator cuff–related issues are extremely common in individuals involved in strength training. This is true at all ages, but it becomes even more prevalent in the mature athlete with age-related changes to the rotator cuff as well as injuries or imbalances that may have accumulated over the years. Exercise remains important for these individuals, but modifications must be incorporated to protect the vulnerable cuff area and to make it less susceptible to repetitive strain or acute injury. A full-body aerobic warm-up should precede any shoulder-related exercise. Proper form is essential, with focus on slow, controlled movements rather than sudden, ballistic, high-force activity. Internal and external rotation exercises for the rotator cuff using elastic bands should be incorporated, and overhead lifts should be modified to avoid the painful arc. Scapular stabilization and shoulder stretching are also added. Some individuals may never be able to return to heavy, full overhead training.

Another extremely common problem in the mature athlete involves patellofemoral joint pain, most commonly related to different stages of osteoarthritis (see chapter 34). Individuals with patellofemoral joint pain are particularly susceptible to problems with exercise routines. In an effort to "strengthen" their legs and knees, they usually rely on traditional squats, lunges, leg extensions, and step work. These exercises are all excellent quadriceps builders, but they also create extreme forces across the patellofemoral joint, with predictable increase in symptoms. Exercise modification therefore is essential for these individuals. For aerobic training, I recommend brisk walking or elliptical trainers and avoid step aerobics or any hill training. When using a stationary bike, these patients should keep the seat relatively high and learn to use toe straps or clips to lessen the load on the anterior knee area. For strength training, they should avoid squats, lunges, and leg extensions, substituting quadriceps isometrics and short-arc isotonic exercises if tolerated. These individuals must be instructed on proper quadriceps and vastus medialis obliquus (VMO) contraction techniques, as many use the anterior hip muscles instead of the quadriceps to initiate the leg lift, and do not even contract the important VMO portion. Core, gluteal, and pelvic area strengthening is important, as well as hamstring, hip, lateral thigh, and iliotibial band stretching. Patients with chronic patellofemoral pain often need permanent modification of their fitness routines.

I have developed specific exercise-related modifications for the 20 most common musculoskeletal and sports medicine conditions[4] as well as advanced certification programs (with the American Council on Exercise) for fitness professionals and personal trainers.[17] It is hoped that these approaches will prevent many of the musculoskeletal injuries commonly associated with exercise. More comprehensive exercise routines modified for individuals with low back,[18] knee,[19] and shoulder[20] ailments also are available. Patients with known cardiopulmonary issues should consult with their primary care physician or a cardiologist so that appropriate modifications can be made.

Recovery is an important area of consideration for the mature athlete. With age, recovery time from vigorous workouts or sports competition is not as rapid as it is in younger athletes or individuals. Whereas a young athlete may be able to go back the next day after a hard workout and perform at close to maximum capability, the mature athlete may take days for optimal recovery. When the body is pushed hard, it is taxed locally (in the body areas directly impacted by the activity) and also systemically from a metabolic standpoint. Both areas need recovery. In fact, fitness gains and body adaptations are made during recovery periods. This is when repair and remodeling occurs. If the athlete does not routinely allow for adequate recovery, then overtraining syndrome and/or overuse injuries will follow. This happens at all ages, but the mature athlete is particularly susceptible. Planned down time and "active" rest (ie, lower intensity, more relaxing activities) are the keys to recovery, in addition to optimal nutrition and hydration around activity. I have found that other stress-relieving activities like guided meditation, yoga, and tai chi can also aid in the process.

The Exercise Mandate

As health care is reformed in the United States, comprehensive strategies must be included to encourage more individuals of all ages to incorporate exercise into their daily routines, a cornerstone of *personal* healthcare reform. Nearly all people, including pregnant women; older people; and people with chronic, degenerative, or handicapping conditions, can benefit from a well-designed individualized exercise program. Physicians and other healthcare professionals should play a critical role in this process. In the foreword to *The Exercise Prescription,* Arnold Schwarzenegger, then chairman of the President's Council on Physical Fitness and Sports, commented on his vision for healthcare providers in relation to exercise prescription. He wrote, "My hope is that each time physicians, regardless of their specialty, meet a patient, a category of treatment in their mental checklist is exercise, and a page of their prescription pad reflects this."[21] With effort, we can reach this goal, and all of our patients, especially the "mature athlete," will reap the benefits.

Summary

The mature athlete is a relatively new phenomenon whose ranks are growing exponentially in number. Being active for life is a laudable goal with countless benefits, and something that all healthcare professionals should promote and enthusiastically endorse. It also, however, brings many challenges, as mature athletes are not just younger athletes who have added a few years, and miles, to their frames. The mature athlete's body has changed in many ways. It is more vulnerable. Also, at some point, despite best efforts, performance will begin to decline. This should not in any way dissuade individuals from pursuing an active, fit lifestyle as long as possible, as this is one of the primary keys to healthy aging and a longer lifespan. Mature athletes can accomplish this by not just relying on their favorite sport or activity, but rather embracing a balanced, year-round fitness program. They need to learn to better listen to their body; find those vulnerabilities or weak links that inevitably will have accumulated after a certain age; and seek professional help to try to resolve them, toughen them, or learn to safely work around them. This may include exercise modifications and the addition of rehabilitation-type exercises to their daily routines. Recovery must be included to optimize their workouts and performance and lessen the risk of down time from overuse or injury. Many inspirational mature athletes are exploring the true capabilities of the human body and spirit at all ages. As a result, "aging" is being redefined, and this, I am certain, will positively impact many individuals for years to come.

References

1. US Department of Health and Human Services: *Physical Activity and Health: A Report of the Surgeon General*. Atlanta, GA, US Department of Health and Human Services, Centers for Disease Control and Prevention, National Center for Chronic Disease Prevention and Health Promotion, 1996.

2. Blair SN, Kohl HW III, Paffenbarger RS Jr, Clark DG, Cooper KH, Gibbons LW: Physical fitness and all-cause mortality: A prospective study of healthy men and women. *JAMA* 1989;262(17):2395-2401.

3. DiNubile NA: Strength training. *Clin Sports Med* 1991;10(1):33-62.

4. DiNubile NA: *FrameWork—Your 7 Step Program for Healthy Muscles, Bones and Joints*. New York, NY, Rodale Books, 2005.

5. DiNubile NA: The role of exercise in the treatment of osteoarthritis. *Am J Med Sports* 1999;1:188-200.

6. Dinubile NA: Osteoarthritis: how to make exercise part of your treatment plan. *Phys Sportsmed* 1997;25(7): 47-56.

7. American College of Sports Medicine: *ACSM's Guidelines for Exercise Testing and Prescription*, ed 7. Baltimore, MD, Lippincott Williams & Wilkins, 2006.

8. Pate RR, Pratt M, Blair SN, et al: Physical activity and public health: A recommendation from the Centers for Disease Control and Prevention and the American College of Sports Medicine. *JAMA* 1995;2/3(5): 402-407.

9. Centers for Disease Control and Prevention (CDC): Prevalence of regular physical activity among adults—United States, 2001 and 2005. *MMWR Morb Mortal Wkly Rep* 2007;56(46):1209-1212.

10. Haskell WL, Lee IM, Pate RR, et al: Physical activity and public health: Updated recommendation for adults from the American College of Sports Medicine and the American Heart Association. *Med Sci Sports Exerc* 2007;39(8):1423-1434.

11. Nelson ME, Rejeski WJ, Blair SN, et al: Physical activity and public health in older adults: Recommendation from the American College of Sports Medicine and the American Heart Association. *Med Sci Sports Exerc* 2007;39(8):1435-1445.

12. Garber CE, Blissmer B, Deschenes MR, et al: American College of Sports Medicine position stand: Quantity and quality of exercise for developing and maintaining cardiorespiratory, musculoskeletal, and neuromotor fitness in apparently healthy adults. Guidance for prescribing exercise. *Med Sci Sports Exerc* 2011;43(7): 1334-1359.

13. Groppel J, DiNubile N: Tennis: For the health of it! *Phys Sportsmed* 2009;37(2):40-50.

14. DiNubile NA: Are you 3-d fit? *Phys Sportsmed* 2009; 37(2):5-6.

15. Fiatarone MA, O'Neill EF, Ryan ND, et al: Exercise training and nutritional supplementation for physical frailty in very elderly people. *N Engl J Med* 1994; 330(25):1769-1775.

16. Hootman JM, Macera CA, Ainsworth BE, Addy CL, Martin M, Blair SN: Epidemiology of musculoskeletal injuries among sedentary and physically active adults. *Med Sci Sports Exerc* 2002;34(5):838-844.

17. DiNubile NA: *Your Client's FrameWork—7 Steps to Healthy Muscles, Bones and Joints*. Online course available through the American Council on Exercise. http://www.acefitness.org/continuingeducation/ continuingeducationcoursedetail.aspx?courseid= 45w32686. Accessed September 21, 2011.

18. DiNubile NA: *FrameWork for the Lower Back: A 6-Step Plan for a Healthy Lower Back*. New York, NY, Rodale Books, 2010.

19. DiNubile NA: *FrameWork for the Knee: A 6-Step Plan for Preventing Injury and Ending Pain*. New York, NY, Rodale Books, 2010.

20. DiNubile NA: *FrameWork for the Shoulder: A 6-Step Plan for Preventing Injury and Ending Pain*. New York, NY, Rodale Books, 2011.

21. DiNubile NA, ed: *The Exercise Prescription*. Philadelphia, PA, Saunders, 1991.

Chapter 10

Cardiovascular Concerns in the Mature Athlete: An Overview for the Orthopaedist

Lawrence W. Gaul, MD

Key Points

- Cardiovascular disease, specifically coronary artery disease (CAD), is the most common cause of sport-related death in athletes older than 35 years.
- Screening of athletes for cardiovascular contraindications to sport has been proven effective, although the specifics are controversial.
- The 36th Bethesda Conference set the general standards for cardiovascular care of athletes in the United States.
- Cardiovascular risk in athletes is often underappreciated.

Introduction

As the baby boomers age, they are continuing the pursuit of health, fitness, and sports that they began during their younger years. The running boom that began in the 1970s, alpine skiing, soccer, and adult league ice hockey are just a few of the activities represented in the explosion in recreational sports. One of the fastest growing sports is ultra-running, a sport I have been involved with personally for 17 years. The musculoskeletal implications for patients who run 100 miles in rugged mountain terrain are obvious; less well appreciated are the cardiovascular concerns. As stated in the 2009 *British Journal of Sports Medicine* special issue on sudden cardiac death (SCD) in athletes, "There is general agreement that vigorous exercise is a trigger for sudden cardiac death in athletes with underlying cardiovascular disease."[1,2]

Many, if not most, older athletes will first present to the orthopaedist or general sports medicine physician. The goal of the sports medicine physician should be to maximize our patients' ability to participate safely in their chosen events as long as possible. Although it is unlikely that the older athlete will need to present for formal medical clearance to be allowed to participate in a sport, the orthopaedist may have a unique opportunity to intervene in a previously underappreciated manner, particularly as most exercise classes and commercially available media for home exercise recommend evaluation by a physician before beginning an exercise program.

Sport-related death has many causes, but cardiovascular causes are the most common. One disease alone, hypertrophic cardiomyopathy (HCM), accounts for 36% of all field deaths in the United States.[3] In recognition of this problem, the April 2011 conference of the International Olympic Committee (IOC), titled "The Prevention of Illness and Injury in Sport,"[4] focused on many cardiovascular issues. The first course and certificates of competency in the interpretation of electrocardiograms (ECGs) in athletes will occur at IOC headquarters in Lausanne, Switzerland, in the fall of 2011. Hopefully, this will not only make interpretation of ECGs more accurate but also help align the guidelines of the European Society of Cardiology (ESC) and the American Heart Association (AHA). The ESC and IOC guidelines are based on the Lausanne recommendations of 2004 on the prevention of sudden cardiovascular death in athletes.[5] These recommendations were in turn based on the work of Pellicia, Corrado, and others in Italy and elsewhere that has reduced sudden death in younger athletes by some 90% since the 1980s through required screening.[6]

Cardiovascular disease and its prevention in sport have come of age, yet little attention has been directed to the mature athlete. This chapter attempts to provide a succinct overview of the cardiovascular issues facing the aging athlete. It also provides a framework that will enable the reader to make a preliminary identification of cardiovascular disease and intervene when faced with not only patients at risk of sudden death but also those with other underlying cardiovascular conditions. Each topic addressed has been written about extensively; selected references are provided.

One central question is whether athletes are at greater risk for cardiovascular problems than the general population. The benefits of a "healthy lifestyle," including regular exercise, have been well documented, yet individuals have an increased risk of sudden death during exercise. This fact was highlighted in an early, frequently referenced study that reviewed the impact of the Italian law requiring preparticipation screening.[6] The incidence of sudden death in *unscreened nonathletes* was 0.8 per 100,000 person-years, whereas it was 4.2 per 100,000 person-years in *unscreened athletes*. Following the institution of mandatory screening beginning in adolescence, the rate of sudden death in athletes decreased to 0.9 per 100,000 person-years. Data from around the world have varied, but a recent study from the United States suggested a much higher rate of SCD: up to 1 per 43,000 person-years in collegiate basketball players of African-American descent, and 1 per 9,000 person-years in military recruits.[7]

Because of the lack of organized, association-controlled sports for older athletes, the incidence of SCD and other significant cardiovascular issues in this population is unknown. Many studies have shown the most common cause of SCD in athletes younger than 35 years is HCM in the United States and arrhythmogenic right ventricular dysplasia or cardiomyopathy (ARVD/C) in Italy. In athletes older than 35 years, the leading cause of SCD in both countries is CAD.

The Preparticipation Examination

The role of the preparticipation examination (PPE) in young athletes has long been both well established and controversial,[1] but in any case the PPE concentrates on the young high school, collegiate, or professional athlete. The ESC and the IOC recommend following the Lausanne recommendations, but the AHA and the American College of Cardiology (ACC) promote a different set of guidelines. The primary difference is in the use of the ECG in the PPE, which is not recommended in the US version.[8] A recent article by Hill et al[9] challenged the utility of ECG screening in young athletes. Careful reading, however, suggests the lack of efficacy is related more to the lack of specific training in interpretation of ECG results than to an inherent limitation of the test. It was reported at the IOC Conference in April 2011 that ECG interpretation by both cardiologists and primary care sports physicians could be improved markedly with the use of a simple 1-page reference sheet.[4]

With regard to the "older" athlete, few studies have evaluated specific PPE recommendations for athletes older than 35 years. Certainly caution must be used to avoid overtesting, which can involve expensive and potentially invasive procedures with inherent risks. On the other hand, undertesting is also a concern. It is easy to fall victim to the belief that participation in competitive vigorous sports confers or implies immunity to SCD.

Although it is unreasonable and impractical for the orthopaedic surgeon to screen every adult who presents with a sport-related injury, a brief review of systems and a family and individual medical history can be obtained in new patients presenting for sport evaluations. The review and history can focus on high-risk and high-prevalence symptoms or diseases (**Table 1**).

Coronary Artery Disease

Because CAD is the most common cause of sudden death overall in the athlete older than 35 years, it is worthwhile to review signs and symptoms the orthopaedic surgeon should be aware of.

Symptoms may include exertional chest pressure or tightness as a description of angina, syncope, or dyspnea. Most of these patients, however, will present to an emergency department or primary care physician office. Perhaps more important for the orthopaedic surgeon seeing these patients in the office setting is the ability to identify elevated risk and encourage appropriate evaluation.

Despite an explosion of information on various minor and debated risk factors (eg, elevated homocysteine, C-reactive protein [CRP], non–high-density-lipoprotein [non-HDL], and lipoprotein(a) [Lp(a)] levels), concentration on the most well established risk factors is prudent. These include the standard AHA controllable risk factors of smoking, hypertension (≥140/90 mm Hg in office), high or abnormal cholesterol level (HDL <40 mg/dL or low-density-lipoprotein [LDL] >100-130 mg/dL), diabetes, obesity, and physical inactivity. Nonmodifiable risks include family history of premature CAD (<55 years in first-degree male relative or <65 years in first-degree female relative) and patient age greater than 44 years for men and 55 years for women.

Tobacco Use

Tobacco use is less likely to be encountered in the athletic patient population, but if it is encountered, it should be strongly discouraged. The single most effective strategy in motivating a smoker to quit has been reported to be a simple recommendation from a physician. Not drugs, not therapy, just a simple statement. This applies to even the "social" or occasional smoker.

Hypertension

Hypertension requires special attention because it is common and increases in prevalence with age but is often clinically silent. In the orthopaedic surgeon's office, staff education is needed regarding proper technique for the use of high-quality automatic blood pressure cuffs. If a patient has blood pressure readings of 140/90 mm Hg or greater on repeat office measurements taken after several minutes' rest or readings of 135/85 mm Hg or greater on serial home measurements with a cuff verified for accuracy, further evaluation by an internist or other primary care provider is warranted. Additionally, if the patient has known hypertension, attention may need to be directed to the response to exercise. Blood pressure commonly increases during exercise, but too often the treating physician does not have data on how high. Increase in blood pressure also varies with the intensity of exercise. Generally, low-intensity aerobic or endurance activity does not exacerbate blood pressure much above a safe limit of 200/100 mm Hg for an extended period. However, exercise at altitude may exacerbate otherwise clinically silent hypertension. It is prudent to obtain exercise data on patients with known or suspected hypertension. How much additional risk these levels of blood pressure place and contribute to long-term risk is unknown, but certainly this issue needs to be recognized.

Physicians who care primarily for musculoskeletal issues also must remain vigilant to the potential worsening of hypertension with even low doses of nonsteroidal anti-inflammatory drugs (NSAIDs). Patients who need such medications are often older, with concomitant elevated risk of hypertension and myocardial infarction. The US Food and Drug Administration (FDA) has mandated identical labeling warning about this risk on all NSAIDs available in the United States. In general, naproxen is thought to be the safest NSAID, but the evidence is relatively weak. The physician also should remember that NSAIDs can alter renal blood flow and may increase the chance of renal failure in patients who participate in endurance sports.

Type 2 Diabetes Mellitus

With the increasing incidence and prevalence of obesity in the United States, the physician is likely to encounter type 2 diabetes mellitus (DM) frequently, as many

---

Table 1: Red Flags for the Orthopaedist That May Warrant Referral to a Cardiologist

Review of Systems

Cardiovascular
Chest pressure or tightness
Palpitations or skipped beats
Lightheadedness with exertion
Murmur (do not ignore even if the patient's physician said "not to worry, it's always been there," as aortic stenosis may present that way)
New pronounced decrease in exercise tolerance

Respiratory
New or unexpected shortness of breath
Cough or wheezing
Asthma

Gastrointestinal
New or unexplained indigestion
Exertional nausea or vomiting

Neurologic
Numbness or tingling
Weakness
Loss of sensation
Unexplained seizure

Ophthalmologic
Partial or temporary loss of vision

Medical History

Cardiovascular
Heart attack or angina
Coronary artery disease with or without PTCA or stent placement
Congestive heart failure
ICD or pacemaker implant
Supraventricular tachycardia or prior ablation
Atrial fibrillation
Wolff-Parkinson-White syndrome
Infection in or around heart
Pericarditis or inflammation of heart
Kawasaki disease

Cardiovascular (continued)
Abnormal cholesterol level, especially very high LDL level or very low HDL level
Stroke or TIA
Hypertension, even if considered controlled
Leg cramps with walking

Pulmonary
Asthma
COPD/recurrent bronchitis
Tobacco use

Family History

Marfan syndrome
Unexplained premature sudden death
Long or short QT syndrome
Abnormal heart rhythms such as atrial fibrillation

Hypertrophic cardiomyopathy
ARVD/C
Brugada syndrome
Ventricular tachycardia

ARVD/C = arrhythmogenic right ventricular dysplasia or cardiomyopathy, COPD = chronic obstructive pulmonary disease, HDL = high-density lipoprotein, ICD = implantable cardioverter-defibrillator, LDL = low-density lipoprotein, PTCA = percutaneous transluminal coronary angioplasty, TIA = transient ischemic attack.

---

people who begin a new sport or exercise program do so to lose weight. A diagnosis of type 2 DM in a patient confers an approximately twofold to threefold increase in the risk of CAD, so this should prompt a cautious approach and may warrant more aggressive screening diagnostics. Referral for evaluation should include at least an ECG, stress testing with imaging if the ECG is abnormal, a lipid panel, a hemoglobin A1c (HbA1c) test, and a comprehensive metabolic panel. Exercise will alter glucose metabolism through modulation of counterregulatory hormones. This often mandates change to medication regimens, especially insulin. Very few physicians have experience managing this in competitive athletes, and often the patient can be the better "doctor." Certainly a referral to a physician with proficiency in the management of diabetes as well as experience with sport and exercise is warranted.

Cholesterol

Managing lipids is not likely to be in the purview of the orthopaedic surgeon, but a general knowledge of the basics is useful. The National Cholesterol Education Project Adult Treatment Program III (ATP-III) guidelines are a good starting point.[10] Total cholesterol level should be less than 200 mg/dL except when due to a very high HDL level; triglycerides should be less than 150 mg/dL; and the LDL level ideally should be less than 100 mg/dL, but certainly less than 130 mg/dL. Unfortunately, although diet and exercise may help lower the LDL level somewhat, medications are usually required if the LDL level is elevated. Recent data have questioned the efficacy of medications in raising HDL, at least with the brand name Niaspan (Abbott Laboratories, Abbott Park, IL).[11] Modification of diet and moderation of alcohol intake will suffice for all but the most elevated triglyceride levels.

Patients should be informed that some anticholesterol medications may be associated with muscular pain or cramping. The orthopaedist should be aware that these medications may be the cause of the pain for which the patient is being evaluated.

Valvular Heart Disease

Many older patients present with acquired valvular heart disease. The most important of these conditions is aortic stenosis, the presence of which is a good reason to examine the heart. Rheumatic fever still causes some cases of aortic stenosis, but calcific disease is a more likely etiology in older individuals. Significant stenosis is manifest clinically by exertional angina or syncope and a harsh systolic murmur that is best heard along the right upper sternal border. However, critical stenosis may present with syncope and no murmur, as there is not enough flow to generate sound. Chronic aortic insufficiency, unless mild, is concerning, and referral to a cardiologist is indicated.

Mitral disease is also sometimes seen in athletes. Dyspnea on exertion, while it can represent many pulmonary or cardiovascular ailments, may be caused by mitral stenosis or regurgitation. Mitral stenosis, which is almost always of rheumatic origin, may trigger atrial fibrillation and may warrant limiting the intensity of the athlete's participation in sports. Patients taking systemic anticoagulants should avoid all competitive sports with any danger of traumatic injury. Mitral regurgitation is common; specific recommendations depend on the underlying cause and severity. A loud, blowing systolic is the murmur most commonly heard by examiners during a PPE, in my experience.

Fortunately, patients with a history of valve replacement (mechanical or bioprosthetic) or repair will already be under the care of a cardiologist. In these patients, the responsibility of the orthopaedic surgeon is to ensure that adequate medical optimization is undertaken prior to exercise participation or surgery.

Arrhythmias

The mature athlete may report symptoms of palpitations during a visit to any sports medicine physician. Again, a history of exertional syncope should prompt a rapid referral to a cardiologist. Often the athlete will mention the palpitations in an offhand manner ("By the way, doctor....."). Although definitive diagnosis requires cardiac monitoring with a looping event recorder or 24-hour ambulatory monitor, the physician can discern the urgency of the condition to some degree from the history. If the patient reports a sense of a rapid, chaotic heartbeat, atrial fibrillation is a likely diagnosis. Atrial fibrillation is more common in athletes who perform at least 1 hour of aerobic exercise 4 days per week, and its prevalence is proportional to advancing age. Stroke is the most serious complication of atrial fibrillation, and therefore atrial fibrillation warrants rapid, although not emergent, identification and evaluation. Depending on the total stroke risk, the patient may need anticoagulation therapy or restriction of activity. Total stroke risk can be based on the CHADS-2 (Congestive heart failure, Hypertension, Age ≥75 years, Diabetes, Stroke or transient ischemic attack) score or a similar scoring system. The modified CHADS-2 from the European Society of Cardiology is an enhanced version of this. Occasional palpitations are generally of little concern, unless they appear to worsen with exercise or cause dyspnea or near-syncope. Many forms of catecholamine-related arrhythmias, including ventricular tachycardia, present with exercise, so this circumstance warrants specialty evaluation.

Summary

Patients often present directly to the orthopaedic surgeon or other sports medicine physician with a sport-related injury or symptoms. The older athlete who may have known cardiovascular disease might have a primary physician but may initially see an orthopaedic surgeon who specializes in sports medicine to allow return to sport. Although these physicians are not expected to be experts in cardiovascular diseases, having a working idea of the major categories of risk is certainly beneficial. My experience helping orthopaedic sports medicine fellows with adolescent PPEs has shown that even a rudimentary knowledge of cardiovascular disease and examination techniques can identify athletes at risk.

The 36th Bethesda Conference is an excellent in-depth review of cardiovascular disease in sport and is generally held to be a basis for standard of care.[12] Physicians caring for athletes should be aware of its contents and general recommendations.

References

1. Drezner J, Pluim B, Engebretsen L: Prevention of sudden cardiac death in athletes: New data and modern perspectives confront challenges of the 21st century. *Br J Sports Med* 2009;43(9):625-626.

2. Corrado D, Basso C, Rizzoli G, Schiavon M, Thiene G: Does sports activity enhance the risk of sudden death in adolescents and young adults? *J Am Coll Cardiol* 2003;42(11):1959-1963.

3. Maron BJ, Doerer JJ, Haas TS, Tierney DM, Mueller FO: Sudden deaths in young competitive athletes: Analysis of 1866 deaths in the United States, 1980-2006. *Circulation* 2009;119(8):1085-1092.

4. Corrado D: ECG interpretation in athletes (video online). *IOC World Conference on Prevention of Injury & Illness in Sport*. Monte Carlo, Monaco, April 7-9, 2011. http://www.ioc-preventionconference.org/OnLPMonaco.php. Accessed October 3, 2011.

5. Corrado D, Pelliccia A, Bjørnstad HH, et al: Cardiovascular pre-participation screening of young competitive athletes for prevention of sudden death: Proposal for a common European protocol. *Eur Heart J* 2005;26(5):516-524.

6. Corrado D, Basso C, Pavei A, Michieli P, Schiavon M, Thiene G: Trends in sudden cardiovascular death in young competitive athletes after implementation of a preparticipation screening program. *JAMA* 2006;296(13):1593-1601.

7. Harmon KG, Asif IM, Klossner D, Drezner JA: Incidence of sudden cardiac death in national collegiate athletic association athletes. *Circulation* 2011;123(15):1594-1600.

8. Chaitman BR: An electrocardiogram should not be included in routine preparticipation screening of young athletes. *Circulation* 2007;116(22):2610-2615.

9. Hill AC, Miyake CY, Grady S, Dubin AM: Accuracy of Interpretation of preparticipation screening electrocardiograms. *J Pediatr* 2011; Jul 9 [Epub ahead of print].

10. National Institutes of Health, National Heart, Lung, and Blood Institute: National Cholesterol Education Program: ATP III Guidelines At-A-Glance Quick Desk Reference. May 2001. http://www.nhlbi.nih.gov/guidelines/cholesterol/atglance.pdf. Accessed September 22, 2011.

11. National Institutes of Health, National Heart, Lung, and Blood Institute: NIH stops clinical trial on combination cholesterol treatment. May 26, 2011. http://public.nhlbi.nih.gov/newsroom/home/GetPressRelease.aspx?id=2792. Accessed September 22, 2011.

12. Mitten MJ, Maron BJ, Zipes DP: Task Force 12: Legal aspects of the 36th Bethesda Conference recommendations. *J Am Coll Cardiol* 2005;45(8):1373-1375.

Chapter 11

Core Stability of the Lumbopelvic-Hip Complex

Rafael F. Escamilla, PhD, PT, CSCS, FACSM

Key Points

- Core exercises activate abdominal muscles and load the lumbar spine in a variety of ways, such as actively flexing the trunk, controlling trunk extension, flexing the hips with posterior pelvic rotation, or a combination of trunk and hip flexion with spinal and pelvic rotations.
- Roll-out exercises are more effective than crunches and sit-ups in activating the rectus abdominis, internal oblique, external oblique, and latissimus dorsi muscles while minimizing lumbar paraspinal and rectus femoris activity.
- Although both the crunch and bent-knee sit-up demonstrate similar amounts of abdominal activity, the crunch may be a safer exercise for individuals with low back pathologies.
- Exercises that effectively activate the rectus abdominis, internal oblique, external oblique, and latissimus dorsi muscles may also produce relatively high rectus femoris or lumbar paraspinal activity, which may be problematic for individuals with lumbar pathologies.
- Exercises that generate high activity from multiple core muscles, such as abdominal bracing, produce high core stability but also produce high lumbar compressive loads that may increase the risk of injury to the lumbar spine.
- Exercises that activate only a few core muscles, such as abdominal hollowing, may not be effective in producing the level of core stability needed for many functional activities, such as lifting, running, and jumping. However, these types of exercises may be appropriate early in a core stabilization program, as well as for individuals that cannot tolerate high lumbar compressive loading.
- The effect of higher level functional exercises on core stability needs to be the focus of future research.

Neither Dr. Escamilla nor any immediate family member has received anything of value from or owns stock in a commercial company or institution related directly or indirectly to the subject of this chapter.

Introduction

This chapter summarizes relevant literature regarding core stability, core muscle activity during common abdominal exercises, and lumbar spinal loading and injury risk during exercises commonly used to enhance core stability. The primary focus is on core exercises used in abdominal strengthening programs. It should be noted that nearly all the data in the literature that focuses on abdominal strengthening programs were from subjects that were younger than

---

40 years. This chapter describes the core and discusses its importance; identifies the core muscles most important for core stability; and describes the benefits and risks of core stabilization exercises, the use of traditional and nontraditional exercises for core stability, and biomechanical differences between abdominal hollowing and bracing exercises, trunk flexion and extension abdominal exercises, and crunch and bent-knee sit-up exercises. The role of nonabdominal core muscles in enhancing core stability also is reviewed.

The Core and Its Importance

The core has been defined as the lumbopelvic-hip complex. The core is important in many functional and athletic activities because it provides proximal stability for distal mobility.[1] As trunk musculature contracts, it helps stabilize the core by compressing and stiffening the spine. This stability is important because the osteoligamentous lumbar spine buckles under compressive loads of only 90 N (approximately 20 lb).[2,3] The core muscles act as guidewires around the human spine to prevent spinal buckling.[2,3] Increased intra-abdominal pressure as core muscles contract has also been shown to further increase spinal stiffness and enhance core stability.[4,5]

The Muscles of the Core

It is currently unclear which core muscles are the most important in optimizing core stability (spinal stabilization). Several studies have suggested that the transversus abdominis and multifidi muscles are key muscles in enhancing spinal stabilization,[6-12] but other studies have questioned the importance of these muscles as major spinal stabilizers.[2,3,13] Isolated contractions from the transversus abdominis have not been demonstrated during higher demand functional activities (such as those that occur during sports) that require all abdominal muscles to become active.[14,15]

Although it has been reported and generally accepted by clinicians that in healthy individuals without lumbar pathology, the transversus abdominis is the first muscle activated and this activation occurs before upper limb motion regardless of the direction of the motion,[10,16] this recently has been challenged. Allison et al[13] reported that transversus abdominis activation is directionally specific and that symmetric, bilateral preactivation of the transversus abdominis does not normally occur during rapid unilateral arm movements in healthy individuals without lumbar pathology. This is important because it is postulated that bilateral preactivation of the transversus abdominis provides lumbar spine stability in anticipation of perturbations of posture.[10] In contrast, transversus abdominis activation is significantly delayed in patients with low back pain with all movements, which indicates a motor control deficit that is believed to result in inefficient muscular stabilization of the spine.[10,17] However, preferential activity of the transversus abdominis has been demonstrated in patients with chronic low back pain during select low-intensity exercises, such as abdominal hollowing (drawing-in) exercises.[18] Moreover, there is limited evidence that exercises that specifically target the deep abdominal muscles (transversus abdominis and internal oblique), such as abdominal hollowing, can train these specific muscles in individuals with chronic low back pain.[19]

For optimal spinal stabilization to occur, it appears that numerous core muscles, including both smaller, deeper core muscles (eg, transversospinalis, transversus abdominis, internal oblique, quadratus lumborum) and larger superficial core muscles (eg, erector spinae, external oblique, rectus abdominis) must contract in sequence with appropriate timing and tension.[2,3] Cholewicki and VanVliet[20] investigated the relative contribution of core muscles to lumbar spine stability and reported that no single core muscle can be identified as most important for lumbar spine stability. They also reported that the relative contribution of each core muscle to lumbar spine stability depended on trunk loading direction (spinal instability was greatest during trunk flexion) and magnitude, and no one muscle contributed more than 30% to overall spine stability. Therefore, they concluded that lumbar stabilization exercises may be most effective when they involve the entire spinal musculature and its motor control under various spine loading conditions.

Benefits and Risks of Core Stabilization Exercises

Strengthening of the muscles of the lumbopelvic region, such as the rectus abdominis, internal oblique, external oblique, transversus abdominis, erector spinae, transversospinalis, quadratus lumborum, and latissimus dorsi, may help decrease the risk of injuries to the lumbar spine by enhancing spinal stability.[21] Core strengthening has been shown to both decrease lower extremity injury risk and enhance performance.[22-24] However, although appropriate spinal loading enhances spinal stability, excessive spinal loading may increase the injury risk to the lumbar spine. Therefore, spinal loading must be adequate for maximal core stability to occur, but excessive spinal loading should be avoided. For example, lumbar compressive forces during lifting (eg, the dead lift) with extremely heavy weights have been estimated to be between 18,000 and 36,000 N.[25,26] These excessively high lumbar compressive forces, which result from both the heavy external load being lifted and the high muscle forces (primarily from the trunk extensors) that are generated during heavy lifting, may be injurious to the lumbar spine.[25,26]

Unfortunately, there is a major void in the literature regarding the efficacy of lumbar stabilization exercises on specific types of lumbar pathology, and future research needs to be conducted to address this deficit.[27] Moreover, although lumbar stabilization exercise programs have been shown to be effective in treating individuals with chronic low back pain, these programs have not conclusively demonstrated that lumbar stabilization programs are more effective in treating individuals with chronic low back pain than is a less specific, more generalized exercise program.[27-29]

Biomechanical Differences Between Exercises

Abdominal Hollowing Versus Abdominal Bracing

Abdominal hollowing (drawing-in maneuver) is typically performed with the athlete supine and with the hips flexed 45° and the knees flexed 90° (hook-lying position).[9,30] The athlete is instructed to take a deep breath and, while exhaling, to pull the navel up and in toward the spine.[9,30] In abdominal bracing, the individual is instructed to globally activate all abdominal and low back muscles by tensing the entire trunk, without drawing in or pushing out the abdominal cavity.[9,15,31,32]

Abdominal hollowing has been shown to be effective in preferential recruitment of the deeper abdominal (transversus abdominis and internal oblique muscles) and lumbar (multifidi) muscles.[9,33,34] Through MRI analysis, Hides et al[34] demonstrated that during abdominal hollowing, the transversus abdominis and internal oblique contract bilaterally to form a musculofascial "corset" that appears to tighten, which may enhance lumbar spine stabilization and decrease injury risk to the lumbar spine. Contractions from the transversus abdominis and internal oblique are also believed to enhance lumbar stability by increasing intra-abdominal pressure and tensioning the thoracolumbar fascia, and additional spinal stability may be provided by the multifidi by directly controlling lumbar intersegmental movement.[4,7,9,11] Moreover, Richardson et al[9] demonstrated that during abdominal hollowing, contraction of the transversus abdominis significantly decreased the laxity of the sacroiliac joint to a greater extent than did abdominal bracing. These data provide limited evidence that abdominal hollowing may enhance spinal stability and be beneficial for individuals with select lumbar pathologies.

Several additional studies have compared abdominal hollowing and abdominal bracing with respect to spinal stability and muscle activity.[9,15,31,32] Using a biomechanical simulation model, Grenier and McGill[15] reported that abdominal hollowing was not as effective as abdominal bracing for increasing lumbar spine stability. Compared with abdominal hollowing, abdominal bracing improved lumbar spine stability by 32%, with only a 15% increase in lumbar spine compression; that is, it had a higher benefit of lumbar stability with a lower risk of lumbar injury. The simulation model also demonstrated that the transversus abdominis alone had very little effect on lumbar spine stability. If the effects of internal oblique and intra-abdominal pressure are combined with the effects of transversus abdominis, however, core stability is improved, and it is enhanced further as more core muscles are activated (such as occurs during abdominal bracing).

Vera-Garcia et al[32] investigated the effectiveness of abdominal hollowing and bracing techniques to control spinal mobility and stability against rapid perturbations. The major finding was that abdominal bracing performed better than abdominal hollowing for spinal stabilization during rapid perturbations. Abdominal bracing actively stabilized the spine and reduced lumbar spine displacement during rapid perturbations, whereas abdominal hollowing was ineffective in spinal stabilization. It can be inferred from these data that abdominal bracing is a more effective technique than abdominal hollowing during functional activities such as lifting, jumping, pushing, and pressing activities in sport or daily living. However, core muscle cocontraction during abdominal bracing significantly increases lumbar compressive loads compared to abdominal hollowing, and this may be problematic in individuals with lumbar pain and pathology. Rectus abdominis and external oblique activity was significantly greater in abdominal bracing than in abdominal hollowing. In addition, abdominal hollowing demonstrated a higher cost (spinal compressive loading) to benefit (spine stability) ratio, which implies that abdominal hollowing resulted in increased spinal compressive loads (resulting in increased injury risk) without reducing spine displacement after perturbation (resulting in decreased spine stability). These authors also reported that during abdominal hollowing, no participant was able to activate the deep abdominal muscles in isolation, but always included substantial activity from both the external oblique and internal oblique.[32]

Stanton and Kawchuk[31] investigated the effect on posteroanterior spinal stiffness of abdominal stabilization contractions during abdominal hollowing and bracing. Compared with abdominal hollowing, abdominal bracing provided significantly greater posterior-anterior spinal stiffness. Further work is needed to assess the long-term effects of abdominal hollowing and abdominal bracing on posterior-anterior spinal stiffness in individuals with low back pain and pathologies.

Several studies have examined the effects of performing abdominal hollowing or bracing techniques immediately before performing core strengthening exercises.[30,33,35] Barnett and Gilleard[33] used abdominal hollowing and bracing techniques with abdominal curl-up and rotation exercises. Compared with the curl-up (crunch) without abdominal hollowing or bracing, the curl-up with hollowing and bracing resulted in the deep abdominal muscles (transversus abdominis and internal oblique) being recruited earlier than the

superficial abdominal muscles (rectus abdominis and external oblique).

Teyhen et al[30] used ultrasound imaging to examine deep abdominal recruitment patterns during numerous abdominal exercises (crunch, sit-back, leg lowering, side plank) and low back exercises (quadruped opposite arm and leg lift) performed immediately after using abdominal hollowing. They reported that the highest recruitment of the transversus abdominis and internal oblique occurred during the side plank. McGill et al[2,36] also reported high activity from several important core muscles (quadratus lumborum, internal oblique, external oblique) during the side plank, resulting in enhanced spinal stability with moderate spinal compressive loading. Moreover, Teyhen et al[30] reported high recruitment of the transversus abdominis and internal oblique and low compressive spinal loading during crunches performed after abdominal hollowing, which is similar to results reported by Axler and McGill.[21] In addition, performing the quadruped opposite arm and leg lift after abdominal hollowing preferentially recruited the transversus abdominis with minimal recruitment of the internal oblique, which provides evidence for its role in early phases of motor control exercise programs that emphasize the firing of the transversus abdominis without concomitant high recruitment from other abdominal muscles. It can be concluded from these data that performing abdominal hollowing before doing abdominal exercises is beneficial to improving core muscle recruitment and spinal stability.

Oh et al[35] investigated the effects of performing abdominal hollowing during prone hip extension exercises on hip and back muscle activity and anterior pelvic tilt. Compared with hip extension without abdominal hollowing, hip extension with abdominal hollowing resulted in significantly less erector spinae activity (17% ± 12% versus 49% ± 14% maximum voluntary isometric contraction [MVIC]) and significantly greater gluteus maximus (52% ± 15% versus 24% ± 8% MVIC) and medial hamstrings (58% ± 20% versus 47% ± 14% MVIC) activity. Moreover, anterior pelvic tilt was significantly greater without abdominal hollowing (10° ± 2°) than with abdominal hollowing (3° ± 1°). From these data, it can be concluded that performing abdominal hollowing with hip extension may be an effective strategy when the goal is to minimize anterior pelvic tilt, lumbar motion, and erector spinae activity and to maximize hip extensor activity.

Traditional Versus Nontraditional Exercises

Several traditional and nontraditional abdominal core exercises used to enhance core stability are illustrated in **Figures 1** through **18**, beginning on p 123. These exercises are primarily used to strengthen abdominal musculature, but they also recruit additional core muscles such as the latissimus dorsi and lumbar paraspinals. Electromyographic (EMG) core muscle activity measured during these exercises is shown in **Tables A-1** through **A-4** in the **Appendix,** beginning on p. 129.

Strong abdominal muscles help stabilize the trunk and unload the lumbar spine.[21,37] Abdominal muscles are commonly activated by actively flexing the trunk by means of a concentric muscle contraction. Trunk flexion occurs during many traditional core exercises, such as the bent-knee sit-up or crunch (**Figures 1** and **2**). During the crunch, the hips remain at a constant angle and the pelvis does not rotate, whereas during the bent-knee sit-up, the hips flex and the pelvis rotates anteriorly.[38] Although the bent-knee sit-up has been shown to be effective in activating rectus abdominis and internal and external oblique musculature,[39-41] the crunch has been recommended in place of the bent-knee sit-up. The crunch has been shown to activate abdominal musculature as effectively as the bent-knee sit-up, but without the relatively high hip flexor activity that occurs during the sit-up, which may increase stress to the lumbar spine.[21,41-43]

Additional traditional abdominal exercises other than the crunch and bent-knee sit-up include the prone plank on toes and side plank on toes (**Figures 3** and **4**). Several studies have reported core muscle activity using EMG during these exercises.[44-47] Escamilla et al[45] examined core muscle activity for the crunch, bent-knee sit-up, prone plank on toes, and side plank on toes (**Table A-4**). The following significant differences were found: (1) Upper rectus abdominis activity was greater in the crunch compared with the prone plank on toes and side plank on toes, and greater in the bent-knee sit-up compared with the side plank on toes. (2) Lower rectus abdominis activity was less in the side plank on toes compared with the other three exercises. (3) Exter-

nal oblique activity was greater in the side plank on toes compared with the other three exercises. (4) Latissimus dorsi activity was greater in the prone plank on toes compared with the crunch and bent-knee sit-up. (5) Lumbar paraspinal activity was greater in the side plank on toes compared with the other three exercises. (6) Rectus femoris activity was greater in the bent-knee sit-up compared with the side plank on toes and crunch, and greater in the prone plank on toes compared with the crunch.

Ekstrom et al[44] also studied the prone plank on toes and side plank on toes and reported rectus abdominis and external oblique activity similar to that reported by Escamilla et al[45] and also reported moderate to high longissimus thoracis, lumbar multifidi, gluteus medius, and gluteus maximus activity during the side plank on toes. Moreover, moderate to high activity of the internal oblique and quadratus lumborum have been demonstrated during the side plank on toes.[36,44-46] It can be concluded from these EMG data that the side plank on toes is a very effective exercise in recruiting core muscles that are important for core stability. However, lumbar compressive force is relatively high in the side plank on toes,[46] which may be problematic for individuals with lumbar pathologies. The prone plank on toes and crunch produce similar amounts of rectus abdominis, internal oblique, and external oblique activity, but the prone plank on toes was more effective in recruiting the latissimus dorsi and rectus femoris muscles compared to the crunch.

Nontraditional core exercises activate abdominal musculature in a different manner than the traditional crunch and bent-knee sit-up. An example of a nontraditional exercise is the reverse crunch (performing the traditional crunch in reverse), which involves flexing the trunk by posteriorly rotating the pelvis (**Figures 5** and **6**). Nontraditional core exercises may also involve controlling or preventing trunk extension (working against the force of gravity acting on the trunk) by isometric or eccentric muscle contractions, such as performing the Swiss ball decline push-up (**Figure 18**) while maintaining a neutral pelvis and spine.

Many nontraditional core exercises also may be performed using the Swiss ball or other commercial devices or machines such as those shown in **Figures 7** through **18**. **Table 1** lists some of these devices and their manu-

Table 1: Devices for Core Strengthening

Device	Manufacturer (Place of Manufacture)
Power Wheel	LifelineUSA (Madison, WI)
Ab Slide	Tianli Hardware Manufacturing Factory (Zhejiang, China)
Torso Track	ATP Direct (West Chester, PA)
Super Abdominal Machine	Not commercially available
Ab Revolutionizer	Wuyi Jielite Tools (Zhejiang, China)
Ab Doer	Zhejiang Raytheon Technology (Zhejiang, China)
Ab Shaper	Wuyi Enpower Fitness Company (Zhejiang, China)
Ab Flex	Zhejiang Boyes Industrial (Zhejiang, China)
Ab Roller	Nantong Tengtai Sporting Fitness (Zhejiang, China)
Ab Rocker	Ningbo Karshall Industry (Zhejiang, China)
Ab Vice	Not commercially available
Ab Twister	Yongkang Huaxi Industry and Trade (Zhejiang, China)

facturers. Some devices or machines allow only uniplanar motion, such as trunk flexion; others allow multiplanar motions, such as trunk flexion and rotation or trunk extension and rotation.[48,49] Adding rotational components to trunk flexion can be advantageous in internal or external oblique recruitment. For example, performing the crunch and Ab Roller crunch with rotation results in simultaneous trunk flexion and rotation. As seen in **Table A-1**, performing these exercises with left rotation (crunch oblique and Ab Roller oblique) resulted in greater right external oblique activity compared with performing them with trunk flexion and no rotation (crunch normal and Ab Roller crunch).[49]

Limited EMG data are available in the scientific literature for nontraditional abdominal exercises, with or without abdominal devices.[42,48-55] Some studies quantified core muscle activity while performing abdominal exercises employing commercial machines or devices, such as the Torso Track, Power Wheel, hanging strap, Super Abdominal Machine, Ab Revolutionizer, Ab Slide, Ab Doer, Ab Shaper, Ab Flex, Ab Roller, Ab Rocker, Ab Vice, and Ab Twister.[42,48-55] Several abdominal devices do not appear to offer any advantage in recruiting abdominal musculature compared to traditional abdominal exercises.[48,49] For example, all exercise variations of the Ab Revolutionizer produced similar abdominal muscle activity compared to the crunch, bent-knee sit-up, and reverse crunch flat.[49] However, one advantage of the Ab Revolutionizer is that external weight can be added, thereby allowing exercise intensity to be varied. The reverse crunch flat and Ab Revolutionizer reverse crunch were performed nearly identical to each other, with the only difference being that the reverse crunch flat was performed without using an abdominal device. In addition, the crunch and Ab Roller crunch, which are performed in a nearly identical manner, produced similar amounts of abdominal activity (**Table A-1**). However, one advantage of the Ab Roller is that the head is supported (**Figure 10**), which may be more comfortable, and therefore many individuals may prefer the Ab Roller crunch over the traditional crunch.

Escamilla et al[49] found that several additional commercial devices, such as the Ab Twister, Ab Doer, and Ab Rocker, demonstrated significantly less abdominal muscle activity compared to the traditional crunch, reverse crunch, and bent-knee sit-up, as well as significantly less abdominal activity compared to other commercial abdominal devices, such as the Torso Track, Ab

Slide, and Ab Roller. Moreover, the Ab Twister, Ab Doer, and Ab Rocker tend to generate relatively high rectus femoris or lumbar paraspinal activity, which may be contraindicated in individuals with lumbar spine pathologies.

Escamilla et al[48,49] also examined core muscle activity in 27 traditional and nontraditional core exercises with and without various commercial abdominal devices and machines. Twelve of the 27 exercises are illustrated in **Figures 2, 5, 6,** and **7** through **14** with their EMG data shown in **Tables A-1** and **A-2**. From these data, it can be concluded that although the traditional crunch and bent-knee sit-up are effective in recruiting abdominal musculature, several exercises are as effective or more effective in abdominal recruitment, such as the Power Wheel roll-out, Power Wheel pike, Power Wheel knee-up, hanging knee-up with straps, reverse crunch inclined 30°, Ab Slide, and Torso Track.

Many of the same exercises performed with commercial abdominal devices or machines can also be performed using a Swiss ball, and several studies have quantified core muscle activity during various Swiss ball exercises.[53,56-64] Escamilla et al[65] quantified core muscle activity for several Swiss ball exercises (**Figures 15** through **18**) and the traditional crunch and bent-knee sit-up (**Figures 1** and **2**). As seen in **Table A-3**, rectus abdominis activity was greatest in the Swiss ball roll-out, Swiss ball pike, and crunch; external and internal oblique activity was greatest in the Swiss ball roll-out, Swiss ball pike, and Swiss ball knee-up; latissimus dorsi activity was greatest in the Swiss ball pike, Swiss ball knee-up, and Swiss ball decline push-up; rectus femoris activity was greatest in the Swiss ball pike, Swiss ball knee-up, and bent-knee sit-up; and lumbar paraspinal activity was relatively low in all exercises. It can be concluded from these data that although rectus abdominis recruitment is similar in the crunch, bent-knee sit-up, and Swiss ball exercises, internal and external oblique activity was generally greater in Swiss ball exercises compared with crunches and bent-knee sit-ups.

Many abdominal exercises traditionally performed on a flat surface can also be performed on a Swiss ball, such as the push-up, bench press, and crunch. Several studies have reported an increase in abdominal muscle activity when the push-up is performed on an unstable surface (eg, Swiss ball) compared with a flat, stable surface.[59,60,66,67] Moreover, an increase in abdominal muscle activity also has been demonstrated when a bench press is performed on a Swiss ball compared with a flat, stable surface.[68,69] In addition, several studies have demonstrated an increase in abdominal muscle activity when the crunch is performed on a Swiss ball compared with on a flat surface.[57,63,64]

Core muscles other than the abdominals are often recruited during many abdominal exercises. The Power Wheel roll-out, Swiss ball roll-out, Power Wheel pike, Swiss ball pike, Power Wheel knee-up, Swiss ball knee-up, hanging knee-up with straps, and reverse crunch inclined 30°, reverse crunch flat, Ab Slide, Torso Track, prone plank on toes, and side plank on toes,[49] in addition to activating abdominal musculature effectively, are also effective for activating the latissimus dorsi[48,49,65] (**Tables A-1** through **A-4**). The latissimus dorsi tenses the thoracolumbar fascia when it contracts and helps stabilize the trunk. Moreover, most of these exercises produce high internal oblique activity, and tension in the thoracolumbar fascia from contractions of the internal oblique (and presumably the transversus abdominis) may further enhance lumbar stability while these exercises are performed. However, all these exercises except for the Power Wheel roll-out, Swiss ball roll-out, Ab Slide, and Torso Track also exhibited significant rectus femoris activity (and to a lesser extent lumbar paraspinal activity), which, because of the tendency of the hip flexors and lumbar extensors to accentuate lumbar lordosis, lumbar compression, and intradiskal pressure, may be problematic for some individuals with low back pathologies.[21,70] Therefore, the Power Wheel roll-out, Swiss ball roll-out, Ab Slide, and Torso Track may be the most effective exercises for recruiting abdominal and latissimus dorsi musculature while minimizing rectus femoris and lumbar paraspinal activity. During these four roll-out exercises, the latissimus dorsi contract eccentrically during the initial roll-out phase to control the rate of shoulder flexion, and they contract concentrically in the return phase as the shoulders extend. Moreover, although it is logical to assume that the rectus femoris contracts eccentrically during the initial roll-out phase (to control the rate of hip extension) and concentrically during the return phase (to flex the hips), rectus femoris activity was very low during these four exercises. This may be explained partially by the neutral pelvic and spine positions that are maintained during these exercises. Workman et al[71] demonstrated that when the pelvis is maintained in neutral or a posteriorly tilted position compared with an anteriorly tilted position, abdominal activity tends to increase and rectus femoris activity tends to decrease. Therefore, the latissimus dorsi (and upper extremity muscles in general) may play a greater role than the hip flexors in both controlling and causing the roll-out and roll-back movements during these exercises.

Many traditional and nontraditional core exercises activate hip flexor and lumbar paraspinal musculature, which is not beneficial in all individuals. Performing exercises that recruit the rectus femoris and lumbar paraspinals may be contraindicated for individuals with weak abdominal muscles or lumbar instability. The forces generated when the hip flexors and lumbar extensors contract anteriorly rotate the pelvis and increase the lordotic curve of the lumbar spine, as well as increase L4-5 disk compression and intradiskal pressure; when coupled with weak abdominal musculature, this increases the risk of low back pathologies.[21,41,72,73] Some individuals with weak abdominal muscles or lumbar instability may want to avoid exercises such as the bent-knee sit-up, Power Wheel pike, Power Wheel knee-up, reverse crunch inclined 30°, and reverse crunch flat because of the significantly greater rectus femoris or lumbar paraspinal activity generated during these exercises compared with other exercises, such as the crunch, Ab Roller, Ab Slide, Torso Track, and Power Wheel roll-out.[48,49] Moreover, it has been demonstrated that during abdominal exercises, the EMG magnitude and recruitment pattern of the psoas and iliacus is similar to (within 10% of) the EMG magnitude and recruitment pattern of the rectus femoris.[47,72,73] This implies that the psoas, iliacus, and rectus femoris may exhibit similar EMG recruitment patterns and magnitudes during the aforementioned abdominal exercises. The psoas muscle, by its attachments into the lumbar spine, attempts to hyperextend the spine as it flexes the hip, and this action may be detrimental to some individuals with lumbar instability. It has also been demonstrated that the psoas muscle can generate lumbar compression and anterior shear force at L5-S1,[41,74] which may be problematic for some individuals with lumbar disk pathologies. Although muscle force from the lum-

bar paraspinals also can increase compression of the lumbar spine, it should be noted that the aforementioned abdominal exercises generate relatively low muscle activity (<10% of an MVIC) from the lumbar paraspinals[48,49] (**Tables A-1** and **A-2**).

Active Hip or Trunk Flexion Versus Controlled Hip or Trunk Extension

Because trunk movements vary among core exercises, not all core exercises are appropriate for every individual. Some core exercises, such as the bent-knee sit-up, cause hip and trunk flexion; other core exercises, such as the Power Wheel or Swiss ball roll-out, control hip and trunk extension. Core exercises that actively flex the trunk, because they increase intradiskal pressure[70] and lumbar spine compression,[21] may be problematic for some individuals with lumbar disk pathologies, as well as for individuals with osteoporosis because of the risk of vertebral compression fractures.[75] In these individuals, it may be more beneficial to maintain a neutral pelvis and spine, such as occurs with the Power Wheel or Swiss ball roll-out, rather than causing forceful flexion of the lumbar spine, such as occurs with the bent-knee sit-up. In contrast, some individuals with facet joint syndrome, spondylolisthesis, and lumbar vertebral or intervertebral foraminal stenosis may not tolerate exercises in which the trunk is maintained in extension, but may better tolerate trunk flexion exercises such as the crunch. In these individuals, trunk flexion–type exercises may decrease facet joint stress and pain and increase vertebral or intervertebral foramina openings, decreasing the risk of spinal cord impingement, nerve root impingement, or facet joint syndrome.

Although roll-out exercises (eg, Power Wheel roll-out, Swiss ball roll-out, Ab Slide, Torso Track) and reverse crunch–type exercises (eg, hanging knee-up with straps, reverse crunch inclined 30°) are all effective in activating abdominal musculature, these two types of exercises are performed differently. During roll-out exercises, the abdominal musculature contracts eccentrically or isometrically to resist the attempt of gravity to extend the trunk and rotate the pelvis. During the return motion, the abdominal muscles contract concentrically or isometrically. If the pelvis and spine are stabilized and maintained in a neutral position throughout the roll-out and return movements, then the abdominal musculature primarily contracts isometrically. While performing roll-out exercises, a relatively neutral pelvis and spine is maintained throughout the movement. In contrast, in reverse crunch–type exercises, such as the hanging knee-up, the abdominal musculature contracts concentrically initially as the hips flex, the pelvis rotates posteriorly, and the lumbar spine flexes. As the knees are lowered and the hips extend, the reverse movements occur, and the abdominal musculature contracts eccentrically to control the rate of return to the starting position.

The hanging knee-up with straps, Swiss ball pike, Power Wheel pike, Swiss ball knee-up, and Power Wheel knee-up are all performed similarly by flexing the hips, posteriorly rotating the pelvis, and flattening the lumbar spine, which is basically the reverse action of what occurs during the bent-knee sit-up, which involves trunk flexion followed by hip flexion.[48,65] One drawback of the hanging knee-up with straps is the relatively high disk compression that occurs at L4-5;[21] however, L4-5 disk compression has been shown to be slightly higher in the bent-knee sit-up than in the hanging knee-up with straps.[21] Furthermore, EMG data from the upper and lower rectus abdominis and internal and external oblique muscles show significantly greater activity during the hanging knee-up with straps than during the bent-knee sit-up.[48] Therefore, the hanging knee-up with straps may be preferred over the bent-knee sit-up for higher level athletes who want to elicit a greater challenge to the abdominal musculature; however, neither exercise may be appropriate for some individuals with lumbar pathologies because of the relatively high L4-5 disk compression.

When the lumbar spine is forcefully flexed, which may occur during commercial abdominal machine exercises such as the Ab Twister, Ab Rocker, and Ab Doer, the anterior fibers of the intervertebral disk are compressed while the posterior fibers are in tension. In addition, in extreme lumbar flexion, intradiskal pressure may increase several times above the normal intradiskal pressure from a resting supine position.[70] Although these stresses on the disk may not be problematic for the normal healthy disk, they may be detrimental to the degenerative disk or pathologic spine.

Crunch Versus Bent-Knee Sit-up

Not all abdominal exercises involve the same degree of lumbar spine flexion. Halpern and Bleck[40] demonstrated that lumbar spinal flexion was only 3° during the crunch but approximately 30° during the bent-knee sit-up. In addition, the bent-knee sit-up has been shown to generate greater lumbar intradiskal pressure[70] and compression[21] compared to exercises similar to the crunch, largely due to increased lumbar flexion.[41,43] This implies that the crunch may be a safer exercise to perform than the bent-knee sit-up for some individuals who need to minimize lumbar spinal flexion or compressive forces because of lumbar pathology.[21]

Although the crunch and bent-knee sit-up are both effective in recruiting abdominal musculature (**Tables A-1** through **A-3**), there are some differences. Several studies have shown external oblique activity and, to a lesser extent, internal oblique activity are significantly greater in the bent-knee sit-up compared with the crunch.[21,41,48,49,72,73] However, upper rectus abdominis (and, to a lesser extent, the lower rectus abdominis) activity has been shown to be greater in the crunch compared with the bent-knee sit-up.[40,42,48,65] In addition, rectus femoris and psoas activity has been shown to be greater in the bent-knee sit-up compared with the crunch.[36,41,43,48,49] Increased muscle activity from the rectus femoris and psoas may exacerbate low back pain in some individuals with low back pathologies.

Abdominal and Oblique Recruitment Between the Crunch and Reverse Crunch

Willett et al[76] presented limited EMG data demonstrating that performing the reverse crunch flat activates the lower abdominals and external oblique to a greater extent than does the crunch. In contrast, Escamilla et al[48,49] and Clark et al[51] reported significantly greater upper and lower rectus abdominis activity in the crunch compared with the reverse crunch flat. These authors also found that external and internal oblique activity for these two exercises did not differ significantly. These discrepancies may be due to methodologic differences among studies. For example, in the study by Willett et al,[76] participants performed the reverse crunch flat by raising the lower half of the body off the table as far as possible; in the studies by Escamilla et al,[48,49] the participants were instructed to maximally posteriorly tilt the pelvis and flex the hips. During the reverse crunch inclined 30°, however, which involved a higher degree of difficulty than both the crunch and reverse crunch flat, there was significantly greater upper rectus abdominis, internal oblique, and external oblique activity compared to the crunch and reverse crunch flat, but there was no significant difference in lower rectus abdominis activity between the reverse crunch inclined 30° and the crunch[48] (**Table A-2**). These data show that the increased difficulty of the reverse crunch inclined 30° results in proportional increases in muscle activity.

Summary

Understanding how different exercises elicit core muscle activity and load in the lumbar spine is useful to physical therapists and other healthcare or fitness specialists who develop specific core exercises for their patients or clients. This chapter summarized relevant literature regarding core stability, core muscle activity during common abdominal exercises, and lumbar spinal loading and injury risk during exercises commonly used to enhance core stability. The core exercises discussed in this chapter activate abdominal muscles and load the lumbar spine in a variety of ways, such as actively flexing the trunk, controlling trunk extension, flexing the hips with posterior pelvis rotation, or a combination of flexing the trunk and flexing the hips with spinal and pelvic rotation. Several nontraditional abdominal exercises generate significantly greater rectus abdominis, internal oblique, and external oblique activity than traditional abdominal exercises like the crunch and bent-knee sit-up. Although both the crunch and bent-knee sit-up demonstrate similar amounts of abdominal activity, the crunch may be a safer exercise for individuals with low back pathologies because relatively high rectus femoris activity and lumbar intradiskal pressure are generated during the bent-knee sit-up. Roll-out exercises (eg, Power Wheel roll-out, Swiss ball roll-out, Ab Slide, and Torso Track) were shown to be the most effective exercise in activating the rectus abdominis, internal oblique, external oblique, and latissimus dorsi muscles while minimizing lumbar paraspinal and rectus femoris activity. The Power Wheel pike, Swiss ball pike, Power Wheel knee-up, Swiss ball knee-up, hanging knee-up with straps, and reverse crunch inclined 30° are effective in activating the rectus abdominis, internal

oblique, external oblique, and latissimus dorsi muscles, but they also produce relatively high rectus femoris or lumbar paraspinal activity, which may be problematic for individuals with lumbar pathologies. Many exercises that generate high activity from multiple core muscles, such as abdominal bracing, also produce the greatest core stability as well as relatively high lumbar compressive loads, which may increase injury risk to the lumbar spine. Exercises that activate only a few muscles, such as abdominal hollowing, may not be effective in producing the level of core stability needed for many functional activities, such as lifting, running, and jumping. However, these types of exercises may be appropriate early in a core stabilization program, as well as for individuals who cannot tolerate high lumbar compressive loading. Many individuals, such as athletes in training for sports, use a wide array of sport-specific functional exercises to develop core muscles and enhance core stability. However, there is a paucity of research in the literature regarding the effect on core stability of performing higher level functional exercises. This should be the focus of future study.

A core training regimen for individuals with lumbar spine pathology should include at least 2 or 3 training sessions per week and should include core exercises that minimize lumbar flexion, maintain the spine in a relatively neutral position, and minimize lumbar spine compressive and shear loading. Good exercises to start with, because they involve low lumbar spine loading, include abdominal hollowing followed by abdominal bracing. These exercises can then be progressed to the prone and side plank on knees and, if tolerated, prone and side plank on toes (**Figures 3** and **4**). These exercises could be progressed by adding more dynamic movements, such as—(from easiest to most difficult)— the Torso Track (**Figure 7**), Ab Slide (**Figure 8**), Swiss ball rollout (**Figure 17**), Power Wheel rollout (**Figure 13**), and Swiss ball decline pushup (**Figure 18**). The rollout type exercises shown in **Figures 7, 8, 13,** and **17** can be progressed by initially rolling out only a short distance, and then progressing to a full rollout. The rollout distance is determined by the ability of the individual to maintain a neutral spine position throughout the entire distance.

A core training regimen for individuals without lumbar spine pathology should include at least 3 or 4 training sessions per week and should include core exercises that both maintain a neutral spine position and also allow lumbar flexion. The progressions described above for individuals with lumbar spine pathology are also appropriate as a starting progression for individuals without lumbar spine pathology. More challenging dynamic exercises can be added later, progressing from easiest to hardest; for example, the Ab Roller (**Figure 10**), crunch (**Figure 2**), reverse crunch flat (**Figure 5**), Swiss ball pike (**Figure 15**), Power Wheel pike (**Figure 11**), Swiss ball knee-up (**Figure 16**), Power Wheel knee-up (**Figure 12**), and finally hanging knee-ups with straps (**Figure 14**).

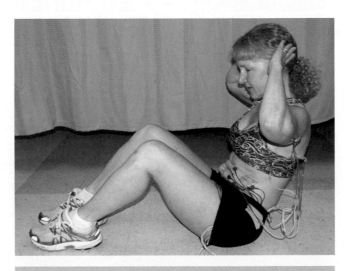

Figure 1   Bent knee sit-up.

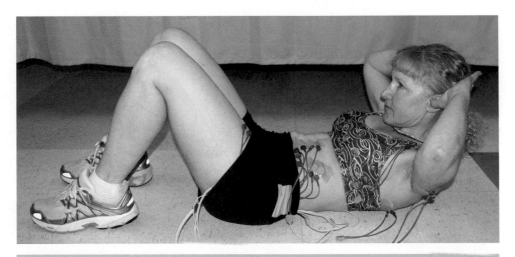

Figure 2   Crunch.

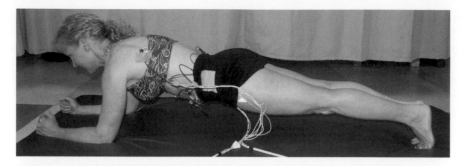

Figure 3 Prone plank on toes.

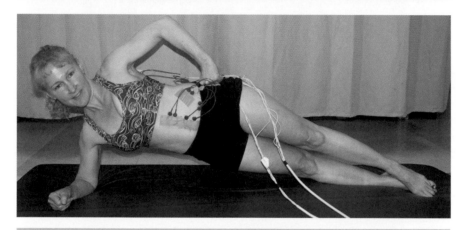

Figure 4 Side plank on toes.

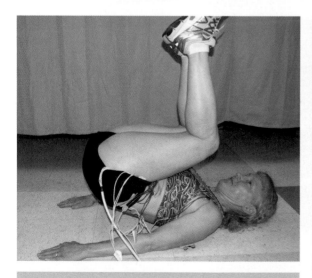

Figure 5 Reverse crunch flat.

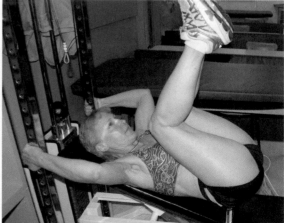

Figure 6 Reverse crunch inclined 30°.

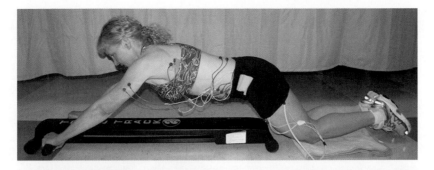

Figure 7   Torso Track.

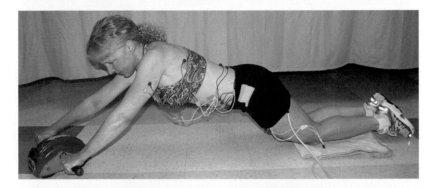

Figure 8   Ab Slide.

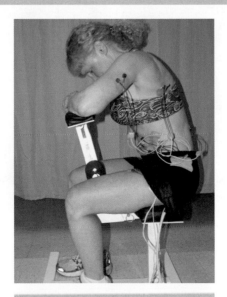

Figure 9   Super Abdominal Machine (SAM).

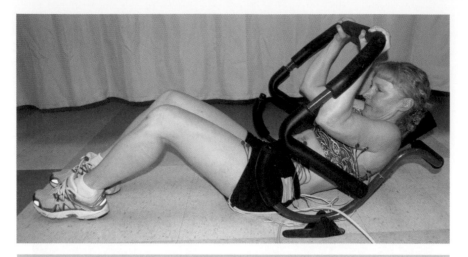

Figure 10   Ab Roller.

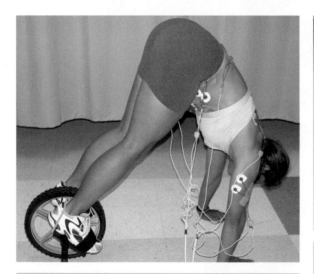

Figure 11   Power Wheel pike. (From Escamilla RF, Babb E, DeWitt R, et al: Electromyographic analysis of traditional and nontraditional abdominal exercises: Implications for rehabilitation and training. *Phys Ther* 2006;86(5):656-671.)

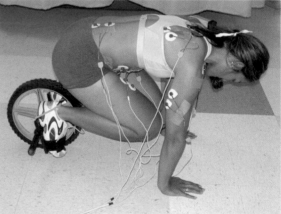

Figure 12   Power Wheel knee-up. (From Escamilla RF, Babb E, DeWitt R, et al: Electromyographic analysis of traditional and nontraditional abdominal exercises: Implications for rehabilitation and training. *Phys Ther* 2006;86(5):656-671.)

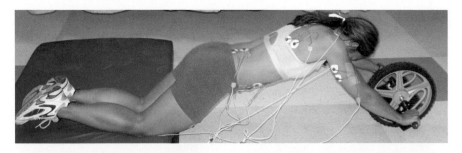

Figure 13 Power Wheel roll-out. (From Escamilla RF, Babb E, DeWitt R, et al: Electromyographic analysis of traditional and nontraditional abdominal exercises: Implications for rehabilitation and training. *Phys Ther* 2006;86(5):656-671.)

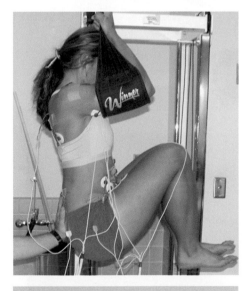

Figure 14 Hanging knee-ups with straps. (From Escamilla RF, Babb E, DeWitt R, et al: Electromyographic analysis of traditional and nontraditional abdominal exercises: Implications for rehabilitation and training. *Phys Ther* 2006;86(5):656-671.)

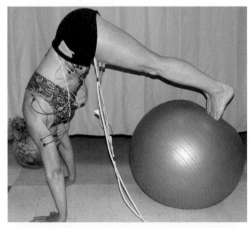

Figure 15 Swiss ball pike.

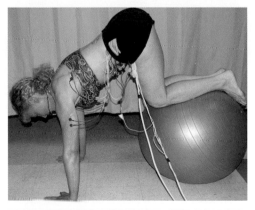

Figure 16 Swiss ball knee-up.

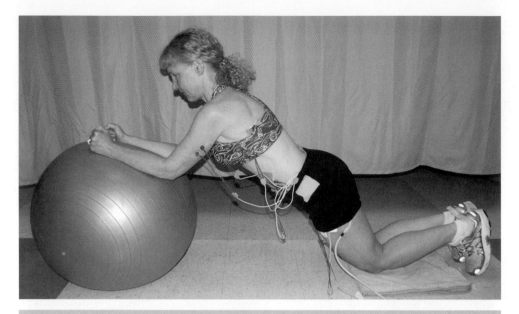

Figure 17   Swiss ball roll-out.

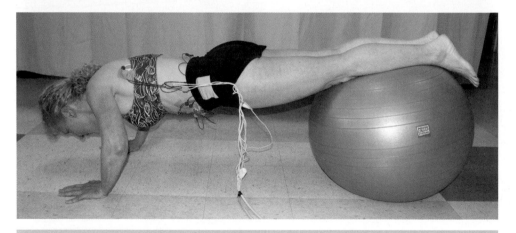

Figure 18   Swiss ball decline push-up.

Appendix

Table A-1: Mean EMG for Abdominal Machines and Traditional Abdominal Crunch and Sit-up Exercises[a]

Exercise	Upper Rectus Abdominis	Lower Rectus Abdominis	Internal Oblique	External Oblique	Latissimus Dorsi	Lumbar Paraspinals	Rectus Femoris
Ab Slide (straight)	67 ± 26	72 ± 19	53 ± 15	40 ± 16	10 ± 4	3 ± 2	5 ± 3^b
Torso Track	67 ± 25	72 ± 17	58 ± 14	32 ± 18	10 ± 5	2 ± 2	6 ± 5^b
Crunch (normal)	51 ± 9	$50 \pm 8^{c,d}$	41 ± 9	$16 \pm 11^{c,e}$	5 ± 1^b	2 ± 1	3 ± 2^b
Crunch (oblique)	50 ± 15	$39 \pm 14^{c,d}$	40 ± 11	32 ± 22	8 ± 5	5 ± 3	3 ± 2^b
Bent-knee sit-up	$38 \pm 12^{c,d}$	$44 \pm 13^{c,d}$	49 ± 21	41 ± 16	6 ± 3^b	4 ± 2	36 ± 16
Super Ab-dominal Machine (SAM)	$42 \pm 17^{c,d}$	$50 \pm 20^{c,d}$	36 ± 13^d	31 ± 21	12 ± 6	4 ± 2	20 ± 15
Ab Roller (crunch)	46 ± 17	$42 \pm 12^{c,d}$	38 ± 9^d	$13 \pm 8^{c,e}$	5 ± 2^b	3 ± 2	1 ± 1^b
Ab Roller (oblique)	49 ± 12	$36 \pm 16^{c,d}$	$25 \pm 11^{c,d,e}$	20 ± 9	6 ± 2^b	3 ± 2	2 ± 2^b

[a]EMG ± SD expressed as a % of maximum isometric voluntary contraction. A significant difference ($P < 0.001$) in electromyographic (EMG) activity between machine and traditional exercises was measured for all muscles. Pairwise comparisons ($P < 0.01$):

[b]Significantly less EMG activity compared with the Super Abdominal Machine.

[c]Significantly less EMG activity compared with the Ab Slide (straight and curved).

[d]Significantly less EMG activity compared with the Torso Track.

[e]Significantly less EMG activity compared with the bent-knee sit-up.

Adapted with permission from Escamilla RF, McTaggart MS, Fricklas EJ, et al: An electromyographic analysis of commercial and common abdominal exercises: Implications for rehabilitation and training. *J Orthop Sports Phys Ther* 2006;36(2): 45-57.

Table A-2: Mean EMG for Power Wheel and Reverse Crunch Exercises and Hanging Knee-up With Straps Compared With Traditional Abdominal Crunch and Sit-up Exercises[a]

Exercise	Upper Rectus Abdominis	Lower Rectus Abdominis	Internal Oblique
Power Wheel roll-out	76 ± 26	81 ± 29	66 ± 25
Power Wheel pike	$41 \pm 11^{e,f,h,i}$	$53 \pm 16^{e,b}$	83 ± 31
Power Wheel knee-up	$41 \pm 18^{e,f,h,i}$	$45 \pm 12^{e,b}$	72 ± 32
Hanging knee-up with straps	69 ± 21	75 ± 16	85 ± 40
Reverse crunch inclined 30°	77 ± 27	$53 \pm 13^{e,b}$	86 ± 37
Reverse crunch flat	$41 \pm 20^{e,f,h,i}$	$30 \pm 13^{b,c,e,f,h,i}$	$52 \pm 24^{b,c,e,f}$
Crunch	$56 \pm 17^{f,h}$	$48 \pm 13^{e,b}$	$42 \pm 10^{b,c,e,f}$
Bent-knee sit-up	$39 \pm 9^{e,f,h,i}$	$38 \pm 11^{b,e,f,h}$	$49 \pm 22^{b,c,e,f}$

[a]EMG ± SD expressed as a % of maximum isometric voluntary contraction. A significant difference ($P < 0.001$) in electromyographic (EMG) activity between machine and traditional exercises was measured for all muscles. Pairwise comparisons ($P < 0.01$):

[b]Significantly less EMG activity compared with the Power Wheel pike.

[c]Significantly less EMG activity compared with the Power Wheel knee-up.

[d]Significantly less EMG activity compared with the reverse crunch flat.

[e]Significantly less EMG activity compared with the hanging knee-up with straps.

[f]Significantly less EMG activity compared with the reverse crunch inclined 30°.

[g]Significantly less EMG activity compared with the bent-knee sit-up.

[h]Significantly less EMG activity compared with the Power Wheel roll-out.

[i]Significantly less EMG activity compared with the crunch.

Adapted with permission from Escamilla RF, Babb E, DeWitt R, et al: Electromyographic analysis of traditional and nontraditional abdominal exercises: Implications for rehabilitation and training. *Phys Ther* 2006;86(5):656-671.

Table A-2: (*continued*)

External Oblique	Latissimus Dorsi	Lumbar Paraspinals	Rectus Femoris
64 ± 27^{b}	$15 \pm 7^{b,c,d}$	$5 \pm 2^{b,c,e,f}$	$6 \pm 4^{b,c,e,f,g}$
96 ± 32	27 ± 16	8 ± 3	26 ± 11^{c}
80 ± 30	25 ± 12	8 ± 4	43 ± 18
79 ± 25	21 ± 12	7 ± 3	$15 \pm 8^{b,c}$
$50 \pm 19^{b,c,e}$	$14 \pm 8^{b,c,d}$	8 ± 4	22 ± 12^{c}
$39 \pm 16^{b,c,e,h}$	23 ± 14	$6 \pm 3^{b,c,f}$	$11 \pm 5^{b,c,f,g}$
$27 \pm 16^{b,c,d,e,f,g,h}$	$5 \pm 3^{b,c,d,e,f,h}$	$3 \pm 1^{b,c,d,e,f,g}$	$3 \pm 3^{b,c,d,e,f,g}$
$50 \pm 16^{b,c,e}$	$6 \pm 3^{b,c,d,e,h}$	$6 \pm 3^{b,c,f}$	22 ± 12^{c}

Table A-3: Mean EMG for Prone Position Swiss Ball Exercises Compared With Traditional Supine Position Abdominal Crunch and Sit-up Exercises[a]

Exercise	Upper Rectus Abdominis	Lower Rectus Abdominis	Internal Oblique	External Oblique	Latissimus Dorsi	Lumbar Paraspinal	Rectus Femoris
Swiss ball roll-out	63 ± 30	53 ± 23	46 ± 21	46 ± 18^b	$12 \pm 9^{b,c}$	6 ± 2	$8 \pm 5^{b,c,d}$
Swiss ball pike	47 ± 18	55 ± 16	56 ± 22	84 ± 37	25 ± 11	8 ± 3	24 ± 6
Swiss ball knee-up	$32 \pm 15^{e,f}$	35 ± 14	41 ± 16	64 ± 39	22 ± 13	6 ± 3	23 ± 8
Crunch	53 ± 19	39 ± 16	33 ± 13^b	$28 \pm 17^{b,c}$	$8 \pm 3^{b,c,g}$	5 ± 2	$6 \pm 4^{b,c,d}$
Bent knee sit-up	40 ± 13^e	35 ± 14	31 ± 11^b	$36 \pm 14^{b,c}$	$8 \pm 3^{b,c,g}$	6 ± 2	23 ± 12
Swiss ball decline push-up	38 ± 20^e	37 ± 16	33 ± 18^b	$36 \pm 24^{b,c}$	18 ± 12	6 ± 2	$10 \pm 6^{b,c,d}$

[a]EMG ± SD expressed as a % of maximum isometric voluntary contraction. A significant difference ($P < 0.001$) in electromyographic (EMG) activity among the exercises was measured for all muscles.

Pairwise comparisons ($P < 0.01$):

[b]Significantly less EMG activity compared with the Swiss ball pike.

[c]Significantly less EMG activity compared with the Swiss ball knee-up.

[d]Significantly less EMG activity compared wtih the bent-knee sit-up.

[e]Significantly less EMG activity compared with the Swiss ball roll-out.

[f]Significantly less EMG activity compared with the crunch.

[g]Significantly less EMG activity compared with the Swiss ball decline push-up.

Adapted with permission from Escamilla RF, Lewis C, Bell D, et al: Core muscle activation during Swiss ball and traditional abdominal exercises. *J Orthop Sports Phys Ther* 2010;40(5):265-276.

Table A-4: Prone and Side-Plank Exercises Compared With Traditional Abdominal Crunch and Sit-up Exercises[a]

Exercise	Upper Rectus Abdominis	Lower Rectus Abdominis	Internal Oblique	External Oblique	Latissimus Dorsi	Lumbar Paraspinal	Rectus Femoris
Prone plank on toes	34 ± 15^b	40 ± 10	29 ± 12	40 ± 21^c	18 ± 12	5 ± 2^c	20 ± 7
Side plank on toes	$26 \pm 15^{b,d}$	$21 \pm 9^{b,d,e}$	28 ± 12	62 ± 37	12 ± 10	29 ± 16	14 ± 4^d
Crunch	53 ± 19	39 ± 16	33 ± 13	28 ± 17^c	8 ± 3^e	5 ± 2^c	$6 \pm 4^{d,e}$
Bent-knee sit-up	40 ± 13	35 ± 14	31 ± 11	36 ± 14^c	8 ± 3^e	6 ± 2^c	23 ± 12

[a]EMG ± SD expressed as a % of maximum isometric voluntary contraction. A significant difference ($P < 0.001$) in electromyographic (EMG) activity among the exercises was measured for all muscles. Pairwise comparisons ($P < 0.01$):
  [b]Significantly less EMG activity compared with the crunch.
  [c]Significantly less EMG activity compared with the side plank on toes.
  [d]Significantly less EMG activity compared with the bent-knee sit-up.
  [e]Significantly less EMG activity compared with the prone plank on toes.
Adapted with permission from Escamilla RF, Lewis C, Bell D, et al: An electromyographic analysis of plank and Swiss ball exercises: Training and rehabilitation implications. *Med Sci Sports Exerc* 2007;39(5):S259.

References

1. Kibler WB, Press J, Sciascia A: The role of core stability in athletic function. *Sports Med* 2006;36(3):189-198.

2. McGill SM: Low back stability: From formal description to issues for performance and rehabilitation. *Exerc Sport Sci Rev* 2001;29(1):26-31.

3. McGill SM, Grenier S, Kavcic N, Cholewicki J: Coordination of muscle activity to assure stability of the lumbar spine. *J Electromyogr Kinesiol* 2003;13(4):353-359.

4. Cresswell AG, Oddsson L, Thorstensson A: The influence of sudden perturbations on trunk muscle activity and intra-abdominal pressure while standing. *Exp Brain Res* 1994;98(2):336-341.

5. Essendrop M, Andersen TB, Schibye B: Increase in spinal stability obtained at levels of intra-abdominal pressure and back muscle activity realistic to work situations. *Appl Ergon* 2002;33(5):471-476.

6. Hodges PW: Is there a role for transversus abdominis in lumbo-pelvic stability? *Man Ther* 1999;4(2):74-86.

7. Hodges PW, Cresswell AG, Daggfeldt K, Thorstensson A: In vivo measurement of the effect of intra-abdominal pressure on the human spine. *J Biomech* 2001;34(3):347-353.

8. Hodges PW, Richardson CA: Transversus abdominis and the superficial abdominal muscles are controlled independently in a postural task. *Neurosci Lett* 1999;265(2):91-94.

9. Richardson CA, Snijders CJ, Hides JA, Damen L, Pas MS, Storm J: The relation between the transversus abdominis muscles, sacroiliac joint mechanics, and low back pain. *Spine (Phila Pa 1976)* 2002;27(4):399-405.

10. Hodges PW, Richardson CA: Inefficient muscular stabilization of the lumbar spine associated with low back pain: A motor control evaluation of transversus

abdominis. *Spine (Phila Pa 1976)* 1996;21(22):2640-2650.

11. Wilke HJ, Wolf S, Claes LE, Arand M, Wiesend A: Stability increase of the lumbar spine with different muscle groups: A biomechanical in vitro study. *Spine (Phila Pa 1976)* 1995;20(2):192-198.

12. Jull GA, Richardson CA: Motor control problems in patients with spinal pain: A new direction for therapeutic exercise. *J Manipulative Physiol Ther* 2000;23(2):115-117.

13. Allison GT, Morris SL, Lay B: Feedforward responses of transversus abdominis are directionally specific and act asymmetrically: Implications for core stability theories. *J Orthop Sports Phys Ther* 2008;38(5):228-237.

14. Davidson KL, Hubley-Kozey CL: Trunk muscle responses to demands of an exercise progression to improve dynamic spinal stability. *Arch Phys Med Rehabil* 2005;86(2):216-223.

15. Grenier SG, McGill SM: Quantification of lumbar stability by using 2 different abdominal activation strategies. *Arch Phys Med Rehabil* 2007;88(1):54-62.

16. Hodges PW, Richardson CA: Feedforward contraction of transversus abdominis is not influenced by the direction of arm movement. *Exp Brain Res* 1997;114(2):362-370.

17. O'Sullivan P, Twomey L, Allison G, Sinclair J, Miller K: Altered patterns of abdominal muscle activation in patients with chronic low back pain. *Aust J Physiother* 1997;43(2):91-98.

18. Teyhen DS, Miltenberger CE, Deiters HM, et al: The use of ultrasound imaging of the abdominal drawing-in maneuver in subjects with low back pain. *J Orthop Sports Phys Ther* 2005;35(6):346-355.

19. O'Sullivan PB, Twomey L, Allison GT: Altered abdominal muscle recruitment in patients with chronic back pain following a specific exercise intervention. *J Orthop Sports Phys Ther* 1998;27(2):114-124.

20. Cholewicki J, VanVliet JJ IV: Relative contribution of trunk muscles to the stability of the lumbar spine during isometric exertions. *Clin Biomech (Bristol, Avon)* 2002;17(2):99-105.

21. Axler CT, McGill SM: Low back loads over a variety of abdominal exercises: Searching for the safest abdominal challenge. *Med Sci Sports Exerc* 1997;29(6):804-811.

22. Hewett TE, Lindenfeld TN, Riccobene JV, Noyes FR: The effect of neuromuscular training on the incidence of knee injury in female athletes: A prospective study. *Am J Sports Med* 1999;27(6):699-706.

23. Myer GD, Chu DA, Brent JL, Hewett TE: Trunk and hip control neuromuscular training for the prevention of knee joint injury. *Clin Sports Med* 2008;27(3):425-448, ix.

24. Willson JD, Dougherty CP, Ireland ML, Davis IM: Core stability and its relationship to lower extremity function and injury. *J Am Acad Orthop Surg* 2005;13(5):316-325.

25. Cholewicki J, McGill SM, Norman RW: Lumbar spine loads during the lifting of extremely heavy weights. *Med Sci Sports Exerc* 1991;23(10):1179-1186.

26. Granhed H, Jonson R, Hansson T: The loads on the lumbar spine during extreme weight lifting. *Spine (Phila Pa 1976)* 1987;12(2):146-149.

27. Standaert CJ, Weinstein SM, Rumpeltes J: Evidence-informed management of chronic low back pain with lumbar stabilization exercises. *Spine J* 2008;8(1):114-120.

28. Rackwitz B, de Bie R, Limm H, von Garnier K, Ewert T, Stucki G: Segmental stabilizing exercises and low back pain: What is the evidence? A systematic review of randomized controlled trials. *Clin Rehabil* 2006;20(7):553-567.

29. Standaert CJ, Herring SA: Expert opinion and controversies in musculoskeletal and sports medicine: Core stabilization as a treatment for low back pain. *Arch Phys Med Rehabil* 2007;88(12):1734-1736.

30. Teyhen DS, Rieger JL, Westrick RB, Miller AC, Molloy JM, Childs JD: Changes in deep abdominal muscle thickness during common trunk-strengthening exercises using ultrasound imaging. *J Orthop Sports Phys Ther* 2008;38(10):596-605.

31. Stanton T, Kawchuk G: The effect of abdominal stabilization contractions on posteroanterior spinal stiffness. *Spine (Phila Pa 1976)* 2008;33(6):694-701.

32. Vera-Garcia FJ, Elvira JL, Brown SH, McGill SM: Effects of abdominal stabilization maneuvers on the control of spine motion and stability against sudden trunk perturbations. *J Electromyogr Kinesiol* 2007;17(5):556-567.

33. Barnett F, Gilleard W: The use of lumbar spinal stabilization techniques during the performance of abdominal strengthening exercise variations. *J Sports Med Phys Fitness* 2005;45(1):38-43.

34. Hides J, Wilson S, Stanton W, et al: An MRI investigation into the function of the transversus abdominis muscle during "drawing-in" of the abdominal wall. *Spine (Phila Pa 1976)* 2006; 31(6):E175-E178.

35. Oh JS, Cynn HS, Won JH, Kwon OY, Yi CH: Effects of performing an abdominal drawing-in maneuver during prone hip extension exercises on hip and back extensor muscle activity and amount of anterior pelvic tilt. *J Orthop Sports Phys Ther* 2007;37(6):320-324.

36. McGill S, Juker D, Kropf P: Quantitative intramuscular myoelectric activity of quadratus lumborum during a wide variety of tasks. *Clin Biomech (Bristol, Avon)* 1996;11(3):170-172.

37. Gardner-Morse MG, Stokes IA: The effects of abdominal muscle coactivation on lumbar spine stability. *Spine (Phila Pa 1976)* 1998;23(1):86-92.

38. Ricci B, Marchetti M, Figura F: Biomechanics of sit-up exercises. *Med Sci Sports Exerc* 1981;13(1):54-59.

39. Godfrey KE, Kindig LE, Windell EJ: Electromyographic study of duration of muscle activity in sit-up variations. *Arch Phys Med Rehabil* 1977;58(3):132-135.

40. Halpern AA, Bleck EE: Sit-up exercises: An electromyographic study. *Clin Orthop Relat Res* 1979;(145):172-178.

41. Juker D, McGill S, Kropf P, Steffen T: Quantitative intramuscular myoelectric activity of lumbar portions of psoas and the abdominal wall during a wide variety of tasks. *Med Sci Sports Exerc* 1998;30(2):301-310.

42. Beim GM, Giraldo JL, Pincivero DM, Borror MJ, Fu FH: Abdominal strengthening exercises: A comparative EMG study. *J Sports Rehabil* 1997;6(1):11-20.

43. Guimaraes AC, Vaz MA, De Campos MI, Marantes R: The contribution of the rectus abdominis and rectus femoris in twelve selected abdominal exercises: An electromyographic study. *J Sports Med Phys Fitness* 1991;31(2):222-230.

44. Ekstrom RA, Donatelli RA, Carp KC: Electromyographic analysis of core trunk, hip, and thigh muscles during 9 rehabilitation exercises. *J Orthop Sports Phys Ther* 2007;37(12):754-762.

45. Escamilla RF, Lewis C, Bell D, et al: Abstract: An electromyographic analysis of plank and Swiss ball exercises: Training and rehabilitation implications. *Med Sci Sports Exerc* 2007;39(5):S259.

46. Kavcic N, Grenier S, McGill SM: Quantifying tissue loads and spine stability while performing commonly prescribed low back stabilization exercises. *Spine (Phila Pa 1976)* 2004;29(20):2319-2329.

47. McGill S, Juker D, Kropf P: Appropriately placed surface EMG electrodes reflect deep muscle activity (psoas, quadratus lumborum, abdominal wall) in the lumbar spine. *J Biomech* 1996;29(11):1503-1507.

48. Escamilla RF, Babb E, DeWitt R, et al: Electromyographic analysis of traditional and nontraditional abdominal exercises: Implications for rehabilitation and training. *Phys Ther* 2006;86(5):656-671.

49. Escamilla RF, McTaggart MS, Fricklas EJ, et al: An electromyographic analysis of commercial and common abdominal exercises: Implications for rehabilitation and training. *J Orthop Sports Phys Ther* 2006;36(2):45-57.

50. Avedisian L, Kowalsky DS, Albro RC, Goldner D, Gill RC: Abdominal strengthening using the AbVice machine as measured by surface electromyographic activation levels. *J Strength Cond Res* 2005;19(3):709-712.

51. Clark KM, Holt LE, Sinyard J: Electromyographic comparison of the upper and lower rectus abdominis during abdominal exercises. *J Strength Cond Res* 2003;17(3):475-483.

52. Demont RG, Lephart SM, Giraldo JL, Giannantonio FP, Yuktanandana P, Fu FH: Comparison of two abdominal training devices with an abdominal crunch using strength and EMG measurements. *J Sports Med Phys Fitness* 1999;39(3):253-258.

53. Hildenbrand K, Noble L: Abdominal muscle activity while performing trunk-flexion exercises using the Ab Roller, ABslide, FitBall, and conventionally performed trunk curls. *J Athl Train* 2004;39(1):37-43.

54. Sternlicht E, Rugg S: Electromyographic analysis of abdominal muscle activity using portable abdominal exercise devices and a traditional crunch. *J Strength Cond Res* 2003;17(3):463-468.

55. Warden SJ, Wajswelner H, Bennell KL: Comparison of Abshaper and conventionally performed abdominal exercises using surface electromyography. *Med Sci Sports Exerc* 1999;31(11):1656-1664.

56. Behm DG, Leonard AM, Young WB, Bonsey WA, MacKinnon SN: Trunk muscle electromyographic activity with unstable and unilateral exercises. *J Strength Cond Res* 2005;19(1):193-201.

57. Cosio-Lima LM, Reynolds KL, Winter C, Paolone V, Jones MT: Effects of physioball and conventional floor

exercises on early phase adaptations in back and abdominal core stability and balance in women. *J Strength Cond Res* 2003;17(4):721-725.

58. Drake JD, Fischer SL, Brown SH, Callaghan JP: Do exercise balls provide a training advantage for trunk extensor exercises? A biomechanical evaluation. *J Manipulative Physiol Ther* 2006;29(5):354-362.

59. Marshall P, Murphy B: Changes in muscle activity and perceived exertion during exercises performed on a swiss ball. *Appl Physiol Nutr Metab* 2006;31(4): 376-383.

60. Marshall PW, Murphy BA: Core stability exercises on and off a Swiss ball. *Arch Phys Med Rehabil* 2005;86(2): 242-249.

61. Mori A: Electromyographic activity of selected trunk muscles during stabilization exercises using a gym ball. *Electromyogr Clin Neurophysiol* 2004;44(1):57-64.

62. Stanton R, Reaburn PR, Humphries B: The effect of short-term Swiss ball training on core stability and running economy. *J Strength Cond Res* 2004;18(3): 522-528.

63. Sternlicht E, Rugg S, Fujii LL, Tomomitsu KF, Seki MM: Electromyographic comparison of a stability ball crunch with a traditional crunch. *J Strength Cond Res* 2007;21(2):506-509.

64. Vera-Garcia FJ, Grenier SG, McGill SM: Abdominal muscle response during curl-ups on both stable and labile surfaces. *Phys Ther* 2000;80(6):564-569.

65. Escamilla RF, Lewis C, Bell D, et al: Core muscle activation during Swiss ball and traditional abdominal exercises. *J Orthop Sports Phys Ther* 2010;40(5): 265-276.

66. Freeman S, Karpowicz A, Gray J, McGill S: Quantifying muscle patterns and spine load during various forms of the push-up. *Med Sci Sports Exerc* 2006;38(3):570-577.

67. Lehman GJ, MacMillan B, MacIntyre I, Chivers M, Fluter M: Shoulder muscle EMG activity during push up variations on and off a Swiss ball. *Dyn Med* 2006;5:7.

68. Marshall PW, Murphy BA: Increased deltoid and abdominal muscle activity during Swiss ball bench press. *J Strength Cond Res* 2006;20(4):745-750.

69. Norwood JT, Anderson GS, Gaetz MB, Twist PW: Electromyographic activity of the trunk stabilizers during stable and unstable bench press. *J Strength Cond Res* 2007;21(2):343-347.

70. Nachemson A: The lumbar spine: An orthopaedic challenge. *Spine (Phila Pa 1976)* 1976;1(1):59-71.

71. Workman JC, Docherty D, Parfrey KC, Behm DG: Influence of pelvis position on the activation of abdominal and hip flexor muscles. *J Strength Cond Res* 2008;22(5):1563-1569.

72. Andersson EA, Ma Z, Thorstensson A: Relative EMG levels in training exercises for abdominal and hip flexor muscles. *Scand J Rehabil Med* 1998;30(3):175-183.

73. Andersson EA, Nilsson J, Ma Z, Thorstensson A: Abdominal and hip flexor muscle activation during various training exercises. *Eur J Appl Physiol Occup Physiol* 1997;75(2):115-123.

74. Santaguida PL, McGill SM: The psoas major muscle: A three-dimensional geometric study. *J Biomech* 1995; 28(3):339-345.

75. Ralston SH, Urquhart GD, Brzeski M, Sturrock RD: Prevalence of vertebral compression fractures due to osteoporosis in ankylosing spondylitis. *BMJ* 1990; 300(6724):563-565.

76. Willett GM, Hyde JE, Uhrlaub MB, Wendel CL, Karst GM: Relative activity of abdominal muscles during commonly prescribed strengthening exercises. *J Strength Cond Res* 2001;15(4):480-485.

Chapter 12

Age- and Sex-Related Performance Decline in Elite Senior Athletes

Brett C. Perricelli, MD
Vonda J. Wright, MD

Key Points

- Age is just a number; physical activity should not cease based on age alone.
- Aging athletes are capable of high levels of physical performance into their 70s.
- Common trends include an earlier performance decline in women than in men and a rapid decline at age 70 in women.
- Both endurance and sprint events demonstrate age-related decline, although it is not clear which type declines first.
- Loss of independence before 70 to 75 years of age is most likely due to the effects of disease, disuse, genetic predisposition, or destructive lifestyle habits.
- Loss of absolute and lean muscle mass occurs in seniors. Implications of muscle loss and when/how to intervene have not yet been clinically determined.

Introduction

It is often said that "Age is just a number." But what does that really mean? In recent years, the world has been shocked by records, feats of endurance, and victories of athletes who have been categorized as exceptional. From George Foreman to Dara Torres to Mark Martin to Nolan Ryan, athletes remind us that the human body is capable of pushing the limits to unfathomable levels. In 2009, less than 1 year after he underwent a total hip arthroplasty and when he was just 2 years away from eligibility for Social Security, Tom Watson made it to a sudden death playoff for the British Open title. These amazing physical feats and endurance performances are not merely the privilege of elite masters athletes (also known as senior athletes and elite senior athletes) but are possible for the thousands of recreational athletes who fill physicians' waiting rooms each day. To keep this motivated group mobile, healthcare providers must not only examine their surgical, rehabilitation, and therapy techniques, but also undergo a paradigm shift in attitude toward the aging athlete.

Most orthopaedic surgeons accept the idea that the older body cannot adjust as fast, heal as well, compete in the same events, or handle adversity as well as the young body. These ideas are talked about in the clinic and in the operating room. Quite often, a patient is called "too old" for a gold standard operation, so a "temporary" operation is proposed as sufficient; or a patient is encouraged to "just stop" a given activity. Although genuine physical changes accompany aging, smart training, experience, and a "feel" for a sport developed over a lifetime can help masters athletes achieve long past the time traditionally thought of as peak performance.

Until recently, relatively little research existed regarding ways to slow or halt the seemingly inexorable decline from vitality to disability that accompanies aging. In the past 15 years, however, great strides have been made toward understanding the positive effects of exercise on health and well being as people age. Masters athletes and senior Olympians perhaps represent the best examples of successful aging. By studying these senior athletes, who continue to exhibit high levels of functional capacity as well as quality of life throughout their lives, information may be gained about the effects of aging, as research outcomes are less likely to be confounded by the variables of disuse or chronic disease. Our 2008 study of senior Olympians[1] found that these athletes are largely white, well educated, and middle class. Therefore, they do not represent a cross section of the aging population and may reflect the health benefits conferred by their socioeconomic status. Most senior Olympians have been active throughout their lives and report better physical and mental health than the general population. They are not immune to chronic illnesses, but they are better able to handle them physically.

Much of the orthopaedic literature has focused on optimizing treatment of bone disease and trauma in the elderly. Little attention has been paid, however, to active aging and healthy bone aging, and there is currently no definition of a healthy, active, aging musculoskeletal system. It is known, however, that human physical performance is notably reduced with sedentary aging.

It is well documented that the prevalence of diabetes, cardiovascular disorders, mental disorders, and certain types of cancer is lower in people who engage in consistent physical activity than in their sedentary counterparts.[2,3] As a result, the incidence of mortality and functional disability also is lower in the active aging population.[4]

Masters athletes and elite senior athletes represent an opportunity to review and compare physical perfor-

mance at its crest, with fewer variables.[5] One of the first reports to analyze records of older athletes was by Archibald Hill[6] in 1925. He examined the records in a variety of sports to explain the physiologic determinants of human performance. In his presidential address to the Section of Physiology of the British Association, Professor Hill noted, "In the study of the physiology of muscular exercise there is a vast store of accurate information in the records of athletic sports and racing." Many physiologic and biologic insights have been gained by analyzing the performance of highly trained athletes, and successful predictions of events and performance have been made.[5,7,8]

Other physiologists have studied the response of the human body to exercise and environmental stress. The body's endurance and strength and its response to heat, cold, and altitude have been studied in athletes, soldiers, aviators, and climbers. Most importantly, records have been used to compare different groups of athletes, athletes of different disciplines, and changes in performance with time.[1,9] The records of elite senior athletes have been studied, and a model for successful aging has emerged.[10-15]

For example, Sydney Maree set the men's collegiate record for the mile at 3:52.44 in 1981. This was only 2 seconds faster than the time recorded by masters athlete Steve Scott, who at the age of 35 clocked in at 3:54.13. At the age 57, Nolan Shaheed recorded a 4:42.7. Yes, these are elite athletes who train. Keep in mind that a time of 6:06 at 17 years of age puts an athlete in the 85th percentile. The human body, when trained, conditioned, and healthy, is capable of amazing feats throughout many decades of life.

For a masters athlete to achieve this level of performance, adequate and regular training, a fortuitous genetic code, and an appropriate lifestyle are required. The genetic code cannot be altered, but training and lifestyle can.

Effects of Age, Sex, and Event Type on Physical Performance
Track-and-Field Athletes
One of the earliest analyses of record data from masters athletes was Moore's[16] 1975 analysis of track-and-field regional records from different age classes. He found an

exponential decline in running speed with age, and performance in the shot put and discus throw declined even more rapidly with advancing age than did performance in running events. Within the running events, the decline is more rapid in sprint events, such as the 200-meter sprint, than in the marathon run. Moore concluded that "strength deteriorates faster than stamina."

In 1994, Fung and Ha[17] used existing track-and-field records to study performance decline with age. The study goal was to identify the running, jumping, and throwing event that was most affected by advancing age among male and female athletes. Results indicated that the 400-meter run and the long jump were most affected by advancing age among both male and female masters athletes. In throwing events, the events most affected were the javelin for men and the discus for women.[17] It was again felt that "strength deteriorates before stamina."

In 2003, Baker et al[18] found different results when they analyzed published masters athlete records in track-and-field events to evaluate the percentage decline in maximum physiologic performance with increasing age. The authors statistically derived that track running records declined with age in a curvilinear fashion, whereas the walking and field events declined in a linear manner. Significant differences were found in the rates of percentage decline in the running events over various distances for both men and women, and significant differences also were found between men and women. Decline with aging was greater for women and for the longer or endurance running events. No differences were found in the rates of decline of function for any of the walking events, and the only jumping event to show a significant difference was the high jump, which showed the slowest decline. The strength-dependent throwing events and the pole vault showed the greatest decline with age. In general terms, men's performance declined to 75% of peak performance in sprint events by the early 70s, in the longer track distances by the mid to late 60s, and in field events by the mid to late 50s. Women's performance declined to a similar extent by the mid 60s in track events and by the late 40s to early 50s in field events.

The work of Baker et al[18] supported the previous work of Stones and Kozma[19] on regional running records, which noted the rate of age-related decline in running performance was greater for middle and longer distance events than for sprints. Both groups of authors, at different time points, suggested that performance in distance events would decline more rapidly with age than sprinting performance. Clearly, there is a dichotomy in the literature as to whether strength or endurance declines faster.

We[1] investigated 2,599 athletes at the 2001 Senior Olympics, analyzing the top eight performances by pentad and comparing the running and sprinting records of contemporary masters athletes. Minimal performance decline was seen from age 50 to 75 years, with less than 2% decline in performance per year for both men and women. At 75 years of age, however, the senior athletes' performance declined dramatically, with performance decreasing approximately 7% per year. Men showed no difference in decline of sprint and endurance events, whereas the decline in the sprint was greater than that in endurance events for women, especially after the age of 75 years (**Figures 1** and **2**).

Marathon Runners

As the number of athletes older than 50 years who participate in high-level sports increases, they also continue to get faster. Jokl et al[20] examined New York City Marathon runners from 1983 to 1999. The authors found that the number of participants older than 50 years is increasing faster than other age groups. Also, the running times showed significantly greater improvement in the masters groups than in the younger age groups, where the results have plateaued.[20]

Leyk et al[21] examined age-related changes in endurance performance of marathon and half-marathon finishers. They found that no significant age-related losses in endurance performance occurred before the age of 50 years. Mean times for the marathon and half marathon were virtually identical for the age groups from 20 to 49 years. Moreover, age-related performance decreases in the 50- to 69-year-old subjects were in the range of only 2.6% to 4.4% per decade. These results corroborate our findings that most older athletes are able to maintain a high degree of physical plasticity. Leyk et al[22] found that lifestyle factors have considerably stronger influences on functional capacity than does age in the physically active and fit elderly.

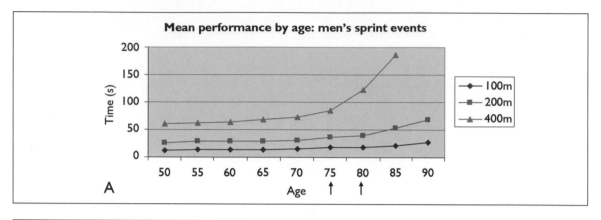

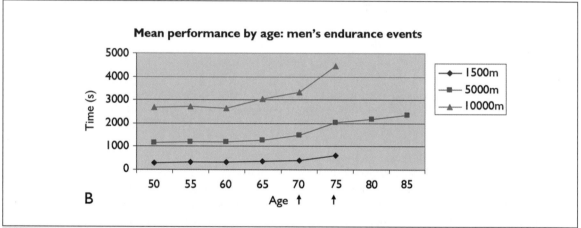

Figure 1 Graph shows mean performance in men's sprint (**A**) and endurance (**B**) track events by age. Data are from the 2001 Senior Olympics. Arrows (↑) indicate ages at which performance times differed significantly (P <0.05) from those of the previous age group. (Adapted with permission from Wright VJ, Perricelli BC: Age-related rates of decline in performance among elite senior athletes. *Am J Sports Med* 2008;36(3):443-450.)

Weight Lifting

The study of senior Olympians and masters athletes is not limited to track-and-field events. Meltzer[23] used two different methods to examine weight-lifting ability as a function of age. First, cross-sectional data corresponding to two separate populations of masters weight lifters were analyzed and a longitudinal study of 64 male US masters weight lifters was performed. Performance-versus-age curves resulting from the two methods were very similar, reflecting approximately 1.0% to 1.5% deterioration per year. Characterization of these curves by common features regarding the rate of decline of muscular power with increasing age was in agreement

with published data regarding masters sprinters and jumpers. Both m ethods produced surprisingly concordant results, demonstrating a progressive diminution of lifting capacity over time. Again, this decline accelerated after the age of 70 years.

Power lifting and weight lifting were further reviewed by Anton et al[24] in 2004. A retrospective regression analysis of weight-lifting and power-lifting records in the oldest age group was performed. The results showed that in both men and women, weight-lifting and power-lifting performance declined curvilinearly and linearly, respectively. The rate and the overall magnitude of decline in performance with age were markedly greater in weight lifting than in power lifting.

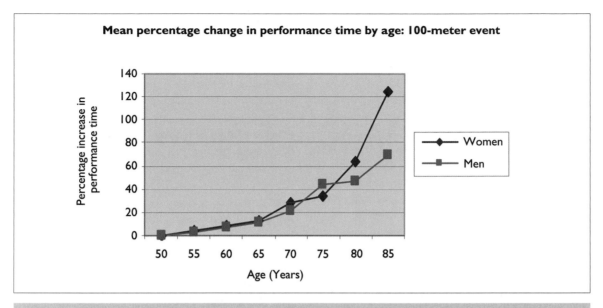

Figure 2 Graph shows mean percentage performance change in the 100-meter event for men and women at various ages. Data are from the 2001 Senior Olympics. (Adapted with permission from Wright VJ, Perricelli BC: Age-related rates of decline in performance among elite senior athletes. *Am J Sports Med* 2008;36(3):443-450.)

In power-lifting events, the rates of age-related decline in muscular power were not different between upper body (bench press) and lower body (squat); in weight-lifting events, the age-related declines were not different between the snatch and the clean-and-jerk. The magnitude of the declines with age was greater in women than in men in weight lifting; no such sex-related differences were observed in power-lifting performance. The authors concluded that (1) peak anaerobic muscular power, as assessed by peak lifting performance, decreases progressively from even earlier ages than previously thought; (2) the overall magnitude of decline in peak muscular power appears to be greater in tasks requiring more complex and powerful movements; (3) the age-related rates of decline are greater in women than in men only in the events that require more complex and explosive power; and (4) upper-body and lower-body muscular power demonstrate similar rates of decline with age.

Pearson et al[25] found that although muscle function in elite masters weight lifters and in healthy control subjects declines at a similar rate with increasing age, the absolute differences between the weight lifters and

the control subjects were significant, such that an 85-year-old weight lifter was as powerful as a 65-year-old control subject. This would therefore represent an apparent age advantage of approximately 20 years for the weight lifters.

The importance of the aging process was further supported by a 2003 study by Thé and Ploutz-Snyder[26] that analyzed Masters Weightlifting Championship data. They reported that the rate of decline in power with advancing age was similar in world record holders, other masters athletes, and healthy untrained individuals.

Swimming

Tanaka and Seals conducted a cross-sectional study of physiologic functional capacity of masters swimmers in 1997[14] and revisited the topic in a longitudinal study in 2003.[27] Studying swimmers has several advantages over studying runners. First, swimming is a nonimpact activity, with a lower rate of injury; thus, the effect of age-related injury as a confounding variable when trying to determine age-related decline is reduced. Second, swimming has a more equal male-to-female ratio.

The 1997 Tanaka and Seals study[14] analyzed the peak exercise performance of swimmers to understand the relationship of age, sex, and exercise task duration with a 5-year retrospective model of freestyle performance from the US Masters Swimming Championships. Analysis of an endurance event (1,500-meter freestyle) revealed that a peak level was reached at 35 to 40 years of age, and performance declined linearly after that until approximately 70 years of age. After age 70, performance declined exponentially. Compared with the 1,500-meter freestyle, performance in the 50-meter freestyle (short-duration task) showed a more modest decline until age 75 years in women and age 80 years in men. The rate and magnitude of declines in both short- and long-duration swimming performance with age were greater in women than in men.

Tanaka and Seals' follow-up longitudinal study in 2003[27] found that (1) swimming performance declines progressively until age 70, when the decrease becomes exponential; (2) the rates of the decline in swimming performance with age are greater in a long-duration event than in a short-duration event, suggesting a relatively smaller loss of anaerobic muscular power with age compared with cardiovascular endurance; (3) the age-related rates of decline are greater in women than in men only in short-duration events; and (4) the variability of the age-related decline in performance increases markedly with advancing age.

Side-by-side comparisons by several authors of the running and swimming models studied by Tanaka et al yielded interesting results.[14,24,29] Both sports demonstrate a curvilinear performance pattern for men and women, but the magnitude of overall reduction of swimming performance compared with running performance is 30% less with advancing age. In swimming, exponential declines in performance occur later, at approximately 70 years instead of 60 years of age. Comparing the data shows that performance can be influenced by tasks performed.

Tennis

Tennis players also have been studied for age-related decline but not in a true physiologic sense. Lobjois et al[30] studied the effect of aging and tennis playing on coincidence-timing accuracy. Three groups of individuals (20-30, 60-69, and 70-79 years of age), some of whom played tennis and others who did not, were asked to synchronize a simple push-button response with a moving stimulus. The older players were as accurate as younger ones, despite less efficient perceptual-motor processes. These results were interpreted to mean that playing tennis is beneficial to older adults.

Effects of Age and Sex

With aging, performance times and percentage change in performance increase for both men and women. This has been shown in multiple types of events. For example, in track athletes, performance times are well maintained until age 50 and then decline modestly until age 75, when performance plummets. Seniors should be able to remain functionally independent until that age. This has been supported by several other studies of senior athletes.[14,21,27-29] The loss of independence before 70 to 75 years of age is most likely due to the effects of disease, disuse, genetic predisposition, or destructive lifestyle habits. These phenomena, which may occur earlier in less active individuals, have key implications for our aging population.[31] The first baby boomers turned 65 in 2011. Physicians have little time to intervene significantly before the elder surge reaches the age of decreased functional capacity.

Rates of performance decline are similar in male and female athletes, as observed in senior athletes in 2001.[1,18] Male American track-and-field record holders, however, declined more slowly than their female counterparts (**Figure 3**). The faster performance decline in record-holding women may have a biologic basis or may reflect the smaller numbers of women continuing to compete at an advanced age. Examples of age-associated declines in activity abound in nature, from insects to humans.[32-35]

In senior Olympians, the rates of decline are more rapid in sprint races in both men and women; in record holders, rates of decline are greater in the endurance races.[1] Several investigators did not observe distance- or time-dependent performance trends in running,[18] but in swimming, the sex differences were greatest in the sprints and smallest in the distance events (endurance).[14] Moore[16] reported a larger decline in performance in the sprint distances, while Stones and Kozma[19] found a larger decline in the endurance races.

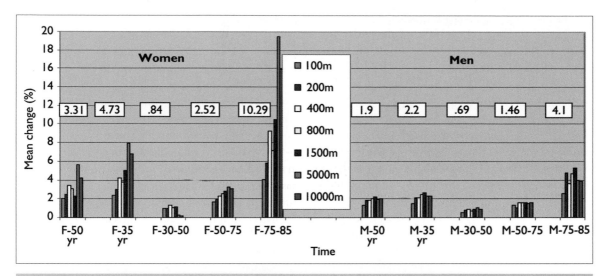

Figure 3   Graph shows mean percentage change in performance time per year during various age spans and over various time periods in American track-and-field record holders. F/M 35 = percentage change per event over 35 years of competition; F/M 50 = percentage change per event over 50 years of competition; F/M 50-75 = percentage change per event from ages 50 to 75 years; F/M 75-85 = percentage change per event from ages 75 to 85 years. (Adapted with permission from Wright VJ, Perricelli BC: Age-related rates of decline in performance among elite senior athletes. *Am J Sports Med* 2008;36(3):443-450.)

Two camps are now evident in the literature: those who postulate that age-related decline is greatest in sports that tax the body's energy resources more ("energy expenditure hypothesis"), such as sprints, and those who propose that energy supply (needed in endurance races) is more important. Perhaps the mechanisms of decline are different for different sports, depending on the specific demands of the event.

Factors Affecting Performance

The functional decline seen in senior athletes has been attributed to multiple age-related factors. These include declines in training intensity, reaction time, joint mobility, skeletal size, body fat composition, anaerobic and aerobic power supply, recovery ability, strength, proprioception, endurance, and coordination.[18,36-41]

Muscle Strength

One important factor in loss of independence is weakness secondary to age-related loss of lean muscle mass, or senile sarcopenia. For most elderly people, the decrease in muscle mass is paralleled by an equal (or greater) decrease in strength and power.[42-46] This is also accompanied by an increase in muscle weakness and fatigability.[47-49] Muscle power is lost at a greater rate than endurance capacity: 3.5% versus 1.8% per year.[50] We know that aged sprinters have 40% shorter stride lengths[51] and therefore require more strides to cover the same distance; this may be the result of a decrease in power. However, when a statistical adjustment is made to account for the variation in an aging runner's velocity, older runners did not have a significantly shorter stride length at any given velocity.[52] Among swimmers, the stroke frequency decline is about 2.5 times the decline in stroke length.[53] These data parallel the results of a longitudinal study of aging skeletal muscle in sedentary adults. Frontera et al[54] found that over a 12-year period beginning at a mean age of 65.4 ± 4.2 years, muscle cross-sectional area in men declined 14.7%. Several studies have documented increased fat infiltration into muscle with age in nonathletes.[43,55,56] Although there is a clinical impression that loss of muscle mass and changes in muscle composition are associated with a functional decline, results have been inconsistent in the literature.

The mass of a given skeletal muscle is the product of the volume of a muscle fiber (fiber length × fiber cross-sectional area) multiplied by the number of fibers present in that muscle. The number of muscle fibers does not increase after skeletal maturity. A change in muscle mass is a direct consequence of either a change in fiber cross-sectional area or a decrease in the number of fibers. It is unknown how much each of these entities contributes to muscle mass decline. Genetics and lifestyle also certainly play a role, although that role is not clearly understood.

Visser et al,[57] in conjunction with the National Institutes of Health's Dynamics of Health, Aging, and Body Composition study, examined healthy 70- to 79-year-old nonathletes. The authors found that smaller muscle mass in the leg and greater fat infiltration in the muscle was associated with poorer lower extremity performance. Baumgartner et al[58] reported that seniors with sarcopenia are three to four times more likely to report disability, have balance abnormalities, and use an assistive device for ambulation. Goodpaster et al[59] reported that high fat infiltration into muscle was associated with poor knee extensor strength and decreased muscle contractility, muscle fiber recruitment, and muscle metabolism. A greater muscle fat content has also been found to be associated with glucose intolerance and diabetes mellitus.[59,60] Several studies have shown a rapid decline in muscular strength in men of up to 2.5% per year after 60 years of age.[54,61,62] Parallel observations have been made by Alway et al,[63] who noted a loss of muscle strength in older endurance-trained athletes relative to untrained younger men. The issue, therefore, is not just loss of absolute muscle mass, but loss of lean muscle mass.

It is encouraging to note that sarcopenia can be modified by physical exercise.[64] Fiatarone et al[65] found that even in people older than 90 years, the supposed age-dependent loss of muscle size and strength can be reversed by high-intensity resistance training. The strength gains were modest, however, compared with those seen in younger individuals.

Short-term muscle power depends on the degradation of adenosine triphosphate (ATP) and its replenishment from phosphocreatine (PCr).[66] The rate of both processes is high, but as PCr stores are limited and need to be replenished by the slower, oxidative metabolism,

the high-phosphate-based power can be sustained for a limited time. Sprinting performance relies on this anaerobic mechanism, whereas endurance performance is usually thought to be limited by aerobic power. In skeletal muscle, power generation in sprinting performance is mainly by type II muscle fibers (anaerobic), whereas type I fibers are responsible for the aerobic power generation in endurance events.

Past cross-sectional studies have suggested that aging involves selective atrophy and loss of type II (fast-twitch) muscle fibers.[45,67-70] Lexell et al[45] presented data from a cross-sectional autopsy study that showed a 10% decline in muscle size between 24 and 50 years of age that increased to a 30% decline between 50 and 80 years of age. With this in mind, one would expect an age-related decrease in metabolic power to be most evident in sprint rather than endurance performance. Lexell et al[45] also found a decline in the absolute number of muscle fibers. Troop[50] reported that muscle fiber number declines modestly until the age of 50 and increases more rapidly thereafter, which parallels the decline in performance reported in our study.[1] Faulkner et al[71] noted that a gradual loss of muscle fibers begins at approximately 50 years of age and continues such that by 80 years of age, approximately 50% of the fibers are lost from the limb muscles. The effect of lost type II fibers may be attenuated by the maintenance of type I (slow-twitch) muscle cells. In fact, the cross-sectional area of type I fibers was unchanged with age, whereas that of type II fibers was reduced in sprint-trained athletes.[72] These durable cells remain constant or may actually expand up to 20% with physical activity.[73]

In contrast, other cross-sectional studies did not find differences in muscle composition between older and younger people.[70,74] Tarpenning et al[75] noted that type I and type II fiber area and distribution did not differ between age groups through the eighth decade. The data suggested that chronic endurance training can delay the age of significant decline in peak torque and changes in muscle morphology characteristics of muscle.

Physical activity impacts the cross-sectional area of the fibers that remain and may even permit hypertrophy.[70,73,76-78] Type II muscle fibers tend to decrease in cross-sectional area with aging, and slow type I fibers tend to maintain their cross-sectional area.[45,70]

Recently, in a longitudinal study, fiber type proportion was assessed in the same individuals at 64 years and then at 75 years of age. The histology demonstrated a decrease from 60% to 40% of type I fiber content.[61]

It has also been shown that sprint-trained athletes experience the typical age-related reduction in the size of fast-twitch fibers, a shift toward a slower myosin-heavy chain (MHC) isoform profile, and a lower maximum shortening velocity of type I MHC fibers, which play a role in the decline in explosive force production. However, the muscle characteristics were found to be preserved at a high level in the oldest runners studied by Korhonen et al.[72] This suggests a favorable impact of sprint exercise on aging muscle.[72] Trappe et al[73] showed that progressive resistance training in elderly men increases muscle cell size, strength, contractile velocity, and power in both slow- and fast-twitch muscle fibers. However, it appears that these changes are more pronounced in the type I MHC muscle fibers.[73]

Endurance-trained athletes have been studied to more closely examine the effect of long-term exercise on age-associated changes in skeletal muscle structure and function. The studies demonstrated that continued endurance training maintains the aerobic capacity of muscle but does not appear to slow age-associated loss of muscle mass, atrophy of type II fibers, or decline in whole-muscle force production.[79-82]

As mentioned earlier, Pearson et al[25] presented evidence that long-term strength training in weight lifters can assist with preservation of the structural and mechanical characteristics of skeletal muscle seen during aging. Klitgaard et al[81] supported this notion with a cross-sectional study of elderly men with 12 to 17 years of strength training who demonstrated muscle fiber size, MHC composition, and muscle force characteristics similar to those of young adult control subjects.

The loss of muscle cells is thought to be secondary to age-related neural degeneration.[69] Muscle cells require stimulation from motor nerve cells and, in the absence of this stimulation, will atrophy. The observation in both humans and rats that the timing and magnitude of the loss of motor units is similar to the loss of muscle fibers suggests that the same mechanism is responsible for the loss of fibers and the loss of whole motor units.

The degree of atrophy of the fibers that remain is largely dependent on the habitual level of physical activity of the individual.[71] Importantly, any loss of muscle fibers due to neuropathic phenomena cannot be reversed.[83]

Resistance training has been found to decrease the shrinkage of type II muscle fibers and increase their capillary blood supply.[84,85] In fact, studies have shown that aerobic exercise alone is not enough to maintain muscle mass. Only strength-trained seniors had muscle mass and composition similar to that of young control subjects. Coggan et al[84] further found that training intensity and duration affect muscle fiber distribution, not aging alone. The success of masters athletes and of previously sedentary elderly who undertake well-designed, carefully administered training programs provides dramatic evidence that age-associated atrophy, weakness, fatigability, muscle morphology, and decline in peak torque can be slowed, but not halted.[71,75] These studies highlight the critical need for resistance training after the age of 50 for maintenance of muscle strength and independence.

Loss of Endurance Capacity

Tanaka and Seals[12] demonstrated that reductions in maximal oxygen uptake or maximal aerobic capacity (VO2 max; the maximum energy production via oxidative pathways) and the decline in lactate threshold may be responsible for the changes in endurance performance with aging. Based on the Fick equation, VO_2 is dependent upon heart rate, cardiac output, and tissue oxygen uptake. One of the primary factors believed to be responsible for functional aging is VO_2 max.[39] Studies have demonstrated that a reduction in maximal heart rate will decrease VO_2 max with age in trained and untrained adults.[86,87] Conversely, other studies have shown that there is no relationship between reduction in maximal heart rate and habitual exercise status.[32,88,89] The remainder of the variables include cardiac output and maximal arteriovenous oxygen difference, which can be altered with stroke volume and skeletal muscle oxidative capacity.

Ogawa et al[90] found that a smaller stroke volume accounted for nearly 50% of age-related differences in VO_2 max, and the remainder was explained by a lower maximal heart rate and reduced oxygen extraction. The decline in VO_2 max may be diminished by 50% by intense habitual exercise. This effect is thought to be due primarily to maintenance of cardiac output through stroke volume. Men and women have relatively similar rates of VO_2 max decline when expressed as a percentage reduction from youth to older adulthood.[33] As training levels decline, so does the VO_2 max. Women, however, appear to experience a greater decline in muscular strength and power (sprinting-type events) with aging.[91,92] Individuals with the greatest decreases in exercise volume and/or intensity will demonstrate the greatest age-associated reduction in maximal aerobic capacity.[12]

As previously discussed, differences by sex in swimming performance were greatest in shorter events and decreased with increasing distance.[14] Physiologically, this may not make much sense, as it has only been observed with swimming events; however, in swimming, smaller body size means less drag, and greater body fat percentage results in greater buoyancy. Shorter legs result in a more horizontal posture and less drag, in addition to quicker flip turns. All of these make the oxygen cost of swimming more economical for women. This may mean that potential energy stores can be conserved for parts later in the race. Conversely, all of the above factors may result in decreased performance for women in other sporting events.

Peak blood lactate concentration can be used as an indirect measure of anaerobic glycolytic activity.[93] Peak blood lactate concentration following activity has been shown to be lower in 20- to 30-year-old men than in 60- to 70-year-old men.[94] In masters athletes, there is an age-related decrease of lactate following maximal activity in both running and swimming.[95,96] Lactate concentration and production are known to be correlated with the total muscle mass engaged in activity.[97] The anaerobic glycolytic energy production probably declines with age as a function of decreases in muscle mass and type II fiber area. Age-related decrease in anaerobic performance in masters athletes can potentially be explained by a shift to a more oxidative pathway given the relative increase in oxidative slow-twitch fibers.

Loss of Exercise Economy

Changes in flexibility, joint motion, and coordination all contribute significantly to declines in exercise economy. Shorter stride lengths and an increase in

ground contact time are found in aged sprinters when compared with their younger counterparts, whereas stride frequency shows only a minor decline and swing time remains relatively unaffected.[51] These changes may be partly due to loss of muscle strength and power. The importance of joint flexibility is often overlooked. With age, connective tissue becomes inherently stiffer and knee motion decreases by up to 33%, from a mean of 123° to a mean of 95°. Assuming that the transition from swing phase to stance phase occurs at 90° of flexion, this transition is near the point of maximum joint flexion in the senior athlete, which slows the power of the free leg to take the next step.[50] Flexibility maintains the stretch/reflex response of muscle and therefore can boost speed. In addition, stretching may reduce delayed-onset exercise soreness.

Summary

Valuable lessons can be learned from aging athletes. Aging alone is not a reason for becoming inactive. Although chronic disease is more prevalent in the aging population, senior athletes are able to maintain an active lifestyle and report a great sense of physical and mental well-being. Performance declines gently after 35 to 40 years of age and is relatively maintained until 70 years of age. Significant loss of function observed before the age of 70 years can likely be attributed to disuse, sedentary lifestyle behaviors, and genetic disposition. The tipping point for a change in physical ability seems to occur around 70 to 75 years of age, when performance typically plummets.

Age-associated decline in performance is generally greater in women. These differences are larger in endurance running and sprint-type swimming events. These differences are less evident with endurance-type swimming events. No clear consensus has been reached as to whether these differences are based on genetic code, social factors, or physiologic reasons.

Maximal aerobic capacity (VO_2 max) declines based on multiple variables. Identification and optimization of these variables can potentially halt or slow the aging process. Individuals who engage in physical exercise are capable of activities that are often not achievable by their sedentary peers. More important, seniors who engage in physical activity have a lower prevalence of diabetes, cardiovascular disorders, mental disorders,

Table 1: Notable Studies of Performance in Masters Athletes

Author(s) (Year)	Population	Key Points
Moore (1975)[16]	US track-and-field regional record holders	Throwing declined more rapidly than running. Decline of running speed with age was noted. "Strength deteriorates faster than stamina."
Stones and Kozma (1980)[19]	US marathoners	Rate of age decline in running performances was greater for middle-distance and longer distance events than for sprints.
Fung and Ha (1994)[17]	Masters athletes	400-meter run and long jump declined the fastest for men and women. Javelin declined the fastest for men and the discus for women. "Strength deteriorates before stamina."
Meltzer (1994)[23]	Masters weight lifters	Olympic weight-lifting ability in trained subjects undergoes a non-linear decline with age.
Tanaka and Seals (1997)[14]	US Masters swimmers	Performance in 50-meter freestyle showed modest decline until 75 to 80 years of age when compared with 1500-meter event. Linear decrease until 70 to 80 years of age, then decline is exponential
Baker et al (2003)[18]	Masters athletes	Track performance declined with age in a curvilinear fashion. Walking and field event performance declined in a linear manner. Decline with aging was greater for women and for endurance running events. Strength-dependent throwing events and pole vault showed the greatest decline with age.
Tanaka and Seals (2003)[12]	US Masters swimmers	Rates of the decline in swimming performance with age are greater in a long-duration than in a short-duration event. Age-related rates of decline are greater in women than in men only in a short-duration event.
Thé and Ploutz-Snyder (2003)[26]	World Masters weight lifters	The rate of decline in power with advancing age is similar and is in agreement with previous reports for world record holders, other masters athletes, and healthy, untrained individuals. High importance of the aging process itself over physical activity history
Anton et al (2004)[24]	US weight-lifting and power-lifting records	Men's and women's weight-lifting and power-lifting performance declined curvilinearly and linearly, respectively. The rate and the overall magnitude of declines in performance with age were markedly greater in weight lifting than in power lifting.
Jokl et al (2004)[20]	US marathoners	Participation in the New York City Marathon is increasing at a higher rate in the masters groups than in other age groups. Male and female masters athletes continued to improve running times at a greater rate than the younger athletes, whose performance levels have plateaued.

Table 1: (*continued*)		
Author(s) (Year)	**Population**	**Key Points**
Leyk et al (2007)[21]	German marathoners	Significant age-related losses in endurance performance did not occur before the age of 50 years.
		Mean marathon and half–marathon times were nearly identical for the age groups from 20-49 years.
		Age-related performance decreases of the 50- to 69-year-old subjects were 2.6% to 4.4%/decade.
Wright and Perricelli (2008)[1]	Senior Olympians and masters athletes	Performance declined (men and women) at 3.4%/year over 35 years of competition.
		Slow decline from age 50 to 75 (1.8%/year for men and 1.9%/year for women)
		Quick decline after age 75 (7.86%/year for men and 7.36%/year for women)
		Men showed no difference in decline of sprint and endurance events; decline in the sprint was greater than in endurance for women, especially after the age of 75 years.
		The healthiest individuals in terms of musculoskeletal aging experienced significant performance declines around 75 years of age.
Leyk et al (2009)[22]	German marathoners	Aging is a natural process that can be considerably accelerated or slowed by lifestyle.
		Age-related marathon performance declines did not occur before the age of 55 years.
		Most middle-aged and elderly athletes have training histories of less than 7 years of running.

and certain types of cancer than their sedentary counterparts.[2,3] Premature mortality and functional disability have a lower incidence[4] in active patients than in their sedentary counterparts.[4]

Table 1 lists key studies of athletic performance in masters athletes. **Table 2** lists key studies of muscle deterioration with age.

Future Directions

Future clinical and translational research on senior athletes should focus on three areas: keeping the senior athlete competitive longer, sustaining the independence of seniors in the community, and monitoring the impact of these programs on health status outcomes and healthcare resource utilization.

Monitoring the effect of self-selection, chronic illness, activity history, or genetic propensity is difficult in a cross-sectional study. Longitudinal studies of this population will clarify these confounding issues.

The role of exercise in prevention of disability in seniors will be of paramount importance to the baby boomer generation and for generations to come. Examining the population of senior athletes who have slowed the disabling effects of aging will provide a valuable means not only to understand this growing population but also to design preventive measures for baby boomers and the general population.

Table 2: Key Studies on Muscle Deterioration

Authors (Year)	Population	Key Points
Lexell et al (1988)[45]	Physically healthy men	Aging atrophy of the vastus lateralis muscle begins around 25 years of age and accelerates thereafter. This atrophy is caused mainly by a loss of fibers, with no predominant effect on any fiber type, and to a lesser extent by a reduction in type II fibers.
Fiatarone et al (1990)[65]	Frail and institutionalized volunteers	High-resistance weight training leads to gains in muscle strength, size, and functional mobility among frail residents of nursing homes up to 96 years of age.
Frontera et al (2000)[61]	Healthy sedentary men	Muscle biopsies taken from vastus lateralis muscles showed a reduction in percentage of type I fibers over 12 years.
Gatta et al (2006)[53]	World Masters Championship swimmers	Decline of stroke frequency was 2.5 times steeper than stroke length. Stroke length is less affected by the aging process.
Korhonen et al (2006)[72]	Male masters sprinters	Sprint-trained athletes experienced the typical age-related reduction in the size of fast fibers, a shift toward a slower myosin-heavy chain isoform profile, and a lower maximum shortening velocity of type I myosin-heavy chain fibers. The muscle characteristics were preserved at a high level in the oldest runners, underlining the favorable impact of sprint exercise on aging muscle.
Faulkner et al (2007)[71]	Masters athletes	Performance of marathon runners and weight lifters declines after 40 years of age, with peak levels of performance decreased by approximately 50% by 80 years of age. For both humans and rats, the timing and magnitude of the loss of motor units is similar to that for muscle fibers. Suggested mechanisms include the loss of fibers and the loss of whole motor units is the same. The degree of atrophy of the fibers that remain is largely dependent on the habitual level of physical activity of the individual.
Korhonen et al (2009)[51]	Competitive runners	Running velocity is related to decrease in stride length with age and increase in ground contact time. An age-related decline occurs in muscle thickness, type II fiber area, and maximal and rapid force-generating capacity of the lower limb muscles..

References

1. Wright VJ, Perricelli BC: Age-related rates of decline in performance among elite senior athletes. *Am J Sports Med* 2008;36(3):443-450.

2. American College of Sports Medicine Position Stand: American College of Sports Medicine Position Stand: Exercise and physical activity for older adults. *Med Sci Sports Exerc* 1998;30(6):992-1008.

3. Powell KE, Thompson PD, Caspersen CJ, Kendrick JS: Physical activity and the incidence of coronary heart disease. *Annu Rev Public Health* 1987;8:253-287.

4. Blair SN, Kohl HW III , Barlow CE, Paffenbarger RS Jr, Gibbons LW, Macera CA: Changes in physical fitness and all-cause mortality: A prospective study of healthy and unhealthy men. *JAMA* 1995;273(14):1093-1098.

5. Di Prampero PE, Capelli C, Pagliaro P, et al: Energetics of best performances in middle-distance running. *J Appl Physiol* 1993;74(5):2318-2324.

6. Hill AV: The physiological basis of athletic records. *Nature* 1925;116(2919):544-548.

7. Capelli C, Schena F, Zamparo P, Monte AD, Faina M, di Prampero PE: Energetics of best performances in track cycling. *Med Sci Sports Exerc* 1998;30(4):614-624.

8. di Prampero PE: Factors limiting maximal performance in humans. *Eur J Appl Physiol* 2003;90(3-4):420-429.

9. Chatterjee S, Laudato M: Gender and performance in athletics. *Soc Biol* 1995;42(1-2):124-132.

10. Lazarus NR, Harridge SD: Inherent ageing in humans: The case for studying master athletes. *Scand J Med Sci Sports* 2007;17(5):461-463.

11. Rittweger J, Kwiet A, Felsenberg D: Physical performance in aging elite athletes—Challenging the limits of physiology. *J Musculoskelet Neuronal Interact* 2004;4(2):159-160.

12. Tanaka H, Seals DR: Invited review: Dynamic exercise performance in Masters athletes: Insight into the effects of primary human aging on physiological functional capacity. *J Appl Physiol* 2003;95(5):2152-2162.

13. Pollock ML, Foster C, Knapp D, Rod JL, Schmidt DH: Effect of age and training on aerobic capacity and body composition of master athletes. *J Appl Physiol* 1987;62(2):725-731.

14. Tanaka H, Seals DR: Age and gender interactions in physiological functional capacity: Insight from swimming performance. *J Appl Physiol* 1997;82(3):846-851.

15. Wiswell RA, Hawkins SA, Jaque SV, et al: Relationship between physiological loss, performance decrement, and age in master athletes. *J Gerontol A Biol Sci Med Sci* 2001;56(10):M618-M626.

16. Moore DH II : A study of age group track and field records to relate age and running speed. *Nature* 1975;253(5489):264-265.

17. Fung L, Ha A: Changes in track and field performance with chronological aging. *Int J Aging Hum Dev* 1994;38(2):171-180.

18. Baker AB, Tang YQ, Turner MJ: Percentage decline in masters superathlete track and field performance with aging. *Exp Aging Res* 2003;29(1):47-65.

19. Stones MJ, Kozma A: Adult age trends in record running performances. *Exp Aging Res* 1980;6(5): 407-416.

20. Jokl P, Sethi PM, Cooper AJ: Master's performance in the New York City Marathon 1983-1999. *Br J Sports Med* 2004;38(4):408-412.

21. Leyk D, Erley O, Ridder D, et al: Age-related changes in marathon and half-marathon performances. *Int J Sports Med* 2007;28(6):513-517.

22. Leyk D, Erley O, Gorges W, et al: Performance, training and lifestyle parameters of marathon runners aged 20-80 years: Results of the PACE-study. *Int J Sports Med* 2009;30(5):360-365.

23. Meltzer DE: Age dependence of Olympic weightlifting ability. *Med Sci Sports Exerc* 1994;26(8):1053-1067.

24. Anton MM, Spirduso WW, Tanaka H: Age-related declines in anaerobic muscular performance: Weightlifting and powerlifting. *Med Sci Sports Exerc* 2004;36(1):143-147.

25. Pearson SJ, Young A, Macaluso A, et al: Muscle function in elite master weightlifters. *Med Sci Sports Exerc* 2002;34(7):1199-1206.

26. Thé DJ, Ploutz-Snyder L: Age, body mass, and gender as predictors of masters Olympic weightlifting performance. *Med Sci Sports Exerc* 2003;35(7):1216-1224.

27. Donato AJ, Tench K, Glueck DH, Seals DR, Eskurza I, Tanaka H: Declines in physiological functional capacity with age: A longitudinal study in peak swimming performance. *J Appl Physiol* 2003;94(2):764-769.

28. Dempsey S: Aging, exercise and cardiopulmonary function, in Lamb DR Gisolfi CV, Nadel E, eds: *Perspectives in Exercise Science and Sports Medicine: Exercise in Older Adults.* Carmel, IN, Cooper Publishing Goup, 1995, vol 8, pp 237-304.

29. Tanaka H, Higuchi M: Age, exercise performance, and physiological functional capacities. *Adv Exerc Sports Physiol* 1998;4:51-56.

30. Lobjois R, Benguigui N, Bertsch J: The effect of aging and tennis playing on coincidence-timing accuracy. *J Aging Phys Act* 2006;14(1):74-97.

31. United States Department of Health and Human Services: *Healthy People 2010: Understanding and Improving Health*, ed rev. Boston, MA, Jones and Bartlett Publishers, 2001.

32. Eskurza I, Donato AJ, Moreau KL, Seals DR, Tanaka H: Changes in maximal aerobic capacity with age in endurance-trained women: 7-yr follow-up. *J Appl Physiol* 2002;92(6):2303-2308.

33. Holloszy JO: *Exercise*. Bethesda, MD, American Physiological Society, 1995.

34. Holloszy JO, Smith EK, Vining M, Adams S: Effect of voluntary exercise on longevity of rats. *J Appl Physiol* 1985;59(3):826-831.

35. Sohal RS, Buchan PB: Relationship between physical activity and life span in the adult housefly, Musca domestica. *Exp Gerontol* 1981;16(2):157-162.

36. Maharam LG, Bauman PA, Kalman D, Skolnik H, Perle SM: Masters athletes: Factors affecting performance. *Sports Med* 1999;28(4):273-285.

37. Joyner MJ: Physiological limiting factors and distance running: Influence of gender and age on record performances. *Exerc Sport Sci Rev* 1993;21:103-133.

38. Joyner MJ: Modeling: Optimal marathon performance on the basis of physiological factors. *J Appl Physiol* 1991;70(2):683-687.

39. Koralewicz LM, Engh GA: Comparison of proprioception in arthritic and age-matched normal knees. *J Bone Joint Surg Am* 2000;82-A(11):1582-1588.

40. Lakatta EG: Alterations in the cardiovascular system that occur in advanced age. *Fed Proc* 1979;38(2):163-167.

41. Pollock ML, Mengelkoch LJ, Graves JE, et al: Twenty-year follow-up of aerobic power and body composition of older track athletes. *J Appl Physiol* 1997;82(5):1508-1516.

42. Bassey EJ, Fiatarone MA, O'Neill EF, Kelly M, Evans WJ, Lipsitz LA: Leg extensor power and functional performance in very old men and women. *Clin Sci (Lond)* 1992;82(3):321-327.

43. Frontera WR, Hughes VA, Lutz KJ, Evans WJ: A cross-sectional study of muscle strength and mass in 45- to 78-yr-old men and women. *J Appl Physiol* 1991;71(2):644-650.

44. Goodpaster BH, Park SW, Harris TB, et al: The loss of skeletal muscle strength, mass, and quality in older adults: The health, aging and body composition study. *J Gerontol A Biol Sci Med Sci* 2006;61(10):1059-1064.

45. Lexell J, Taylor CC, Sjöström M: What is the cause of the ageing atrophy? Total number, size and proportion of different fiber types studied in whole vastus lateralis muscle from 15- to 83-year-old men. *J Neurol Sci* 1988;84(2-3):275-294.

46. Young A, Stokes M, Crowe M: The size and strength of the quadriceps muscles of old and young men. *Clin Physiol* 1985;5(2):145-154.

47. Brooks SV, Faulkner JA: Forces and powers of slow and fast skeletal muscles in mice during repeated contractions. *J Physiol* 1991;436:701-710.

48. Brooks SV, Faulkner JA: Skeletal muscle weakness in old age: Underlying mechanisms. *Med Sci Sports Exerc* 1994;26(4):432-439.

49. Faulkner JA, Brooks SV: Muscle fatigue in old animals: Unique aspects of fatigue in elderly humans. *Adv Exp Med Biol* 1995;384:471-480.

50. Troop B: *Training for Masters Athletes*. London, United Kingdom, Peak Performance Publishing, 2004.

51. Korhonen MT, Mero AA, Alén M, et al: Biomechanical and skeletal muscle determinants of maximum running speed with aging. *Med Sci Sports Exerc* 2009;41(4):844-856.

52. Conoboy P, Dyson R: Effect of aging on the stride pattern of veteran marathon runners. *Br J Sports Med* 2006;40(7):601-604.

53. Gatta G, Benelli P, Ditroilo M: The decline of swimming performance with advancing age: A cross-sectional study. *J Strength Cond Res* 2006;20(4):932-938.

54. Frontera WR, Hughes VA, Fielding RA, Fiatarone MA, Evans WJ, Roubenoff R: Aging of skeletal muscle: A 12-yr longitudinal study. *J Appl Physiol* 2000;88(4):1321-1326.

55. Borkan GA, Hults DE, Gerzof SG, Robbins AH, Silbert CK: Age changes in body composition revealed by computed tomography. *J Gerontol* 1983;38(6):673-677.

56. Overend TJ, Cunningham DA, Paterson DH, Lefcoe MS: Thigh composition in young and elderly men determined by computed tomography. *Clin Physiol* 1992;12(6):629-640.

57. Visser M, Kritchevsky SB, Goodpaster BH, et al: Leg muscle mass and composition in relation to lower extremity performance in men and women aged 70 to 79: The health, aging and body composition study. *J Am Geriatr Soc* 2002;50(5):897-904.

58. Baumgartner RN, Koehler KM, Gallagher D, et al: Epidemiology of sarcopenia among the elderly in New Mexico. *Am J Epidemiol* 1998;147(8):755-763.

59. Goodpaster BH, Carlson CL, Visser M, et al: Attenuation of skeletal muscle and strength in the elderly: The Health ABC Study. *J Appl Physiol* 2001;90(6):2157-2165.

60. Jacob S, Machann J, Rett K, et al: Association of increased intramyocellular lipid content with insulin resistance in lean nondiabetic offspring of type 2 diabetic subjects. *Diabetes* 1999;48(5):1113-1119.

61. Aniansson A, Hedberg M, Henning GB, Grimby G: Muscle morphology, enzymatic activity, and muscle strength in elderly men: A follow-up study. *Muscle Nerve* 1986;9(7):585-591.

62. Frontera WR, Hughes VA, Krivickas LS, Kim SK, Foldvari M, Roubenoff R: Strength training in older women: Early and late changes in whole muscle and single cells. *Muscle Nerve* 2003;28(5):601-608.

63. Alway SE, Siu PM, Murlasits Z, Butler DC: Muscle hypertrophy models: Applications for research on aging. *Can J Appl Physiol* 2005;30(5):591-624.

64. Ryan AS, Nicklas BJ: Age-related changes in fat deposition in mid-thigh muscle in women: Relationships with metabolic cardiovascular disease risk factors. *Int J Obes Relat Metab Disord* 1999;23(2):126-132.

65. Fiatarone MA, Marks EC, Ryan ND, Meredith CN, Lipsitz LA, Evans WJ: High-intensity strength training in nonagenarians: Effects on skeletal muscle. *JAMA* 1990;263(22):3029-3034.

66. di Prampero PE: Energetics of muscular exercise. *Rev Physiol Biochem Pharmacol* 1981;89:143-222.

67. Larsson L: Morphological and functional characteristics of the ageing skeletal muscle in man: A cross-sectional study. *Acta Physiol Scand Suppl* 1978;457:1-36.

68. Larsson L: Histochemical characteristics of human skeletal muscle during aging. *Acta Physiol Scand* 1983;117(3):469-471.

69. Macaluso A, De Vito G: Muscle strength, power and adaptations to resistance training in older people. *Eur J Appl Physiol* 2004;91(4):450-472.

70. Lexell J: Human aging, muscle mass, and fiber type composition. *J Gerontol A Biol Sci Med Sci* 1995;50(Spec No):11-16.

71. Faulkner JA, Larkin LM, Claflin DR, Brooks SV: Age-related changes in the structure and function of skeletal muscles. *Clin Exp Pharmacol Physiol* 2007;34(11):1091-1096.

72. Korhonen MT, Cristea A, Alén M, et al: Aging, muscle fiber type, and contractile function in sprint-trained athletes. *J Appl Physiol* 2006;101(3):906-917.

73. Trappe S, Williamson D, Godard M, Porter D, Rowden G, Costill D: Effect of resistance training on single muscle fiber contractile function in older men. *J Appl Physiol* 2000;89(1):143-152.

74. Porter MM, Vandervoort AA, Lexell J: Aging of human muscle: Structure, function and adaptability. *Scand J Med Sci Sports* 1995;5(3):129-142.

75. Tarpenning KM, Hamilton-Wessler M, Wiswell RA, Hawkins SA: Endurance training delays age of decline in leg strength and muscle morphology. *Med Sci Sports Exerc* 2004;36(1):74-78.

76. Trappe S, Godard M, Gallagher P, Carroll C, Rowden G, Porter D: Resistance training improves single muscle fiber contractile function in older women. *Am J Physiol Cell Physiol* 2001;281(2):C398-C406.

77. Grimby G, Saltin B: The ageing muscle. *Clin Physiol* 1983;3(3):209-218.

78. Lexell J, Taylor CC: Variability in muscle fibre areas in whole human quadriceps muscle: Effects of increasing age. *J Anat* 1991;174:239-249.

79. Harridge S, Magnusson G, Saltin B: Life-long endurance-trained elderly men have high aerobic power, but have similar muscle strength to non-active elderly men. *Aging (Milano)* 1997;9(1-2):80-87.

80. Proctor DN, Sinning WE, Walro JM, Sieck GC, Lemon PW: Oxidative capacity of human muscle fiber types: Effects of age and training status. *J Appl Physiol* 1995;78(6):2033-2038.

81. Klitgaard H, Mantoni M, Schiaffino S, et al: Function, morphology and protein expression of ageing skeletal muscle: A cross-sectional study of elderly men with different training backgrounds. *Acta Physiol Scand* 1990;140(1):41-54.

82. Widrick JJ, Trappe SW, Blaser CA, Costill DL, Fitts RH: Isometric force and maximal shortening velocity of single muscle fibers from elite master runners. *Am J Physiol* 1996;271(2 Pt 1):C666-C675.

83. Narici MV, Maganaris CN: Adaptability of elderly human muscles and tendons to increased loading. *J Anat* 2006;208(4):433-443.

84. Coggan AR, Spina RJ, King DS, et al: Skeletal muscle adaptations to endurance training in 60- to 70-yr-old men and women. *J Appl Physiol* 1992;72(5):1780-1786.

85. Orlander J, Aniansson A: Effect of physical training on skeletal muscle metabolism and ultrastructure in 70 to 75-year-old men. *Acta Physiol Scand* 1980;109(2):149-154.

86. Hagberg JM: Effect of training on the decline of VO2max with aging. *Fed Proc* 1987;46(5):1830-1833.

87. Heath GW, Hagberg JM, Ehsani AA, Holloszy JO: A physiological comparison of young and older endurance athletes. *J Appl Physiol* 1981;51(3):634-640.

88. Fitzgerald MD, Tanaka H, Tran ZV, Seals DR: Age-related declines in maximal aerobic capacity in regularly exercising vs. sedentary women: A meta-analysis. *J Appl Physiol* 1997;83(1):160-165.

89. Pimentel AE, Gentile CL, Tanaka H, Seals DR, Gates PE: Greater rate of decline in maximal aerobic capacity with age in endurance-trained than in sedentary men. *J Appl Physiol* 2003;94(6):2406-2413.

90. Ogawa T, Spina RJ, Martin WH III , et al: Effects of aging, sex, and physical training on cardiovascular responses to exercise. *Circulation* 1992;86(2):494-503.

91. Phillips SK, Rook KM, Siddle NC, Bruce SA, Woledge RC: Muscle weakness in women occurs at an earlier age than in men, but strength is preserved by hormone replacement therapy. *Clin Sci (Lond)* 1993;84(1):95-98.

92. Skelton DA, Greig CA, Davies JM, Young A: Strength, power and related functional ability of healthy people aged 65-89 years. *Age Ageing* 1994;23(5):371-377.

93. Lacour JR, Bouvat E, Barthélémy JC: Post-competition blood lactate concentrations as indicators of anaerobic energy expenditure during 400-m and 800-m races. *Eur J Appl Physiol Occup Physiol* 1990;61(3-4):172-176.

94. Makrides L, Heigenhauser GJ, Jones NL: High-intensity endurance training in 20- to 30- and 60- to 70-yr-old healthy men. *J Appl Physiol* 1990;69(5):1792-1798.

95. Korhonen MT, Suominen H, Mero A: Age and sex differences in blood lactate response to sprint running in elite master athletes. *Can J Appl Physiol* 2005;30(6):647-665.

96. Benelli P, Ditroilo M, Forte R, De Vito G, Stocchi V: Assessment of post-competition peak blood lactate in male and female master swimmers aged 40-79 years and its relationship with swimming performance. *Eur J Appl Physiol* 2007;99(6):685-693.

97. Stainsby WN, Brooks GA: Control of lactic acid metabolism in contracting muscles and during exercise. *Exerc Sport Sci Rev* 1990;18:29-63.

Chapter 13
The Psychology of the Aging Athlete

Daniel Fulham O'Neill, MD, EdD

Key Points

- Physical injury is always accompanied by some level of psychologic injury.
- Baby boomers are engaging in riskier sports, with a resultant increase in injuries.
- Athletic identity, social networks, and exercise history most often determine a person's activity profile.
- Athletic activity often serves as a coping mechanism for the aging athlete; therefore, it is incumbent upon doctors, therapists, and athletic trainers to provide support while a patient recovers from injury.
- The physiology, psychology, and sociology of aging, activity, sports, and injury are intimately intertwined.

Introduction

The old joke about the doctor who tells a patient, "If it hurts when you do that, then don't do that" is not just a joke. This remains the philosophy of many healthcare practitioners, especially when dealing with older patients. Fortunately, with the dawn of sports medicine and the demands of the baby boomer generation, this attitude is steadily changing. Unfortunately, real physiologic changes occur during aging, and they separate the older, or masters, athlete from the younger athlete. Interruptions in an older athlete's usual activities can lead to unique biologic and, just as important, psychologic issues. In younger athletes, injury might lead to concerns about losing a position on a team or an athletic scholarship.

In older athletes, the stakes are potentially greater, as the injury may raise psychologic issues of entrenched athletic identity[1] in addition to very real fears of mortality.

In the past century, such drastic changes in life expectancy, medical care, job descriptions, and leisure activities have occurred that sociologists as well as physicians and athletic trainers have found it difficult to chart and respond to developing trends.[2] The number of people 65 years and older in the United States is expected to double from the beginning of this century to the year 2030, twice as fast as the rest of the population,[3] with similar trends seen in the worldwide population.[4] These millions of seniors might be retiring from their jobs, but they are not retiring from their avocations—including sports and other sometimes physically risky leisure pursuits. In fact, with encouragement from marketing firms, family members, doctors, athletic trainers, and physical therapists, many people are just beginning their sports careers and aggressive physical activities at an advanced age.[5]

Although it is known that young athletes respond psychologically to injury at all levels of competition[6,7] and the rehabilitation of the psychologic injury has been shown to be an important aspect of successful rehabilitation from physical injury when returning any athlete to his or her previous level of performance,[1] there is a dearth of data on the psychology of the aging athlete. Thus, despite the difference of goals and motives for the older athlete, it might be prudent for a sports medicine provider to assume that the psychologic response of an older athlete to injury is at least as serious as it would be in a younger athlete. For younger athletes recovering from injury, coping mechanisms, time management, and social support are keys for a successful return to sport. In contrast, many older patients use athletics *for* coping, time management, and social support, so when this activity is not available, the psychologic effect can be devastating.

Pursuing athletic activities into old age, whether after a lifetime of athletic participation or as a newcomer to exercise, is the classic double-edged sword.[8,9] Multiple studies extol the health benefits, both physical and psychologic, of regular exercise,[10-12] but almost all studies acknowledge an increase in injury rates in adults who pursue an active lifestyle.[13-15] Data collected at the 2001 National Senior Olympic Games showed that 17% of participants had undergone knee surgery.[9]

This chapter is organized into four sections: (1) the nexus of physical activity and psychology, (2) the psychology of injury, (3) self-efficacy and the aging athlete, and (4) the psychology of recovery.

The Nexus of Physical Activity and Psychology

In his 1993 memoir *Life Work*,[16] the poet Donald Hall describes the shock of New Hampshire farmers at the turn of the last century when a factory opened in their town. Suddenly men were "only working 6 days a week."

The work week was six days, 6:00 A.M. to 6:00 P.M., and apparently the farmboys who worked there could hardly believe their good fortune: no work on Sunday, and only twelve hours on weekdays! Around 1900 the bosses, overcome by benignity, cut Saturday afternoons so that the shop's saws ran only from 6:00 A.M. until noon on the sixth day. Old timers muttered, "*That's* not a week's wuk!"[16]

Finding physical work was not an issue in the industrial and agricultural societies of 100 years ago, but the introduction of sophisticated machines into every aspect of life has altered this drastically. There are too many differences between the lives of our ancestors just three generations ago and our own to make valid comparisons regarding health indices, but it seems clear that physical activity is a prerequisite for healthy living and aging. The landmark longitudinal Survey in Europe on Nutrition and the Elderly, a Concerted Action (SENECA; named for the philosopher who asked, "You want to live—but do you know how to live?"), which evaluated more than 2,000 subjects older than 70 years across 9 countries in Western Europe, showed that inactive smokers with poor diets had more health issues and increased mortality compared with active, nonsmoking, healthier-eating control groups.[10] Similar data were recorded in an American study that noted that physical activity delayed all-cause mortality, mostly due to decreases in death from cardiovascular disease and cancer.[17] Although neither study looked specifically at the psychology of these aging seniors, physical activity has been linked directly to psychologic health in several other studies.[12,18,19]

In 1948, the World Health Organization defined health as "a state of complete physical, mental and social well-being, and not merely the absence of disease or infirmity."[10] Aging, as it relates to a living creature, can be defined as "universal, decremental, progressive, and intrinsic."[20] In these and other definitions offered after World War II, health and aging were already cast as multidimensional entities including biologic, psychologic, and sociologic factors. Although an interest in the psychology of aging is just over a century old,[21] perhaps because before the 1900s people simply did not live consistently to an old age, the phrases "aging athlete," "aging gracefully," and "active retirement" did not start appearing in the literature of the United States and Western Europe until the present era of relative prosperity.

Some reference appears almost daily in the popular media regarding the nexus of physical activity and psychology. Although most of these reports take the form of testimonials, good evidence links physical fitness to improved mood, reduced depression, and increased perceived wellness.[12,18,19] *Mood* or *affect* refers to a combination of anxiety and depression. Mood is generally considered more transient, whereas affect tends to refer to a long-term state of being. Although theories linking psychologic improvements with physical activity involve multiple concepts such as "filling time,"[22] endorphin release,[23] self-efficacy,[24] sense of belonging,[11] societal approval,[22] and maintaining mobility,[12] it is still not entirely clear why this link is noted consistently across different cultures. Perhaps it is because the biochemical response of the human brain to stressful stimuli is the same as it has been for hundreds of thousands of years, as evidenced by the feeling experienced when one is startled by thunder or stuck in traffic.[25] Besides the fact that the human sympathetic nervous system still has a "fight or flight" response, other primitive areas of our brain may respond with a positive psychology to physical activity.[26] The biology is still uncertain, but multiple clinical studies point to this connection between physical and psychologic fitness.[3,27]

Just as physical activity has been linked to positive effects on the psyche, lack of physical activity has been linked to depression. A European study of more than 1,500 subjects followed over 5 years found that increasing age and lack of physical activity were risk factors for depression.[27] In many societies, increasing age is often accompanied by financial difficulties, illness, and decrease in activity.[27] In other words, various age-related factors are constantly interacting; age is accompanied by loss of balance, loss of balance leads to injury, injury (and fear of injury) leads to decreased activity, decreased activity leads to somatic problems, somatic illness leads to depression, and on and on in a vicious cross-pollinating cycle. Camacho et al[23] conducted a similar study in the United States but followed their subjects over a longer time period, almost 20 years. They

also found a connection between inactivity and depression.

Anyone older than 30 years, even the most athletic among us, begins to understand the physical ravages of age. This observation is backed, unfortunately, by numerous studies.[9,28-30] Many of these studies looked at long-distance runners because many masters athletes participate in running, making large groups available for analysis.[31-33] Although aging and some decline in physiology is inevitable, perhaps this should not be automatically classified as pathologic.[20] One source of frustration when assessing the effects of aging is that organ systems age at different rates. One person might be limited by a damaged heart, and another patient may have a perfectly healthy heart but be limited by knee arthritis. Situations might even be reversed in two people in the same family who share many of the same genes. For these reasons, designing studies and putting together control groups to account for so many variables, including other risk factors, cultural background, economics, and past activity, is incredibly difficult.

Senior athletes actually perform better than their younger counterparts in several aspects of sport, usually aspects related to experience. These usually involve mental and emotional elements such as self-understanding, motivation, more efficient training methods, and tactical experience.[20,34-36] This is cold comfort, however, for senior athletes trying to keep up with younger counterparts on a club bike ride!

Most research points to healthier and seemingly happier aging through activity, so it does appear that the risks of injury are worth the physical and psychologic rewards. Consequently, two questions arise: (1) How does the health care professional keep an already athletic patient participating safely? and, perhaps a tougher problem, (2) How can a nonathletic patient be motivated to start moving? Health and performance can be improved with age if the patient is given adequate education and then makes even a modest effort.[37] Unfortunately, the effectiveness of this depends in part on prior exercise behavior and strong support from the patient's social network.[38] Individuals for whom getting their heart rate over 150 beats/min is not their idea of fun can still benefit from moderate exercise. Some evidence exists that great physical gains or even big physical effort is not required for a person to enjoy psychologic benefits from activity.[3,11] One thing that is known is that people who exercise early in life tend to keep exercising.[14,15,37] One thing that is *not* known is how the loss of physical education programs in our schools and the obesity crisis in many developed countries will affect not just the physical health but also the mental health of adults in the decades to come.

The Psychology of Injury

One lesson learned from both the scientific literature and anecdotally from patients, teammates, and the sports pages is that athletes, be they world class or sandlot, incur some psychologic injury when they sustain physical trauma.[6,7] Although this might seem obvious in a professional athlete with a family to support or a high school prospect hoping for a scholarship, the issue is no less real with recreational athletes, including masters athletes.

Gould et al[39] describe various stress sources that athletes might have to deal with when recovering from injury. They list three particularly significant stressors, including (1) "a major life event change," referring to the loss of career and paycheck; (2) "chronic stress," both physical and psychologic, due to injury; and (3) "daily hassles," due to physical immobility. I would contend that except for the monetary issue, these stressors play a huge part in the psychology of the older athlete, especially those who are retired from work and whose children have left the home. For these individuals, their athletic activity, whether it is competitive, social, or simply walking the dog in the woods, is a major part of their health. Older athletes are often one significant injury or illness away from disability, and this fact is not lost on them.

Brewer et al[40] define athletic identity as "the degree to which an individual identifies with the athlete role." This self-evaluation often remains throughout a lifetime. Such evaluations are influenced by past achievements, family, friends, and no doubt certain intrinsic motivations. Simply getting old does not change this attitude. On the positive side, this influence is also thought to help individuals continue some type of physical activity into old age.[30,41] Perhaps not surprisingly, however, when an individual who identifies with the role of athlete, whether young or old, sustains a significant injury, medical caregivers must be alert to a possible negative psychologic response. As noted earlier, many of these patients use athletics for coping, time structure, and social support. What are their coping mechanisms?[42] What do they see as alternatives to their previous activities while they are recovering or if they never recover? What alternatives do they have for this lost social support? When older athletes are injured and cannot walk the dog or attend ski races, triathlons, and lawn-bowling matches, a tremendous void is created in their lives.[34] Healthcare providers must be part of the new "coping mechanism" to help them through this period.

The blow to athletic identity with injury and illness is often accompanied by mood disturbance, lowered self-esteem, and even thoughts of mortality.[7,43,44] Recovery from injury ideally follows these steps: (1) injury, (2) healing, (3) rehabilitation, and (4) gradual return to sports. Psychologic recovery, however, might not proceed in such a stepwise fashion.[1,44] Many of these patients will not respond to psychologic support without a physical outlet. Physicians must suggest new, safe outlets for the physical needs of these patients while they recover from injury. Ideally, these activities will satisfy the competitive and social aspects provided by their former sports. Thankfully, individuals with athletic backgrounds tend to be more compliant with rehabilitation and cope better after injury than do nonathletes.[45]

In addition to considering the psychologic response to an injury, factors that caused the injury in the first place should be considered, as social psychology might be an important factor. Physicians and society encourage people to remain active into old age, and some patients take the idea of fighting the ravages of aging a step too far and look to risk-taking activities for their recreation.[46] Although a minority of these seniors are risk takers by nature, most are simply trying to continue their usual activities (ie, activities they engaged in before osteoporosis, arthritis, Achilles tendon rupture, etc) that have now become not only unhealthy but also potentially dangerous. Aggressive singles tennis, mogul skiing, and competitive basketball with college kids might not be recommended or advisable after a significant musculoskeletal problem.[47] Unfortunately, seniors often receive significant encouragement from society, as a glance at the evening news just about any night will show their peers being lauded for such behavior. George H.W. Bush jumping out of an airplane at age 85 and being clapped on the back for it is just one example. The marathon runner who continues to participate despite knee replacements is another. The extreme sports mentality is reaching across all age groups. Whether the individual is "keeping up with the grandchildren," taking the sport to the next level because time and resources allow it (eg, climbing Mt. Everest when older than 60), or trying to maintain athletic identity,[48] physicians need to help patients separate the psychologic risk/reward from the physical risk/reward. Before Mr. Bush made his jump, every precaution was taken. Most patients, however, do not have access to that level of planning. The positive aspects of activity should be encouraged, but it is equally important to minimize the risks.

Self-Efficacy and the Aging Athlete

The first Senior Olympic Games, with participants aged 50 or older, was held in 1970 and attracted some 200 competitors. This event now registers more than 10,000 athletes.[9,20] Clearly, many seniors participate seriously in athletics and make such activities and competitions a focal point of their lives. Many of these seniors are participating regularly for the first time in their lives, perhaps because their lifestyle and finances now allow such interests. By consistently participating in such activities, these patients can see enormous benefits as they improve body composition, fitness, longevity, personal care abilities, and the management of chronic illness.[3] Because an active lifestyle slows the effects of aging,[31] it can also be a factor in the development of self-efficacy and thus psychologic health. *Self-efficacy*, a term made famous by Bandura[49] in 1977, is a person's belief that he or she can successfully perform an action. Such an action can be anything from winning gold at the Senior Olympics, to hitting a tennis serve, to seemingly mundane but vital activities of daily living such as bringing in the groceries.[50] The loss of self-efficacy is one of the hallmarks of aging and is particularly evident in individuals who test themselves in athletics. The bunkers one used to clear, the fly balls one used to run down, or the peleton in which one used to ride seemingly become unattainable overnight. Thus, one of the keys to caring for aging athletes is to help

them periodically reassess their goals (ie, balance the risk/reward portfolio) regarding their activities. McAuley et al[50] looked at previously inactive subjects with a mean age of 65 years. Most made initial improvements in self-efficacy in the 6-month study period, and affect improved during the physical activity. Despite this, many seniors stopped doing the activity when they were no longer directed. This is the opposite problem from what is seen in most masters athletes, for whom not being able to participate in their exercise program or seeing a diminution in their abilities is a source of anxiety. One charge for doctors caring for these patients is to help them maintain a high level of physiologic and psychologic skill in the face of injury and progressive change. This would also be a time to enlist the help of therapists, trainers, and possibly a sport psychologist to participate in the care of these patients.

Loss of fitness and performance is not just a function of physiology but often is a matter of decreasing interest or a change of emphasis. We see these same changes in younger athletes, but on a different scale. Such losses can be due to decreased competitiveness, injury, cognition, or intrinsic motivation; or they may be caused by family and job pressures.[4,28,51] Certainly anything that interferes with aggressive training will have an effect on an older athlete's performance, just as young athletes must maintain a high level of intense training for top results. Diminishing motivation for physical activity with aging is not unique to human beings; it is also seen, for example, in insects, rodents, and the family dog. This loss of motivation may be due in part to cognitive changes that accompany the changes in cardiovascular, musculoskeletal, and other physical systems.[29]

As any physician knows from observing family, friends, and patients, aging is a complex biosocial and personal process that does not inevitably bring uniform deteriorating physical changes, although certainly after the age of 30 the general trend is downward. Sports can bring psychosocial well-being and social connectedness that reinforce the participant's commitment and can alleviate many of the health conditions that accompany old age.[34] For example, one study found that Australian golfers seemed to enjoy the game more when they changed their competitive attitudes toward golf, with the result that their game did not deteriorate significantly.[35] A similar positive change of attitude was seen in a study of Italian cyclists. These athletes continued a tradition of long rides through the seasons, noting that their attention to physical activity carried over to their diet and a generally healthier lifestyle. This added up to a life of improved physical and mental well-being.[34] Although they could not ride as fast as they once could, knowing the course, refining their technique, and participating consistently led to self-efficacy, not just during sport, but in all aspects of their lives.

The Psychology of Recovery

Many people see athletics as their ticket to a longer life, but not everyone views sports participation so pragmatically. An intense competitive drive can be present at all ages, even at the masters level. Many patients will roll their eyes if you suggest that during recovery they consider bridge, chess, or billiards. For these patients, competition at a high physical level seems to be as crucial to their sense of well-being as the physical outlet. Many famous athletes (for example, Michael Jordan, Lance Armstrong, and Brett Favre) clearly compete because they love the way competing in athletics makes them feel, both mentally and physically. Many higher level athletes continue to participate in sports after their professional athletic careers are over, even if just on a recreational level.[52,53]

Part of the physician's job is to recognize and educate patients in the muscle qualities that lead to health (balance, coordination, strength, flexibility, endurance, speed, and quickness). Although alternative activities may not satisfy the competitive urge, they still can fulfill physical needs. Pilates, yoga, water aerobics, cycling, swimming, golf, and other "soft" workouts are all great substitutes for or, better still, additions to the more pounding activities that wear down the body as we age. To make these alternatives more appealing, rather than telling a runner with arthritis to dust off the old bike stored in the back of the garage, the physician might recommend looking into the great new technologies available, from lightweight bikes to computers providing calorie and heart rate information to perspiration-wicking clothing. It is in the best interest of these patients to have the best experience possible so they will enjoy the sport and thus continue the activity. No one would go for another hike if the first one was to the bottom of the Grand Canyon in sneakers! Properly

fitting high-quality equipment, attention to safety precautions, coaching or lessons from a professional, and a personal trainer to modify the program are all keys to getting a patient to commit to a new fitness program to attain the psychologic benefits without incurring physical harm. The mature athlete must work *smarter* to achieve the same goals that were achieved when younger. Healthcare providers must continually help patients rebalance the portfolio of injury risk and fun.

Discussion

Participating in any physical activity carries the risk of injury, but this risk appears to be offset by the positive psychologic and physical gains. With proper exercise, older patients show greater aerobic power, strength, and flexibility than do people 10 to 20 years younger.[2] Such changes invariably have an effect on the psyche of the aging athlete. Although the proportion of elderly individuals in developed countries continues to increase, the fitness revolution has not attracted everyone. Health care providers should encourage such behavior, as it will ultimately save substantial healthcare dollars, particularly as the baby boomer generation ages. There is good evidence that a habit of exercise that is established at a young age will carry into adulthood.[33,41,54,55] Physicians should help expedite this attainment of overall health while discouraging behavior that might undermine this goal, by encouraging patients to avoid obvious risk and discouraging participation in marathons after joint arthroplasties or return to cutting sports after multiple knee ligament reconstructions. The attitude that "when something breaks, we just fix it," has become fashionable but does not ultimately promote physical or psychologic health.[56] The goal of healthcare providers should be to keep the patient active and upright, but not to the point of harm. It is good medicine to talk to all patients about pursuing alternative activities as they age, but particularly the athletes whose identities are wrapped up in sports.

Unfortunately, "aging gracefully" has not just been promoted by modern medicine as a way to maintain health; it also has been championed by Madison Avenue to sell products. The question must be asked if an activity is being done for health, enjoyment, and entertainment or because of a strong advertising campaign. Risks are inherent in any type of physical activity, but healthcare providers should be able to recommend ways to keep these risks to a minimum. Societal pressures (or pressure from grandchildren!) can encourage individuals to engage in behavior that goes beyond healthy activity and toward behavior that perhaps no person should undertake, and certainly not a senior citizen.[57] These less healthy motivations can lead to not only serious injury but also decreased psychologic motivation because of fear or, often, simply lack of fun. Moreover, overcommitted masters athletes also may fail to find pleasure in their activities.[20] Thus, the physiology, psychology, and sociology of aging and injury are intertwined.

One question that has not been addressed in the literature is just who the aging athlete is. Are these the same people who were active in youth and continued into adulthood, or are a significant proportion relatively new converts to their sports because they now have more time and resources? Contrarily, many people simply eschew almost all forms of exercise. Is this due to psychology or physiology? In other words, are there specific physiologies that enjoy exercise more? We know that all animals, including humans, need some form of activity; thus, should we find something for these "less active physiologies" to do in order to access the health benefits of movement into old age? What would such a program look like? Such questions will be answered as more studies are done on the baby boomer generation and are important for the medical practitioner to keep in mind when dealing with these patients.

Competing in sports into old age has obvious health advantages. Another advantage of competing as a mature athlete is that age categories apply. As a result, one sees golfers coming out of retirement to complete on the champions' (senior) tour. Cyclists, runners, and triathletes look forward to the birthday that allows them to participate in the higher age group. They might not be able to beat their 20-year-old rivals to the finish line, but once the field is leveled by age, one's sense of self-efficacy and achievement can soar.

A final intangible but no less real benefit of staying active into old age is the pride one derives from having friends and family bragging about what "Uncle Artie can do at the age of 80" (although Artie might point out he's closer to 85!). Human beings not only have the need to perform their activities of daily living but also

have a psychologic desire to stay active. Older athletes take these primitive drives a step further by participating at a competitive level, and they lead happier, healthier lives because of it. Although motivations can further extend to sociologic and aesthetic, they need to be generally encouraged by the medical community—with the caveats discussed previously.[58] Retirement from the workplace is often accompanied by a sense of decline and uselessness.[34] Exercise and competition help people deal with feelings of social isolation, role changes, declining fitness, loss of productivity, and myriad other emotions.[59] As the US population ages and society recognizes these changes, plans should be made to encourage healthy behavior by building bicycle and walking paths, providing public transportation to senior centers, and developing other ways to keep seniors active, productive members of society.[60,61] Although the last generation of doctors said "If it hurts, don't do it," most of us now would say "If it feels good, continue to do it." Twenty-two percent of Americans already have made exercise a habit.[25] The physical and emotional benefits these people are receiving should be respected by physicians, who should find ways to help them continue.[62] Perhaps a harder task is figuring out why, with all of the obvious benefits of exercise, it is so difficult to get the other 78% on board.

References

1. Brewer BW: Review and critique of models of psychological adjustment to athletic injury. *J Appl Sport Psychol* 1994;6:87-100.

2. Doyle T: *2007-1998 Participation by 45-54 Yr Olds.* National Sporting Goods Association. http://www.nsga.org/i4a/pages/index.cfm?pageid=4133. Accessed March 9, 2011.

3. Arent SM, Landers DM, Etnier JL: The effects of exercise on mood in older adults: A meta-analytic view. *J Aging Phys Act* 2000;8:407-430.

4. Tanaka H, Seals DR: Invited review: Dynamic exercise performance in Masters athletes. Insight into the effects of primary human aging on physiological functional capacity. *J Appl Physiol* 2003;95(5):2152-2162.

5. Roberts R: Getting their game on: Why should kids have all the fun? Adults are getting back in the game and taking to sports fields. *Parks Recreat* March 2009:23-26.

6. Heil J: Sport psychology, the athlete at risk, and the sports medicine team, in Heil J, ed: *Psychology of Sport Injury*. Champaign, IL, Human Kinetics, 1993, pp 1-13.

7. Brewer BW, Linder DE, Phelps CM: Situational correlates of emotional adjustment to athletic injury. *Clin J Sport Med* 1995;5(4):241-245.

8. Nicholas JA, Friedman MJ: Orthopaedic problems in middle-aged athletes. *Phys Sportsmed* 1979;7:39-46.

9. Wright VJ, Perricelli BC: Age-related rates of decline in performance among elite senior athletes. *Am J Sports Med* 2008;36(3):443-450.

10. Haveman-Nies A, de Groot LC, van Staveren WA: Dietary quality, lifestyle factors and healthy ageing in Europe: The SENECA study. *Age Ageing* 2003;32(4):427-434.

11. Bailey M, McLaren S: Physical activity alone and with others as predictors of sense of belonging and mental health in retirees. *Aging Ment Health* 2005;9(1):82-90.

12. Kolt GS, Driver RP, Giles LC: Why older Australians participate in exercise and sport. *J Aging Phys Act* 2004;12(2):185-198.

13. Parkkari J, Kannus P, Natri A, et al: Active living and injury risk. *Int J Sports Med* 2004;25(3):209-216.

14. Hubert HB, Fries JF: Predictors of physical disability after age 50: Six-year longitudinal study in a runners club and a university population *Am Epidemiol* 1994;4(4)285-294.

15. Maharam LG, Bauman PA, Kalman D, Skolnik H, Perle SM: Masters athletes: Factors affecting performance. *Sports Med* 1999;28(4):273-285.

16. Hall D: *Life Work*. Boston, MA, Beacon Press, 1993, p 31.

17. Blair SN, Kohl HW III, Paffenbarger RS Jr, Clark DG, Cooper KH, Gibbons LW: Physical fitness and all-cause mortality: A prospective study of healthy men and women. *JAMA* 1989;262(17):2395-2401.

18. Laukkanen P, Kauppinen M, Heikkinen E: Physical activity as a predictor of health and disability in 75- and 80-year old men and women: A five year longitudinal study. *J Aging Phys Act* 1998;6:141-156.

19. Folkins CH, Sime WE: Physical fitness training and mental health. *Am Psychol* 1981;36(4):373-389.

20. Menard D, Stanish WD: The aging athlete. *Am J Sports Med* 1989;17(2):187-196.

21. White SH: G. Stanley Hall: From philosophy to developmental psychology, in Parke RD, Ornstein PA, Rieser JJ, Zahn-Waxler C, eds: *A Century of Developmental Psychology*. Washington, DC, American Psychological Association, 1994, pp 103-125.

22. Stathi A, Fox KR, McKenna J: Physical activity and dimensions of subjective well-being in older adults. *J Aging Phys Act* 2002;10:76-92.

23. Camacho TC, Roberts RE, Lazarus NB, Kaplan GA, Cohen RD: Physical activity and depression: Evidence from the Alameda County Study. *Am J Epidemiol* 1991;134(2):220-231.

24. Davis-Berman J: Physical self-efficacy, perceived physical status, and depressive symptomatology in older adults. *J Psychol* 1990;124(2):207-215.

25. Lieberman DE: Human evolution, endurance running and injury. *Joseph B. Wolffe Memorial Lecture, ACSM 56th Annual Meeting*. Seattle, WA, 2009.

26. O'Neill DF: Injury contagion in alpine ski racing: The effect of injury on teammates' performance. *J Clin Sport Psychol* 2008;2:278-292.

27. Weyerer S, Eifflaender-Gorfer S, Köhler L, et al: Prevalence and risk factors for depression in non-demented primary care attenders aged 75 years and older. *J Affect Disord* 2008;111(2-3):153-163.

28. Tanaka H, Seals DR: Endurance exercise performance in Masters athletes: Age-associated changes and underlying physiological mechanisms. *J Physiol* 2008;586(1):55-63.

29. Hogan MH: Physical and cognitive activity and exercise for older adults: A review. *Int J Aging Hum Dev* 2005;60(2):95-126.

30. Trappe SW, Costill DL, Vukovich MD, Jones J, Melham T: Aging among elite distance runners: A 22-yr longitudinal study. *J Appl Psysiol* 1996;80(1):285-290.

31. Jokl P, Sethi PM, Cooper AJ: Master's performance in the New York City Marathon 1983-1999. *Br J Sports Med* 2004;38(4):408-412.

32. Morley JE: The aging athlete. *J Gerontol A Biol Sci Med Sci* 2000;55(11):M627-M629.

33. Morgan WP, Costill DL: Selected psychological characteristics and health behaviors of aging marathon runners: A longitudinal study. *Int J Sports Med* 1996;17(4):305-312.

34. Whitaker ED: The bicycle makes the eyes smile: Exercise, aging, and psychophysical well-being in older Italian cyclists. *Med Anthropol* 2005;24(1):1-43.

35. Over R, Thomas P: Age and skilled psychomotor performance: A comparison of younger and older golfers . *Int J Aging Hum Dev* 1995;41(1):1-12.

36. Schulz R, Musa D, Staszewski J, Siegler RS: The relationship between age and major league baseball performance: Implications for development. *Psychol Aging* 1994;9(2):274-286.

37. Seeman TE, Berkman LF, Charpentier PA, Blazer DG, Albert MS, Tinetti ME: Behavioral and psychosocial predictors of physical performance: MacArthur studies of successful aging. *J Gerontol A Biol Sci Med Sci* 1995;50(4):M177-M183.

38. Martin JC, Farrar RP, Wagner BM, Spirduso WW: Maximal power across the lifespan. *J Gerontol A Biol Sci Med Sci* 2000;55(6):M311-M316.

39. Gould D, Urdy E, Bridges D, Beck L: Stress sources encountered when rehabilitating from season-ending ski injuries. *Sport Psychol* 1997;11:361-378.

40. Brewer BW, Van Raalte J, Linder DE: Athletic identity: Hercules' muscle or Achilles heel? *Int J Sport Psychol* 1993;24:237-254.

41. Marks BL: Health benefits for veteran (senior) tennis players. *Br J Sports Med* 2006;40(5):469-476.

42. Gould D, Urdy E, Bridges D, Beck L: Coping with season-ending injuries. *Sport Psychol* 1997;11:379-399.

43. Smith AM, Scott SG, Wiese DM: The psychological effects of sports injuries: Coping. *Sports Med* 1990;9(6):352-369.

44. Wiese-Bjornstal DM, Smith AM, Shaffer SM, Morrey MA: An integrated model of response to sport injury: Psychological and sociological dynamics. *J Appl Sport Psychol* 1998;10:46-69.

45. Johnston LH, Carroll D: Coping, social support, and injury: Changes over time and the effects of level of sports involvement. *J Sport Rehabil* 2000;9(4):290-300.

46. Tedrick T: Seniors set sights on staying competitive. *National Recreation and Parks Association.* http://www.nrpa.org/content/default.aspx?documentId=1404. Accessed April 22, 2009.

47. O'Neill DF: *Knee Surgery: The Essential Guide to Total Knee Recovery.* St. Martin's Press, New York, NY, 2009, pp 171-196.

48. Bianco T, Malo S, Orlick T: Sport injury and illness: Elite skiers describe their experiences. *Res Q Exerc Sport* 1999;70(2):157-169.

49. Bandura A: Self-efficacy: Toward a unifying theory of behavioral change. *Psychol Rev* 1977;84(2):191-215.

50. McAuley E, Jerome GJ, Marquez DX, Elavsky S, Blissmer B: Exercise self-efficacy in older adults: Social, affective, and behavioral influences. *Ann Behav Med* 2003;25(1):1-7.

51. Bird S, Balmer J, Olds T, Davison RC: Differences between the sexes and age-related changes in orienteering speed. *J Sports Sci* 2001;19(4):243-252.

52. Weiss MR: Psychological aspects of sport-injury rehabilitation: A developmental perspective. *J Athl Train* 2003;38(2):172-175.

53. Brewer BW, Cornelius AE, Van Raalte JL, et al: Age-related differences in predictors of adherence to rehabilitation after anterior cruciate ligament reconstruction. *J Athl Train* 2003;38(2):158-162.

54. Bäckmand H, Kaprio J, Kujala U, Sarna S: Personality and mood of former elite male athletes—A descriptive study. *Int J Sports Med* 2001;22(3):215-221.

55. Kerr JH, Fujiyama H, Campano J: Emotion and stress in serious and hedonistic leisure sport activities. *J Leisure Res* 2002;34:272-289.

56. Sarmiento A: Is Socrates dying? *J Bone Joint Surg Am* 2008;90(3):675-676.

57. Boman S: *How Much is Too Much?* http://www.masters-athlete.com/public/93.cfm. Accessed April 22, 2008.

58. Stempel C: Adult participation sports as cultural capital: A test of Bourdieu's theory of the field of sports. *Int Rev Sociol Sport* 2005;40(4):411-432.

59. Janke M, Davey A, Kleiber D: Modeling change in older adults' leisure activities. *Leisure Sci* 2006;28: 285-303.

60. Kemperman A, Timmermans H: Influences of the built environment on walking and cycling of latent segments of the aging population. *Proceedings of the 88th Annual Meeting of the Transportation Research Board.* Washington, DC, 2009.

61. Sallis JF, Bauman A, Pratt M: Environmental and policy interventions to promote physical activity. *Am J Prev Med* 1998;15(4):379-397.

62. Orsega-Smith E, Payne LL, Godbey G: Physical and psychosocial characteristics of older adults who participate in a community-based exercise program. *J Aging Phys Act* 2003;11(4):516-531.

SECTION 3

UPPER EXTREMITY

John M. Tokish, MD
Section Editor

Chapter 14

Nonsurgical Rehabilitation Guidelines for the Mature Patient With Rotator Cuff Pathology

Kevin Wilk, PT, DPT
Leonard C. Macrina, MSPT, SCS, CSCS

Key Points

- Nonsurgical intervention for rotator cuff pathology is often used to treat impingement syndrome.
- Correct recognition and classification will assist the clinician in attaining the best outcomes.
- Rehabilitation for shoulder impingement must address multiple factors.
- Criteria-based rehabilitation allows individualization for each patient.
- The primary goals of rehabilitation are to restore pain-free range of motion (ROM) and improve strength, endurance, and function.

Portions of this chapter are adapted with permission from Reinold MM, Macrina LC, Wilk KE, Andrews JR: Rehabilitation of micro-instability, in Ellenbecker TS, ed: Shoulder Rehabilitation: Non-Operative Treatment. New York, NY, Thieme Medical Publishers, 2006. www.thieme.com.

Introduction

Shoulder impingement is often seen in the orthopaedic and sports medicine setting. The glenohumeral joint requires tremendous amounts of mobility to function, thus making it inherently unstable and prone to injuries. Furthermore, a wide range of shoulder impingements exist,[1] from subacromial impingement in the general orthopaedic patient to internal impingement, which is often observed in the overhead athlete. Often, these conditions can be treated nonsurgically. Each type of impingement occurs in different patient populations and is treated quite differently. This chapter provides an overview of the classification and mechanism of glenohumeral impingement syndrome and discusses the specific rehabilitation principles and guidelines used to treat this patient population.

Biomechanics and Pathoanatomy

Functional stability of the shoulder is achieved through the precise interaction of the static and dynamic stabilizing systems of the glenohumeral joint. Static stability is accomplished via the joint geometry, capsule, glenohumeral ligaments, and labrum. The large amount of motion required at the shoulder, particularly in the overhead athlete, may stretch the static stabilizers, demanding a greater amount of dynamic stability to remain asymptomatic. If the dynamic stabilizers are overstressed, pathology may develop.

The underlying causes of rotator cuff pathology, listed in **Table 1**, may

Table 1: Classification of Rotator Cuff Disease

Primary compressive disease

Instability with secondary compressive disease

Primary tensile overload

Tensile overload due to capsular instability

Rotator cuff tear

Primary internal impingement

Calcific tendinitis

PASTA (partial articular-sided tendon avulsion) lesion

PAINT (partial articular tear with intratendinous extension) lesion

Secondary internal impingement with primary hypermobility

Secondary tensile overload with primary hypermobility

be classified in various ways. Primary compressive rotator cuff pathology has been recognized by numerous authors;[1-4] it also may be a source of subacromial impingement. This is the most common form of rotator cuff pathology in the general orthopaedic population. Rockwood et al[5] defined this as encroachment of the rotator cuff on the acromion, coracoacromial ligament, coracoid process, and/or the acromioclavicular (AC) joint during flexion and rotation. It is believed that the rotator cuff lesion is an extra-articular failure of the tendon caused by repetitive compressive loads.[4] Symptoms commonly associated with this pathology include pain with active elevation that worsens with repetitive overhead movements. Primary structural factors that may contribute to the onset of rotator cuff impingement may differ in clinical presentation. Oftentimes, the patient may have a hooked acromion that is detectable on plain radiographs. This hooked acromion is the result of repetitive loading of the acromion in which a bone spur eventually develops and decreases the subacromial space. The AC joint also may be a source of impingement of the rotator cuff. Bone spurs can develop along the inferior aspect as a result of chronic,

repetitive stresses or from a previous sprain and additionally narrow the subacromial space.[3,4]

Secondary factors also may contribute to development of subacromial impingement. Issues of capsular hypomobility or hypermobility may result in altered glenohumeral arthrokinematics.[6-8] The altered mechanics may overstress the surrounding soft-tissue structures, particularly the rotator cuff, and cause tendinopathy. The position of the scapula on the rib cage also has been implicated as a source of glenohumeral dysfunction.[9-13] The term *scapular dyskinesis* describes an alteration in the normal position or motion of the scapula during coupled scapulohumeral movements.[11] An altered scapular position may contribute to pathology of the rotator cuff, bursa, and surrounding structures. Rehabilitation is directed toward improving the position of the scapula and allowing a normal scapulohumeral coupling motion, particularly with overhead movements.

Dynamic stability is achieved through the precise neuromuscular interaction of the force couples of the rotator cuff and the shoulder musculature.[8,14] Inman et al[15] described two force couples of the glenohumeral joint. The first force couple involves the subscapularis and the posterior rotator cuff, which is composed of the infraspinatus and teres minor. The second force couple of the glenohumeral joint involves the deltoid and the entire rotator cuff complex. These force couples are active throughout the entire range of shoulder motion and provide a dynamic symmetry of joint forces.[8]

Speer and Garrett[16] described the force couples of the glenohumeral joint differently, as including the prime movers of the shoulder counterbalanced by the combined effects of the rotator cuff musculature. The larger prime mover muscles move the shoulder and position the upper extremity, and the rotator cuff steers and compresses the humeral head into the glenoid fossa to avoid detrimental translation from the shear forces produced by the deltoid and other large muscles.[17]

Thus, the role of the surrounding glenohumeral musculature in dynamic stabilization is multifactorial. The precise interaction of the anterior and posterior rotator cuff musculature as well as the prime movers and the stabilizing rotator cuff musculature is vital for normal glenohumeral arthrokinematics. Muscle weakness or strength imbalances may have a deleterious

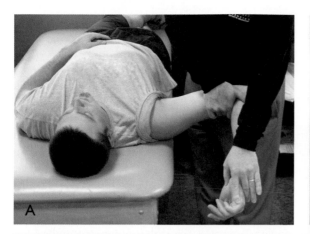 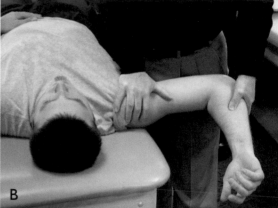

Figure 1   A, Internal impingement sign indicative of posterior rotator cuff tendinitis. **B,** Relocation maneuver, in which a posteriorly directed force is applied to determine if the symptoms are due to excessive anterior translation.

effect on shoulder mechanics. Posterior rotator cuff weakness is commonly observed in patients with various types of glenohumeral impingement.[18] The need for greater motion in the shoulder, compared with a more stable joint like the hip, requires the dynamic stabilizers to perform efficiently, particularly near the available end range of motion, where static stability is most compromised.

Finally, mature overhead athletes with microinstability often present with internal impingement. Meister et al[19] originally described the internal impingement sign, in which the patient is positioned supine with the humerus at 90° of abduction (**Figure 1**, *A*). The examiner passively rotates the shoulder into maximal external rotation until symptoms are elicited. Rather than feeling symptoms in the anterior aspect of the shoulder, which is common in patients with classic impingement, the patient with internal impingement will have symptoms located specifically over the posterosuperior aspect of the shoulder. A relocation maneuver is then performed while the shoulder is in maximal external rotation. The examiner provides a posterior force to relocate the humeral head within the glenoid. If this effectively alleviates symptoms, the relocation maneuver is positive, suggesting that the symptoms were related to anterior translation (**Figure 1**, *B*).

Rehabilitation Program for Overhead Patients With Impingement

Rehabilitation for shoulder impingement must address the multiple factors that cause the impingement, so an accurate diagnosis of all contributing factors is key to a successful outcome. The clinician must systematically progress the patient through a functional rehabilitation. The rehabilitation process for patients with glenohumeral impingement must restore range of motion, muscular strength, and endurance, as well as gradually restore proprioception, dynamic stability, and neuromuscular control. As the patient advances, sport-specific drills are emphasized to prepare for a gradual return to competition through an interval sport program. Neuromuscular control drills are performed throughout and advanced as the athlete progresses to provide continuous challenges to the dynamic stabilizers and neuromuscular system. This section provides an overview of a functional rehabilitation progression for patients with rotator cuff impingement that incorporates the previously discussed principles and guidelines. The program is divided into four separate phases: the acute phase, the intermediate phase, the advanced phase, and the return to activity phase. Each has specific goals and criteria to be met before advancing to the next phase. The use of a criteria-based rehabilitation pro-

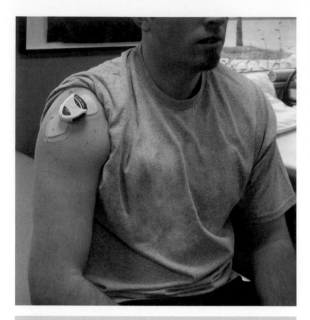

Figure 2 Iontophoresis is applied to the supraspinatus tendon to decrease inflammation.

gram allows for individualization to each patient. It is imperative to modify the program based on the extent of the particular pathology. Alterations in exercise activities, positioning, and rate of progression are based on the type of injury, healing constraints, and the tissues that are being stressed during rehabilitation.

Acute Phase

The acute phase of rehabilitation begins immediately following the injury or when symptoms arise. The duration of the acute phase is dependent on the healing constraints of the involved pathologic tissues and the degree of the injury. The initial goals of the acute phase are to diminish pain and inflammation, normalize motion and muscular balance, and restore baseline proprioception and kinesthetic awareness.

The patient usually presents with pain and inflammation as a result of bursitis. A chronic, persistent pain lasting weeks to months is usually a result of tendinosis. The clinician must distinguish each presentation to develop the proper plan of care, including the choice of modalities to use. The application of ice or cold therapy is the most common modality used by clinicians treating acute rotator cuff injuries. Clinically, the primary

goal of cryotherapy is the prevention of swelling by blocking the histamine response and impeding edematous fluids from building up at the injury site as well as any secondary injury that may have occurred due to surrounding tissue hypoxia. The body's response to cryotherapy application includes vasoconstriction, decreased cellular metabolism and temperature, decreased peripheral nerve conduction, and a decrease in pain. An adjunct modality that may be used for an acute injury is iontophoresis (**Figure 2**). Iontophoresis involves the delivery of a charged medication through the skin and into underlying tissue by using direct-current electrical stimulation. Glass et al[20] reported the depth of penetration of dexamethasone with iontophoresis to be 13 to 18 mm in the hip region. Gangarosa et al[21] reported a 1- to 3-cm depth of penetration of lidocaine. A recent study performed by Anderson et al[22] showed the depth of penetration of dexamethasone using iontophoresis to be 12 mm following administration of a standard dose.

For more chronic issues involving the shoulder, moist heat is often used. Through conduction, moist heat is capable of reaching subcutaneous tissues to a depth of 1 cm or less. The application of heat causes vasodilation with resultant increases in local circulation, thus increasing oxygen and nutrients delivered to the area. Another option in treating chronic rotator cuff pathologies is therapeutic ultrasound, a deep heating modality that penetrates tissue deeper than superficial hot packs or warm whirlpools.

One of the primary goals during the acute phase is to normalize total motion bilaterally. This often requires the addition of passive range-of-motion and flexibility exercises for internal and external rotation in a restricted range of motion based on the theory that motion assists in the enhancement and organization of collagen tissue, stimulates joint mechanoreceptors, and may assist in the neuromodulation of pain. The rehabilitation program should allow for progressive applied loads, beginning with gentle passive range of motion. Active-assisted range-of-motion exercises are performed by the patient and can include using a cane or L-Bar (Breg, Vista, CA) for flexion, external rotation, and internal rotation. As the patient advances, flexion progresses as tolerated and shoulder rotation range of motion is progressed from 0° of abduction to 30°, 45°, and 90° of abduction. Also, pendulum and rope-and-pulley exer-

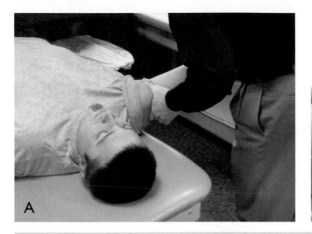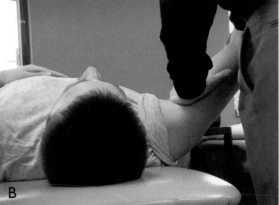

Figure 3 Joint mobilization. **A,** Inferior glide. **B,** Posterior glide.

cises may be used as needed to facilitate additional motion.

The clinician also should assess joint mobility, as this can be a cause of range-of-motion loss, pain, and shoulder tightness. An arthrokinematic assessment may reveal a pathologic condition in which excessive tightness on one side of the capsule,[8] particularly the inferior aspect, may result in superior migration of the humeral head. With this finding, the goal of rehabilitation is to balance the capsule through joint mobilization, self-performed stretching of the capsule, and gentle passive range of motion. Joint mobilization techniques should focus on restoring the normal amount of capsular laxity. Careful attention should also be paid to the anterior aspect of the shoulder because the pectoralis major and minor can become tight, which can alter the scapulohumeral rhythm. The inferior capsule mobility must be restored to ensure normal and asymptomatic shoulder range of motion (**Figure 3,** *A*). Posterior capsular hypomobility also exists, although we anecdotally observe this less frequently than most other capsular contractions. The clinician uses a posterolateral force with the mobilization technique to allow the humeral head to clear the posterior rim of the glenoid and allow true capsular stretching to occur (**Figure 3,** *B*). Because of the natural version of the glenoid, a true posterior force would result only in the humeral head abutting the posterior glenoid rim, a hard end-feel, and an incorrect assessment and treatment of this portion of the capsule.

Strengthening begins with submaximal, pain-free isometrics for shoulder flexion, extension, abduction, external rotation, internal rotation, and elbow flexion. Isometrics are used to slow or prevent muscular atrophy and restore voluntary muscular control while avoiding detrimental shoulder forces. Isometrics should be performed at multiple angles throughout the available range of motion. Particular emphasis is placed on contraction at the end of the currently available range of motion.

Intermediate Phase

The intermediate phase begins once the patient has regained near-normal passive motion and sufficient muscular strength of the shoulder. The goals of the intermediate phase are to enhance functional dynamic stability, re-establish neuromuscular control, restore muscular strength and balance, and maintain full range of motion.

Range-of-motion exercises are continued and the patient is encouraged to perform active-assisted range of motion with a cane or L-Bar to maintain motion. Joint mobility is continually assessed and joint mobilizations and self-capsular stretches may be performed to prevent asymmetric glenohumeral joint capsular tightness.

Strengthening exercises are advanced to include external and internal rotation with exercise tubing at 0° of abduction and active range-of-motion exercises against gravity. These exercises initially include standing scap-

Thrower's Ten Program

The Thrower's Ten Program is designed to exercise the major muscles necessary for throwing. The Program's goal is to be an organized and concise exercise program. In addition, all exercises included are specific to the thrower and are designed to improve strength, power and endurance of the shoulder complex musculature.

1A. Diagonal Pattern D2 Extension: Involved hand will grip tubing handle overhead and out to the side. Pull tubing down and across your body to the opposite side of leg. During the motion, lead with your thumb. Perform _____ sets of _____ repetitions _____ daily.

1B. Diagonal Pattern D2 Flexion: Gripping tubing handle in hand of involved arm, begin with arm out from side 45° and palm facing backward. After turning palm forward, proceed to flex elbow and bring arm up and over involved shoulder. Turn palm down and reverse to take arm to starting position. Exercise should be performed _____ sets of _____ repetitions _____ daily.

2A. External Rotation at 0° Abduction: Stand with involved elbow fixed at side, elbow at 90° and involved arm across front of body. Grip tubing handle while the other end of tubing is fixed. Pull out arm, keeping elbow at side. Return tubing slowly and controlled. Perform _____ sets of _____ repetitions _____ times daily.

2B. Internal Rotation at 0° Abduction: Standing with elbow at side fixed at 90° and shoulder rotated out. Grip tubing handle while other end of tubing is fixed. Pull arm across body keeping elbow at side. Return tubing slowly and controlled. Perform _____ sets of _____ repetitions _____ times daily.

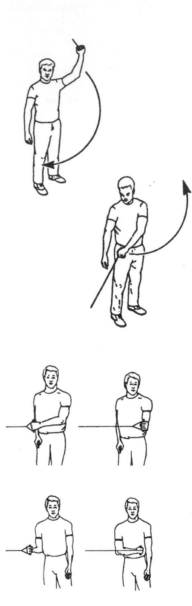

Figure 4   The Thrower's Ten Program, used to improve strength of the shoulder joint complex. (Adapted with permission from Wilk KE, Obma P, Simpson CD, et al: Shoulder injuries in the overhead athlete. *J Orthop Sports Phys Ther* 2009;39(2):38-54.)

2C. (Optional) **External Rotation at 90°
Abduction:** Stand with shoulder abducted
90°. Grip tubing handle while the other end
is fixed straight ahead, slightly lower than
the shoulder. Keeping shoulder abducted,
rotate shoulder back keeping elbow at 90°.
Return tubing and hand to start position.
I. <u>Slow Speed Sets:</u> (Slow and Controlled)
Perform _____ sets of _____ repetitions
_____ times daily.
II. <u>Fast Speed Sets:</u> Perform _____ sets of
_____ repetitions _____ times daily.

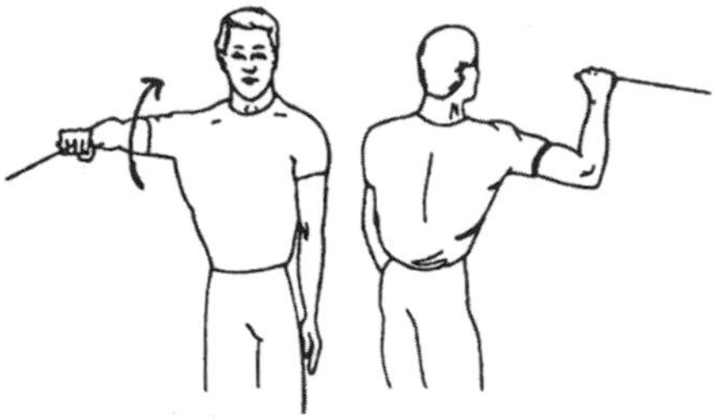

2D. (Optional) **Internal Rotation at 90°
Abduction:** Stand with shoulder abducted
to 90°, externally rotated 90° and elbow bent
to 90°. Keeping shoulder abducted, rotate
shoulder forward, keeping elbow bent at 90°.
Return tubing and hand to start position.
I. <u>Slow Speed Sets:</u> (Slow and Controlled)
Perform _____ sets of _____ repetitions
_____ times daily.
II. <u>Fast Speed Sets:</u> Perform _____ sets of
_____ repetitions _____ times daily.

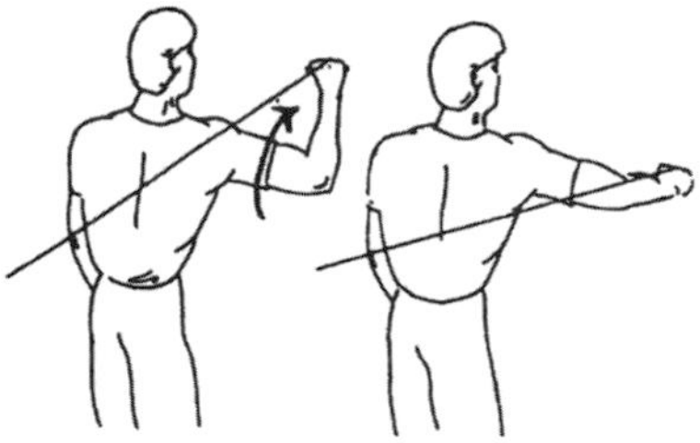

3. **Shoulder Abduction to 90°:** Stand with
arm at side, elbow straight, and palm
against side. Raise arm to the side, palm
down, until arm reaches 90° (shoulder level).
Perform _____ sets of _____ repetitions
_____ times daily.

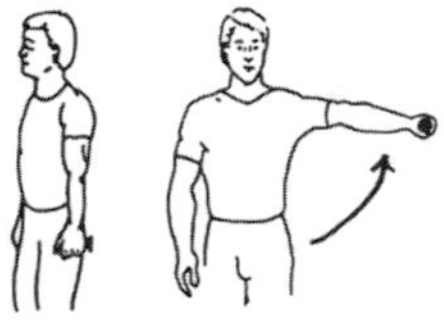

4. **Scaption, External Rotation:** Stand
with elbow straight and thumb up. Raise
arm to shoulder level at 30° angle in front of
body. Do not go above shoulder height.
Hold 2 seconds and lower slowly. Perform
_____ sets of _____ repetitions _____ times
daily.

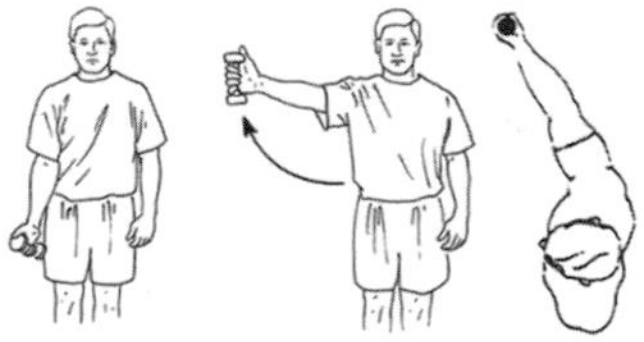

5. **Sidelying External Rotation:** Lie on
uninvolved side, with involved arm at side of
body and elbow bent to 90°. Keeping the
elbow of involved arm fixed to side, raise
arm. Hold seconds and lower slowly.
Perform _____ sets of _____ repetitions
_____ times daily.

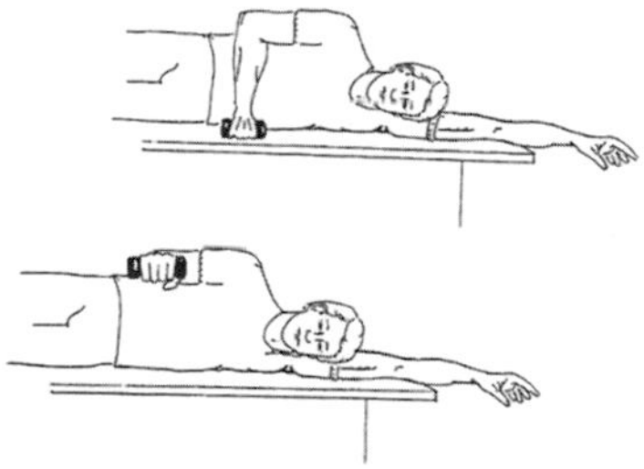

Figure 4 The Thrower's Ten Program (*continued*).

6A.   Prone   Horizontal   Abduction (Neutral): Lie on table, face down, with involved arm hanging straight to the floor, and palm facing down. Raise arm out to the side, parallel to the floor. Hold 2 seconds and lower slowly. Perform _____ sets of _____ repetitions _____ times daily.

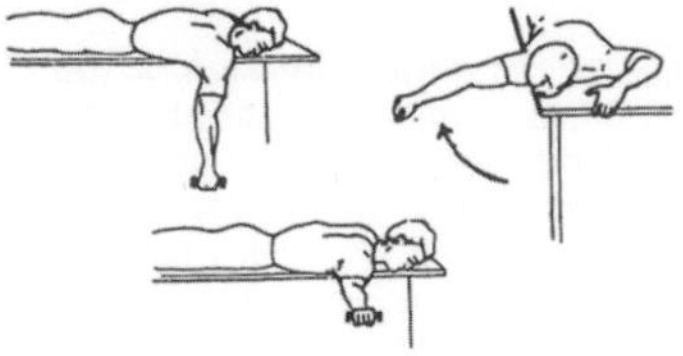

6B. Prone Horizontal Abduction (Full ER, 100° ABD): Lie on table face down, with involved arm hanging straight to the floor, and thumb rotated up (hitchhiker). Raise arm out to the side with arm slightly in front of shoulder, parallel to the floor. Hold 2 seconds and lower slowly. Perform _____ sets of _____ repetitions _____ times daily.

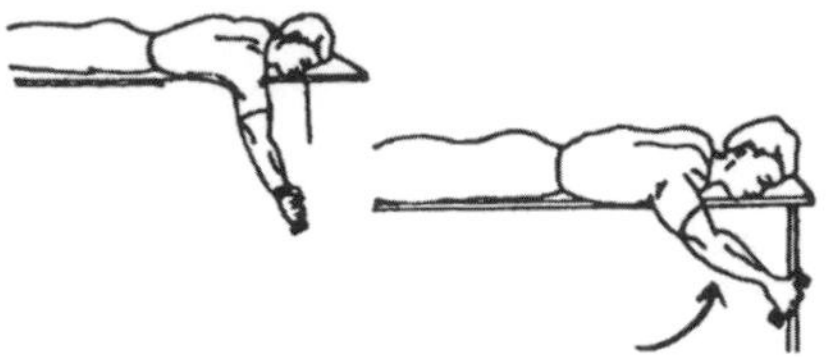

6C. Prone Rowing: Lying on your stomach with your involved arm hanging over the side of the table, dumbbell in hand and elbow straight. Slowly raise arm, bending elbow, and bring dumbbell as high as possible. Hold at the top for 2 seconds, then slowly lower. Perform _____ sets of _____ repetitions _____ times daily.

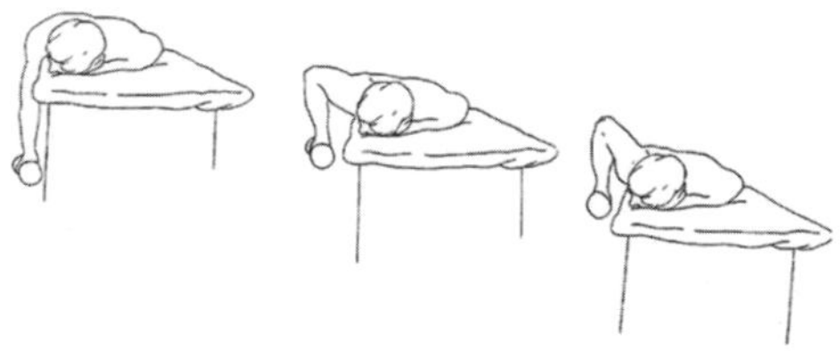

6D.   Prone   Rowing   into   External Rotation: Lying on your stomach with your involved arm hanging over the side of the table, dumbbell in hand and elbow straight. Slowly raise arm, bending elbow, up to the level of the table. Pause one second. Then rotate shoulder upward until dumbbell is even with the table, keeping elbow at 90°. Hold at the top for 2 seconds, then slowly lower taking 2 – 3 seconds. Perform _____ sets of _____ repetitions _____ times daily.

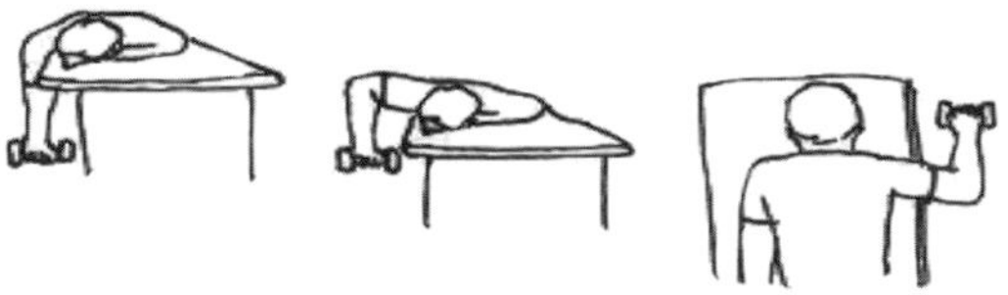

7. Press-ups: Seated on a chair or table, place both hands firmly on the sides of the chair or table, palm down and fingers pointed outward. Hands should be placed equal with shoulders. Slowly push downward through the hands to elevate your body. Hold the elevated position for 2 seconds and lower body slowly. Perform _____ sets of _____ repetitions _____ times daily.

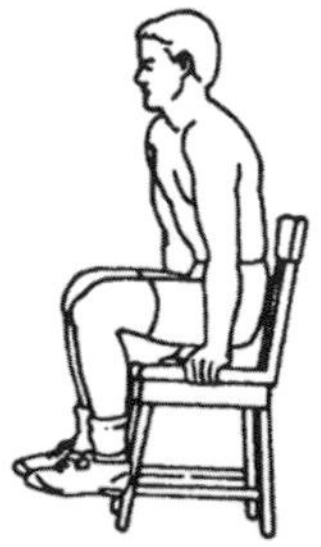

Figure 4 The Thrower's Ten Program (*continued*).

8. **Push-ups:** Start in the down position with arms in a comfortable position. Place hands no more than shoulder width apart. Push up as high as possible, rolling shoulders forward after elbows are straight. Start with a push-up into wall. Gradually progress to table top and eventually to floor as tolerable. Perform _____ sets of _____ repetitions _____ times daily.

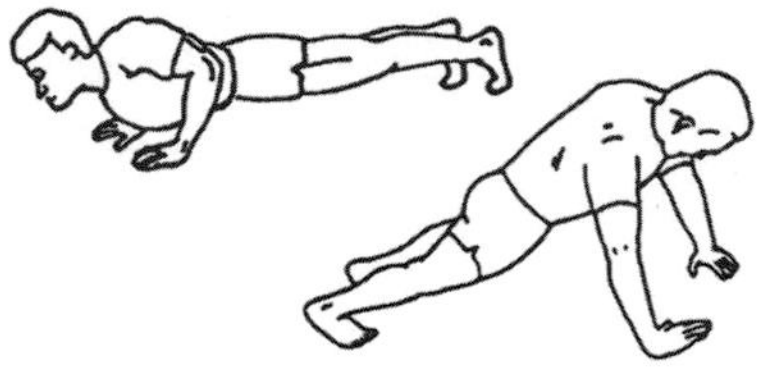

9A. **Elbow Flexion:** Standing with arm against side and palm facing inward, bend elbow upward turning palm up as you progress. Hold 2 seconds and lower slowly. Perform _____ sets of _____ repetitions _____ times daily.

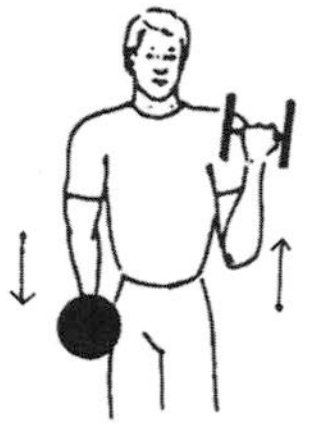

9B. **Elbow Extension (Abduction):** Raise involved arm overhead. Provide support at elbow from uninvolved hand. Straighten arm overhead. Hold 2 seconds and lower slowly. Perform _____ sets of _____ repetitions _____ times daily.

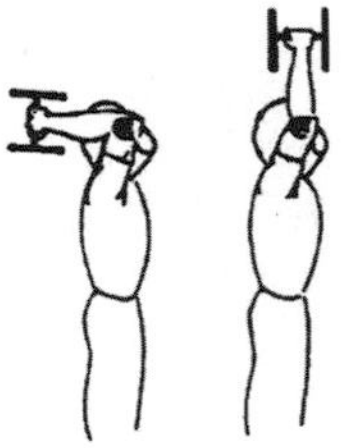

10A. **Wrist Extension:** Supporting the forearm and with palm facing downward, raise weight in hand as far as possible. Hold 2 seconds and lower slowly. Perform _____ sets of _____ repetitions _____ times daily.

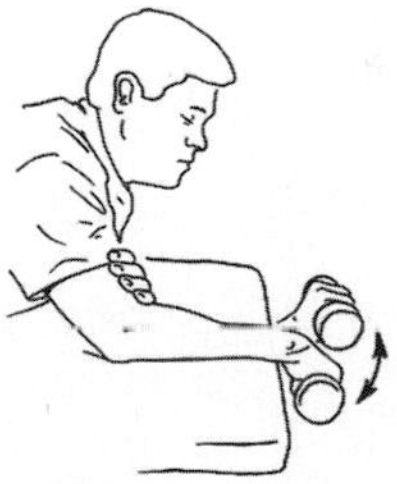

10B. **Wrist Flexion:** Supporting the forearm and with palm facing upward, lower a weight in hand as far as possible and then curl it up as high as possible. Hold for 2 seconds and lower slowly.

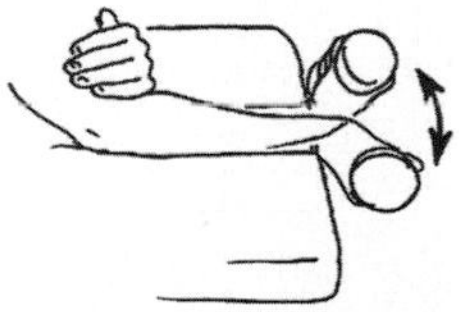

Figure 4 The Thrower's Ten Program (continued).

10C. **Supination:** Forearm supported on table with wrist in neutral position. Using a weight or hammer, roll wrist taking palm up. Hold for a 2 count and return to starting position. Perform _____ sets of _____ repetitions _____ times daily.

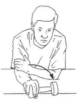

10D. **Pronation:** Forearm should be supported on a table with wrist in neutral position. Using a weight or hammer, roll wrist taking palm down. Hold for a 2 count and return to starting position. Perform _____ sets of _____ repetitions _____ times daily.

Figure 4 The Thrower's Ten Program (*continued*).

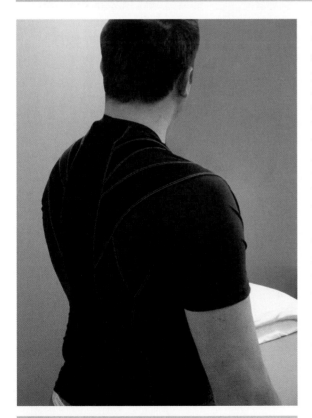

Figure 5 Scapular postural shirt.

tion in external rotation ("full can"), standing abduction, side-lying external rotation, and prone rowing. As strength returns, the program may be advanced to a program that includes full upper extremity strengthening with emphasis on posterior rotator cuff and scapular strengthening, such as the Thrower's Ten program (**Figure 4**). This program has been designed based on electromyographic studies to elicit activity of the muscles most needed to provide dynamic stability.[23,24] Although this program was designed for a younger, elite throwing population, its principles may be applied to the mature ovethead athlete with shoulder issues as well.

Scapular strengthening and neuromuscular control are also critical to regaining full dynamic stability of the glenohumeral joint. The clinician should focus on restoring normal scapular position through various strengthening techniques. Using MRI techniques, Solem-Bertoft et al[25] demonstrated an increase in subacromial space with increased scapular retraction. Lukasiewicz et al[26] analyzed scapular position and orientation in subjects with impingement and compared them with a control group. The impingement group demonstrated decreased posterior tilting and increased scapular elevation, which may indicate altered lower trapezius recruitment. We often use scapular taping or a scapular brace to reposition the scapula and to produce soft-tissue stretching as well (**Figure 5**). Kibler noted that the clinician should emphasize the retractors, depressors, and protractors during the rehabilitation progression.[10,11] We believe patients should initially focus on the scapular retractors and depressors. Exercises to improve middle trapezius function may include prone horizontal abduction and seated rowing.[27] To improve lower trapezius function, the clinician should include a prone full-can exercise, side-lying scapular depression, and wall pushes with retraction.[23,26-29] Several authors have reported that neuromuscular control of the glenohumeral joint may be negatively affected by joint pathology. A decrease in neuromuscular control has also been associated with muscular fatigue. Carpenter et al[30] investigated the ability to detect passive motion of shoulders positioned in 90° of abduction and 90° of external rotation. The authors measured a decrease in detection of both internal and external rotation movement following an isokinetic fatigue protocol. Voight et al[31] examined joint angle replication following an isokinetic fatigue protocol. A significant decrease in accuracy of both active and passive joint angle reproduction was reported following muscle fatigue. Myers et al[32] studied the effects of fatigue using the active angle-reproduction test. The authors reported that fatigue of the shoulder rotators resulted in decreased accuracy at both the midrange and end range of motion. Lower extremity, core, and trunk strength are critical to efficiently perform upper extremity activities by transferring and dissipating forces in a coordinated fashion. Core stabilization drills are used to further enhance proximal stability with distal mobility of the upper extremity. Core stabilization is used, based on the kinetic chain concept in which imbalance within any point of the kinetic chain may result in pathology throughout. Performing movement patterns such as throwing requires a precise interaction of the entire body kinetic chain. An imbalance of strength, flexibility, endurance, or stability may result in fatigue, abnormal arthrokinematics, and subsequent compensation. Therefore, full lower extremity strengthening and core stabilization activities are also performed during the intermediate phase. Basic exercises such as abdominal crunches and pelvic tilts are initiated during the late acute to early intermediate phase and progressed to include crunches with an altered center of gravity and with medicine ball throws.

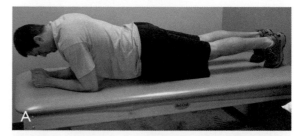

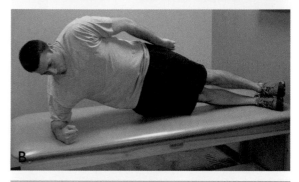

Figure 6   Core and scapular stabilization exercises. **A,** Prone bilateral planks. **B,** Side-lying unilateral planks.

Double- and single-leg balance exercises on unstable surfaces such as foam or a balance beam also are performed. Prone and side-lying planks (**Figure 6**) also may be included to further strengthen the patient's core musculature while also forcing the patient to dynamically stabilize in a closed kinetic chain position. As core stability progresses, upper extremity movement and medicine ball throws may be included to alter the athlete's center of gravity and train the athlete to control unexpected forces.

Advanced Phase

During the advanced phase of rehabilitation, full motion and capsular mobility are maintained through range of motion and self-stretching techniques, including manual stretching and L-Bar exercises. Specific emphasis is placed on ensuring that total motion remains equal bilaterally as the patient progresses throughout the rehabilitation program.

The focus of rehabilitation includes activities to improve collagen regeneration and alignment. Modalities to promote a heating effect and improve blood flow

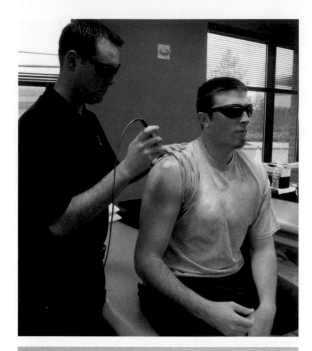

Figure 7   Laser treatment is applied to the shoulder to increase cellular activity and promote healing.

such as continuous ultrasound, hot packs, and tranverse friction massage are often used. Tendon loading by eccentric exercise and strength training has been shown to improve results in this patient population by increasing collagen synthesis[33] and realigning fiber orientation.[34-36] Other modalities, such as cold laser therapy[37-40] (**Figure 7**) and extracorporeal shock wave therapy,[41-43] have shown promising results as well.

Strengthening exercises, including the Thrower's Ten program as well as exercises for the lower extremities and trunk, are continued with a gradual increase in resistance. Exercises such as internal and external rotation with exercise tubing at 90° of abduction may be progressed to also incorporate eccentric and high-speed contractions.

Aggressive strengthening of the upper body also may be initiated, depending on the needs of the individual patient. Common exercises include isotonic weight machine exercises such as bench press, seated row, and latissimus dorsi pull-downs within a restricted range of motion. During bench press and seated row exercises, the patient is instructed to not extend the upper ex-

tremities beyond the plane of the body, to minimize stress on the shoulder capsule. Latissimus dorsi pull-downs are performed in front of the head, and the athlete is instructed to avoid full extension of the arms to minimize the amount of traction force applied to the upper extremities.

Dynamic stabilization and neuromuscular control drills are progressed to include reactive neuromuscular control drills and functional, sport-specific positions. Concentric and eccentric manual resistance may be applied as the athlete performs external rotation with exercise tubing with the arm at 0° of abduction. Rhythmic stabilizations may be included at end range to challenge the athlete to stabilize against the force of the tubing as well as the therapist. Lower extremity and core strengthening and stability are continued. Exercises are progressed to provide further challenge and to include sport-specific positions. An unstable surface such as a stability ball or a balance beam may be used while performing upper extremity isotonic, manual resistance, and plyometric exercises to challenge core stability.

Near the end of the advanced phase, the patient may begin basic sport-specific drills, if that is part of his or her individual goals. Various activities such as underweight and overweight medicine ball throwing may be performed to simulate a more functional activity.

Return to Activity Phase

Upon completion of the previously outlined rehabilitation program and a successful evaluation of the shoulder, the patient may begin the final phase of the rehabilitation program, the return to activity phase. Specific findings on clinical examination that are required before beginning an interval sport program include minimal reports of pain or tenderness; full range of motion; balanced capsular mobility; adequate proprioception, dynamic stabilization, and neuromuscular control; and full muscular strength and endurance. If the patient is an overhead athlete, such as a baseball or tennis player, we routinely perform a combination of isokinetic testing.

Interval sport programs are designed to gradually return motion, function, and confidence in the upper extremity after injury or surgery by slowly progressing through graduated sport-specific activities.[44] These programs are intended to gradually return the overhead athletes to full athletic competition as quickly and safely as possible.

Summary

The mature patient with rotator cuff pathology is often seen in the rehabilitation setting. The rehabilitation specialist must be able to recognize the pathology and develop a comprehensive program designed to establish full range of motion, balanced capsular mobility, and maximal muscular strength and endurance. A functional approach to rehabilitation using specific positions and movement patterns will ensure a gradual return to function. This is necessary to minimize injury so that the patient can safely develop and withstand forces at the glenohumeral joint.

References

1. Hawkins RJ, Abrams JS: Impingement syndrome in the absence of rotator cuff tear (stages 1 and 2). *Orthop Clin North Am* 1987;18(3):373-382.

2. Codman EA, Akerson IB: The Pathology associated with rupture of the supraspinatus tendon. *Ann Surg* 1931;93(1):348-359.

3. Neer CS II: Impingement lesions. *Clin Orthop Relat Res* 1983;173:70-77.

4. Neer CS II: Anterior acromioplasty for the chronic impingement syndrome in the shoulder: A preliminary report. *J Bone Joint Surg Am* 1972;54(1):41-50.

5. Rockwood CA, Matsen FA III, Wirth MA, Lippitt SB, eds: *The Shoulder*, ed 2. Philadelphia, PA, Saunders, 1998, vol 2, p 1341.

6. Harryman DT II, Sidles JA, Clark JM, McQuade KJ, Gibb TD, Matsen FA III: Translation of the humeral head on the glenoid with passive glenohumeral motion. *J Bone Joint Surg Am* 1990;72(9):1334-1343.

7. Speer KP, Deng X, Borrero S, Torzilli PA, Altchek DA, Warren RF: Biomechanical evaluation of a simulated Bankart lesion. *J Bone Joint Surg Am* 1994;76(12):1819-1826.

8. Wilk KE, Arrigo CA, Andrews JR: Current concepts: The stabilizing structures of the glenohumeral joint. *J Orthop Sports Phys Ther* 1997;25(6):364-379.

9. Kibler WB: The role of the scapula in athletic shoulder function. *Am J Sports Med* 1998;26(2):325-337.

10. Kibler WB: Role of the scapula in the overhead throwing motion. *Contemp Orthop* 1991;22:525-532.

11. Kibler WB, McMullen J: Scapular dyskinesis and its relation to shoulder pain. *J Am Acad Orthop Surg* 2003;11(2):142-151.

12. Burkhart SS, Morgan CD, Kibler WB: The disabled throwing shoulder: Spectrum of pathology Part III. The SICK scapula, scapular dyskinesis, the kinetic chain, and rehabilitation. *Arthroscopy* 2003;19(6):641-661.

13. Paine RM: The role of the scapula in the shoulder, in Andrews JR, Wilk KE, eds: *The Athlete's Shoulder*. New York, NY, Churchill Livingstone, 1994, pp 495-512.

14. Wilk KE, Arrigo C: Current concepts in the rehabilitation of the athletic shoulder. *J Orthop Sports Phys Ther* 1993;18(1):365-378.

15. Inman VT, Saunders JB, Abbott LC: Observations of the function of the shoulder joint. 1944. *Clin Orthop Relat Res* 1996;(330):3-12.

16. Speer KP, Garret WE: Muscular control of motion and stability about the pectoral girdle, in Matsen FA, Fu FH, Hawkins JR, eds: *The Shoulder: A Balance of Mobility and Stability*. Rosemont, IL, American Academy of Orthopedic Surgeons, 1993, pp 162-164.

17. Wuelker N, Wirth CJ, Plitz W, Roetman B: A dynamic shoulder model: Reliability testing and muscle force study. *J Biomech* 1995;28(5):489-499.

18. McClure PW, Michener LA, Karduna AR: Shoulder function and 3-dimensional scapular kinematics in people with and without shoulder impingement syndrome. *Phys Ther* 2006;86(8):1075-1090.

19. Meister K, Buckley B, Batts J: The posterior impingement sign: Diagnosis of rotator cuff and posterior labral tears secondary to internal impingement in overhand athletes. *Am J Orthop (Belle Mead NJ)* 2004;33(8):412-415.

20. Glass JM, Stephen RL, Jacobson SC: The quantity and distribution of radiolabeled dexamethasone delivered to tissue by iontophoresis. *Int J Dermatol* 1980;19(9):519-525.

21. Gangarosa LP Sr, Ozawa A, Ohkido M, Shimomura Y, Hill JM: Iontophoresis for enhancing penetration of dermatologic and antiviral drugs. *J Dermatol* 1995;22(11):865-875.

22. Anderson CR, Morris RL, Boeh SD, Panus PC, Sembrowich WL: Effects of iontophoresis current magnitude and duration on dexamethasone deposition and localized drug retention. *Phys Ther* 2003;83(2):161-170.

23. Reinold MM, Wilk KE, Fleisig GS, et al: Electromyographic analysis of the rotator cuff and deltoid musculature during common shoulder external rotation exercises. *J Orthop Sports Phys Ther* 2004; 34(7):385-394.

24. Reinold MM, Macrina LC, Wilk KE, et al: Electromyographic analysis of the supraspinatus and deltoid muscles during 3 common rehabilitation exercises. *J Athl Train* 2007;42(4):464-469.

25. Solem-Bertoft E, Thuomas KA, Westerberg CE: The influence of scapular retraction and protraction on the width of the subacromial space: An MRI study. *Clin Orthop Relat Res* 1993;(296):99-103.

26. Lukasiewicz AC, McClure P, Michener L, Pratt N, Sennett B: Comparison of 3-dimensional scapular position and orientation between subjects with and without shoulder impingement. *J Orthop Sports Phys Ther* 1999;29(10):574-586.

27. Moseley JB Jr, Jobe FW, Pink M, Perry J, Tibone J: EMG analysis of the scapular muscles during a shoulder rehabilitation program. *Am J Sports Med* 1992;20(2): 128-134.

28. Ekstrom RA, Soderberg GL, Donatelli RA: Normalization procedures using maximum voluntary isometric contractions for the serratus anterior and trapezius muscles during surface EMG analysis. *J Electromyogr Kinesiol* 2005;15(4):418-428.

29. Wilk KE, Macrina LC, Reinold MM: Non-operative rehabilitation for traumatic and atraumatic glenohumeral instability. *N Am J Sports Phys Ther* 2006;1(1):16-31.

30. Carpenter JE, Blasier RB, Pellizzon GG: The effects of muscle fatigue on shoulder joint position sense. *Am J Sports Med* 1998;26(2):262-265.

31. Voight ML, Hardin JA, Blackburn TA, Tippett S, Canner GC: The effects of muscle fatigue on and the relationship of arm dominance to shoulder proprioception. *J Orthop Sports Phys Ther* 1996;23(6): 348-352.

32. Myers JB, Guskiewicz KM, Schneider RA, Prentice WE: Proprioception and neuromuscular control of the shoulder after muscle fatigue. *J Athl Train* 1999;34(4): 362-367.

33. Langberg H, Ellingsgaard H, Madsen T, et al: Eccentric rehabilitation exercise increases peritendinous type I collagen synthesis in humans with Achilles tendinosis. *Scand J Med Sci Sports* 2007;17(1):61-66.

34. Shalabi A, Kristoffersen-Wilberg M, Svensson L, Aspelin P, Movin T: Eccentric training of the gastrocnemius-soleus complex in chronic Achilles tendinopathy results in decreased tendon volume and intratendinous signal as evaluated by MRI. *Am J Sports Med* 2004;32(5):1286-1296.

35. Alfredson H, Pietilä T, Jonsson P, Lorentzon R: Heavy-load eccentric calf muscle training for the treatment of chronic Achilles tendinosis. *Am J Sports Med* 1998; 26(3):360-366.

36. Clement DB, Taunton JE, Smart GW: Achilles tendinitis and peritendinitis: Etiology and treatment. *Am J Sports Med* 1984;12(3):179-184.

37. Bjordal JM, Lopes-Martins RA, Iversen VV: A randomised, placebo controlled trial of low level laser therapy for activated Achilles tendinitis with microdialysis measurement of peritendinous prostaglandin E2 concentrations. *Br J Sports Med* 2006;40(1):76-80.

38. England S, Farrell AJ, Coppock JS, Struthers G, Bacon PA: Low power laser therapy of shoulder tendonitis. *Scand J Rheumatol* 1989;18(6):427-431.

39. Lam LK, Cheing GL: Effects of 904-nm low-level laser therapy in the management of lateral epicondylitis: A randomized controlled trial. *Photomed Laser Surg* 2007;25(2):65-71.

40. Stergioulas A, Stergioula M, Aarskog R, Lopes-Martins RA, Bjordal JM: Effects of low-level laser therapy and eccentric exercises in the treatment of recreational athletes with chronic achilles tendinopathy. *Am J Sports Med* 2008;36(5):881-887.

41. Ko JY, Chen HS, Chen LM: Treatment of lateral epicondylitis of the elbow with shock waves. *Clin Orthop Relat Res* 2001;(387):60-67.

42. Wang CJ, Chen HS: Shock wave therapy for patients with lateral epicondylitis of the elbow: A one- to two-year follow-up study. *Am J Sports Med* 2002;30(3): 422-425.

43. Wang CJ, Ko JY, Chen HS: Treatment of calcifying tendinitis of the shoulder with shock wave therapy. *Clin Orthop Relat Res* 2001;(387):83-89.

44. Reinold MM, Wilk KE, Reed J, Crenshaw K, Andrews JR: Interval sport programs: Guidelines for baseball, tennis, and golf. *J Orthop Sports Phys Ther* 2002;32(6): 293-298.

Chapter 15

Arthroscopic Approach to Glenohumeral Arthritis

Brett A. Sweitzer, MD
Richard J. Hawkins, MD

Key Points

- In younger athletes with glenohumeral arthritis, sparing the cartilage is a priority.
- Capsular release is often the best approach in the active mature athlete.
- Microfracture and débridement may be useful adjuncts.
- Interposition arthroplasty may have some potential benefit.
- In older athletes, shoulder arthroplasty results in pain relief and functional improvement (to a greater extent with total shoulder arthroplasty than with hemiarthroplasty).
- Rigorous evidence regarding the efficacy of an arthroscopic approach to glenohumeral arthritis is lacking.

Introduction

According to the Centers for Disease Control and Prevention (CDC), more than 50 million adults in the United States are living with arthritis symptoms, based on a 2007-2009 National Health Interview Survey.[1] In 2006, the CDC reported that nearly 8% of people aged 45 to 64 years and more than 50% of those older than 65 years were affected by arthritis.[2] Those numbers are surely increasing as the baby boomer generation ages. Similarly, because increasing numbers of these mature athletes wish to remain active as they move along in years, the burden on the healthcare system and the role of the sports medicine healthcare provider will expand greatly.

Currently, arthritis is the leading cause of disability in the United States, and it can have a devastating impact on an athlete's ability to perform his or her sport.[3] With the common arthritides, the weight-bearing joints of the knee and hip are most affected, and most literature and investigational research to date has focused on management of these diseases in the lower extremity. Thus, there is a paucity of published studies addressing the treatment of arthritides of the upper extremity. Total joint arthroplasty is often the only surgical treatment suggested for patients afflicted with these arthritic conditions, especially those with glenohumeral arthritis. In 2004, an estimated 41,934 shoulder arthroplasty procedures were performed in the United States alone, and an even greater number were performed in Europe and developed countries elsewhere.[4] The challenge for those who provide health care to athletes is to keep these younger athletes with arthritis active throughout their adult lives, without the encumbrance of weight and activity restrictions. Certainly more research is needed, but based on current literature, an appropriately applied and carefully planned cartilage-sparing arthroscopic approach to shoulder arthritis in the mature athlete is of paramount importance.

Nonsurgical Treatment

Physical therapy, including stretching and strengthening of rotator cuff and scapular stabilizing muscles, along with appropriate prescription of nonsteroidal anti-inflammatory drugs are currently the mainstay of nonsurgical management of arthritis. Judicious use of corticosteroid injections and/or off-label use of hyaluronic acid injections may be considered. In addition, although glucosamine supplements are not recommended by the American Academy of Orthopaedic Surgeons,[5] it is the expert opinion of the senior author (R.J.H.) that these supplements may be of some benefit.

Traditionally, intra-articular corticosteroid injections have been administered to provide short-term pain relief (typically, 3 to 4 months) for arthritic joints.[6-8] Furthermore, when the shoulder is injected with a local anesthetic, a diagnostic test may be performed, providing useful information regarding the etiology of the patient's pain. However, there is no consensus among experts as to the most reliable and effective method for intra-articular glenohumeral joint injection, and the supporting literature on this topic is sparse. Injections may be given through a posterior approach, an anterior approach, or the Neviaser portal. The posterior approach, as described by Andrews et al,[9] is through a "soft point" 2 cm inferior and 2 cm medial to the posterolateral corner of the acromion, directed toward the corocoid. The anterior approach is through the rotator cuff interval just lateral to the tip of the coracoid, aiming toward the posterior joint line.[10] The Neviaser injection is given through the supraclavicular fossa in the superior soft spot surrounded by the clavicle anteriorly, the medial acromion, and the spine of the scapula posteriorly. The needle is inserted 1 cm medial

to the medial border of the acromion and is advanced at a 30° angle laterally and slightly posteriorly into the glenohumeral joint.[11] Sethi et al[12] assessed the accuracy of anterior glenohumeral joint injections in awake patients without radiographic assistance and found that only 26.8% of injections successfully reached their target. The authors concluded it is unlikely that an anteriorly placed intra-articular glenohumeral injection will be accurately placed in awake patients. In a cadaveric study performed by the same authors, anterior injections proved more accurate than posterior injections.[10] The accuracy of injections through the Neviaser portal has not been reported. However, unpublished data from an ongoing study at our institution by Tobola et al suggest that anterior injections are more accurate than posterior and Neviaser injections. This study suggests that all three injection approaches are less accurate than is desirable. The use of radiographic guidance (fluoroscopy or ultrasound) might be considered. The Neviaser portal lends itself to AP fluoroscopy for reliability.

Surgical Treatment

Unfortunately, other than studies of arthroplasty, little has been published in the peer-reviewed literature to direct the surgical treatment of glenohumeral arthritis using an evidence-based approach. A wide variety of surgical options is available, including cartilage-sparing procedures (arthroscopic débridement, microfracture, capsular release, interposition arthroplasty, resurfacing) and cartilage-replacing procedures (hemiarthroplasty and total joint arthroplasty).

Cartilage-sparing procedures are directed at preserving what is left of healthy functioning cartilage, possibly stimulating regeneration of new "repair" cartilage, and improving range of motion. These procedures are of critical importance in the management of the younger athlete with arthritis.

Cartilage-replacing procedures are directed at replacing painful degenerated joint cartilage surfaces with prostheses that preserve motion and function. These procedures are reserved for patients who have failed other nonsurgical treatment options, particularly older athletes with significant pain.

Limited-Resurfacing Arthroplasty

In advanced stages of osteoarthritis or osteonecrosis of the humeral head, shoulder arthroplasty procedures, either hemiarthroplasty or total shoulder arthroplasty, have been the commonly accepted treatment.[13-18] Recently, limited-resurfacing arthroplasty procedures have been popularized as a minimally invasive means of replacing joint surfaces that have degenerated as a result of osteonecrosis, thus preserving unaffected healthy cartilage and bone stock. Proponents of the HemiCAP (Arthrosurface, Franklin, MA) suggest its use as an alternative to traditional arthroplasty procedures in younger patients. In this procedure, only a partial humeral head resurfacing is performed, and the glenoid is not addressed. Patient selection criteria include middle-aged to older patients with large unstable Outerbridge grade IV cartilage loss that is posttraumatic or is due to degenerative joint disease or osteonecrosis and has resulted in significant subchondral bone exposure. In addition, nonsurgical treatment should have been exhausted, and future arthroplasty procedures should be likely.[19] However, there is a paucity of literature on partial humeral head resurfacing in the setting of arthritis. Recently, Uribe and Botto-van Bemden[20] presented their results in 12 shoulders with osteonecrosis treated with partial humeral head resurfacing in a prospective series. Of the 12 shoulders, 11 were Cruess stage III or IV, with only one patient having osteoarthritis (stage V). Promising results were reported, with all patients showing improvements in pain and function, including a mean improvement in the Western Ontario Osteoarthritis of the Shoulder Index (WOOSI) of 1,421 preoperatively to 471 postoperatively. The single patient in this series with osteoarthritis had only modest improvement. It is difficult to draw any definitive conclusions regarding treatment of osteoarthritis in the setting of advanced osteonecrosis of the humeral head with limited-resurfacing arthroplasty based on these limited data.

Arthroscopic Débridement

Arthroscopic débridement is perhaps the simplest surgical treatment of arthritis. Surgical time, blood loss, and invasiveness are typically minimal. In addition, surgical outcomes in carefully selected patients have been good.[21,22] Weinstein et al[22] evaluated the 2-year follow-up of 25 patients undergoing arthroscopic débridement for glenohumeral joint osteoarthritis, with treatment consisting of lavage of the glenohumeral joint, débridement of labral tears and chondral lesions, loose body removal, and partial synovectomy and subacromial bursectomy. In their series, 8% excellent, 72% good, and 20% unsatisfactory results were obtained, as determined by the following criteria: Results were rated as excellent if the patient had no pain and had full use of the extremity and essentially normal motion and strength. Results were classified as good if the patient was satisfied and had only occasional or mild pain in the shoulder, had elevation of more than 130°, and had full strength. All patients had at least 7 months of significant pain relief. Although no significant correlation was demonstrated between radiographic grade or degree of damage to articular cartilage at time of arthroscopy and clinical outcome, the authors concluded that this procedure is not recommended in patients with severe joint incongruity, significant loss of joint space, or large osteophytes. However, arthroscopic débridement was deemed to be a reasonable approach in patients with early osteoarthritis in the setting of a concentric glenohumeral joint and minimal joint space narrowing.[22] Rigorous evidence to support this recommendation is lacking.

Microfracture

The evidence supporting the use of microfracture in the shoulder is sparse, despite the proven efficacy of the microfracture technique for articular cartilage repair in other joints when used in appropriate situations.[23-36] Specifically, as shown in a recent systematic review of microfracture in the knee by Mithoefer et al,[23] microfracture provides effective short-term functional improvement of knee function, especially in physiologically younger patients (<40 years) having shorter duration of antecedent symptoms (<12 months), higher preoperative activity levels (Tegner score >4), lower body mass index (<30 kg/m^2), smaller lesions (<4 cm^2), primary microfracture, and better repair cartilage volume. However, further long-term studies are necessary to further validate the durability of microfracture. In addition, there exists some variability in technique and other confounding factors, such as limited hyaline repair tissue and cartilage volume, which may result in possible functional deterioration.

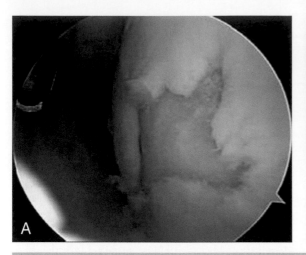 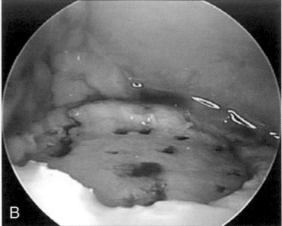

Figure 1   Arthroscopic views of microfracture in the shoulder. **A,** Grade IV chondral lesion on the humeral head measuring approximately 1.5 × 1.5 cm. **B,** Completed microfracture of chondral lesion showing holes and extravasating blood. (Reproduced with permission from Millett PJ, Huffard BH, Horan MP: Outcomes of full-thickness articular cartilage injuries of the shoulder treated with microfracture. *Arthroscopy* 2009;25(8):856-863. http://sciencedirect.com/science/journal/07498063/25/8.)

A microfracture technique similar to that described in the knee may have some promise in the shoulder. A systematic approach is used, starting with gentle débridement of an isolated and well-contained full-thickness cartilage defect on either the glenoid or humeral articular surface, establishing a stable cartilage margin (**Figure 1,** *A*). The underlying calcified cartilage layer is carefully removed with a curet, and an awl is used to microfracture the subchondral bone. These micropenetrations are meticulously made to a depth of 3 to 4 mm and are equally spaced with a bony bridge of 3 to 4 mm between each penetration. Resultant extravasation of bone marrow elements and formation of a mesenchymal clot is confirmed upon lowering of the intra-articular pressure (**Figure 1,** *B*).

Millett et al[37] recently reported on outcomes of full-thickness articular cartilage injuries of the shoulder treated with microfracture using this technique. In this series, 31 shoulders in patients with a mean age of 43 years were examined a minimum of 2 years after the procedure. Fifty percent of the patients were mature athletes, and as a group they demonstrated improvement in pain scores (the score on the visual analog scale decreased from 3.8 to 1.6), improved function (the

American Shoulder and Elbow Surgeons [ASES] score increased from 60 to 80), and overall satisfaction. The authors concluded that the greatest improvement was seen for smaller lesions of the humerus, and the worst results were seen in patients with bipolar lesions. Microfracture probably is of little benefit for diffuse grade IV changes. Prospective studies are currently underway to further assess the efficacy of microfracture in the shoulder.

Arthroscopic Capsular Release

Capsular contracture (and the resultant "stiff" shoulder) is an important component of pain and disability in the arthritic shoulder. In the expert opinion of the senior author (R.J.H.), capsular contracture results in increased pressures within the glenohumeral joint and accelerates the osteoarthritic process through a shear/compression process driven by the dynamic forces of the rotator cuff musculature in the tight shoulder. This situation is a downward spiral, with the osteoarthritis leading to stiffness and the stiffness worsening the osteoarthritis. As such, capsular release may be an effective treatment in slowing the arthritic process of this shear/compression phenomenon and, more important to the patient, allowing for improved function and decreased pain in the arthritic shoulder by increasing joint volume and diminishing glenohumeral joint pressure (**Figure 2**).

In a study of ten patients with an internal rotation contracture and pain after an anterior repair for recurrent dislocation of the shoulder, MacDonald et al[38] demonstrated that treatment with release of the subscapularis muscle can result in decreased pain and improved range of motion. Osteoarthritic changes were evident on the preoperative radiographs of all patients; six demonstrated severe osteoarthritic changes. The release was done an average of 11 years after the original procedure, which for most patients was a Putti-Platt repair. After release of the subscapularis, each patient had less pain (mild pain at average 3.5-year follow-up) in the shoulder and an average increase of 27° of external rotation. An open technique was used, performing a coronal Z-plasty lengthening of the subscapularis tendon with concomitant vertical anterior capsular release as indicated. The authors concluded that release of the subscapularis and capsule can offer relief of pain and of functional limitations associated with the symptoms caused by an internal rotation contracture. This study introduced us to the advantages of releases for stiff shoulders with osteoarthritis. Today, capsular releases are generally performed arthroscopically. In our opinion, the patient with isolated loss of external rotation following anterior stabilization, even with minimal osteoarthritic changes, is well served by restoration of external rotation using arthroscopic procedures.

Warner et al[39] demonstrated the use and efficacy of arthroscopic capsular release of postoperative capsular contracture of the shoulder in 18 patients, in all of whom a mean of 8 months of supervised physical therapy had failed to restore an adequate range of functional motion. All of the patients had painful and limited motion of the shoulder. An arthroscopic technique of selective anterior and/or posterior capsular release and gentle manipulation was used. Postoperatively, patients showed significant improvement in motion and Constant scores. The authors concluded that arthroscopic capsular release is a reliable method for restoring motion with minimal morbidity in carefully selected patients who have postoperative stiffness of the shoulder, pointing out that it can easily be converted to an open release if necessary.

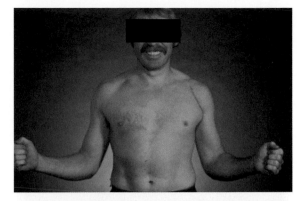

Figure 2   A 40-year-old man presented with external rotation limited to 0° following open Bankart surgery 10 years previously. He underwent arthroscopic capsular release of the left shoulder. Clinical photograph shows improved range of motion.

In a study of 61 patients with grade IV osteochondral lesions of the glenohumeral articular surfaces who were treated with arthroscopic débridement with or without arthroscopic capsular release, Cameron et al[40] demonstrated encouraging results at a minimum 2-year follow-up. Twenty-two patients (36%) had an associated stiff shoulder, which was defined as a loss of motion of at least 15° in any plane. Selective arthroscopic capsular release of the affected portion of the capsule, followed by arthroscopic débridement of any osteochondral lesion, was performed. In the group of 39 patients without stiff shoulders, arthroscopic débridement without capsular release was performed. At 2-year follow-up, 88% of patients reported significant pain relief. However, the investigators did note that osteochondral lesion size greater than 2 cm^2 may be predictive of return of pain and clinical failure. In addition, capsular release is probably critical to improved results in the group with stiff shoulders.

In treatment of osteoarthritis of the shoulder through capsular release (**Figure 3**), success depends on the degree of arthritis and the magnitude of limitation in motion. In the appropriately selected patient, release can effectively restore motion, improve function, and lessen pain. In addition, release may slow the progression of the degenerative process and delay the need for arthroplasty.

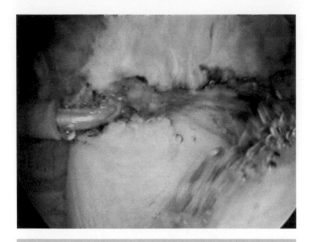

Figure 3 Arthroscopic view of a stiff shoulder shows capsular release with electrocautery.

The ideal patient for an arthroscopic approach emphasizing capsular releases is one with mild to moderate glenohumeral arthritis, mild joint space narrowing, and significant limitation of motion in all planes. In the patient with these characteristics but good motion, the only option is débridement, which in our experience has far less rewarding results.

Summary

In summary, clear and decisive evidence is lacking to guide treatment of glenohumeral arthritis, particularly in athletes. However, an appropriately applied and carefully thought-out arthroscopic approach may be of some benefit.

References

1. Centers for Disease Control and Prevention (CDC): Data and Statistics: National Statistics. www.cdc.gov/arthritis/data_statistics.htm.

2. Hootman J, Bolen J, Helmick C, Langmaid G, Centers for Disease Control and Prevention (CDC): Prevalence of doctor-diagnosed arthritis and arthritis-attributable activity limitation—United States, 2003-2005. *MMWR Morb Mortal Wkly Rep* 2006;55(40):1089-1092.

3. American Academy of Orthopaedic Surgeons: Your Orthopaedic Connection: Arthritis. www.orthoinfo.aaos.org/menus/arthritis.cfm.

4. *The Burden of Musculoskeletal Diseases in the United States: Prevalence, Societal and Economic Cost.*

5. American Academy of Orthopaedic Surgeons: *Clinical Practice Guideline on the Treatment of Glenohumeral Joint Osteoarthritis.* Rosemont, IL, American Academy of Orthopaedic Surgeons, December 2009. http://www.aaos.org/research/guidelines/gloguideline. Accessed October 6, 2011..

6. Raynauld JP, Buckland-Wright C, Ward R, et al: Safety and efficacy of long-term intraarticular steroid injections in osteoarthritis of the knee: A randomized, double-blind, placebo-controlled trial. *Arthritis Rheum* 2003;48(2):370-377.

7. Lambert RG, Hutchings EJ, Grace MG, Jhangri GS, Conner-Spady B, Maksymowych WP: Steroid injection for osteoarthritis of the hip: A randomized, double-blind, placebo-controlled trial. *Arthritis Rheum* 2007; 56(7):2278-2287.

8. Friedman DM, Moore ME: The efficacy of intraarticular steroids in osteoarthritis: A double-blind study. *J Rheumatol* 1980;7(6):850-856.

9. Andrews JR, Carson WG Jr, Ortega K: Arthroscopy of the shoulder: Technique and normal anatomy. *Am J Sports Med* 1984;12(1):1-7.

10. Sethi PM, El Attrache N: Accuracy of intra-articular injection of the glenohumeral joint: A cadaveric study. *Orthopedics* 2006;29(2):149-152.

11. Neviaser TJ: Arthroscopy of the shoulder. *Orthop Clin North Am* 1987;18(3):361-372.

12. Sethi PM, Kingston S, Elattrache N: Accuracy of anterior intra-articular injection of the glenohumeral joint. *Arthroscopy* 2005;21(1):77-80.

13. Hattrup SJ: Indications, technique, and results of shoulder arthroplasty in osteonecrosis. *Orthop Clin North Am* 1998;29(3):445-451.

14. Hattrup SJ, Cofield RH: Osteonecrosis of the humeral head: Results of replacement. *J Shoulder Elbow Surg* 2000;9(3):177-182.

15. Mansat P, Huser L, Mansat M, Bellumore Y, Rongières M, Bonnevialle P: Shoulder arthroplasty for atraumatic avascular necrosis of the humeral head: Nineteen shoulders followed up for a mean of seven years. *J Shoulder Elbow Surg* 2005;14(2):114-120.

16. Orfaly RM, Rockwood CA Jr, Esenyel CZ, Wirth MA: Shoulder arthroplasty in cases of avascular necrosis of the humeral head. *J Shoulder Elbow Surg* 2007; 16(3 Suppl):S27-S32.

17. Parsch D, Lehner B, Loew M: Shoulder arthroplasty in nontraumatic osteonecrosis of the humeral head. *J Shoulder Elbow Surg* 2003;12(3):226-230.

18. Smith RG, Sperling JW, Cofield RH, Hattrup SJ, Schleck CD: Shoulder hemiarthroplasty for steroid-associated osteonecrosis. *J Shoulder Elbow Surg* 2008;17(5):685-688.

19. Scalise JJ, Miniaci A, Ianotti JP: Resurfacing arthroplasty of the humerus: Indications, surgical technique, and clinical results. *Tech Shoulder Elbow Surg* 2007;8(3):152-160.

20. Uribe JW, Botto-van Bemden A: Partial humeral head resurfacing for osteonecrosis. *J Shoulder Elbow Surg* 2009;18(5):711-716.

21. Kerr BJ, McCarty EC: Outcome of arthroscopic débridement is worse for patients with glenohumeral arthritis of both sides of the joint. *Clin Orthop Relat Res* 2008;466(3):634-638.

22. Weinstein DM, Bucchieri JS, Pollock RG, Flatow EL, Bigliani LU: Arthroscopic debridement of the shoulder for osteoarthritis. *Arthroscopy* 2000;16(5):471-476.

23. Mithoefer K, McAdams T, Williams RJ, Kreuz PC, Mandelbaum BR: Clinical efficacy of the microfracture technique for articular cartilage repair in the knee: An evidence-based systematic analysis. *Am J Sports Med* 2009;37(10):2053-2063.

24. Bae DK, Yoon KH, Song SJ: Cartilage healing after microfracture in osteoarthritic knees. *Arthroscopy* 2006;22(4):367-374.

25. Blevins FT, Steadman JR, Rodrigo JJ, Silliman J: Treatment of articular cartilage defects in athletes: An analysis of functional outcome and lesion appearance. *Orthopedics* 1998;21(7):761-768.

26. Gill TJ: The treatment of articular cartilage defects using microfracture and debridement. *Am J Knee Surg* 2000;13(1):33-40.

27. Kon E, Gobbi A, Filardo G, Delcogliano M, Zaffagnini S, Marcacci M: Arthroscopic second-generation autologous chondrocyte implantation compared with microfracture for chondral lesions of the knee: Prospective nonrandomized study at 5 years. *Am J Sports Med* 2009;37(1):33-41.

28. Gobbi A, Nunag P, Malinowski K: Treatment of full thickness chondral lesions of the knee with microfracture in a group of athletes. *Knee Surg Sports Traumatol Arthrosc* 2005;13(3):213-221.

29. Gudas R, Kalesinskas RJ, Kimtys V, et al: A prospective randomized clinical study of mosaic osteochondral autologous transplantation versus microfracture for the treatment of osteochondral defects in the knee joint in young athletes. *Arthroscopy* 2005;21(9):1066-1075.

30. Knutsen G, Drogset JO, Engebretsen L, et al: A randomized trial comparing autologous chondrocyte implantation with microfracture: Findings at five years. *J Bone Joint Surg Am* 2007;89(10):2105-2112.

31. Mithoefer K, Williams RJ III, Warren RF, et al: The microfracture technique for the treatment of articular cartilage lesions in the knee: A prospective cohort study. *J Bone Joint Surg Am* 2005;87(9):1911-1920.

32. Rodrigo JJ, Steadman JR, Silliman JJ, Fulstone HA: Improvement of full-thickness chondral defect healing in the human knee after debridement and microfracture using continuous passive motion. *Am J Knee Surg* 1994;7(3):109-116.

33. Steadman JR, Briggs KK, Rodrigo JJ, Kocher MS, Gill TJ, Rodkey WG: Outcomes of microfracture for traumatic chondral defects of the knee: Average 11-year follow-up. *Arthroscopy* 2003;19(5):477-484.

34. Steadman JR, Miller BS, Karas SG, Schlegel TF, Briggs KK, Hawkins RJ: The microfracture technique in the treatment of full-thickness chondral lesions of the knee in National Football League players. *J Knee Surg* 2003;16(2):83-86.

35. Philippon MJ, Schenker ML, Briggs KK, Maxwell RB: Can microfracture produce repair tissue in acetabular chondral defects? *Arthroscopy* 2008;24(1):46-50.

36. Crawford K, Philippon MJ, Sekiya JK, Rodkey WG, Steadman JR: Microfracture of the hip in athletes. *Clin Sports Med* 2006;25(2):327-335, x.

37. Millett PJ, Huffard BH, Horan MP, Hawkins RJ, Steadman JR: Outcomes of full-thickness articular cartilage injuries of the shoulder treated with microfracture. *Arthroscopy* 2009;25(8):856-863.

38. MacDonald PB, Hawkins RJ, Fowler PJ, Miniaci A: Release of the subscapularis for internal rotation contracture and pain after anterior repair for recurrent anterior dislocation of the shoulder. *J Bone Joint Surg Am* 1992;74(5):734-737.

39. Warner JJ, Allen AA, Marks PH, Wong P: Arthroscopic release of postoperative capsular contracture of the shoulder. *J Bone Joint Surg Am* 1997;79(8):1151-1158.

40. Cameron BD, Galatz LM, Ramsey ML, Williams GR, Iannotti JP: Non-prosthetic management of grade IV osteochondral lesions of the glenohumeral joint. *J Shoulder Elbow Surg* 2002;11(1):25-32.

Chapter 16

Total and Reverse Shoulder Arthroplasty

Frederick S. Song, MD
Rob Bell, MD

Key Points

- Glenohumeral osteoarthritis is a growing problem as the active baby boomer population ages.
- The number of total shoulder arthroplasty (TSA) procedures has continued to increase rapidly to meet this demand.
- Complications with TSA have continued to decrease with advances in materials and techniques, especially on the glenoid side.
- Alternative procedures are currently being investigated for the treatment of younger, more active patients with glenohumeral osteoarthritis.
- Although reverse shoulder arthroplasty (RSA) has been shown to be efficacious in treating rotator cuff tear arthropathy (RCTA) in the low-demand older patient, it is not recommended in the baby boomer athlete because of its high complication rate.

Introduction

Much of the emphasis on joint arthroplasty and osteoarthritis (OA) in the baby boomer population has focused on the hip and the knee. Prosthetic replacement of the shoulder is less commonly performed than hip and knee arthroplasty, but shoulder disorders, including glenohumeral osteoarthritis, rheumatoid arthritis, and RCTA, are a growing problem in the baby boomer population. The number of shoulder arthroplasties, both hemiarthroplasties and TSAs, performed in the United States has doubled in one decade, from approximately 10,000 in 1990 to 20,000 in 2000.[1] With the growing popularity of sports such as golf and tennis among the boomer population, these numbers continue to grow. In the past, older patients with these shoulder conditions were advised to modify their activities, but active patients no longer will settle for this and want treatment that allows them to continue to participate. Shoulder arthroplasty has evolved over time and has proven to be an excellent procedure to enhance the quality of life of these patients.

RCTA has proved difficult to treat in the aging population. Although standard TSA has been a viable solution for rheumatoid arthritis and osteoarthritis affecting the glenohumeral joint, it has not been shown to be as effective in treating RCTA. The reverse ball-and-socket prosthesis, used in a procedure called a reverse shoulder arthroplasty, or RSA, is another tool in the shoulder surgeon's armamentarium for treating this difficult problem. This prosthesis has been used routinely in Europe for the past 2 decades and has been growing in popularity in the United States, with numerous manufacturers developing their own versions. Although outcomes have been favorable with regard to pain relief and restoration of function, a high complication rate has limited the use of the reverse ball-and-socket prosthesis to older, less active patients.[2-8]

Most of this chapter focuses on TSA, as it is more relevant to the active baby boomer population. RSA is discussed briefly, although its use has been reserved for older patients (>65 years) who are less active, so it is less applicable to this population.

Preoperative Clinical Assessment

History and Physical Examination

The preoperative assessment in patients with an arthritide in whom a standard TSA or an RSA is being considered begins with a thorough history and physical examination. In the history, it is important to ascertain the duration of the current disease process, changes in function, alterations in lifestyle, and, most importantly, patient expectations. Prior surgeries and trauma as well as previous treatments, including medications, physical therapy, and/or injections, should be recorded. Shoulder pain in a mature athlete often is an insidious, progressive process that has recently caused the patient to discontinue participation in favorite activities such as tennis, golf, or swimming.

The physical examination commences with a careful inspection, looking for prior incisions and deltoid asymmetry or atrophy. Neurovascular status is assessed. Range of motion, both passive and active, is carefully assessed and compared with the contralateral side, noting planes in which the greatest discrepancies exist and absences that have developed. It is important to differentiate contracture versus motor weakness attributable to either neurologic or rotator cuff deficiencies. Patients with more progressive glenohumeral osteoarthritis typically have a decreased arc of motion with respect to internal and external rotation. These motions are often limited and painful in this patient population.

In patients with massive rotator cuff tears, elevation may be severely limited. If the humeral head exhibits anterosuperior escape when the patient attempts forward elevation, it is indicative of underlying RCTA. This should lead the examiner to give further consideration to RSA over standard TSA. Studies have shown that the RSA procedure has been relatively successful in treating pseudoparesis of the shoulder and restoring shoulder function.[2-8]

Rotator cuff strength is determined by assessing resisted motion in the appropriate planes and comparing it with the contralateral side. Because it is rare for a patient with pure glenohumeral osteoarthritis to have a significant rotator cuff tear, strength typically will be quite good in all planes unless intra-articular pain causes limited motion that mimics weakness. In contrast, individuals with advanced rheumatoid arthritis often have weakness in scapular elevation, indicating supraspinatus compromise. Furthermore, weakness in external rotation would imply extension of the rotator cuff defect posteriorly into the infraspinatus and possibly the teres minor. Tests for subscapularis function include the belly-press and lift-off tests. A recent study has shown that the belly-press test is more specific for the upper subscapularis, and the lift-off test is more specific for the lower subscapularis.[9] Significant weakness with any of these maneuvers, either individually or collectively, may indicate compromise of the rotator cuff and warrants delineation of the tendon status with appropriate MRI and/or neurodiagnostics.

Determining whether a patient's weakness is due to pain or mechanical problems (eg, rotator cuff tear) can be difficult. A diagnostic subacromial injection can help to differentiate the two etiologies. If the pain is relieved after the injection but the weakness remains, there should be a high suspicion for a tear. Cervical range of motion and pain also should be assessed, as the presence of an upper trunk lesion of the brachial plexus or cervical radiculopathy may produce functional weakness of the shoulder as well.

Diagnostic Imaging

Preoperative radiographic assessment begins with a three-view trauma series consisting of a true AP scapular view, an outlet view, and the essential axillary view. On the AP scapular view, attention is directed to the degree of humeral head flattening, decrease in the acromiohumeral interval, status of the acromioclavicular joint, presence of humeral osteophytes and loose bodies, and humeral shaft alignment. This view is the best one for evaluating the status of the rotator cuff, with any signs of a high-riding head or acetabularization of the acromion (indicative of pseudoarticulations of the humeral head on the coracoacromial arch) indicating a massive cuff tear. The axillary view is critical for determining the relationship of the humeral head to the glenoid and the presence of glenoid erosion and version changes. In the osteoarthritic patient, there is a tendency for anterior capsular tightness to develop as a result of foreshortening of the subscapularis and anterior capsular tissues. This results in increased posteriorly directed forces on the humeral head and posterior subluxation, which in turn often leads to a biconcave glenoid as described by Walch et al.[10] This must be addressed at the time of glenoid preparation.

Ideally, patients with significant glenoid changes appreciated on routine radiographs should be evaluated with a preoperative CT scan to assess glenoid retroversion and glenoid vault volume. Individuals with retroversion exceeding 20° may need to be considered for bone graft augmentation of the posterior glenoid at the time of arthroplasty.

MRI is becoming a more common diagnostic tool in the armamentarium of shoulder arthroplasty surgeons, especially to evaluate the status of the rotator cuff in individuals with osteoarthritis and a recent deterioration in function with increasing pain. MRI is especially useful for evaluating any fatty infiltration or muscular atrophy of the rotator cuff musculature. In evaluating this, it is important to instruct the MRI technologist to image medially enough to evaluate the muscle bellies of the rotator cuff musculature. Studies have demonstrated inferior results with both TSA and RSA with increasing amounts of fatty infiltration of the cuff musculature.[11,12] Furthermore, MRI is useful to stage the changes of osteonecrosis and thereby assist with decision making as to the need for glenoid resurfacing. Finally, MRI is used to determine the degree of involvement of the cervical spine in rheumatoid arthritis as it pertains to preoperative clearance and cervical stability for intubation during any other procedures.

Indications

For any TSA candidate, it is important that nonsurgical measures be exhausted before surgical treatment is undertaken. In addition, the shoulder pain must be adversely affecting the patient's activities of daily living as defined by the patient. The common indications for standard TSA, accepted by most shoulder surgeons, include (1) primary glenohumeral osteoarthritis in a patient older than 50 years, (2) a patient with rheumatoid arthritis who has sufficient glenoid bone stock to support glenoid resurfacing and an intact or reparable rotator cuff, and (3) A patient with posttraumatic arthrosis or osteonecrosis with glenoid involvement.

Contraindications

The most common contraindication to TSA is severe bony deficiency, especially on the glenoid side.[13] This is a problem that is common in the setting of longstanding rheumatoid arthritis, as poor bone quality can preclude proper implantation of components and lead to early loosening and failure. A prior history of shoulder infection in the face of persistently elevated C-reactive protein level and/or erythrocyte sedimentation rate represents another contraindication and requires further evaluation before surgical intervention. Additional potential contraindications include deltoid dysfunction and neuropathic arthropathy. Patients who manifest weakness not attributable to rotator cuff disease should have a thorough evaluation of the cervical spine with documentation of range of motion, deep tendon reflexes, and the presence of sensory changes. Any evidence of cervical disk disease should be investigated with appropriate imaging and neurodiagnostics. Relative contraindications include poorly controlled seizure disorders and/or Parkinson disease.

Many individuals who present with arthritic changes of the shoulder will have coexistent disease of the lower extremities necessitating arthroplasty. If current shoulder function and pain level are tolerable, it is preferable to proceed with lower extremity arthroplasties before proceeding with shoulder arthroplasty so as to avoid excessive loads being applied to the shoulder arthroplasty during the postoperative period for hip or knee arthroplasty, when a walker or crutches is used. Following the lower extremity arthroplasties, once the patient is independent with ambulation, shoulder arthroplasty may be considered.

Outcomes

Survivorship of TSA

Many studies have demonstrated successful results of TSA in the short and long term, with longer than 10-year follow-up.[14-31] Evaluation of 419 TSAs performed at the Mayo Clinic revealed the following implant survivorship: 96% at 2 years, 92% at 5 years, and 88% at 10 years.[32] Sperling et al[33] evaluated 62 Neer hemiarthroplasties and 29 Neer TSAs with a minimum 15-year follow-up and found that implant survival was superior with TSA (97% at 10 years and 84% at 20 years) versus hemiarthroplasty (82% at 10 years and 75% at 20 years).

A recent study by Deshmukh et al[19] that evaluated 319 unconstrained TSAs yielded similar implant survivorship for TSAs. Their survivorship analysis, with revision as the end point, revealed a survivorship of 98% at 5 years, 93% at 10 years, 88% at 15 years, and 85% at 20 years. Most of the prostheses used (287) were the Neer II implant. With advances in biomechanics and implant design, as well as enhancements in surgical techniques, it is anticipated that implant survival will only improve over time.

Hemiarthroplasty Versus TSA

Many publications have evaluated the outcomes of TSA versus hemiarthroplasty. The initial prevailing thought was that hemiarthroplasty would be better suited for the younger (<50 years), more active patient population. This was based on the fear that increased loads seen in the more active patients would lead to early glenoid component loosening and/or accelerated wear. Additionally, hemiarthroplasty is a technically less demanding procedure than TSA because glenoid resurfacing is not required. Currently, however, most of the literature suggests that shoulder arthroplasty with glenoid resurfacing (ie, TSA) is the best, and most predictable, form of treatment for glenohumeral osteoarthritis in patients older than 50 years.[15,16,20,23,29,30,33] Chapter 17 goes into more detail regarding hemiarthroplasty, its relevance to the baby boomer population, and how the procedure compares with TSA.

Alternative Procedures

In the younger, higher demand boomer population with glenohumeral osteoarthritis refractory to nonsurgical treatment, the surgeon may consider alternatives to TSA because TSA in this patient population has a higher incidence of glenoid component loosening and/or accelerated wear. Matsen and associates reported on a procedure that includes replacement of the humeral head with a prosthesis and nonprosthetic glenoid arthroplasty, known as the "ream and run" procedure.[34,35] Lynch et al[34] reviewed 38 patients with a mean age of 57 years at an average follow-up of 2.7 years (range, 2 to 4 years) who were treated with the ream-and-run procedure and found a significant improvement in function with no surgical complications and no revisions to TSA. In a similar study, Clinton et al[35] compared 35 patients with an average age of 56 years to a case-matched control group of TSA patients. They found that in the short term, the TSA patients had better functional outcomes, but over time, at an average of 12 to 18 months, the "ream and run" patients achieved similar shoulder function.

Another alternative is humeral hemiarthroplasty combined with biologic resurfacing of the glenoid. It is believed that this technique allows for aggressive postoperative activities such as weight lifting and manual labor without the fear of glenoid component complications. Krishnan et al[36] reviewed 34 patients with an average age of 51 years who were managed with this technique. Anterior capsule grafts, autologous fascia lata grafts, and Achilles tendon allografts were used. After a minimum 2-year follow-up (mean, 7 years), patients had a mean increase in American Shoulder and Elbow Surgeons score from 39 points to 91 points. According to Neer's criteria, the procedure resulted in an excellent outcome for 18 patients, satisfactory for 13, and unsatisfactory for 5. Other studies using similar techniques, including lateral meniscal allograft, have demonstrated varying results and typically higher complication rates compared with standard TSA.[37-41] Although the above-described procedures have had some success in the high-demand, younger patient population and are viable options, results have varied and long-term outcomes are lacking. In most cases relating to the baby boomer population, it appears that standard TSA will likely yield the best, most predictable outcomes. In the case of unipolar disease with isolated lesions of the humeral head, humeral head resurfacing may be considered. This bone-conserving procedure gives the patient more options for future arthroplasty and can "buy time," giving the patient the option to continue many high-level sports activities. Long-term results are still pending for humeral head resurfacing.

Indications for RSA have evolved during its brief period of use in the United States and even more so during its nearly 20 years of use in Europe. The higher complication rate and semiconstrained nature of the articulation have resulted in most surgeons limiting its use to two situations: patients older than 65 years with lower functional demand, and revision of failed TSAs. RSA is seldom indicated in younger, more active baby boomer patients because these patients are more likely to apply greater loads to this type of replacement, thereby potentiating mechanical failure and need for revision.

Disease-Specific Considerations

Osteoarthritis

Osteoarthritis is a disease that may result in significant damage to the articular surfaces of the shoulder, as well as to the soft tissues. Typically, patients with osteoarthritis develop an internal rotation contracture due to capsular irritation and contracture, with associated subscapularis shortening. Both lead to increased loads across the glenohumeral articulation, secondary compression of the humeral head, inferior osteophyte formation, and resultant posterior humeral subluxation on the glenoid. Because of the aforementioned changes, certain steps are necessary at the time of arthroplasty to address the deformity and provide appropriate soft-tissue releases and a balanced arthroplasty. Anterior structures can be lengthened via one of two routes: (1) a lateral release of the subscapularis with medial reattachment; or (2) a more medial vertical capsulotomy, complete mobilization of the subscapularis, and anatomic repair at closure, without medialization. In the first option, the subscapularis and underlying capsule are released subperiosteally from the lesser tuberosity and repaired at the time of closure to the margin of the humeral osteotomy using transosseous sutures placed about the humeral component stem. The second approach involves a vertical incision of the subscapularis

and capsule 1.5 cm medial to the bicipital groove, release of the subscapularis circumferentially, and repair to its lateral stump of tissue. Both approaches achieve approximately 2 cm of lengthening and readily improve external rotation.

The osteoarthritic humeral head typically demonstrates characteristic changes, including flattening of the head, large secondary osteophytes about the margin of the articular surface, and even larger osteophytes forming a shelf along the inferior margin of the head (the so-called "goat's beard"). After humeral head osteotomy, these inferior osteophytes are resected, taking the bone back to native bone from the anterior aspect of the head inferiorly, all the way to the posterior aspect of the humeral head. Any appreciable changes in glenoid version are addressed with appropriate surface reamers and rarely with bone graft. In more advanced cases with posterior capsular laxity, a concomitant posterior capsular plication may be needed to ensure stability.

Rheumatoid Arthritis

Rotator cuff tears have been reported in 30% to 50% of patients with rheumatoid arthritis. These tears should be assessed preoperatively with MRI and treated at the time of arthroplasty surgery. Although studies have demonstrated good outcomes with concomitant rotator cuff repair and TSA,[12] care must be taken not to extrapolate these results in rheumatoid patients, as their tissues tend to be of lesser quality. In the absence of extensive fatty infiltration and/or atrophy of the cuff musculature, careful repair can be attempted. Because bone quality is compromised in these patients, a press fit of the humeral component may be inadequate, requiring the use of cement. Additionally, the glenoid is often somewhat medialized; this is best evaluated with preoperative CT imaging. Occasionally, glenoid wear will leave inadequate glenoid bone stock for cement fixation, in which case alternative treatment options, such as hemiarthroplasty or RSA, should be considered.

Capsulorrhaphy Arthropathy

Historically, anterior shoulder instability was treated with several nonanatomic repairs, including the Bristow, Putti-Platt, and Magnuson-Stack procedures. These techniques provided anterior capsular shortening with the hope of stabilizing the glenohumeral articula-

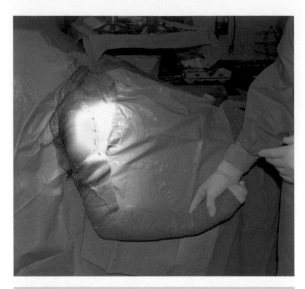

Figure 1 Patient positioning and draping for total shoulder arthroplasty (TSA), allowing the extremity to be brought into full extension.

tion. Unfortunately, many of these techniques resulted in excessive loads across the glenohumeral articulation with the consequent development of chondrolysis and traumatic arthropathy.[41] These patients represent a significant surgical challenge because of severe anterior soft-tissue contracture with resultant loss of external rotation. If the patient presents prior to severe degenerative changes, coronal Z-plasty lengthening of the subscapularis and anterior capsule may be attempted. The results of hemiarthroplasty alone, especially if done in patients with eccentric glenoid wear, have been poor. In response, several authors have attempted to address this issue with humeral head resurfacing combined with biologic resurfacing of the glenoid, as described previously in this chapter. Results pertaining to this treatment method have varied, but technical improvements are constantly being made.[35-40]

Surgical Technique for TSA

Patient Positioning

The patient is placed in the beach chair position and brought to the lateral aspect of the table. The patient's head is stabilized with flexible tape in a neutral position. A 250-mL intravenous bag is placed beneath the in-

volved scapula, and the pelvis is stabilized. This position allows the arm to be brought into full extension, thereby providing exposure of the humeral shaft for humeral component preparation (**Figure 1**). The entire arm is draped free, and a positioning device or a padded Mayo stand is used to hold the arm during various stages of the procedure.

Incision

An oblique 4- to 5-in skin incision is made beginning 3 cm medial to the acromioclavicular joint and proceeding distally over the coracoid process to just lateral to the anterior axillary fold (**Figure 2,** *A*). The deltopectoral interval is identified, and the cephalic vein is mobilized laterally with the deltoid, thereby preserving the many small perforating vessels from the deltoid. A self-retaining retractor is placed deep to the deltoid, on the superficial surface of the conjoined tendon medially, thereby protecting the underlying musculocutaneous nerve. The musculocutaneous nerve should be palpated to ensure proper placement of the medial retractor. A blunt retractor is placed in the subacromial space, allowing visualization of the rotator interval, the anterior border of the supraspinatus, and the biceps tendon (**Figure 2,** *B*). The coracoacromial ligament is routinely released, thereby decompressing the subacromial space and providing additional exposure of the rotator interval.

Capsulotomy and Humeral Exposure

One of the key components of a shoulder arthroplasty is the anterior humeral capsulotomy and subsequent humeral exposure. Although several different approaches may be implemented, all of them are determined by the preoperative and intraoperative examination of the patient's shoulder. If external rotation exceeds 15° to 20°, a standard vertical capsulotomy is made through the subscapularis and capsule. If a significant internal rotation contracture is present that precludes passive external rotation to 15° to 20°, consideration should be given to more aggressive soft-tissue releases and treatment of the subscapularis. After the subscapularis and capsule are incised, a capsulotomy is made, similar to an open Bankart exposure, from the superior border of the subscapularis down to the inferior margin of the capsule at the 6-o'clock position. This capsulotomy can be

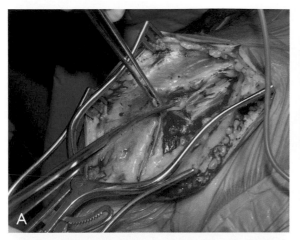
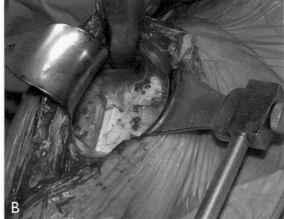

Figure 2   Incision for a TSA. **A,** The standard deltopectoral incision with cephalic vein exposure. Mobilizing the vein laterally with the deltoid preserves the many small perforating vessels from the deltoid. **B,** Blunt retractors are placed in the subacromial space, freeing up any adhesions and allowing visualization of the rotator interval, the biceps tendon, and the anterior edge of the supraspinatus.

carried around further posteriorly if necessary. Additional dissection is performed to release the superficial and superior aspects of the subscapularis. Finally, the release extends to the inferior margin of the subscapularis. The axillary nerve is identified and protected, and the inferior border of the subscapularis muscle is released from lateral to medial. In most cases, the intra-articular capsulotomy, the superior coracohumeral release, and superficial surface release of the subscapularis will help lengthen the subscapularis approximately 2 cm and improve external rotation 20° to 40°. The arm is then gently externally rotated, and the inferior capsule, which has enveloped the inferior osteophytes, is released subperiosteally (**Figure 3**). This dissection is carried around to the posterior aspect of the humeral head.

Humeral Osteotomy

The humeral head is gently delivered from the wound by extending and externally rotating the arm. A retractor is placed on the posterosuperior aspect of the humeral head to protect the supraspinatus and infraspinatus, and a blunt retractor is placed along the medial shaft, just beneath the inferior humeral osteophytes, to protect the axillary nerve. The arm is placed in approximately 30° of external rotation (**Figure 4,** *A*). The

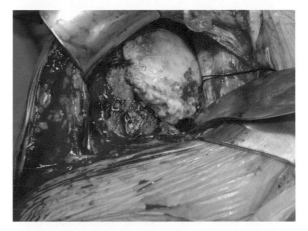

Figure 3   Subperiosteal release of the inferior capsule, which is imperative for humeral head exposure. Note the prominent inferior humeral head osteophytes.

humeral cutting guide is then placed on the anterior aspect of the humeral shaft in line with the humeral shaft and at a height that corresponds to the anatomic neck of the humerus. It is imperative that this cut be dictated not by the humeral osteophyte shelf but by the humeral cutting guide and its alignment with the humeral shaft (**Figure 4,** *B*).

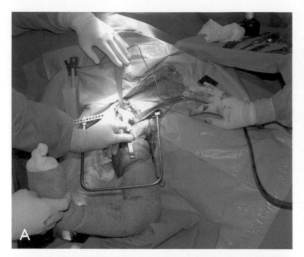

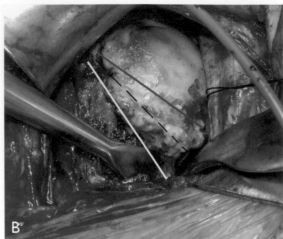

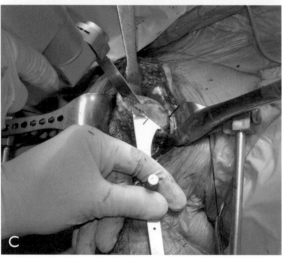

Figure 4   Proximal humeral osteotomy for TSA. **A,** The humerus is positioned in 30° of external rotation while the osteotomy is made. **B,** The yellow line represents a cut that is too steep; the blue line represents a cut that is too shallow; the dashed line represents the ideal plane of osteotomy. **C,** A properly angled proximal humeral osteotomy is made using the cutting guide. This cut is made in 30° of retroversion in routine TSA cases.

A humeral osteotomy cut made too acutely (too steep) will result in medialization of the humeral component and prominence of the greater tuberosity. A cut that is too oblique (too flat) will result in a proud humeral component, compromising the subacromial space. Strict attention to the degree of arm external rotation and alignment of the humeral shaft with the humeral cutting guide will preclude such errors (**Figure 4,** C). The appropriate amount of retroversion is determined by this cut. We usually cut the proximal humerus in 30° of retroversion if no instability exists preoperatively or intraoperatively. With the humeral head removed, the deep surface of the supraspinatus is readily visualized, as is the biceps tendon, as it inserts on the superior labrum and supraglenoid tubercle. The biceps is then tenotomized and the intra-articular portion is resected. The residual portion of the tendon is tenodesed at the inferior aspect of the bicipital groove at the time of closure. Releasing the biceps tendon not only improves visualization but also lessens tension on the soft tissues at the time of retractor placement.

Glenoid Preparation and Placement

Adequate soft-tissue releases on the humeral side, especially along the metaphyseal flare of the proximal humerus, will facilitate glenoid exposure with appropriate retractor placement.

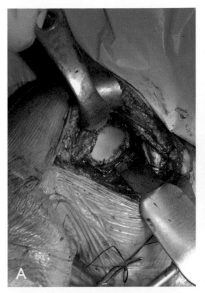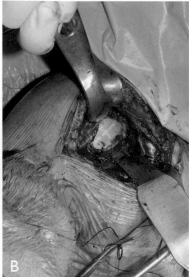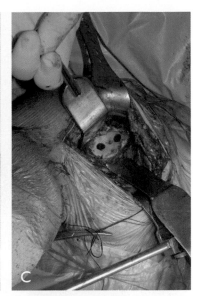

Figure 5   Glenoid preparation in TSA. **A,** Retractors are used to push the humeral head posterolaterally to facilitate glenoid exposure. **B,** Glenoid preparation starts with removal of the labrum, followed by creation of a centering hole. **C,** After templating the glenoid for the appropriate component, peg holes are drilled.

With the soft-tissue releases complete, attention is turned to the glenoid. A spiked retractor is placed on the anterior glenoid neck and a curved retractor is placed posteriorly, pushing the humeral head laterally and posteriorly (**Figure 5,** *A*). The residual labrum is resected and a centering hole is created, followed by reaming and preparation of the glenoid face (**Figure 5,** *B*). In situations of excessive glenoid retroversion (>15°) and/or a biconcave glenoid, additional reaming may be necessary to take down the high anterior wall of the glenoid. Care is taken to define the amount of retroversion preoperatively with appropriate diagnostic studies and imaging, specifically CT scans and three-dimensional reconstructions. Although the vast majority of osteoarthritic shoulders can be addressed with surface reaming alone, with more significant retroversion, posterior glenoid bone graft may be considered, and, in more advanced situations, even reverse arthroplasty. The glenoid is templated for an appropriately sized implant, and peg holes are created into which a trial component is placed (**Figure 5,** *C*). Incomplete seating or toggling of the glenoid trial is unacceptable; if

this occurs, either the surface needs additional reaming or the depth of the peg holes should be increased. Once the trial component is stable, the holes are packed with thrombin-soaked gel foam and a half batch of methyl methacrylate is prepared (**Figure 6,** *A*). The gel foam is removed, and the glenoid component is inserted using modern, standard cementing techniques (**Figure 6,** *B*).

Humeral Preparation

The humeral canal is prepared with sequential reaming only to the point where light cortical contact is noted. In contrast to the cortex of the femur, the cortex of the humerus is often quite thin, especially in patients with rheumatoid arthritis, and avoidance of excessive reaming that may lead to cortical thinning or breach is key. If the cortex is thinned or breached, cement application is warranted. A cement restrictor is placed 1 cm distal to the stem tip. Following reaming, sequential broaching is done, and the final broach is left in place for modular head trialing (**Figure 7**). The modular head size is determined by measuring the diameter of the resected head, taking osteophyte formation into consideration.

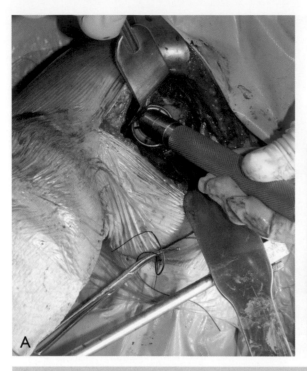

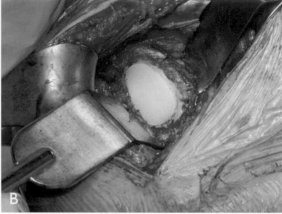

Figure 6   Glenoid component placement in TSA. **A,** The glenoid component is trialed. A flush fit without any toggling is imperative. **B,** The glenoid component is inserted using modern cementing techniques.

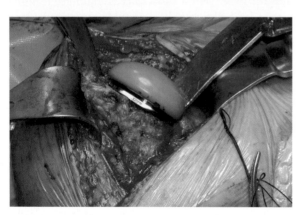

Figure 7   The humeral modular component is trialed.

Head thickness equals the thickness of the resected head minus 4 mm to allow for the thickness of the glenoid component. Various offsets of the modular head taper

allow for a multitude of positioning options and proper tensioning of the soft tissues as well as complete coverage of the proximal humerus.

Assessing Rotator Cuff and Capsular Tension

A critical part of a shoulder arthroplasty is proper component selection and position, to optimize tension of the rotator cuff and capsule. Oversized components will result in overstuffing and diminished function with increased pain and arthroplasty failure. Conversely, undersizing can result in instability, inadequate tensioning of the rotator cuff, and diminished function. Five tests are used to assess rotator cuff and capsular tension following modular head placement and reduction of the shoulder: (1) internal rotation to the abdomen without excessive tension, (2) 90° of external rotation without dislocation, (3) capsular closure with 45° of external rotation, (4) 30% to 40% translation of head on glenoid, and (5) head height at or greater than greater tuberosity (**Table 1**).

Table 1: Tests to Assess Tension of the Rotator Cuff and Capsule

Test	Description
Internal rotation to the abdomen without excessive tension	The surgeon should be able to bring the arm into full internal rotation to the abdomen without evidence of significant posterior capsular tightness. If this is not achievable, it is likely that the head size needs to be decreased or the version altered.
90° of external rotation without dislocation	The surgeon brings the arm into 90° of external rotation and 45° of abduction, holding the arm with only a hand beneath the outer aspect of the elbow and allowing the humeral head to gently lever anteriorly on the glenoid component. If modular head size and soft-tissue balancing are appropriate, the head will subluxate but not dislocate. If the head does dislocate, humeral version may need to be reevaluated and adapted accordingly.
Capsular closure with 45° of external rotation	With the arm in slight abduction and 45° of external rotation, the mobilized subscapularis and capsule are brought out laterally to their original site of attachment. If this cannot be achieved, either additional mobilization of the subscapularis is needed or the subscapularis will need to be repaired to the osteotomy with transosseous sutures. Adequate soft-tissue release at the time of exposure should result in sufficient soft-tissue lengthening to allow this to occur.
30% to 40% translation of head on glenoid	A load-and-shift maneuver is performed on the glenohumeral articulation with the arm in slight external rotation and 20° of abduction. If appropriately sized components have been chosen, there should be a residual amount of laxity built into the construct that allows the humeral head to translate smoothly on the glenoid component by 30% to 40% both anteriorly and posteriorly and a minimal amount inferiorly.
Head height at or greater than greater tuberosity	Optimal head height in shoulder arthroplasty is at, or slightly higher than, the greater tuberosity at its apex. If the apex of the head is lower than the greater tuberosity, there is a risk of tuberosity impingement. Conversely, if the head is significantly higher than the greater tuberosity, the rotator cuff will be overtensioned and compromised.

Bone Graft Preparation

More than 90% of all humeral components may readily be press fit. To enhance the likelihood of bony incorporation, it is recommended that autograft be used in all cases. Autograft is readily available from the resected humeral head, which is cut into 3 × 3 × 30 mm cancellous matchsticks with a microsagittal saw (**Figure 8**). Any residual cortical or chondral tissue is removed from the matchsticks, and they are incorporated with the placement of the humeral component.

Humeral Component Placement and Closure

If a significant internal rotation contracture was identified preoperatively and the capsule and subscapularis were released subperiosteally from their insertions onto the lesser tuberosity, it may be desirable to reattach them at the margin of the humeral osteotomy. To achieve this requires that sutures be placed before component placement. Drill holes (1/8-in) are made 7 to 8 mm apart along the anterior inferior aspect of the

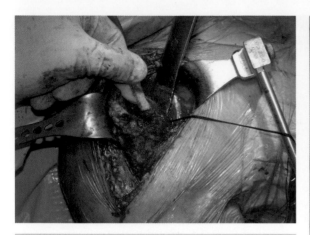

Figure 8 Cancellous bone graft matchsticks created from the resected proximal humeral head are incorporated with the press-fit humeral stem to enhance fixation and bony ingrowth.

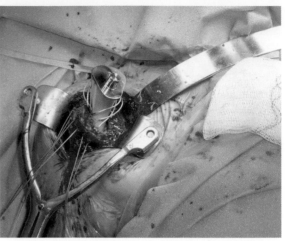

Figure 9 Subscapularis sutures are placed through bony tunnels looped around the humeral stem to negate the risk of suture cut-out.

humeral shaft, through which No. 2 braided high-strength sutures are passed. As each suture is placed, a loop is created with the suture material through which the humeral component will be placed, thereby obviating any risk of suture cut-out (**Figure 9**). Prior to the component being placed, the cancellous graft is placed along the medial calcar. The component is then positioned within the loop created by the sutures and driven down into the canal in a press-fit fashion. If osteotomy sutures have not been used, grafting and component placement are done in a normal fashion. The trunion is then cleaned and the previously determined modular head is gently placed on the trunion, rotated into appropriate position, and impacted. The shoulder is reduced, the capsulotomy is repaired, and the aforementioned stability tests are repeated to ensure that the final component position, size, and version are correct.

Postoperative Considerations

Rehabilitation

Postoperatively, the patient receives a cryothermal unit. The patient is then placed into a shoulder immobilizer with slight external rotation to bring the arm into a more neutral position. The patient is discharged 1 to 2 days following arthroplasty and instructed on gentle active elbow and wrist range-of-motion exercises.

Shoulder shrugs and pendulum exercises also are started immediately. Formal physical therapy is started 1 week postoperatively after confirming wound status, component position, and comfort level. Most of the postoperative exercises are either active or active-assisted, thereby facilitating a more rapid return of proprioceptive input. The limiting factor in the rehabilitation after TSA is the healing of the subscapularis tendon. Postoperative rehabilitation following TSA is dictated in great part by subscapularis quality and mobilization achieved intraoperatively. In patients with mild internal rotation contractures (external rotation >20° to 30° preoperatively), we initiate active and passive external rotation in the first week, allowing them to regain 40° of external rotation during the first 4 to 6 weeks. Patients with more severe contractures (external rotation <20°) in whom an aggressive subscapularis release and mobilization was needed require a more controlled postoperative program, limiting external rotation to only neutral for the first 3 weeks, and progressing to 30° over weeks 4 through 6. In both groups of patients, light, progressive resistance exercises are added at 6 weeks, when the patient has regained a moderate amount of active motion and the subscapularis repair is stable.

Adequate healing of the subscapularis repair is paramount to the success of the procedure. Physical therapy is continued as needed, and the patients are told that they will be allowed to resume everyday activities, such as driving, when they are able to actively forward elevate to at least 90° and externally rotate at least 30°, and have discontinued the use of all narcotics.

Boardman et al[42] evaluated the outcomes of a home-based therapy program after TSA. At a mean follow-up of 4.1 years (range, 2 to 7.1 years), the patients maintained 70% of forward elevation and 90% of external rotation compared with what was possible intraoperatively. Approximately 80% of motion is achieved by 3 months postoperatively. At this point, patients can resume their approved sports activities in a progressive fashion, including chipping and putting for golf or hitting short ground strokes in tennis. Such activities are allowed based on the patient's comfort level, range of motion, strength restoration, and stability.

Return to Activities

No clear guidelines exist regarding the timing of return to sports after shoulder arthroplasty, or even if a patient may safely return to specific sports. Jensen and Rockwood[43] retrospectively evaluated 26 shoulder arthroplasties (6 hemiarthroplasties, 20 TSAs) in 24 patients with respect to their return to golf. They found that 23 of 24 patients (96%) were able to return to golf. Three of the patients in their study underwent bilateral TSA. On average, patients were able to return to golf 4.5 months after surgery. In addition, the 18 patients who reported a preoperative handicap averaged a five-stroke improvement. It is important to note that when the authors compared their golfing patients with patients undergoing TSA who did not golf, there was no increase in radiolucent lines.

One important indicator of a patient's safe return to sport after shoulder arthroplasty appears to be the prior skill level. For example, a patient who is an exceptional tennis player with excellent form will have a higher likelihood of safely returning to tennis after surgery than the occasional player. It may not be advisable for patients undergoing shoulder arthroplasty to attempt sports with which they have no prior experience.

Recommendations on return to sports after shoulder arthroplasty are described more fully in chapter 27.

Complications

Despite promising long-term results with TSA, many complications can require revision surgery. Reported complication rates have been quite variable, ranging from 0% to 62%, with mean complication rates ranging from 10% to 16%.[45-47] A recent review by Bohsali et al[48] revealed 414 complications in 2,810 shoulders (14.7%). In this review, the most common complications, in order of frequency, were component loosening, instability, periprosthetic fracture, rotator cuff tears, neural injury, infection, and deltoid muscle dysfunction.

Failure of the glenoid component is one of the most common complications and accounts for most of the unsatisfactory results following TSA. The reported incidence of radiolucency at the glenoid-cement interface has ranged from 30% to 96%.[14,17,18,21,49-52] In addition, glenoid loosening is the most common reason for prosthesis-related revision surgery.[47,53-55] Several studies have evaluated glenoid component design and implantation techniques to determine the best fixation.[56-73] After comparing keeled versus pegged glenoids and metal-backed uncemented versus all-polyethylene cemented glenoid components, it appears that the current fixation method of choice is a pegged, all-polyethylene component fixed using modern cementing techniques. Nyffeler et al[74] demonstrated that cementing the pegged glenoid component under pressure using a syringe, as well as applying cement to the back of the component, yielded stronger fixation than finger pressure and no cement on the back of the glenoid. In addition, glenoid components with a radius of curvature greater than that of the humeral component have been shown to have lower rates of loosening.[67,68,75-79]

A study performed at the Mayo Clinic reviewed the contemporary complications and their frequency in 431 Cofield TSAs (Smith & Nephew, Memphis, TN) with an average 4.2-year follow-up.[80] In their review, the authors concluded that the frequency of complications has decreased dramatically, as has the number of major complications and the revision rate, with more current arthroplasty designs and techniques. They did, however, find that intraoperative periprosthetic humeral fractures were more common with more modern techniques. The authors speculated that this may be due to the shift away from the anteromedial exposure with release of the anterior deltoid to the long deltopectoral exposure, which necessitates increased extension and external rotation torque on the humerus.

Summary

TSA has been proven in the literature to be a predictable, successful, and reliable treatment for most cases of glenohumeral OA. The preponderance of major complications has been on the glenoid side, but with improvement in techniques and prosthetic materials, the complication rate has declined. Careful attention must be paid to the soft-tissue aspect of the procedure to ensure proper tensioning and stability. Many baby boomers can return to their sports activities after TSA, although recommendations and evidence in the literature are sparse. It seems that a patient's prior skill level is a significant factor in the return to sport after TSA, as is the initial shoulder pathology.

Patients with RCTA do not do as well with standard TSA. To address this difficult problem, the reverse ball-and-socket prosthesis has been developed and has demonstrated success in both pain relief and restoration of function. Caution must be exercised when using this prosthesis, as the complication rate in short-term follow-up has been quite high. This prosthesis is usually reserved for the older, less active patient population, although with technologic advancements in prosthetic design and technique, the indications will continue to expand.

References

1. Jain N, Pietrobon R, Hocker S, Guller U, Shankar A, Higgins LD: The relationship between surgeon and hospital volume and outcomes for shoulder arthroplasty. *J Bone Joint Surg Am* 2004;86-A(3):496-505.

2. Boileau P, Watkinson D, Hatzidakis AM, Hovorka I: Neer Award 2005: The Grammont reverse shoulder prosthesis. Results in cuff tear arthritis, fracture sequelae, and revision arthroplasty. *J Shoulder Elbow Surg* 2006;15(5):527-540.

3. Cuff D, Pupello D, Virani N, Levy J, Frankle M: Reverse shoulder arthroplasty for the treatment of rotator cuff deficiency. *J Bone Joint Surg Am* 2008; 90(6):1244-1251.

4. Frankle M, Siegal S, Pupello D, Saleem A, Mighell M, Vasey M: The Reverse Shoulder Prosthesis for glenohumeral arthritis associated with severe rotator cuff deficiency: A minimum two-year follow-up study of sixty patients. *J Bone Joint Surg Am* 2005;87(8): 1697-1705.

5. Guery J, Favard L, Sirveaux F, Oudet D, Molé D, Walch G: Reverse total shoulder arthroplasty: Survivorship analysis of eighty replacements followed for five to ten years. *J Bone Joint Surg Am* 2006;88(8): 1742-1747.

6. Sirveaux F, Favard L, Oudet D, Huquet D, Walch G, Molé D: Grammont inverted total shoulder arthroplasty in the treatment of glenohumeral osteoarthritis with massive rupture of the cuff: Results of a multicentre study of 80 shoulders. *J Bone Joint Surg Br* 2004;86(3):388-395.

7. Wall B, Nové-Josserand L, O'Connor DP, Edwards TB, Walch G: Reverse total shoulder arthroplasty: A review of results according to etiology. *J Bone Joint Surg Am* 2007;89(7):1476-1485.

8. Werner CM, Steinmann PA, Gilbart M, Gerber C: Treatment of painful pseudoparesis due to irreparable rotator cuff dysfunction with the Delta III reverse-ball-and-socket total shoulder prosthesis. *J Bone Joint Surg Am* 2005;87(7):1476-1486.

9. Tokish JM, Decker MJ, Ellis HB, Torry MR, Hawkins RJ: The belly-press test for the physical examination of the subscapularis muscle: Electromyographic validation and comparison to the lift-off test. *J Shoulder Elbow Surg* 2003;12(5):427-430.

10. Walch G, Boulahia A, Boileau P, Kempf JF: Primary glenohumeral osteoarthritis: Clinical and radiographic classification. The Aequalis Group. *Acta Orthop Belg* 1998;64(Suppl 2):46-52.

11. Simovitch RW, Helmy N, Zumstein MA, Gerber C: Impact of fatty infiltration of the teres minor muscle on the outcome of reverse total shoulder arthroplasty. *J Bone Joint Surg Am* 2007;89(5):934-939.

12. Edwards TB, Boulahia A, Kempf JF, Boileau P, Némoz C, Walch G: The influence of rotator cuff disease on the results of shoulder arthroplasty for primary osteoarthritis: Results of a multicenter study. *J Bone Joint Surg Am* 2002;84-A(12):2240-2248.

13. Bell RH, Noble JS: The management of significant glenoid deficiency in total shoulder arthroplasty. *J Shoulder Elbow Surg* 2000;9(3):248-256.

14. Barrett WP, Franklin JL, Jackins SE, Wyss CR, Matsen FA III: Total shoulder arthroplasty. *J Bone Joint Surg Am* 1987;69(6):865-872.

15. Boyd AD Jr, Thomas WH, Scott RD, Sledge CB, Thornhill TS: Total shoulder arthroplasty versus hemiarthroplasty: Indications for glenoid resurfacing. *J Arthroplasty* 1990;5(4):329-336.

16. Bryant D, Litchfield R, Sandow M, Gartsman GM, Guyatt G, Kirkley A: A comparison of pain, strength, range of motion, and functional outcomes after hemiarthroplasty and total shoulder arthroplasty in patients with osteoarthritis of the shoulder: A systematic review and meta-analysis. *J Bone Joint Surg Am* 2005;87(9):1947-1956.

17. Neer CS II, Watson KC, Stanton FJ: Recent experience in total shoulder replacement. *J Bone Joint Surg Am* 1982;64(3):319-337.

18. Cofield RH: Total shoulder arthroplasty with the Neer prosthesis. *J Bone Joint Surg Am* 1984;66(6):899-906.

19. Deshmukh AV, Koris M, Zurakowski D, Thornhill TS: Total shoulder arthroplasty: Long-term survivorship, functional outcome, and quality of life. *J Shoulder Elbow Surg* 2005;14(5):471-479.

20. Gartsman GM, Roddey TS, Hammerman SM: Shoulder arthroplasty with or without resurfacing of the glenoid in patients who have osteoarthritis. *J Bone Joint Surg Am* 2000;82(1):26-34.

21. Hawkins RJ, Bell RH, Jallay B: Total shoulder arthroplasty. *Clin Orthop Relat Res* 1989;(242): 188-194.

22. Kelly IG, Foster RS, Fisher WD: Neer total shoulder replacement in rheumatoid arthritis. *J Bone Joint Surg Br* 1987;69(5):723-726.

23. Lo IK, Litchfield RB, Griffin S, Faber K, Patterson SD, Kirkley A: Quality-of-life outcome following hemiarthroplasty or total shoulder arthroplasty in patients with osteoarthritis: A prospective, randomized trial. *J Bone Joint Surg Am* 2005;87(10):2178-2185.

24. McCoy SR, Warren RF, Bade HA III, Ranawat CS, Inglis AE: Total shoulder arthroplasty in rheumatoid arthritis. *J Arthroplasty* 1989;4(2):105-113.

25. Norris TR, Iannotti JP: Functional outcome after shoulder arthroplasty for primary osteoarthritis: A multicenter study. *J Shoulder Elbow Surg* 2002; 11(2):130-135.

26. Orfaly RM, Rockwood CA Jr, Esenyel CZ, Wirth MA: A prospective functional outcome study of shoulder arthroplasty for osteoarthritis with an intact rotator cuff. *J Shoulder Elbow Surg* 2003;12(3):214-221.

27. Neer CS: Glenohumeral arthroplasty, in Neer CS, ed: *Shoulder Reconstruction.* Philadelphia, PA, WB Saunders, 1990, pp 143-272.

28. Neer CS II: Replacement arthroplasty for glenohumeral arthritis. *J Bone Joint Surg Am* 1974;56(1):1-13.

29. Radnay CS, Setter KJ, Chambers L, Levine WN, Bigliani LU, Ahmad CS: Total shoulder replacement compared with humeral head replacement for the treatment of primary glenohumeral osteoarthritis: A systematic review. *J Shoulder Elbow Surg* 2007;16(4): 396-402.

30. Sperling JW, Cofield RH, Schleck CD, Harmsen WS: Total shoulder arthroplasty versus hemiarthroplasty for rheumatoid arthritis of the shoulder: Results of 303 consecutive cases. *J Shoulder Elbow Surg* 2007;16(6): 683-690.

31. Torchia ME, Cofield RH, Settergren CR: Total shoulder arthroplasty with the Neer prosthesis: Long-term results. *J Shoulder Elbow Surg* 1997;6(6):495-505.

32. Cofield RH: Revision procedure for shoulder arthroplasty, in Morrey BF, An KN, Cabanells ME, eds: *Reconstructive Surgery of the Joints,* ed 2. New York, NY, Churchill Livingstone, 1996, p 789.

33. Sperling JW, Cofield RH, Rowland CM: Minimum fifteen-year follow-up of Neer hemiarthroplasty and total shoulder arthroplasty in patients aged fifty years or younger. *J Shoulder Elbow Surg* 2004;13(6):604-613.

34. Lynch JR, Franta AK, Montgomery WH Jr, Lenters TR, Mounce D, Matsen FA III: Self-assessed outcome at two to four years after shoulder hemiarthroplasty with concentric glenoid reaming. *J Bone Joint Surg Am* 2007;89(6):1284-1292.

35. Clinton J, Franta AK, Lenters TR, Mounce D, Matsen FA III: Nonprosthetic glenoid arthroplasty with humeral hemiarthroplasty and total shoulder arthroplasty yield similar self-assessed outcomes in the management of comparable patients with glenohumeral arthritis. *J Shoulder Elbow Surg* 2007;16(5):534-538.

36. Krishnan SG, Nowinski RJ, Harrison D, Burkhead WZ: Humeral hemiarthroplasty with biologic resurfacing of the glenoid for glenohumeral arthritis: Two to fifteen-year outcomes. *J Bone Joint Surg Am* 2007;89(4):727-734.

37. Ball C, Galatz L, Yamaguchi K: Meniscal allograft interposition arthroplasty for the arthritic shoulder:

Description of a new surgical technique. *Tech Shoulder Elbow Surg* 2001;2:247-254.

38. Burkhead WZ Jr, Hutton KS: Biologic resurfacing of the glenoid with hemiarthroplasty of the shoulder. *J Shoulder Elbow Surg* 1995;4(4):263-270.

39. Nicholson GP, Goldstein JL, Romeo AA, et al: Lateral meniscus allograft biologic glenoid athroplasty in total shoulder arthroplasty for young shoulders with degenerative joint disease. *J Shoulder Elbow Surg* 2007;16(5 Suppl):S261-S266.

40. Nowinski RJ, Newark OH, Burkhead WZ Jr: Hemiarthroplasty with biologic glenoid resurfacing: 5-13 year outcomes, in: Bioleau P, ed: *Shoulder Arthroscopy & Arthroplasty: Current Concepts.* Montpellier, France, Sauramps Medical, 2004, pp 354-360.

41. Hawkins RJ, Angelo RL: Glenohumeral osteoarthrosis: A late complication of the Putti-Platt repair. *J Bone Joint Surg Am* 1990;72(8):1193-1197.

42. Boardman ND III, Cofield RH, Bengtson KA, Little R, Jones MC, Rowland CM: Rehabilitation after total shoulder arthroplasty. *J Arthroplasty* 2001;16(4): 483-486.

43. Jensen KL, Rockwood CA Jr: Shoulder arthroplasty in recreational golfers. *J Shoulder Elbow Surg* 1998;7(4): 362-367.

44. Healy WL, Iorio R, Lemos MJ: Athletic activity after joint replacement. *Am J Sports Med* 2001;29(3): 377-388.

45. Wirth MA, Rockwood CA Jr: Complications of total shoulder-replacement arthroplasty. *J Bone Joint Surg Am* 1996;78(4):603-616.

46. Matsen FA III, Rockwood CA Jr, Wirth MA, Lippitt SB, Parsons M: Glenohumeral arthritis and its management, in Rockwood CA Jr, Matsen FA III, Wirth MA, Lippitt SB, eds: *The Shoulder*, ed 3. Philadelphia, PA, WB Saunders, 2004, pp 879-1008.

47. Wirth MA, Rockwood CA Jr: Complications of shoulder arthroplasty. *Clin Orthop Relat Res* 1994;(307): 47-69.

48. Bohsali KI, Wirth MA, Rockwood CA Jr: Complications of total shoulder arthroplasty. *J Bone Joint Surg Am* 2006;88(10):2279-2292.

49. Bade H, Warren R, Ranawat C, et al: Long term results of Neer total shoulder replacement, in Bateman J, Welsh R, eds: *Surgery of the Shoulder.* St. Louis, MO, Mosby, 1984, pp 249-252.

50. Boileau P, Walch G, Noël E, Liotard JP: Neer's shoulder prosthesis: Results according to etiology. *Rev Rhum Ed Fr* 1994;61(9):607-618.

51. Boyd AD, Thornhill TS: Glenoid resurfacing in shoulder arthroplasty, in Freidman RJ, ed: *Arthroplasty of the Shoulder.* New York, NY, Thieme, 1994, pp 306-316.

52. Brenner BC, Ferlic DC, Clayton ML, Dennis DA: Survivorship of unconstrained total shoulder arthroplasty. *J Bone Joint Surg Am* 1989;71(9):1289-1296.

53. Brems J: The glenoid component in total shoulder arthroplasty. *J Shoulder Elbow Surg* 1993;2(1):47-54.

54. Mestdagh H, Boileau P, Walch G: Intra and postoperative complications of shoulder arthroplasty, in Walch G, Boileau P, eds: *Shoulder Arthroplasty.* Berlin, Germany, Springer-Verlag, 1999, pp 163-167.

55. Rodosky MW, Bigliani LU: Indications for glenoid resurfacing in shoulder arthroplasty. *J Shoulder Elbow Surg* 1996;5(3):231-248.

56. Wirth MA, Korvick DL, Basamania CJ, Toro F, Aufdemorte TB, Rockwood CA Jr: Radiologic, mechanical, and histologic evaluation of 2 glenoid prosthesis designs in a canine model. *J Shoulder Elbow Surg* 2001;10(2):140-148.

57. Gunther SB, Graham J, Norris TR, Ries MD, Pruitt L: Retrieved glenoid components: A classification system for surface damage analysis. *J Arthroplasty* 2002;17(1): 95-100.

58. Cheung EV, Sperling JW, Cofield RH: Polyethylene insert exchange for wear after total shoulder arthroplasty. *J Shoulder Elbow Surg* 2007;16(5): 574-578.

59. Hopkins AR, Hansen UN, Amis AA, et al: Wear in the prosthetic shoulder: Association with design parameters. *J Biomech Eng* 2007;129(2):223-230.

60. Gupta S, van der Helm FC, van Keulen F: Stress analysis of cemented glenoid prostheses in total shoulder arthroplasty. *J Biomech* 2004;37(11):1777-1786.

61. Martin SD, Zurakowski D, Thornhill TS: Uncemented glenoid component in total shoulder arthroplasty: Survivorship and outcomes. *J Bone Joint Surg Am* 2005;87(6):1284-1292.

62. Boileau P, Avidor C, Krishnan SG, Walch G, Kempf JF, Molé D: Cemented polyethylene versus uncemented metal-backed glenoid components in total

shoulder arthroplasty: A prospective, double-blind, randomized study. *J Shoulder Elbow Surg* 2002;11(4): 351-359.

63. Wallace AL, Phillips RL, MacDougal GA, Walsh WR, Sonnabend DH: Resurfacing of the glenoid in total shoulder arthroplasty: A comparison, at a mean of five years, of prostheses inserted with and without cement. *J Bone Joint Surg Am* 1999;81(4):510-518.

64. Hopkins AR, Hansen UN, Amis AA, Emery R: The effects of glenoid component alignment variations on cement mantle stresses in total shoulder arthroplasty. *J Shoulder Elbow Surg* 2004;13(6):668-675.

65. Swieszkowski W, Bednarz P, Prendergast PJ: Contact stresses in the glenoid component in total shoulder arthroplasty. *Proc Inst Mech Eng H* 2003;217(1):49-57.

66. Wallace AL, Walsh WR, Sonnabend DH: Dissociation of the glenoid component in cementless total shoulder arthroplasty. *J Shoulder Elbow Surg* 1999;8(1):81-84.

67. Anglin C, Wyss UP, Nyffeler RW, Gerber C: Loosening performance of cemented glenoid prosthesis design pairs. *Clin Biomech (Bristol, Avon)* 2001;16(2): 144-150.

68. Anglin C, Wyss UP, Pichora DR: Mechanical testing of shoulder prostheses and recommendations for glenoid design. *J Shoulder Elbow Surg* 2000;9(4):323-331.

69. Szabo I, Buscayret F, Edwards TB, Nemoz C, Boileau P, Walch G: Radiographic comparison of flat-back and convex-back glenoid components in total shoulder arthroplasty. *J Shoulder Elbow Surg* 2005;14(6): 636-642.

70. Iannotti JP, Spencer EE, Winter U, Deffenbaugh D, Williams G: Prosthetic positioning in total shoulder arthroplasty. *J Shoulder Elbow Surg* 2005;14(1, Suppl S):111S-121S.

71. Lazarus MD, Jensen KL, Southworth C, Matsen FA III: The radiographic evaluation of keeled and pegged glenoid component insertion. *J Bone Joint Surg Am* 2002;84-A(7):1174-1182.

72. Klepps S, Chiang AS, Miller S, Jiang CY, Hazrati Y, Flatow EL: Incidence of early radiolucent glenoid lines in patients having total shoulder replacements. *Clin Orthop Relat Res* 2005;(435):118-125.

73. Gartsman GM, Elkousy HA, Warnock KM, Edwards TB, O'Connor DP: Radiographic comparison of pegged and keeled glenoid components. *J Shoulder Elbow Surg* 2005;14(3):252-257.

74. Nyffeler RW, Meyer D, Sheikh R, Koller BJ, Gerber C: The effect of cementing technique on structural fixation of pegged glenoid components in total shoulder arthroplasty. *J Shoulder Elbow Surg* 2006; 15(1):106-111.

75. Karduna AR, Williams GR, Iannotti JP, Williams JL: Total shoulder arthroplasty biomechanics: A study of the forces and strains at the glenoid component. *J Biomech Eng* 1998;120(1):92-99.

76. Karduna AR, Williams GR, Williams JL, Iannotti JP: Glenohumeral joint translations before and after total shoulder arthroplasty: A study in cadavera. *J Bone Joint Surg Am* 1997;79(8):1166-1174.

77. Severt R, Thomas BJ, Tsenter MJ, Amstutz HC, Kabo JM: The influence of conformity and constraint on translational forces and frictional torque in total shoulder arthroplasty. *Clin Orthop Relat Res* 1993; (292):151-158.

78. Terrier A, Büchler P, Farron A: Influence of glenohumeral conformity on glenoid stresses after total shoulder arthroplasty. *J Shoulder Elbow Surg* 2006; 15(4):515-520.

79. Walch G, Edwards TB, Boulahia A, Boileau P, Molé D, Adeleine P: The influence of glenohumeral prosthetic mismatch on glenoid radiolucent lines: Results of a multicenter study. *J Bone Joint Surg Am* 2002;84-A(12): 2186-2191.

80. Chin PY, Sperling JW, Cofield RH, Schleck C: Complications of total shoulder arthroplasty: Are they fewer or different? *J Shoulder Elbow Surg* 2006;15(1): 19-22.

Chapter 17

Hemiarthroplasty Versus Total Shoulder Arthroplasty

David M. Lutton, MD
Evan L. Flatow, MD

Key Points

- The term "mature athlete" describes an expanding cohort of individuals who are typically between the ages of 40 and 60 and who maintain a very active lifestyle, including participation in sports. Treatment options for glenohumeral arthritis in this population can be less straightforward than in an older, more sedentary population.
- Nonsurgical treatment options such as nonsteroidal anti-inflammatory drugs (NSAIDs) and local corticosteroid injections should be considered.
- A variety of surgical options are available, including arthroscopic procedures and arthroplasty. Each has its advantages and disadvantages.
- Total shoulder arthroplasty (TSA) has proved to be an effective and reliable surgical option.
- The treatment algorithm must be tailored to the individual patient with respect to severity of symptoms, functional demand, patient expectations, and medical comorbidities.

Dr. Flatow or an immediate family member serves as a board member, owner, officer, or committee member of the American Shoulder and Elbow Surgeons, the Arthroscopy Association of North America, and the Mt. Sinai Medical Center; has received royalties from Innomed and Zimmer; serves as a paid consultant to or is an employee of Wyeth; serves as an unpaid consultant to Zimmer; and has received research or institutional support from Zimmer. Neither Dr. Lutton nor any immediate family member has received anything of value from or owns stock in a commercial company or institution related directly or indirectly to the subject of this chapter.

Introduction

As medical care improves and life expectancy increases, the term "mature athlete" is being redefined. A paradigm shift is emerging as many patients are maintaining an athletic lifestyle far beyond conventional norms and expectations.[1] Unfortunately, these patients may have a variety of shoulder ailments with the end point of painful arthrosis. In concert with the epidemiologic change, the indications, techniques, and prostheses for shoulder arthroplasty have advanced and may afford these mature athletes more options for pain relief. Patients with symptoms that are refractory to nonsurgical and/or arthroscopic measures may benefit from prosthetic replacement. Hemiarthroplasty (humeral head replacement), TSA, and biologic resurfacing have proven to be viable options for these patients.[2-5]

Etiology

Painful arthrosis of the glenohumeral joint can be caused by a variety of pathologic processes: degenerative osteoarthritis, osteonecrosis, sequelae of proximal humerus fractures, post-traumatic arthritis, and inflamma-

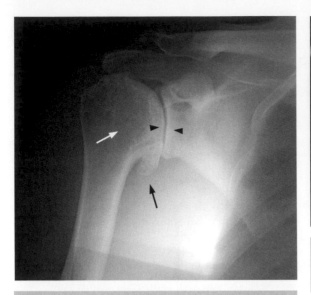

Figure 1 True AP view demonstrates the typical pattern of osteoarthritis—inferior osteophytes (black arrow), subchondral sclerosis (arrowheads), and cystic formation (white arrow).

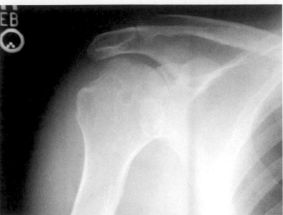

Figure 2 AP view of a rheumatoid shoulder demonstrates medialization of the humeral head, osteopenia, and erosions.

tory arthritis. Understanding the etiology and pathophysiology of each disease can aid the clinician in appropriately managing patients with these ailments. These patients may benefit from surgical intervention—not limited to prosthetic replacement, but also including appropriate capsular releases and soft-tissue balancing as dictated by the site of capsular contractures and laxity unique to each disease process.

Osteoarthritis often affects the glenohumeral joint, although it is not as common as in the hip or knee. In the early phases of the disease, patients with glenohumeral arthritis report pain with activities of daily living, pain at night, and limited internal rotation. Radiographic evaluation demonstrates joint space narrowing, sclerosis, subchondral cysts, inferior humeral osteophytes, and glenoid erosion[6] (**Figure 1**). Glenoid wear is typically most severe in the posterosuperior quadrant.[7] Medical management is palliative; to date, no pharmacologic or physical therapy modality has been proven to alter disease progression. Surgical management is aimed at releasing capsular contractures, correcting glenoid version, and recentering the humeral head.

Rheumatoid arthritis is the most common inflammatory arthropathy affecting the shoulder. Glenohumeral pathology is a common finding in the rheumatoid patient; 65% to 90% of patients will report shoulder pain and/or loss of function during their lifetime.[8] Shoulder involvement is typically associated with polyarthropathy.[9] Rheumatoid arthritis has a 3:1 female-to-male prevalence. The typical patient who presents with rheumatoid arthritis is a woman between 35 and 50 years of age.[8] These patients may have variable rotator cuff integrity. Radiographs demonstrate osteopenia, medial (but variable) glenoid wear, and possibly mild proximal humeral migration from thinning of the rotator cuff (**Figure 2**). Medical management with disease-modifying antirheumatic drugs may slow the progression of glenohumeral arthrosis; however, once the disease process has advanced, early surgical intervention may be indicated, as it can provide pain relief as well as prevent further bony or tendinous destruction.

Osteonecrosis of the humeral head is associated with a variety of disease processes and may occur after trauma,[10] high doses of systemic corticosteroids, alcohol use, sickle cell disease, lupus erythematosus, hemophilia, Caisson disease, lipidoses, subtle coagulation abnormalities such as protein C and S deficiency, and idiopathic causes. Osteonecrosis often presents with progressive pain and loss of range of motion. The soft

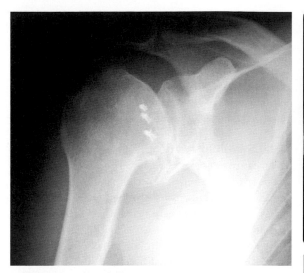

Figure 3   AP view demonstrates postcapsulorraphy glenohumeral arthritis. Patients may demonstrate significant posterior wear.

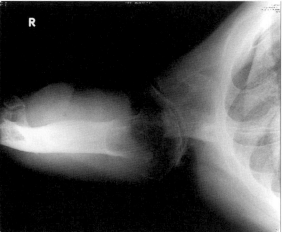

Figure 4   Axillary lateral view of the shoulder of a patient who had undergone a Putti-Platt procedure 30 years earlier demonstrates severe postcapsulorraphy glenohumeral arthritis and posterior wear with associated humeral head subluxation.

tissues about the glenohumeral joint become globally scarred. Radiographic evidence of osteonecrosis of the humeral head mirrors that seen in the femoral head, as described by Merle D'Aubigné et al.[11] Cruess[12] was the first to propose a radiographic classification of osteonecrosis progression of the glenohumeral joint: subchondral resorption, subchondral collapse, humeral head collapse, and, finally, glenoid involvement. MRI can show initial increased signal intensity on T2-weighted images, which may enable an attempt of nonsurgical management or minimally invasive techniques. Unfortunately, once radiographic evidence of osteonecrosis is present, it is often too late to salvage the humeral head. Surgical treatment at this time may consist of pancapsular release, humeral head resurfacing, or hemiarthroplasty, if the condition is addressed before glenoid involvement has occurred.

Instability-associated glenohumeral arthrosis has several etiologies, including recurrent dislocations, hardware complications, infection, postoperative chondrolysis,[13] and tightness after capsulorraphy[14,15] (**Figure 3**); however, it is most often multifactorial. Neer et al[16] were the first to describe overtightening of the anterior structures as a major cause of postcapsulorraphy arthritis. Unlike patients with osteoarthritis, these patients often present at a younger age, frequently younger than 40 years. Bigliani et al[14] found that symptomatic arthrosis required prosthetic replacement, on average 16 years after initial shoulder stabilization. Postcapsulorraphy arthritis results in pain and a severe internal rotation contracture. Radiographs demonstrate subchondral sclerosis, cysts, and osteophytes associated with posterior subluxation of the humeral head, with reciprocal severe posterior glenoid wear (**Figure 4**). Treatment of this disease is focused on anterior releases and recentering the humeral head on the glenoid. If postcapsulorraphy arthritis is identified early enough, an anterior arthroscopic release or coronal lengthening of the subscapularis may reduce the severity of disease. Unfortunately, this disease often presents after significant glenoid arthrosis and posterior wear has occurred. Adequate surgical treatment may require posterior glenoid augmentation and immobilization in a gunslinger brace for 2 to 4 weeks postoperatively. It is hoped that the more recent developments in anatomic instability reconstruction will decrease the rates of postcapsulorraphy arthritis.

Nonsurgical Management

Regardless of treatment modality, the goals of treatment of glenohumeral arthrosis are relief of pain and restoration of function.[7] Nonsurgical management depends on whether the pain is acute or chronic. An isolated, acute inflammatory flare may be treated with a brief period of rest, cryotherapy, analgesics, and an oral anti-inflammatory medication. Nonselective nonsteroidal anti-inflammatory drugs have been proven to be more effective than acetaminophen and codeine for symptomatic inflammatory arthritidies;[17] however, they also carry the inherent risks of bleeding, ulcers, and nephropathy. Modalities such as cortisone phonophoresis have not yet been proven to be beneficial, but their use is reasonable in refractory cases. Unfortunately, prolonged rest and immobilization can be detrimental, leading to stiffness and muscle atrophy. We do not routinely use intra-articular injections for symptomatic osteoarthritis; rather, we limit the use of these injections to patients who are either unwilling or unable to undergo definitive treatment. Infrequently, we will use cortisone injections in rheumatoid patients, as these injections may provide substantial and long-lasting relief. We avoid nontherapeutic intra-articular injections because of the inherent risk of septic arthritis. Although intra-articular cortisone injections may be diagnostic with shoulder arthritis, it is unusual for the diagnosis to be unclear. Studies have not shown viscosupplementation to be clearly beneficial for shoulder arthritis, and it has not yet been approved by the US Food and Drug Administration (FDA) for use in the shoulder.[18] Chronic pain can be managed medically with heat, hydrotherapy, and ultrasound. It is thought that these modalities may assuage pain and improve joint mobility by improving blood flow to the soft tissues surrounding the glenohumeral joint.

We do not believe that formal physical therapy provides demonstrable benefit with glenohumeral osteoarthritis, as it does in most other shoulder conditions. Simple use of the shoulder with activities of daily living and gentle exercises to maintain range of motion and muscle tone are typically sufficient. Motion maintains a supple joint and provides nutrition to the limited articular cartilage remaining on the humerus and glenoid.

Surgical Considerations in the Mature Athlete

The treatment approach to glenohumeral arthrosis in the mature athlete is predicated upon etiology, postoperative demands, and physiologic age. Several treatment options exist, including TSA, hemiarthroplasty, arthroscopic techniques, and interposition arthroplasty.

Total Shoulder Arthroplasty

For most pathologies, TSA has demonstrated clear superiority for pain relief, function, and patient satisfaction; however, concerns of prosthetic loosening and/or failure in the young patient may drive treating surgeons to search for alternative treatment options. Levy and Copeland[2] reported results for cementless prosthetic resurfacing of the humeral head and found they were comparable to those for stemmed arthroplasty. Humeral head resurfacing can be done with or without glenoid resurfacing. Maintenance of bone stock may make revision surgery, if needed, less difficult. Uribe and Botto-van Bemden[19] reported good results with partial humeral head resurfacing for a group of 11 patients with Cruess stage III, IV, or V osteonecrosis of the humeral head. At a mean follow-up of 30 months, the authors noted statistically significant ($P < 0.001$) improvements in pain, forward elevation, external rotation, and functional scores, including Western Ontario Osteoarthritis of the Shoulder, Shoulder Score Index, and Constant scores.

Hemiarthroplasty

Hemiarthroplasty is the undisputed treatment of choice in patients, regardless of age, who have unreconstructable humeral head disease without glenoid arthrosis, such as is seen in osteonecrosis, severe proximal humerus fractures, and tumor. Controversy still exists in defining the exact indications for resurfacing of the glenoid in glenohumeral arthrosis, however. Advocates of hemiarthroplasty cite reduced surgical complexity, reduced surgical time, reduced blood loss, and prevention of osteolysis and glenoid component loosening as reasons for leaving the native glenoid. Classic indications for a hemiarthroplasty center around isolated humeral head disease with normal or near-normal glenoid cartilage, as is seen with acute fractures, tumors, and early-stage osteonecrosis without glenoid wear. Additional indications for hemiarthroplasty focus on the inability to implant or maintain a well-fixed glenoid, as seen in irreparable rotator cuff tears with arthritis, insufficient glenoid bone stock to accept a glenoid prosthesis, and in the active laborer.[20] If an arthritic glenoid is to be left unresurfaced, several authors recommend that the glenoid not be completely ignored. Copeland[21] recommend drilling the surface to incite a fibrocartilaginous response similar to that seen after arthroscopic microfracture. Matsen et al[22] advocated the "ream-and-run" technique. The key to success with this technique is correction of glenoid version and concavity and soft-tissue releases.

As surgeons expand their indications for hemiarthroplasty, they may encounter patients who experience inconsistent pain relief and progressive glenoid erosion. In contrast, TSA has proven to provide more reliable pain relief and restoration of motion in osteoarthritis as well as in posttraumatic arthrosis,[23] osteonecrosis,[24] and rheumatoid arthritis.[25] Sperling et al[26] found that in the patient with rheumatoid arthritis and an intact rotator cuff, TSA provided significantly better pain relief and function than hemiarthroplasty.

Arthroscopic Treatment Options

In patients with involvement of both the humeral head and the glenoid, treatment should be dictated by the physiologic age of the patient. Arthritis with contracture is particularly amenable to an arthroscopic release to lengthen capsuloligamentous structures and decompress the joint. Resection of an inferior humeral head osteophyte (goat's beard) may additionally decompress the glenohumeral joint and allow greater motion. The results of simple arthroscopic glenohumeral débridement are unclear. Results in the knee literature seem fraught with significant placebo effect;[27,28] however, the knee is a weight-bearing joint that may behave differently than the glenohumeral joint. Kerr and McCarty[29] retrospectively reviewed 19 patients (20 shoulders) who underwent glenohumeral débridement for osteoarthritis. The patients were all younger than 55 years. All patients had improved validated outcome scores at 12 months. The authors concluded that although the grade of lesion did not influence the outcome scores, reciprocal change on both the glenoid and humerus was a poor prognostic factor. Other authors

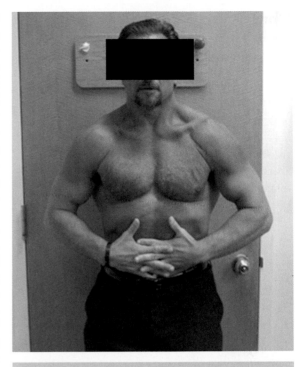

Figure 5 Photograph of an active 53-year-old male body builder who presented with glenohumeral arthritis and had the goal of continuing heavy lifting. At the time of this photograph, he had undergone a left resurfacing with lateral meniscal allograft. He has since undergone bilateral resurfacings.

also have reported improvement in postoperative pain and function following arthroscopic glenohumeral débridement.[30,31] Recent advancements in arthroscopy have allowed arthroscopic interpositional biologic resurfacing; however, we are not aware of long-term studies of this technique.

Resurfacing Options

Patients between the ages of 40 and 60 present a management crossroads. Establishing transparency in patient goals and postoperative expectations is essential to postoperative patient satisfaction. The 50-year-old competitive weight lifter is clearly a different patient than the 50-year-old weekend golfer. Patients who wish to resume impact loading activities (weight lifting, boxing, construction work, etc) after their treatment may be better served with a humeral resurfacing or hemi-

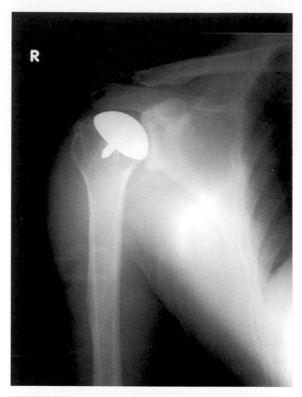

Figure 6   Postoperative AP view of the shoulder of a 52-year-old weight lifter who presented with glenohumeral arthrosis. His postoperative goal was pain relief and to resume heavy weight lifting. A metallic humeral resurfacing was performed to complement a glenoid resurfacing with lateral meniscal allograft.

arthroplasty and possibly a fascial interposition[32] (**Figure 5**). Biologic resurfacing of the glenoid with or without humeral resurfacing was developed as an alternative to TSA (**Figure 6**). The goal of this procedure is to bridge the gap between minimally invasive techniques and TSA for the young active patient to avoid osteolysis and glenoid loosening. This technique has been pioneered by Burkhead, Krishnan, and others.[32-35] Anterior capsule autograft,[36] Achilles tendon allograft,[32] lateral meniscal allograft,[37] and dermal allografts[35] have been used, with varying success. Krishnan et al[5] recently published their results at 24 to 180 months (mean, 84 months) of follow-up in patients with a mean age of 51 years. In the 36 shoulders

evaluated, the etiologies of arthrosis were degenerative osteoarthritis, postcapsulorraphy arthritis, posttraumatic arthritis, and osteonecrosis. Mean postoperative American Shoulder and Elbow Surgeons (ASES) scores increased by 52 points; 18 of 36 shoulders were rated as excellent, 13 satisfactory, and 5 unsatisfactory. Comparing studies of hemiarthroplasty and TSA in the same age group,[38] biologic resurfacing of the glenoid with hemiarthroplasty demonstrates very reasonable outcomes considering the demanding patient population in Krishnan's study. Patients must understand that this is a temporizing measure to allow them to resume their strenuous activities and that the data are inconsistent. Other authors have reported unsatisfactory results of biologic glenoid resurfacing. In a recent article, Elhassan et al[39] noted that 10 of 13 patients who underwent biologic resurfacing in combination with humeral head arthroplasty required revision surgery because of pain and decreased range of motion. Radiographic evidence of decreased joint space and erosion of the glenoid accompanied the clinical findings.

Outcomes

Patients who are able to modify their goals and accept limiting their activities to mild to moderate loading exercises such as tennis and golf are well served with a TSA. They can expect excellent pain relief, function, and resumption of normal activities of daily life. In fact, McCarty et al[40] reported that 71% of patients who participated in sports preoperatively experienced an improvement in their ability to participate. Swimmers, tennis players, and golfers had the highest rate of return to sport; softball players had the lowest. Mean time to full return was 5.8 months. Jensen and Rockwood[41] reported on a series in which 23 of 24 shoulder arthroplasty patients who regularly played golf preoperatively were able to return to recreational golf at a higher level following surgery. No differences were noted between the hemiarthroplasty and TSA groups, but the mean follow-up was only 53.4 months, potentially negating the issue of implant longevity. The literature supports better outcomes and better longevity at 20 years with a TSA over a hemiarthroplasty for this age group (40 to 60 years). Concern for conversion to TSA is legitimate. If the patient outlives the lifespan of the TSA, revising a simple loose glenoid may be easier than addressing severe glenoid bone loss associated with a failed hemiarthroplasty.

The treatment algorithm is less confusing in the arthritic patient older than 60 years, as TSA is the clear treatment of choice. TSA provides predictable, highly effective results, mirroring results reported for total hip arthroplasty and total knee arthroplasty in this age bracket. With increasing age, patients place diminishing loads on their shoulders, protecting the prosthesis. Although glenoid loosening is the major reason for revision TSA, a loose glenoid will often be asymptomatic.

Retrospective clinical outcome studies and meta-analyses have shown that for primary osteoarthritis, TSA is superior to hemiarthroplasty.[42-44] In a multicenter study, Edwards et al[44] demonstrated that TSA provides statistically superior results when directly comparing pain relief, active range of motion, and patient satisfaction. In a smaller study, Bell and Gschwend[45] compared their results for 11 TSAs and 17 hemiarthroplasties. The authors recentered the humeral head on the glenoid with a glenoid osteotomy in 5 of the 17 patients in their hemiarthroplasty cohort. Using this surgical technique, the authors demonstrated improved average elevation and pain relief with the addition of glenoid prosthetic resurfacing. Bryant et al[43] reviewed the literature and found statistical significance with respect to better pain relief with TSA than with hemiarthroplasty at 2 years, but further investigation may be necessary to determine clinical significance, and the authors cautioned that longer term follow-up would be needed to determine whether these results are maintained over time. Prospective randomized trials also have supported the superiority of TSA for the treatment of osteoarthritis. Gartsman et al[33] prospectively followed 51 shoulders with primary osteoarthritis and demonstrated that the TSA group had significantly greater improvement in pain relief and functional range of motion than did the hemiarthroplasty patients. To examine quality of life outcomes after shoulder arthroplasty, Lo et al[4] prospectively followed 42 patients randomized to TSA or hemiarthroplasty. At a minimum of 2 years after surgery, although no statistical differences were found between groups, there was a trend toward superior outcomes in the TSA cohort.

Studies have begun to show that the results of hemiarthroplasty for osteoarthritis deteriorate over time, mainly due to glenoid wear and progressive pain. In the younger patient population, some studies have shown loss of joint space in as little as 3 years.[46] Cofield et al[47] reported on the Mayo experience with conversion of hemiarthroplasty to TSA. At mean 9.3-year follow-up, 51% of patients had unsatisfactory results stemming from glenoid wear. Unfortunately, conversion of a hemiarthroplasty to a TSA often does not result in the same rate of satisfaction as an index TSA procedure. Carroll et al[42] reviewed their experience with conversion and concluded that on the basis of both the complexity of the revision surgery and the resultant 47% unsatisfactory rate, salvage TSA is inferior to primary TSA.

Unfortunately, few studies have directly compared hemiarthroplasty and TSA for glenohumeral arthritis in the young patient. Studies that have attempted comparison suffer from limited patient populations and antiquated surgical implants and technique.[48,49] Sperling et al[38] retrospectively reviewed 62 Neer hemiarthroplasties and 29 Neer TSAs in patients 50 years or younger performed between 1976 and 1985. During that time period, surgeons used first-generation implants and first-generation cementation techniques. Indications for arthroplasty included osteoarthritis, rheumatoid arthritis, osteonecrosis, and postinfectious or posttraumatic arthritis. At a minimum 15-year follow-up, TSA outperformed hemiarthroplasty with respect to implant survival, patient satisfaction, and pain relief. At 10-year and 20-year follow-up, hemiarthroplasty demonstrated a higher rate of revision, usually to address glenoid arthrosis. No difference was observed in functional range of motion between the two groups. Previous shoulder surgery was associated with postoperative patient dissatisfaction and need for revision. Unfortunately, Sperling found that the rates of good to excellent outcomes were low in both the hemiarthroplasty and TSA groups and therefore recommended that alternative methods of treatment be exhausted before resorting to shoulder arthroplasty in patients 50 years or younger.

Concern for implant failure due to loosening or wear is appropriate when considering arthroplasty in a younger patient.[1] Despite a high incidence of radio-

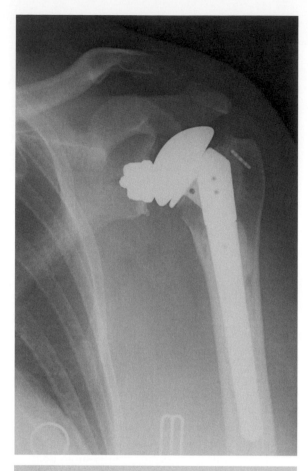

Figure 7   Postoperative AP view of the shoulder of an extremely active 53-year-old woman who underwent TSA with an ingrowth glenoid for glenohumeral osteoarthritis.

graphic lucent lines, however, evidence of clinically significant glenoid loosening is not common. Implant manufacturers have focused on improving glenoid prosthetic design to minimize shear forces and maximize implant strength. Newer designs use ongrowth or ingrowth potential to theoretically decrease glenoid loosening (**Figure 7**). It has not yet been proven whether the theoretical advantages will translate into clinical reality; however, it is reasonable to expect that with pressurized cementation technique and improved implant technology, the durability of TSA should only improve.

Several treatment options exist for the minority of patients who demonstrate clinically significant glenoid

loosening. Fortunately, even in the face of symptomatic aseptic loosening, most patients will report less pain than before the index procedure. If patients decide to live with the symptoms, nonsurgical management may be chosen. If patients are unwilling to undergo invasive surgery or are poor surgical candidates, arthroscopic removal of an all-polyethylene glenoid prosthesis is a valuable technique. Many patients will have significant improvement of their symptoms with simple glenoid component removal, effectively converting the TSA to a hemiarthroplasty.[50] If patients are willing to undergo revision arthroplasty, it may actually be easier to revise a loose glenoid with a simple central contained defect than to reconstruct a hemiarthroplasty with significant glenoid wear.

Summary

The etiology of the condition and the patient's postoperative expectations and physiologic age play crucial roles in choosing an optimal treatment algorithm tailored to the mature athlete with glenohumeral arthrosis. Many treatment options exist, running the full spectrum from nonsurgical medical management to arthroscopy to various arthroplasty techniques.

In most circumstances, surgeons should attempt to treat glenohumeral arthritis in patients younger than 40 years with either nonsurgical management or arthroscopic techniques. Arthritic contractures are ideal for arthroscopic release and decompression. Patients between the ages of 40 and 60 present a more complicated treatment paradigm. The mature athlete who desires to resume impact activities may be best treated with a hemiarthroplasty, with or without biologic glenoid resurfacing. Patients must have the clear understanding that the goal of treatment is pain relief and temporization of their disease until they modify their activities to allow for stable fixation of a prosthetic glenoid component.

Severe osteoarthritis in patients older than 60 years, with rare exception, should be managed with TSA, which offers patients predictable pain relief and postoperative function. With advancing age, prosthetic loosening becomes less of a concern, and even in the face of overt glenoid loosening, patients are often still less symptomatic than before their index procedure.

Acknowledgment

The authors acknowledge the assistance of Daniel L. Aaron, MD, who made several helpful edits to the final manuscript.

References

1. Bishop JY, Flatow EL: Humeral head replacement versus total shoulder arthroplasty: Clinical outcomes—A review. *J Shoulder Elbow Surg* 2005; 14(1 Suppl S):141S-146S.

2. Levy O, Copeland SA: Cementless surface replacement arthroplasty (Copeland CSRA) for osteoarthritis of the shoulder. *J Shoulder Elbow Surg* 2004;13(3):266-271.

3. Neer CS II: Neer hemiarthroplasty and Neer total shoulder arthroplasty in patients fifty years old or less: Long-term results. *J Bone Joint Surg Am* 1999;81(2): 295-296.

4. Lo IK, Litchfield RB, Griffin S, Faber K, Patterson SD, Kirkley A: Quality-of-life outcome following hemiarthroplasty or total shoulder arthroplasty in patients with osteoarthritis: A prospective, randomized trial. *J Bone Joint Surg Am* 2005;87(10):2178-2185.

5. Krishnan SG, Nowinski RJ, Harrison D, Burkhead WZ: Humeral hemiarthroplasty with biologic resurfacing of the glenoid for glenohumeral arthritis: Two to fifteen-year outcomes. *J Bone Joint Surg Am* 2007;89(4):727-734.

6. Walch G, Badet R, Boulahia A, Khoury A: Morphologic study of the glenoid in primary glenohumeral osteoarthritis. *J Arthroplasty* 1999;14(6): 756-760.

7. Neer CS II: Replacement arthroplasty for glenohumeral osteoarthritis. *J Bone Joint Surg Am* 1974;56(1):1-13.

8. Cuomo F, Greller MJ, Zuckerman JD: The rheumatoid shoulder. *Rheum Dis Clin North Am* 1998;24(1):67-82.

9. Barrett WP, Thornhill TS, Thomas WH, Gebhart EM, Sledge CB: Nonconstrained total shoulder arthroplasty in patients with polyarticular rheumatoid arthritis. *J Arthroplasty* 1989;4(1):91-96.

10. Hertel R, Hempfing A, Stiehler M, Leunig M: Predictors of humeral head ischemia after intracapsular fracture of the proximal humerus. *J Shoulder Elbow Surg* 2004;13(4):427-433.

11. Merle D'Aubigné R, Postel M, Mazabraud A, Massias P, Gueguen J, France P: Idiopathic necrosis of the femoral head in adults. *J Bone Joint Surg Br* 1965; 47(4):612-633.

12. Cruess RL: Rheumatoid arthritis of the shoulder. *Orthop Clin North Am* 1980;11(2):333-342.

13. Saltzman M, Mercer D, Bertelsen A, Warme W, Matsen F: Postsurgical chondrolysis of the shoulder. *Orthopedics* 2009;32(3):215.

14. Bigliani LU, Weinstein DM, Glasgow MT, Pollock RG, Flatow EL: Glenohumeral arthroplasty for arthritis after instability surgery. *J Shoulder Elbow Surg* 1995;4(2):87-94.

15. Hawkins RJ, Angelo RL: Glenohumeral osteoarthrosis: A late complication of the Putti-Platt repair. *J Bone Joint Surg Am* 1990;72(8):1193-1197.

16. Neer CS II, Watson KC, Stanton FJ: Recent experience in total shoulder replacement. *J Bone Joint Surg Am* 1982;64(3):319-337.

17. Kaplan SR, Lally EV: Steroids, NSAIDs, gold and D-penicillamine, and antimalarials: Decision points in the management of rheumatoid arthritis. *J Musculoskeletal Med* 1986;46-50.

18. Valiveti M, Reginato AJ, Falasca GF: Viscosupplementation for degenerative joint disease of shoulder and ankle. *J Clin Rheumatol* 2006;12(3): 162-163.

19. Uribe JW, Botto-van Bemden A: Partial humeral head resurfacing for osteonecrosis. *J Shoulder Elbow Surg* 2009;18(5):711-716.

20. Boileau P, Sinnerton RJ, Chuinard C, Walch G: Arthroplasty of the shoulder. *J Bone Joint Surg Br* 2006;88(5):562-575.

21. Copeland SA: Cementless total shoulder replacement, in Post M, Morrey BF, Hawkins RJ, eds: *Surgery of the Shoulder.* St. Louis, MO, Mosby, 1990, pp 289-293.

22. Matsen FA III, Bicknell RT, Lippitt SB: Shoulder arthroplasty: The socket perspective. *J Shoulder Elbow Surg* 2007;16(5 Suppl):S241-S247.

23. Boileau P, Coste JS, Ahrens PM, Staccini P: Prosthetic shoulder replacement for fracture: Results of the multicentre study, in Walch G, Boileau P, Molé D, eds: *2000 Shoulder Prostheses: Two to Ten Year Follow-Up.* Montpellier, France, Sauramps Médical, 2001, pp 561-578.

24. Nové-Josserand L: Prothéses d'épaule sur ostéonécrose avasculaire: Synthèse concernant les indications et résultats, in Walch G, Boileau P, Molé D, eds: *2000 Shoulder Prostheses: Two to Ten Year Follow-Up.*

Montpellier, France, Sauramps Médical, 2001, pp 149-155.

25. Rydholm U, Sjögren J: Surface replacement of the humeral head in the rheumatoid shoulder. *J Shoulder Elbow Surg* 1993;2(6):286-295.

26. Sperling JW, Cofield RH, Schleck CD, Harmsen WS: Total shoulder arthroplasty versus hemiarthroplasty for rheumatoid arthritis of the shoulder: Results of 303 consecutive cases. *J Shoulder Elbow Surg* 2007;16(6): 683-690.

27. Moseley JB, O'Malley K, Petersen NJ, et al: A controlled trial of arthroscopic surgery for osteoarthritis of the knee. *N Engl J Med* 2002;347(2):81-88.

28. Moseley JB Jr, Wray NP, Kuykendall D, Willis K, Landon G: Arthroscopic treatment of osteoarthritis of the knee: A prospective, randomized, placebo-controlled trial. Results of a pilot study. *Am J Sports Med* 1996;24(1):28-34.

29. Kerr BJ, McCarty EC: Outcome of arthroscopic débridement is worse for patients with glenohumeral arthritis of both sides of the joint. *Clin Orthop Relat Res* 2008;466(3):634-638.

30. Weinstein DM, Bucchieri JS, Pollock RG, Flatow EL, Bigliani LU: Arthroscopic debridement of the shoulder for osteoarthritis. *Arthroscopy* 2000;16(5):471-476.

31. Ogilvie-Harris DJ, D'Angelo G: Arthroscopic surgery of the shoulder. *Sports Med* 1990;9(2):120-128.

32. Krishnan SG, Reineck JR, Nowinski RJ, Harrison D, Burkhead WZ: Humeral hemiarthroplasty with biologic resurfacing of the glenoid for glenohumeral arthritis: Surgical technique. *J Bone Joint Surg Am* 2008;90(Suppl 2 Pt 1):9-19.

33. Gartsman GM, Roddey TS, Hammerman SM: Shoulder arthroplasty with or without resurfacing of the glenoid in patients who have osteoarthritis. *J Bone Joint Surg Am* 2000;82(1):26-34.

34. Nicholson GP, Goldstein JL, Romeo AA, et al: Lateral meniscus allograft biologic glenoid arthroplasty in total shoulder arthroplasty for young shoulders with degenerative joint disease. *J Shoulder Elbow Surg* 2007; 16(5 Suppl):S261-S266.

35. Burkhead WZ Jr, Krishnan SG, Lin KC: Biologic resurfacing of the arthritic glenohumeral joint: Historical review and current applications. *J Shoulder Elbow Surg* 2007;16(5 Suppl):S248-S253.

36. Font-Rodriguez DE, Baghain S, Williams GR: Abstract: Soft-tissue interposition without hemiarthroplasty as an alternative for degenerative arthritis in young, active patients. *Annual Meeting Proceedings*. Rosemont, IL, American Academy of Orthopaedic Surgeons, 2003, pp 544-545.

37. Ball C, Galatz L, Yamaguchi K: Meniscal allograft interposition arthroplasty for the arthritic shoulder: Description of a new surgical technique. *Tech Shoulder Elbow Surg* 2001;2(4):247-254.

38. Sperling JW, Cofield RH, Rowland CM: Neer hemiarthroplasty and Neer total shoulder arthroplasty in patients fifty years old or less: Long-term results. *J Bone Joint Surg Am* 1998;80(4):464-473.

39. Elhassan B, Ozbaydar M, Diller D, Higgins LD, Warner JJ: Soft-tissue resurfacing of the glenoid in the treatment of glenohumeral arthritis in active patients less than fifty years old. *J Bone Joint Surg Am* 2009; 91(2):419-424.

40. McCarty EC, Marx RG, Maerz D, Altchek D, Warren RF: Sports participation after shoulder replacement surgery. *Am J Sports Med* 2008;36(8):1577-1581.

41. Jensen KL, Rockwood CA Jr: Shoulder arthroplasty in recreational golfers. *J Shoulder Elbow Surg* 1998;7(4): 362-367.

42. Carroll RM, Izquierdo R, Vazquez M, Blaine TA, Levine WN, Bigliani LU: Conversion of painful hemiarthroplasty to total shoulder arthroplasty: Long-term results. *J Shoulder Elbow Surg* 2004;13(6): 599-603.

43. Bryant D, Litchfield R, Sandow M, Gartsman GM, Guyatt G, Kirkley A: A comparison of pain, strength, range of motion, and functional outcomes after hemiarthroplasty and total shoulder arthroplasty in patients with osteoarthritis of the shoulder: A systematic review and meta-analysis. *J Bone Joint Surg Am* 2005;87(9):1947-1956.

44. Edwards TB, Kadakia NR, Boulahia A, et al: A comparison of hemiarthroplasty and total shoulder arthroplasty in the treatment of primary glenohumeral osteoarthritis: Results of a multicenter study. *J Shoulder Elbow Surg* 2003;12(3):207-213.

45. Bell SN, Gschwend N: Clinical experience with total arthroplasty and hemiarthroplasty of the shoulder using the Neer prosthesis. *Int Orthop* 1986;10(4):217-222.

46. Parsons IM IV, Millett PJ, Warner JJ: Glenoid wear after shoulder hemiarthroplasty: Quantitative radiographic analysis. *Clin Orthop Relat Res* 2004;421: 120-125.

47. Cofield RH, Frankle MA, Zuckerman JD: Humeral head replacement for glenohumeral arthritis. *Semin Arthroplasty* 1995;6(4):214-221.

48. Raiss P, Aldinger PR, Kasten P, Rickert M, Loew M: Total shoulder replacement in young and middle-aged patients with glenohumeral osteoarthritis. *J Bone Joint Surg Br* 2008;90(6):764-769.

49. Sperling JW, Cofield RH, Rowland CM: Minimum fifteen-year follow-up of Neer hemiarthroplasty and total shoulder arthroplasty in patients aged fifty years or younger. *J Shoulder Elbow Surg* 2004;13(6):604-613.

50. O'Driscoll SW, Petrie RS, Torchia ME: Arthroscopic removal of the glenoid component for failed total shoulder arthroplasty: A report of five cases. *J Bone Joint Surg Am* 2005;87(4):858-863.

Chapter 18

Management of Adhesive Capsulitis in the Mature Athlete

Alexis Colvin, MD
Evan L. Flatow, MD

Key Points

- Adhesive capsulitis can be idiopathic (primary) or due to a known intrinsic, extrinsic, or systemic cause (secondary). Proper treatment begins with a thorough examination to determine if an underlying cause can be identified.
- In addition to physical therapy, rehabilitation for the mature athlete may include an alternative sport-specific training regimen to prevent deconditioning.
- When surgical treatment is indicated, a 360° arthroscopic capsular release, followed by manipulation under anesthesia (MUA), facilitates a precise resection of the capsule and prevents capsular tears that may lead to scarring.

Dr. Flatow or an immediate family member serves as a board member, owner, officer, or committee member of the American Shoulder and Elbow Surgeons, the Arthroscopy Association of North America, and Mt. Sinai Medical Center; has received royalties from Innomed and Zimmer; serves as a paid consultant to or is an employee of Wyeth; serves as an unpaid consultant to Zimmer; and has received research or institutional support from Zimmer. Neither Dr. Colvin nor any immediate family member has received anything of value from or owns stock in a commercial company or institution related directly or indirectly to the subject of this chapter.

Introduction

Adhesive capsulitis (also called stiff shoulder or frozen shoulder) is a common disorder that is marked by the loss of both active and passive motion.[1] Adhesive capsulitis can be divided into two types: primary (idiopathic) and secondary (having a known intrinsic, extrinsic, or systemic cause).[2] Adhesive capsulitis affects 2% to 3% of the general population, with a higher percentage (10% to 18%) seen in patients with diabetes.[3] Other risk factors include age greater than 40 years,[4,5] nondominant extremity,[5] trauma, diabetes,[4,6,7] prolonged immobilization, thyroid disease,[5,8] stroke or myocardial infarction, and autoimmune diseases.[1] In patients with diabetes, the severity of adhesive capsulitis is associated with a longer duration of diabetes and tends to be more resistant to nonsurgical treatment (ie, manipulation alone).[4,6,7]

Determination of any underlying cause for the stiffness will facilitate appropriate treatment. Posttraumatic stiffness can result from soft-tissue contracture, bone deformity, pain inhibition/guarding, and articular incongruity. It is imperative to determine whether the soft-tissue contracture is intra-articular, extra-articular (strap muscles or subscapularis), from muscle/tendon scarring (rotator cuff), or due to secondary disuse. Bone deformity resulting from fracture malunion can result in impingement of the greater tuberosity on the acromion or the glenoid, or angulation and/or rotation of the surgical neck, although this is usually less important than scar tissue. Articular incongruity can result from posttraumatic arthritis or osteonecrosis, intra-articular fracture, dislocation (especially posterior), or heterotopic bone formation.

Pathogenesis

Both synovial hyperplasia and capsular fibrosis have been implicated in primary adhesive capsulitis;[9,10] they also are seen in secondary adhesive capsulitis, but are not requisite. Fibroblasts and myofibroblasts form a dense matrix of type I and type III collagen within the capsule, leading to adhesive capsulitis.[11] Fibrogenic growth factors are also increased in adhesive capsulitis tissues.[10,11] Histology demonstrates fibrosis, hyalinization, and fibrinoid degeneration, as well as fibrosis of the subsynovial tissue and lack of a synovial cell layer on the joint side of the rotator interval.[12] Additionally, multiple biochemical abnormalities are seen in patients with diabetes, including altered collagen synthesis, increased glycosylation of collagenous proteins, and increased accumulation of advanced glycosylation end products, which may contribute to the pathogenesis of diabetic adhesive capsulitis.[13-15]

Four stages of adhesive capsulitis have been described.[16] Stage I, the preadhesive stage, is characterized by a fibrinous synovial inflammation that is detectable by arthroscopy. There is essentially no limitation in range of motion. Patients in this stage typically present with pain alone.[1] The goal of treatment at this stage is to decrease pain and inflammation, with a combination of nonsteroidal anti-inflammatory drugs, intra-articular corticosteroid injection, activity modification, and/or therapy.[1] In stage II, the "freezing" stage, patients present with restricted range of motion with pain at the extremes of motion.[1] This stage is characterized by early adhesions and a proliferative synovitis.[16] Treatment in this stage continues to be focused on decreasing pain and inflammation as well as minimizing capsular adhesions and maintaining range of motion. The maturation stage, stage III, is characterized by less synovitis and loss of the axillary fold. Patients in this "frozen" phase typically have less pain but significant restrictions in motion.[1] Finally, in stage IV, known as chronic, the adhesions have fully matured and are restrictive.[16] During this "thawing" phase, the patient typically has less pain and has progressive improvement in range of motion.[1] The goal of treatment in stages III and IV is to increase range of motion.

Gross findings include a thickened capsule, proliferative synovium, patchy synovitis, and reduced joint volume, regardless of the etiology.[17,18]

Evaluation

Important factors to note in the patient with suspected adhesive capsulitis include the onset of symptoms and history of trauma (anywhere in the ipsilateral limb), prior shoulder surgery, or any period of immobility. Other surgeries, such as in the cervical spine, should also be taken into account. A review of systems assessing for diseases such as diabetes mellitus and thyroid disorders should also be conducted. Finally, in throwing athletes, any history of posterior capsular tightness should be elicited.

Physical Examination

Physical examination of the stiff shoulder starts with visual inspection, assessing for muscle atrophy and surgical scars. Next, palpation should be performed, eliciting any tenderness, such as of the acromioclavicular joint. Range of motion should be evaluated both actively and passively. Documentation of forward elevation, abduction, internal rotation behind the back, and external and internal rotation with the shoulder abducted 90° (or at maximal abduction if 90° is unattainable) allows for comparison on subsequent visits. Further testing, including strength testing and provocative tests such as those for impingement and apprehension, is often not helpful in stiff shoulders because of the patient's inability to move the arm into a testable position.

Imaging and Laboratory Tests

Radiographs and CT can be helpful for identifying bony malunion. MRI is useful for assessing the rotator cuff. Occasionally, electromyography may be necessary to rule out nerve injury. Blood tests, including a white blood cell count, C-reactive protein level, and erythrocyte sedimentation rate, are indicated if a postoperative infection is suspected.

Treatment

The duration of the recovery phase of adhesive capsulitis has varied in the literature. Patients have been observed to become pain free and recover full movement in as few as 12 months[5] or up to 2 years.[19] Duration of symptoms may also be correlated with duration of recovery.[20] Several other reviews have found that patients continue to have an objective limitation in motion, but this is not a functional limitation.[5,21,22]

Initial treatment of adhesive capsulitis should involve activity modification, heat, nonsteroidal anti-inflammatory medication, and stretching, with or without a supervised physical therapy program. Patients treated with a minimum 3-month supervised physical therapy program had a 90% satisfactory outcome at an average 22-month follow-up.[22] In the mature athlete, an alternative training regimen, in addition to physical therapy, may be beneficial to prevent deconditioning.[23]

Refractory shoulder stiffness is often seen in patients who have diabetes, complex regional pain syndrome, a failed manipulation or capsular release, or stiffness that is posttraumatic or postoperative. Open treatment is indicated for patients with malunion that requires osteotomy, osteonecrosis or arthritis that requires arthroplasty, or those with prior open procedures, as they are most likely to have major extra-articular adhesions. Arthroscopic release can typically be used in patients with no malunion, no significant arthritis, and no prior open procedures. The advantages of arthroscopic release include a better ability to release the posterior capsule and no need to protect a lengthened and/or repaired subscapularis tendon postoperatively.[24] Furthermore, concomitant pathology, such as acromioclavicular arthritis or calcific deposits, can be identified and treated.[25]

A comparison of arthroscopic capsular release for patients with idiopathic versus postoperative adhesive capsulitis demonstrated that both groups had similar improvements in range of motion but the postoperative group had less subjective improvement.[26] Patients who have had prior open procedures (eg, Magnuson-Stack, Putti-Platt) typically have scarring of the subscapularis tendon, which should be released through an open procedure that may necessitate coronal lengthening of the subscapularis tendon.[27] Arthroscopic capsular release for refractory adhesive capsulitis (ie, adhesive cap-

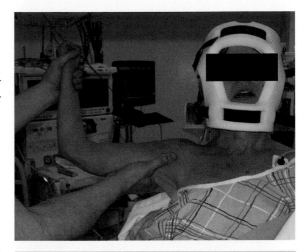

Figure 1   Shoulder range of motion is examined under anesthesia before surgery for adhesive capsulitis.

sulitis that persists despite more than 6 months of nonsurgical treatment) has been shown to result in improved range of motion and functional outcome scores.[24,25] Furthermore, a difference between outcomes in diabetics and nondiabetics has not been found.[24]

Candidates for arthroscopic capsular release are patients who fit the above-mentioned criteria, with a minimum of 6 months of nonsurgical treatment and continued restricted range of motion. Our preferred method of treatment is to perform an arthroscopic 360° capsular release followed by MUA to avoid problems with visualization during the arthroscopy due to bleeding. Capsular release performed prior to MUA allows for more precision when removing the strip of capsule. MUA also should not be performed before arthroscopy, to prevent capsular tears that can lead to scarring. Once the capsular release is performed, a gentle MUA will release any remaining extra-articular adhesions.

The patient is positioned in the beach chair position and the range of motion of both shoulders is examined under anesthesia (**Figure 1**). The posterior portal is initially established with a gentle, superior joint entry, taking care to avoid a "transosseous" portal. The anterior portal is established once the triangle formed by the biceps tendon, glenoid, and subscapularis is visualized. First, tissue around the anterior portal is débrided.

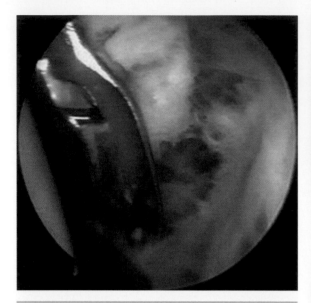

Figure 2 Arthroscopic view shows the glenohumeral joint starting to open as the anteroinferior capsule is resected.

Using a thermal ablation device, the entire rotator interval is opened so that the strap muscles are visible. Next, using the capsular biter through the anterior portal, a 5-mm strip of anterior capsule is resected just lateral to the labrum down to the 5 o'clock position in a right shoulder or the 7 o'clock position in a left shoulder. The glenohumeral joint will start to open as the capsule is resected (**Figure 2**). Adequate hemostasis should be achieved with cautery. After the anteroinferior capsule is resected, the anterosuperior capsule should be addressed. This is accomplished by coming above the biceps tendon and using a capsular biter through the capsule, deep to the supraspinatus and infraspinatus tendons. Resection can safely begin at the glenoid margin if there is no rotator cuff tear. In the setting of a retracted rotator cuff tear, however, care should be taken to avoid injury to the retracted tendon. As the tissue is released, the muscles of the rotator cuff become exposed. Once the superior capsule is resected, the arthroscope is then switched to the anterior portal. Using cautery, the posterior capsule is resected. The capsular biter is then used to resect a strip of the posterior capsule and to connect it with the superior capsulotomy. Once the posterior capsule has been re-

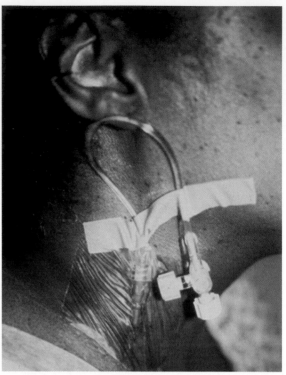

Figure 3 Photograph shows an indwelling interscalene catheter in place.

leased to a 7 o'clock position in a right shoulder and a 5 o'clock position in a left shoulder, an accessory inferior portal can be established. A capsular punch is used to complete the inferior capsulotomy. Caution should be exercised in this area because of the proximity of the axillary nerve. Furthermore, with extensive scarring or in the setting of prior surgery, such as capsular shift or arthroplasty, the axillary nerve may be adherent to the anteroinferior or inferior capsule.

Postoperative Treatment

An indwelling interscalene catheter is useful because it can provide continuous regional anesthesia and provide a full sympathetic block (**Figure 3**). This facilitates rehabilitation and therapy. The catheter is typically left in for 2 days and pulled before the patient is discharged. Cohen et al[28] reported on their experiences with an indwelling interscalene catheter that remained in for an average of 3 days. At an average 3-year follow-up, 95%

of the elevation and 79% of the external rotation achieved intraoperatively was maintained.

Patients are seen while in the recovery room by the physical therapist, who begins terminal stretching in all planes with no limitations. The patient is admitted overnight and undergoes two therapy sessions the following day. Outpatient therapy is then continued 5 days a week for the next 2 weeks, and then decreased to three times a week. Patients who demonstrate loss of motion at 4 to 6 weeks may benefit from MUA and cortisone injection. Shoulder continuous passive motion is not used. The subacromial bursa is examined and resected only if adhesions are present. In patients with rotator cuff changes on MRI in whom secondary stiffness is present, physical therapy usually resolves the stiffness. A subacromial decompression can then be performed without the need for an additional capsular release. Patients are usually allowed to return to sports when they have pain-free range of motion and near-normal motor control and strength. This typically takes 3 to 6 months.

References

1. Hannafin JA, Chiaia TA: Adhesive capsulitis: A treatment approach. *Clin Orthop Relat Res* 2000;(372): 95-109.

2. Tasto JP, Elias DW: Adhesive capsulitis. *Sports Med Arthrosc* 2007;15(4):216-221.

3. Bridgman JF: Periarthritis of the shoulder and diabetes mellitus. *Ann Rheum Dis* 1972;31(1):69-71.

4. Boyle-Walker KL, Gabard DL, Bietsch E, Masek-VanArsdale DM, Robinson BL: A profile of patients with adhesive capsulitis. *J Hand Ther* 1997;10(3): 222-228.

5. Shaffer B, Tibone JE, Kerlan RK: Frozen shoulder: A long-term follow-up. *J Bone Joint Surg Am* 1992;74(5): 738-746.

6. Arkkila PE, Kantola IM, Viikari JS, Rönnemaa T: Shoulder capsulitis in type I and II diabetic patients: Association with diabetic complications and related diseases. *Ann Rheum Dis* 1996;55(12):907-914.

7. Janda DH, Hawkins RJ: Shoulder manipulation in patients with adhesive capsulitis and diabetes mellitus: A clinical note. *J Shoulder Elbow Surg* 1993;2(1):36-38.

8. Cakir M, Samanci N, Balci N, Balci MK: Musculoskeletal manifestations in patients with thyroid disease. *Clin Endocrinol (Oxf)* 2003;59(2):162-167.

9. Neviaser J: Adhesive capsulitis of the shoulder: A study of the pathological findings in periarthritis of the shoulder. *J Bone Joint Surg* 1945;27:211-222.

10. Rodeo SA, Hannafin JA, Tom J, Warren RF, Wickiewicz TL: Immunolocalization of cytokines and their receptors in adhesive capsulitis of the shoulder. *J Orthop Res* 1997;15(3):427-436.

11. Bunker TD, Reilly J, Baird KS, Hamblen DL: Expression of growth factors, cytokines and matrix metalloproteinases in frozen shoulder. *J Bone Joint Surg Br* 2000;82(5):768-773.

12. Ozaki J, Nakagawa Y, Sakurai G, Tamai S: Recalcitrant chronic adhesive capsulitis of the shoulder: Role of contracture of the coracohumeral ligament and rotator interval in pathogenesis and treatment. *J Bone Joint Surg Am* 1989;71(10):1511-1515.

13. Cagliero E, Apruzzese W, Perlmutter GS, Nathan DM: Musculoskeletal disorders of the hand and shoulder in patients with diabetes mellitus. *Am J Med* 2002;112(6): 487-490.

14. Kohn RR, Hensse S: Abnormal collagen in cultures of fibroblasts from human beings with diabetes mellitus. *Biochem Biophys Res Commun* 1977;76(3):365-371.

15. McCully SP, Kumar N, Lazarus MD, Karduna AR: Internal and external rotation of the shoulder: Effects of plane, end-range determination, and scapular motion. *J Shoulder Elbow Surg* 2005;14(6):602-610.

16. Neviaser RJ, Neviaser TJ: The frozen shoulder: Diagnosis and management. *Clin Orthop Relat Res* 1987;(223):59-64.

17. Nicholson GP: Arthroscopic capsular release for stiff shoulders: Effect of etiology on outcomes. *Arthroscopy* 2003;19(1):40-49.

18. Wiley AM: Arthroscopic appearance of frozen shoulder. *Arthroscopy* 1991;7(2):138-143.

19. Grey RG: The natural history of "idiopathic" frozen shoulder. *J Bone Joint Surg Am* 1978;60(4):564.

20. Reeves B: The natural history of the frozen shoulder syndrome. *Scand J Rheumatol* 1975;4(4):193-196.

21. Binder AI, Bulgen DY, Hazleman BL, Roberts S: Frozen shoulder: A long-term prospective study. *Ann Rheum Dis* 1984;43(3):361-364.

22. Griggs SM, Ahn A, Green A: Idiopathic adhesive capsulitis: A prospective functional outcome study of nonoperative treatment. *J Bone Joint Surg Am* 2000; 82-A(10):1398-1407.

23. Galloway MT, Jokl P: Aging successfully: The importance of physical activity in maintaining health and function. *J Am Acad Orthop Surg* 2000;8(1):37-44.

24. Harryman DT II, Matsen FA III, Sidles JA: Arthroscopic management of refractory shoulder stiffness. *Arthroscopy* 1997;13(2):133-147.

25. Pollock RG, Duralde XA, Flatow EL, Bigliani LU: The use of arthroscopy in the treatment of resistant frozen shoulder. *Clin Orthop Relat Res* 1994;(304):30-36.

26. Holloway GB, Schenk T, Williams GR, Ramsey ML, Iannotti JP: Arthroscopic capsular release for the treatment of refractory postoperative or post-fracture shoulder stiffness. *J Bone Joint Surg Am* 2001; 83-A(11):1682-1687.

27. Warner JJ, Allen A, Marks PH, Wong P: Arthroscopic release for chronic, refractory adhesive capsulitis of the shoulder. *J Bone Joint Surg Am* 1996;78(12):1808-1816.

28. Cohen NP, Levine WN, Marra G, et al: Indwelling interscalene catheter anesthesia in the surgical management of stiff shoulder: A report of 100 consecutive cases. *J Shoulder Elbow Surg* 2000;9(4): 268-274.

Chapter 19

Biceps Tendon Pathology and Associated SLAP Lesions

Ben C. Robinson, MD
John M. Tokish, MD

Key Points

- Biceps tendon pathology presents differently in the mature athlete than in the younger athlete: superior labrum anterior-to-posterior (SLAP) lesions are more commonly part of a larger disease process.
- Biceps tendon pathology is more variable in the mature athlete. It may occur at the insertion, in the groove, or in both locations.
- SLAP lesions in the mature athlete are perhaps better treated with tenotomy or tenodesis than with SLAP repair.
- Outcomes for SLAP tears in older patients are better when other pathology is addressed than when the tear is treated in isolation.
- Tenotomy and tenodesis are both effective treatments for biceps tendon pathology in mature athletes, but tenodesis may have a lower risk of cosmetic deformity, fatigue pain, and strength loss.

Introduction

Injuries to the long head of the biceps tendon in athletes older than 40 years differ from those seen in younger patients. All athletes subject the biceps tendon to extreme stresses and biomechanical demands in overhead sports activity, with the potential for injury. However, the level of overall fitness and health of the athlete, time devoted to sport participation and training, and quality of individual tissue are all contributing factors to the possibility of biceps injury in the mature athlete during play. Younger athletes typically injure the biceps acutely by throwing or in a traumatic event during play that more commonly is associated with SLAP lesions. In the mature athlete, the process of injury to the tendon may occur acutely, but it more commonly occurs secondary to deconditioning of the periscapular musculature, muscle imbalance, and poor overhead mechanics, leading to scapular dyskinesia and subacromial impingement, rotator cuff tears, and subsequently biceps tendinopathy or disruption. Like the rotator cuff, the biceps undergoes a degenerative process with aging. The presentation and physical examination findings vary, because the mature athlete often has concomitant cuff pathology in the shoulder; however, most patients report pain. MRI has improved the ability to diagnose SLAP or biceps tendon lesions, but arthroscopy remains the most definitive diagnostic tool. However, there is significant interobserver and intraobserver variability among shoulder surgeons in the diagnosis and treatment of these lesions. Isolated repair of SLAP lesions is rarely the optimal treatment in the mature patient. More commonly, treatment of associated pathology such as rotator cuff tears or subacromial impingement, coupled with biceps tenotomy or tenodesis, leads to improved pain and shoulder function. Spontaneous biceps rupture is not uncommon in the mature athlete, but it is seldom a problem. It often occurs in conjunction with a cuff deficiency.

Anatomy and Pathology of the Biceps Tendon and Superior Labral Complex

The biceps has two heads. The short head originates from the coracoid process along with the coracobrachialis to form the conjoined tendon. The long head originates in the glenohumeral joint, traveling beneath the coracohumeral ligament, through the rotator interval, and into the bicipital groove. At this point, it passes under the transverse humeral ligament between the greater and lesser tuberosities and then beneath an aponeurotic expansion of the pectoralis major called the falciform process.[1] It combines with the short head at the level of the deltoid insertion.

The tendon of the long head, along with the medial attachment of the superior labrum, forms a subsynovial recess that extends for several millimeters from the edge of the superior glenoid.[1,2] The origin of the long head is variable. Traditional teaching is that the tendon originates at the supraglenoid tubercle, but Habermeyer et al[3] reported that the tendon originated from the posterior labrum 48% of the time, from the supraglenoid tubercle only 20% of the time, and from both locations 28% of the time. Vangsness et al[4] demonstrated in a cadaveric study that 50% of the tendons originated from the superior glenoid labrum, with the remaining tendons attached to the supraglenoid tubercle. Most shoulders in which the biceps originates in the labrum have an entirely posterior or a posterior-dominant labral insertion, but the attachment is variable; it may be entirely posterior, posterior-dominant, or equally anterior and posterior into the superior labrum.[2]

Pathology of the biceps tendon is commonly thought to be inflammatory, although a true inflammatory component has not been clearly demonstrated.[5] A more appropriate description is tendinosis, or tendon degeneration.[1] Microscopic studies typically show atrophy and irregular patterns of collagen fibers, as well as fibrocyte proliferation and fibrinoid necrosis.[5]

The biceps tendon can be subject to injury at any location along its course proximally. Disorders at the origin are associated with SLAP lesions. Snyder et al[6] originally described the SLAP lesion and classified it into four types[7] (**Figure 1**). Type I lesions are characterized by an intact biceps origin and labral fraying. In type II lesions, biceps–superior labrum origin is detached. Type III lesions are characterized by an intact biceps anchor and a bucket-handle tear of the superior labrum. Type IV lesions have a bucket-handle tear of the labrum that extends into the biceps tendon. Additional types have been described. Morgan et al[8] divided type II lesions into predominantly anterior, posterior, or combined anterior and posterior. Maffet et al[9] described three additional types: type V lesions, which they defined as SLAP tears combined with a Bankart lesion; type VI lesions, which include an unstable flap tear of the labrum; and type VII lesions, which involve continuation of the defect into the middle glenohumeral ligament origin. Andrews et al[10] described a similar disorder of the biceps origin and superior labrum that results from overhead athletic activity. The authors thought that injury occurred as a result of the eccentric overload placed on the biceps origin and superior labrum complex by the sudden deceleration of elbow extension by the biceps during the follow-through phase of throwing. In younger athletes, SLAP lesions are more commonly the result of excessive forces being placed on the biceps origin and superior labral complex during throwing, a fall on an outstretched arm, or direct trauma. In older athletes, however, many authors believe that SLAP lesions can develop or propagate from repetitive overuse with overhead activities or as a natural process of degeneration and aging.[1,6,11] Snyder et al[6] reported the occurrence of several SLAP lesions as a result of repetitive overhead activity. Eakin et al[1] described a cycle established by destabilization of the biceps anchor in athletes. Older athletes who participate in recreational overhead sports may have decreased

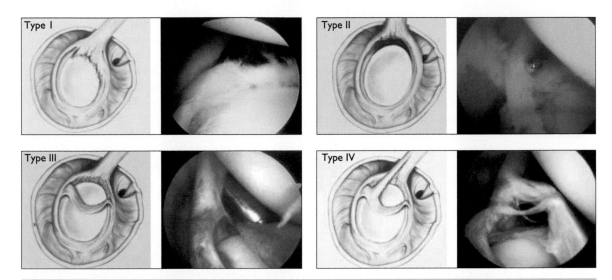

Figure I   Illustrations and representative arthroscopic images of Snyder's four types of SLAP lesions. (Illustrations copyright Stephen J. Snyder, MD, Van Nuys, CA. Arthroscopic images reproduced from Mileski RA, Snyder SJ: Superior labral lesions in the shoulder: Pathoanatomy and surgical management. *J Am Acad Orthop Surg* 1998;6(2):121-131.)

periscapular muscle strength and poor shoulder mechanics, conditioning, or imbalance, which can cause biceps anchor disruption. Biceps anchor disruption leads to increased humeral head translation, which can in turn lead to increased strain on the static humeral head restraints, resulting in glenohumeral joint laxity and/or instability. Glenohumeral laxity further destabilizes the biceps origin, completing the cycle.[1] Degeneration occurs in the biceps, paralleling that of the rotator cuff.

Because of the close anatomic relationship between the biceps tendon and the rotator cuff, the principal aspect of biceps tendon degeneration is related to rotator cuff tearing and subsequent mechanical irritation of the tendon on the coracoacromial arch. Neer[12] reported that biceps tendon disruption rarely occurred without an associated supraspinatus tear. Others have reported the occurrence of biceps tendon subluxation after isolated subscapularis tear.[13] Walch et al[14] described biceps tendon pathology associated with supraspinatus tears and the rotator interval, which is called the "hidden lesion." They described biceps tendon subluxation associated with loss or degeneration of the coracohumeral ligament and the superior glenohumeral ligament, which forms a sling on which the biceps tendon travels

in the interval. Both rotator interval and rotator cuff disease are more common in older patients and athletes.

Factors such as hypovascularity, hypoxia, and primary fiber failure are less understood but potentially contribute to biceps tendon pathology in the aging athlete. Hypoxia as a result of hypovascularity has been shown to be a factor in the development of rotator cuff tears.[15] Additionally, tendon pathology within the groove can develop as a result of osteophyte formation and resultant groove narrowing that commonly occurs with aging.[13] With persistent overhead athletic participation in the face of biceps tendon degeneration, pain and possibly tendon rupture may occur.

The Role of the Biceps in Shoulder Stability/Biomechanics

The exact role of the long head of the biceps tendon in shoulder biomechanics is not completely known. Multiple authors have suggested that the long head of the biceps has a stabilizing effect on the glenohumeral joint.[16-19] Kumar et al[20] showed the biceps tendon to be a static restraint to humeral head superior migration, and Warner and McMahon[21] showed the biceps to be a dynamic depressor of the humeral head. In a cadaveric study, Pagnani et al[18] demonstrated that loading the long head of the biceps significantly decreased humeral head translation, particularly at lower angles of elevation. At 45° of elevation and neutral rotation, loading the long head of the biceps significantly decreased anterior, inferior, and superior humeral head translation.[18] Additionally, it has been shown that detachment of the biceps anchor is associated with increased strain on the inferior glenohumeral ligament.[22] Jobe et al[23] showed that the biceps was active during the late cocking phase of throwing and that it contributed to deceleration of the forearm. Warner and McMahon[21] showed that the biceps tendon provided superior stabilization to the glenohumeral joint with the shoulder abducted.

Using electromyography (EMG) to evaluate athletes with a diagnosis of glenohumeral joint instability, Glousman et al[24] showed increased biceps activity during arm acceleration, indicating that the biceps-labrum complex has at least some role in humeral head stability during throwing.

In another study using EMG to analyze the throwing shoulder, Gowan et al[25] compared the shoulders of amateur and professional athletes and showed that amateurs required more biceps function to accelerate the arm than did professionals. Professionals were able to selectively recruit the subscapularis for arm acceleration. Additionally, amateurs required more biceps function for deceleration during follow-through, placing greater demands on this tendon.

It is clear that an athlete's shoulder is under maximal stress during overhead throwing activities. These stresses are magnified in mature athletes who may have underlying tissue pathology, shoulder stiffness, and compromised biomechanics.

Patient Evaluation of Biceps Tendon Disorders and SLAP Lesions

The diagnosis of superior labral and biceps anchor or tendon pathology can be challenging because associated shoulder injuries are common. The reported incidence of isolated SLAP lesions ranges from 2% to 30%,[6,26-28] but the reported incidence of SLAP lesions associated with other pathology is much higher. In a study evaluating findings during arthroscopy of 544 shoulders, 25% were diagnosed with SLAP lesions; 88% of these

had coexistent pathology.[26] Additionally, current examination techniques lack sensitivity and specificity.[27]

There is also great variability in presentation of patients with SLAP lesions. Younger athletes often present after sustaining a traumatic injury, whereas older patients commonly experience a more insidious onset. SLAP lesions most often occur from traction injuries, falling onto an outstretched arm, compression-type injuries, or from a direct blow. Pain is often the reason for initial presentation, but the location and pattern can be variable, mimicking other types of shoulder pathology.[2,26,29] Snyder et al,[6] in their original description of the SLAP lesion, noted that the most common mechanism of injury was a compression force to the shoulder after falling onto an outstretched arm with the shoulder abducted and slightly forwardly flexed at the time of impact. The most common symptoms reported by patients in their study were pain, especially with overhead activities, and painful "popping" and "catching" in the shoulder. Other authors have suggested that common etiologies of SLAP tears are traction on the biceps tendon or tension on the biceps-labral complex with throwing, or that the lesion is secondary to "peel-back" of the superior labrum as the arm is brought into abduction and external rotation during throwing.[9,10,30] In a series of 139 patients treated for SLAP tears, Kim et al[26] reported that sports activity was the most common cause of injury, accounting for 25% of SLAP lesions in their series. The study also showed that patients with type II SLAP lesions who are younger than 40 years are more likely to have an associated Bankart lesion, whereas those older than 40 are more likely to have an associated supraspinatus tear.

Athletes may report a painful, deep click in the shoulder or a sensation of "giving way" with overhead or other rotational movements of the shoulder. Throwers may report loss of velocity and control and pain occurring in the late cocking and early acceleration phases. The older athlete may report weakness or a sensation of weakness from associated pain that may be due to rotator cuff pathology or subacromial impingement. Instability is more commonly reported by younger athletes and may be associated with a history of traumatic shoulder dislocation. In a study that examined 30 patients with a mean age of 47.8 years who presented with labral or SLAP lesions, 24 had acute onset of symptoms and 6 had insidious onset.[31] Eleven injuries were sports-related, and 11 occurred from falls. The predominant report of all patients was pain.

Patients with biceps tendon pathology often report pain in the anterior region of the shoulder over the bicipital groove; however, this can be highly variable, depending on whether associated pathology exists in the shoulder.

A thorough history should be taken to determine if the pain originated from athletic participation or another traumatic event and if the pain worsened with sports activity. Athletes should be asked whether the pain diminishes their desired performance level. Popping, clicking, or grinding can be associated with the origin of the tendon, such as in SLAP lesions. If an athlete reports a sensation of snapping with certain shoulder motions, this should be differentiated from proximal biceps instability at the bicipital groove.

Physical examination should include careful inspection for shoulder asymmetry, muscle atrophy, or signs of cuff pathology. The shoulder should be palpated for local tenderness. Active and passive range of motion should be documented. Internal and external rotation with the shoulder abducted 90° should be documented. Younger athletes (eg, pitchers) often have increased external and decreased internal rotation of the dominant shoulder, but if the internal rotation side-to-side difference is greater than 25°, the athletes may have glenohumeral internal rotation deficit, which may predispose them to SLAP tears and internal impingement.[32,33]

Rotator cuff musculature, including the supraspinatus, infraspinatus/teres minor, and subscapularis, should be evaluated and compared with the contralateral side. The mature athlete may show weakness on examination, which may indicate rotator cuff pathology or pain from subacromial impingement, which are often associated pathologies.

Numerous special tests exist for the evaluation of SLAP lesions and biceps tendon pathology. The Yergason and Speed tests should be performed to check for biceps tendinopathy, although these tests may be positive in the presence of a SLAP tear as well. The O'Brien test, anterior apprehension test, compression-relocation test, Whipple test, biceps load tests I and II, Jobe relocation, crank test, pain provocation, internal rotation resistance strength test, passive compression test, anterior slide test, and resisted supination-external rotation tests all have been described to detect SLAP lesions.[2,27,34-42] Although most authors report good results with their respective tests, independent researchers who compared examination and intraoperative findings concluded that clinical findings alone are not reliable in diagnosing SLAP lesions.[43,44] Oh et al[27] evaluated the sensitivity and specificity of 10 different examinations for the diagnosis of SLAP lesions. Their results showed the Whipple, O'Brien, anterior apprehension, and compression-rotation tests all had sensitivities just over 60%; the Whipple test was the most sensitive, at 65%. The specificities of the Yergason, biceps load II, and anterior slide tests were over 70%; the Yergason test had the highest specificity, at 87%. No test showed both high sensitivity and specificity. Performing a combination of two of the three relatively sensitive tests and one of the three relatively specific tests improved the sensitivity and specificity to 70% and 95%, respectively. Similar results were seen in patients younger and older than 40 years of age. Standard imaging of the shoulder should be performed, including AP, scapular Y, and axillary lateral views. The bicipital groove view, as described by Cone et al,[45] and the Fisk view can be obtained to more thoroughly evaluate the bicipital groove for osteophytes or narrowing. MRI is the imaging study of choice in the detection of SLAP lesions and other shoulder disorders, although some question its accuracy.[2,46-49] Chandnani et al[50] performed a blind prospective MRI analysis of 20 asymptomatic volunteers using 20 symptomatic patients as controls. Despite the fact that the rotator cuffs and labrums of all of the asymptomatic shoulders were intact, 6 of the rotator cuffs and 10 of the labrums had abnormal internal signal intensity on MRI, leading the authors to conclude that MRI lacks specificity and to recommend that imaging findings should be correlated with physical examination to avoid false-positive interpretations. Whether the imaging study should be magnetic resonance arthrography with contrast or a noncontrast study is debatable and therefore is left to surgeon preference. However, Applegate et al[51] showed that magnetic resonance arthrography had 100% sensitivity, 88% specificity, and 92% accuracy in diagnosing chronic labral tears. Although subtleties exist, magnetic

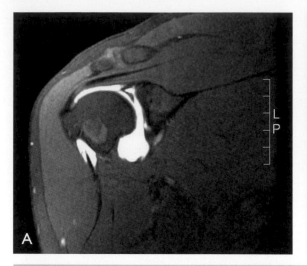
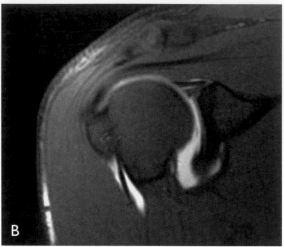

Figure 2   Magnetic resonance arthrograms of SLAP tears. **A,** A type II SLAP tear in a 49-year-old recreational baseball player. **B,** A type III SLAP tear in a 47-year-old patient with a chief report of catching.

resonance arthrography can be definitive in confirming a clinical diagnosis of a SLAP lesion (**Figure 2**).

Arthroscopy is the diagnostic method of choice for SLAP lesions. However, Gobezie et al[52] had 73 surgeons considered specialists in shoulder surgery review 22 clinical vignettes on video. They found substantial interobserver and intraobserver variability even among these expert shoulder specialists regarding the diagnosis and, therefore, the treatment of SLAP lesions when using the Snyder classification. The surgeons had difficulty distinguishing type II SLAP lesions from normal shoulders and distinguishing type III and IV lesions from one another. The study also found that the treatment of type III SLAP lesions was more variable than for other types.

Treatment of Biceps Tendon Pathology and SLAP Lesions

A nonsurgical approach using rest, ice, and nonsteroidal anti-inflammatory drugs is the first line of treatment of the mature athlete with physical examination findings consistent with biceps pathology. Biceps pain may be intra-articular or from the groove. Throwing athletes may improve with periods of rest followed by gradual progression back into sport. Diagnostic injections into the glenohumeral joint or the bicipital groove can help differentiate the location of the primary pathology. A

corticosteroid can be added for therapeutic purposes and may provide relief for athletes who desire to participate in their sport until the end of the season. To prevent the possibility of tendon rupture when injecting steroids into the bicipital groove, care must be taken to ensure the injection is extratendinous.[1]

With resolution of the acute symptoms, rehabilitation can be initiated and should be focused on range of motion followed by strengthening the rotator cuff and scapular stabilizers. Eakin et al[1] recommended initial emphasis on rehabilitation of the internal and external rotators. The internal rotators work eccentrically during the late cocking phase to prevent overstraining the anterior static restraints of the glenohumeral joint. Biceps activity increases in follow-through as the external rotators fatigue. The trapezius and serratus anterior should be rehabilitated to prevent or improve scapular dyskinesia. Next, biceps strengthening can be initiated. If the biceps is degenerative, it is difficult to rehabilitate the biceps itself. With improvement, overhead activity is begun with graduated progression to sports participation. With appropriate nonsurgical treatment and rehabilitation, most athletes respond favorably and are able to return to competition.

Surgical intervention is indicated if symptoms persist despite nonsurgical treatment. The decision as to which procedure is best is somewhat controversial and is multifactorial, depending on where the pathology exists, the age of the athlete, and the functional requirements.

The treatment of SLAP lesions in the younger athlete is dependent on the type of lesion present. Most lesions treated are type II lesions. Snyder et al,[6] in their original description of SLAP lesions, recommended débridement back to a stable labrum for type I and type III lesions. Type II lesions were treated by reattachment of the superior labrum. Type IV lesions were treated with reattachment of the labrum and partial débridement of the split portion of the biceps tendon. If more than 50% of the biceps tendon was involved, tenodesis was performed.

Over time, numerous different methods and products for fixation have been available to fix SLAP lesions, including biodegradable tacks and suture anchors. Outcomes vary depending on the type of lesion treated and any associated shoulder pathology, as well as the type of fixation used for repair. Success rates with biodegradable tacks are reported as 71% to 88%.[22,41,53,54] Return-to-sport rates have not been as successful, however; one study reported that more than 40% of patients had persistent night pain with this type of fixation.[54] Suture anchor fixation has achieved better results, with good to excellent success rates of 90% to 97% reported.[8,55,56] Return to preinjury level of athletic activity also improved with suture anchors, with rates reported as 75% to 91%. Nevertheless, considerable controversy remains as to the best treatment of isolated SLAP lesions. Boileau et al[57] recently compared biceps tenodesis with SLAP repair in patients with isolated SLAP lesions. The authors found that although the tenodesis group was, in general, older than their repair group, clinical outcomes after tenodesis were substantially better than after SLAP repair.[57]

These findings highlight the fact that surgical treatment of biceps pathology and SLAP lesions is different for the older athlete. Isolated SLAP lesions or biceps tendinopathy is uncommon in this population. More commonly, years of athletic participation lead to rotator cuff injury, subacromial impingement, and other pathology in or about the shoulder joint. Snyder et al[58] reported their intraoperative findings at the time of SLAP repair and found that in a group with an average

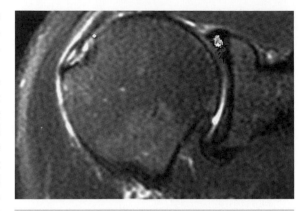

Figure 3   T2-weighted magnetic resonance arthrogram demonstrates a type II SLAP lesion with rotator cuff pathology in a 52-year-old softball player.

age near 40 years, 29% of patients had partial rotator cuff tearing, 11% had full-thickness rotator cuff tears, and 22% had Bankart lesions. Additionally, 47% of the patients in this series had positive tests for subacromial impingement. The presence of additional pathology in the setting of a SLAP tear is common as patients age (**Figure 3**).

Little has been written about the repair of SLAP lesions in older patients. Franceschi et al[59] performed a randomized controlled trial comparing the outcomes of 31 patients treated with arthroscopic fixation for type II SLAP lesions and rotator cuff tears with those of 32 patients treated with biceps tenotomies and rotator cuff repairs. All patients were older than 50 years (mean age, 63 years). Patients were followed for an average of 5.2 years. University of California, Los Angeles (UCLA) scores and range-of-motion values were compared. Patients treated with biceps tenotomy and rotator cuff repair had statistically significant improved outcomes compared with patients treated with repair of a SLAP lesion and rotator cuff tear.

In another study, Voos et al[31] retrospectively evaluated the results in 30 patients with an average age of 47.8 years who were treated arthroscopically for combined rotator cuff and labral lesions. Fourteen patients had SLAP lesions and 16 had Bankart lesions. Eleven of the patients (mean age, 43 years) had a sports-related injury. The mean follow-up was 2.7 years. Significant improvements were noted in shoulder range of motion, and L'Insalata and American Society of Shoulder and Elbow Surgeons (ASES) scores were 92.9 and 94.3, respectively. Additionally, 90% of patients reported good or excellent satisfaction levels, and 77% returned to their preinjury sports activities. Nine of the 11 patients with sports-related lesions were able to return to their preinjury level of athletic participation.

Another study evaluating the outcomes of repair of type II SLAP lesions alone compared with repair of SLAP lesions and acromioplasty reported that 81% of patients in the combined treatment group had good or excellent satisfaction ratings compared with only 65% in the SLAP group.[60] Additionally, 21% of patients in the isolated SLAP repair group had postoperative impingement, compared with none in the combined group. Enad and Kurtz[61] also showed better ASES scores for patients treated for SLAP plus another pathology compared with those treated for SLAP alone.

More has been written about the treatment of biceps tendon pathology in the mature athlete than about repair of SLAP lesions. Gill et al[62] studied the effect of biceps tenotomy for treatment of isolated bicipital pathology (bicipital tenosynovitis, dislocation, or partial rupture) using the ASES shoulder evaluation form in 30 consecutive patients. The procedures were performed arthroscopically, and patients were followed for an average of 19 months. A mean postoperative ASES score of 82 and a significant reduction in pain and improvement in function was reported after release.

Walch et al[63] examined tenotomy of the long head of the biceps tendon in the treatment of large and massive rotator cuff tears. Arthroscopic biceps tenotomy was performed in 307 patients with full-thickness rotator cuff tears that were irreparable or in patients who were older and not willing to participate in the necessary rehabilitation following rotator cuff repair. Patients were followed for a mean of 57 months postoperatively. The mean Constant score improved significantly, from 48.4 preoperatively to 67.6 postoperatively; 87% of patients were satisfied or very satisfied with their outcomes.

Boileau et al[64] retrospectively evaluated the outcomes of 68 consecutive patients with 72 massive irreparable rotator cuff tears treated with isolated arthroscopic biceps tenotomy (39 shoulders) or tenodesis (33 shoulders). The mean age was 68 years. Patients

were evaluated for a mean of 35 months postoperatively; at follow-up, 78% of patients were satisfied with the surgical outcome. The mean Constant score increased from 46.3 preoperatively to 66.5 postoperatively. The results did not differ between the tenotomy and tenodesis groups. The so-called "Popeye" deformity was noted by the surgeon postoperatively in 62% of those treated with tenotomy, but only 41% of the patients noticed the deformity and none of the patients who noted the deformity reported concerns.

The advantages of arthroscopic tenotomy are that the procedure is simple and quick and has minimal morbidity.[62] No postoperative restrictions need be placed on the shoulder, such as those required in tenodesis to allow for healing of the tendon. Simple tenotomy avoids possible problems associated with tenodesis such as tendon pull-out, hardware failure, and pain. Gill et al[62] reported that the average return to work or sport in their series of 30 patients was 1.9 weeks.

The potential disadvantages of tenotomy include the Popeye deformity, fatigue discomfort, loss of flexion and supination strength, and pain with supination. Kelly et al[65] reported that the Popeye deformity developed in 83% of men and 37% of women following biceps tenotomy, and 38% of patients had fatigue discomfort associated with tenotomy. However, Osbahr et al,[66] in a comparison of tenotomy versus tenodesis, showed no statistically significant differences in anterior shoulder pain, muscle spasms in the biceps, and cosmetic deformity of the biceps. Mariani et al[67] showed a 21% loss of supination and 8% loss of elbow flexion strength in patients treated nonsurgically for proximal biceps tendon ruptures compared with those surgically repaired. No differences in range of motion or arm pain were reported in this series.

The advantages of tenodesis over tenotomy are the potentially lower risk of cosmetic deformity, as well as less flexion and supination strength loss. Although the literature does not declare a clear victor in this regard,[65,66] numerous choices are available for location of the tenodesis and type of fixation (**Figure 4**).

In the longest follow-up study reported, Becker and Cofield[68] evaluated the outcomes of tenodesis for chronic tendinitis of the long head of the biceps in 54 shoulders (51 patients) at a mean follow-up of 13 years. At 6 months postoperatively, 51 of the 54 shoulders

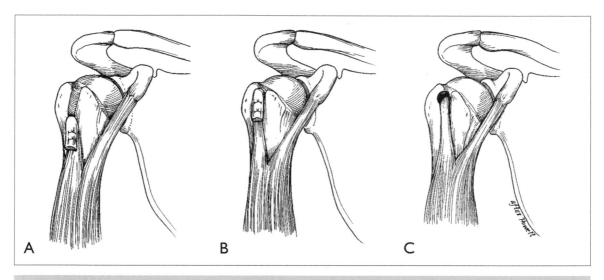

Figure 4   Techniques for biceps tenodesis. **A,** In the two-pronged staple technique, the tendon is pulled proximally to the appropriate tension and then secured with a staple. The proximal free edge of the tendon is pulled distally over the staple (not shown) and sewn to itself. **B,** In the tunnel technique, a burr is used to create a tunnel approximately 2 cm in length. The tendon is delivered into the distal hole and pulled out the proximal hole to the appropriate tension. The free edge of the tendon is then sewn back onto itself to secure it. **C,** In the keyhole technique, the free edge of the tendon is knotted and sutured. A burr is used to create a keyhole that is wider proximally to accommodate the knotted tendon and narrows distally. The knotted tendon is inserted into the keyhole under slight tension, locking it into place. (Adapted with permission from Hawkins RJ, Bell RH, Lippitt SB, eds: *Atlas of Shoulder Surgery.* St Louis, Mosby, 1996, p 145.)

showed improvement. However, with longer follow-up, a satisfactory result was seen in only 50% of patients, with 15% requiring additional surgery. The authors concluded that tenodesis was not an appropriate treatment of chronic biceps tendinitis as an isolated procedure, although it may be considered as part of a larger procedure such as rotator cuff repair.

Isolated biceps tendon pathology in the mature athlete is an unlikely clinical finding. However, it is a common source of pain in this population in conjunction with rotator cuff or other shoulder pathology. Both tenotomy and tenodesis show improved postoperative outcomes. The advantages and disadvantages of each should be understood by the surgeon and discussed with the patient. Patient age, participation in overhead sports activity, cosmetic concerns, and level of competition should all be considered when deciding which option is best for each patient. Tenotomy is simple. Tenodesis can be performed by various methods—intra-articular, subpectoral or supra-

pectoral, arthroscopic or open—with different methods of fixation.

Conclusions

The diagnosis of an isolated SLAP lesion in the mature athlete should rarely be made; it is likely that additional pathology exists. Whether clinical improvement occurs secondary to treatment of other lesions, alone or in combination with SLAP repair, remains to be completely understood. It is clear, however, that older athletes treated for isolated SLAP lesions do worse than those treated for SLAP lesions combined with other shoulder pathology.

Biceps tendon pathology is a common finding in an older athletic population. Clinicians should be aware of the presenting symptoms, physical examination findings, and radiologic evaluation for these patients. Nonsurgical treatment is often effective. Associated pathology such as rotator cuff dysfunction is important to recognize and treat as well. Emerging research continues to address the best surgical treatment of biceps lesions in the older athlete. It would appear that biceps tenotomy is simple and successful but that tenodesis can avoid the Popeye deformity and may result in less strength loss and fatigue. Further study is required to elucidate the indications for each procedure.

References

1. Eakin CL, Faber KJ, Hawkins RJ, Hovis WD: Biceps tendon disorders in athletes. *J Am Acad Orthop Surg* 1999;7(5):300-310.

2. Keener JD, Brophy RH: Superior labral tears of the shoulder: pathogenesis, evaluation, and treatment. *J Am Acad Orthop Surg* 2009;17(10):627-637.

3. Habermeyer P, Kaiser E, Knappe M, Kreusser T, Wiedemann E: Functional anatomy and biomechanics of the long biceps tendon. *Unfallchirurg* 1987;90(7):319-329.

4. Vangsness CT Jr, Jorgenson SS, Watson T, Johnson DL: The origin of the long head of the biceps from the scapula and glenoid labrum: An anatomical study of 100 shoulders. *J Bone Joint Surg Br* 1994;76(6):951-954.

5. Claessens H, Snoeck H: Tendinitis of the long head of the biceps brachii. *Acta Orthop Belg* 1972;58(1):124-128.

6. Snyder SJ, Karzel RP, Del Pizzo W, Ferkel RD, Friedman MJ: SLAP lesions of the shoulder. *Arthroscopy* 1990;6(4):274-279.

7. Mileski RA, Snyder SJ: Superior labral lesions in the shoulder: Pathoanatomy and surgical management. *J Am Acad Orthop Surg* 1998;6(2):121-131.

8. Morgan CD, Burkhart SS, Palmeri M, Gillespie M: Type II SLAP lesions: Three subtypes and their relationships to superior instability and rotator cuff tears. *Arthroscopy* 1998;14(6):553-565.

9. Maffet MW, Gartsman GM, Moseley B: Superior labrum-biceps tendon complex lesions of the shoulder. *Am J Sports Med* 1995;23(1):93-98.

10. Andrews JR, Carson WG Jr, McLeod WD: Glenoid labrum tears related to the long head of the biceps. *Am J Sports Med* 1985;13(5):337-341.

11. Jobe FW, Kvitne RS, Giangarra CE: Shoulder pain in the overhand or throwing athlete: The relationship of anterior instability and rotator cuff impingement. *Orthop Rev* 1989;18(9):963-975.

12. Neer C: *Shoulder Reconstruction.* Philadelphia, PA, WB Saunders, 1990.

13. Bell RH: Biceps disorders, in Hawkins RJ, ed: *Shoulder Injuries in the Athlete: Surgical Repair and Rehabilitation.* New York, NY, Churchill Livingstone, pp 267-282.

14. Walch G, Nove-Josserand L, Levigne C, Renaud E: Tears of the supraspinatus tendon associated with "hidden" lesions of the rotator interval. *J Shoulder Elbow Surg* 1994;3:353-360.

15. Iannotti J: Lesions of the rotator cuff: Pathology and pathogenesis, in Matsen FA FF, Hawkins RJ, eds: *The Shoulder: A Balance of Mobility and Stability.* Rosemont, IL American Academy of Orthopaedic Surgeons, 1993, pp 239-251.

16. Hitchcock HH, Bechtol CO: Painful shoulder: Observations on the role of the tendon of the long head of the biceps brachii in its causation. *J Bone Joint Surg Am* 1948;30A(2):263-273.

17. Itoi E, Kuechle DK, Newman SR, Morrey BF, An KN: Stabilising function of the biceps in stable and unstable shoulders. *J Bone Joint Surg Br* 1993;75(4):546-550.

18. Pagnani MJ, Deng XH, Warren RF, Torzilli PA, O'Brien SJ: Role of the long head of the biceps brachii in glenohumeral stability: A biomechanical study in cadavera. *J Shoulder Elbow Surg* 1996;5(4):255-262.

19. Rodosky MW, Harner CD, Fu FH: The role of the long head of the biceps muscle and superior glenoid labrum in anterior stability of the shoulder. *Am J Sports Med* 1994;22(1):121-130.

20. Kumar VP, Satku K, Balasubramaniam P: The role of the long head of biceps brachii in the stabilization of the head of the humerus. *Clin Orthop Relat Res* 1989;(244):172-175.

21. Warner JJ, McMahon PJ: The role of the long head of the biceps brachii in superior stability of the glenohumeral joint. *J Bone Joint Surg Am* 1995;77(3):366-372.

22. Pagnani MJ, Deng XH, Warren RF, Torzilli PA, Altchek DW: Effect of lesions of the superior portion of the glenoid labrum on glenohumeral translation. *J Bone Joint Surg Am* 1995;77(7):1003-1010.

23. Jobe FW, Moynes DR, Tibone JE, Perry J: An EMG analysis of the shoulder in pitching: A second report. *Am J Sports Med* 1984;12(3):218-220.

24. Glousman R, Jobe F, Tibone J, Moynes D, Antonelli D, Perry J: Dynamic electromyographic analysis of the

throwing shoulder with glenohumeral instability. *J Bone Joint Surg Am* 1988;70(2):220-226.

25. Gowan ID, Jobe FW, Tibone JE, Perry J, Moynes DR: A comparative electromyographic analysis of the shoulder during pitching: Professional versus amateur pitchers. *Am J Sports Med* 1987;15(6):586-590.

26. Kim TK, Queale WS, Cosgarea AJ, McFarland EG: Clinical features of the different types of SLAP lesions: An analysis of one hundred and thirty-nine cases. *J Bone Joint Surg Am* 2003;85A(1):66-71.

27. Oh JH, Kim JY, Kim WS, Gong HS, Lee JH: The evaluation of various physical examinations for the diagnosis of type II superior labrum anterior and posterior lesion. *Am J Sports Med* 2008;36(2):353-359.

28. Parentis MA, Glousman RE, Mohr KS, Yocum LA: An evaluation of the provocative tests for superior labral anterior posterior lesions. *Am J Sports Med* 2006;34(2):265-268.

29. Nam EK, Snyder SJ: The diagnosis and treatment of superior labrum, anterior and posterior (SLAP) lesions. *Am J Sports Med* 2003;31(5):798-810.

30. Burkhart SS, Morgan CD: The peel-back mechanism: Its role in producing and extending posterior type II SLAP lesions and its effect on SLAP repair rehabilitation. *Arthroscopy* 1998;14(6):637-640.

31. Voos JE, Pearle AD, Mattern CJ, Cordasco FA, Allen AA, Warren RF: Outcomes of combined arthroscopic rotator cuff and labral repair. *Am J Sports Med* 2007;35(7):1174-1179.

32. Burkhart SS, Morgan CD, Kibler WB: The disabled throwing shoulder: Spectrum of pathology Part III. The SICK scapula, scapular dyskinesis, the kinetic chain, and rehabilitation. *Arthroscopy* 2003;19(6):641-661.

33. Myers JB, Laudner KG, Pasquale MR, Bradley JP, Lephart SM: Glenohumeral range of motion deficits and posterior shoulder tightness in throwers with pathologic internal impingement. *Am J Sports Med* 2006;34(3):385-391.

34. Berg EE, Ciullo JV: A clinical test for superior glenoid labral or 'SLAP' lesions. *Clin J Sport Med* 1998;8(2):121-123.

35. Kim SH, Ha KI, Ahn JH, Kim SH, Choi HJ: Biceps load test II: A clinical test for SLAP lesions of the shoulder. *Arthroscopy* 2001;17(2):160-164.

36. Kim SH, Ha KI, Han KY: Biceps load test: A clinical test for superior labrum anterior and posterior lesions in shoulders with recurrent anterior dislocations. *Am J Sports Med* 1999;27(3):300-303.

37. Kim YS, Kim JM, Ha KY, Choy S, Joo MW, Chung YG: The passive compression test: A new clinical test for superior labral tears of the shoulder. *Am J Sports Med* 2007;35(9):1489-1494.

38. O'Brien SJ, Pagnani MJ, Fealy S, McGlynn SR, Wilson JB: The active compression test: A new and effective test for diagnosing labral tears and acromioclavicular joint abnormality. *Am J Sports Med* 1998;26(5):610-613.

39. Kibler WB: Specificity and sensitivity of the anterior slide test in throwing athletes with superior glenoid labral tears. *Arthroscopy* 1995;11(3):296-300.

40. Myers TH, Zemanovic JR, Andrews JR: The resisted supination external rotation test: A new test for the diagnosis of superior labral anterior posterior lesions. *Am J Sports Med* 2005;33(9):1315-1320.

41. Rhee YG, Lee DH, Lim CT: Unstable isolated SLAP lesion: Clinical presentation and outcome of arthroscopic fixation. *Arthroscopy* 2005;21(9):1099.

42. Zaslav KR: Internal rotation resistance strength test: A new diagnostic test to differentiate intra-articular pathology from outlet (Neer) impingement syndrome in the shoulder. *J Shoulder Elbow Surg* 2001;10(1):23-27.

43. McFarland EG, Kim TK, Savino RM: Clinical assessment of three common tests for superior labral anterior-posterior lesions. *Am J Sports Med* 2002;30(6):810-815.

44. Parentis MA, Mohr KJ, ElAttrache NS: Disorders of the superior labrum: Review and treatment guidelines. *Clin Orthop Relat Res* 2002;(400):77-87.

45. Cone RO, Danzig L, Resnick D, Goldman AB: The bicipital groove: Radiographic, anatomic, and pathologic study. *AJR Am J Roentgenol* 1983;141(4):781-788.

46. Bencardino JT, Beltran J, Rosenberg ZS, et al: Superior labrum anterior-posterior lesions: Diagnosis with MR arthrography of the shoulder. *Radiology* 2000;214(1):267-271.

47. Connell DA, Potter HG, Wickiewicz TL, Altchek DW, Warren RF: Noncontrast magnetic resonance imaging of superior labral lesions: 102 cases confirmed at arthroscopic surgery. *Am J Sports Med* 1999;27(2):208-213.

48. Jee WH, McCauley TR, Katz LD, Matheny JM, Ruwe PA, Daigneault JP: Superior labral anterior posterior (SLAP) lesions of the glenoid labrum: Reliability and

accuracy of MR arthrography for diagnosis. *Radiology* 2001;218(1):127-132.

49. Tung GA, Entzian D, Green A, Brody JM: High-field and low-field MR imaging of superior glenoid labral tears and associated tendon injuries. *AJR Am J Roentgenol* 2000;174(4):1107-1114.

50. Chandnani V, Ho C, Gerharter J, et al: MR findings in asymptomatic shoulders: A blind analysis using symptomatic shoulders as controls. *Clin Imaging* 1992;16(1):25-30.

51. Applegate GR, Hewitt M, Snyder SJ, Watson E, Kwak S, Resnick D: Chronic labral tears: Value of magnetic resonance arthrography in evaluating the glenoid labrum and labral-bicipital complex. *Arthroscopy* 2004;20(9):959-963.

52. Gobezie R, Zurakowski D, Lavery K, Millett PJ, Cole BJ, Warner JJ: Analysis of interobserver and intraobserver variability in the diagnosis and treatment of SLAP tears using the Snyder classification. *Am J Sports Med* 2008;36(7):1373-1379.

53. Samani JE, Marston SB, Buss DD: Arthroscopic stabilization of type II SLAP lesions using an absorbable tack. *Arthroscopy* 2001;17(1):19-24.

54. Cohen DB, Coleman S, Drakos MC, et al: Outcomes of isolated type II SLAP lesions treated with arthroscopic fixation using a bioabsorbable tack. *Arthroscopy* 2006;22(2):136-142.

55. Ide J, Maeda S, Takagi K: Sports activity after arthroscopic superior labral repair using suture anchors in overhead-throwing athletes. *Am J Sports Med* 2005;33(4):507-514.

56. Kim SH, Ha KI, Kim SH, Choi HJ: Results of arthroscopic treatment of superior labral lesions. *J Bone Joint Surg Am* 2002;84A(6):981-985.

57. Boileau P, Parratte S, Chuinard C, Roussanne Y, Shia D, Bicknell R: Arthroscopic treatment of isolated type II SLAP lesions: Biceps tenodesis as an alternative to reinsertion. *Am J Sports Med* 2009;37(5):929-936.

58. Snyder SJ, Banas MP, Karzel RP: An analysis of 140 injuries to the superior glenoid labrum. *J Shoulder Elbow Surg* 1995;4(4):243-248.

59. Franceschi F, Longo UG, Ruzzini L, Rizzello G, Maffulli N, Denaro V: No advantages in repairing a type II superior labrum anterior and posterior (SLAP) lesion when associated with rotator cuff repair in patients over age 50: A randomized controlled trial. *Am J Sports Med* 2008;36(2):247-253.

60. Coleman SH, Cohen DB, Drakos MC, et al: Arthroscopic repair of type II superior labral anterior posterior lesions with and without acromioplasty: A clinical analysis of 50 patients. *Am J Sports Med* 2007;35(5):749-753.

61. Enad JG, Kurtz CA: Isolated and combined Type II SLAP repairs in a military population. *Knee Surg Sports Traumatol Arthrosc* 2007;15(11):1382-1389.

62. Gill TJ, McIrvin E, Mair SD, Hawkins RJ: Results of biceps tenotomy for treatment of pathology of the long head of the biceps brachii. *J Shoulder Elbow Surg* 2001;10(3):247-249.

63. Walch G, Edwards TB, Boulahia A, Nové-Josserand L, Neyton L, Szabo I: Arthroscopic tenotomy of the long head of the biceps in the treatment of rotator cuff tears: Clinical and radiographic results of 307 cases. *J Shoulder Elbow Surg* 2005;14(3):238-246.

64. Boileau P, Baqué F, Valerio L, Ahrens P, Chuinard C, Trojani C: Isolated arthroscopic biceps tenotomy or tenodesis improves symptoms in patients with massive irreparable rotator cuff tears. *J Bone Joint Surg Am* 2007;89(4):747-757.

65. Kelly AM, Drakos MC, Fealy S, Taylor SA, O'Brien SJ: Arthroscopic release of the long head of the biceps tendon: Functional outcome and clinical results. *Am J Sports Med* 2005;33(2):208-213.

66. Osbahr DC, Diamond AB, Speer KP: The cosmetic appearance of the biceps muscle after long-head tenotomy versus tenodesis. *Arthroscopy* 2002;18(5):483-487.

67. Mariani EM, Cofield RH, Askew LJ, Li GP, Chao EY: Rupture of the tendon of the long head of the biceps brachii: Surgical versus nonsurgical treatment. *Clin Orthop Relat Res* 1988;(228):233-239.

68. Becker DA, Cofield RH: Tenodesis of the long head of the biceps brachii for chronic bicipital tendonitis: Long-term results. *J Bone Joint Surg Am* 1989;71(3):376-381.

Chapter 20

Rotator Cuff Tears: Open Versus Arthroscopic Repair

Alexis Colvin, MD
Evan L. Flatow, MD

Key Points

- Regardless of the rotator cuff repair technique used, tendon integrity is one of the most important factors in patient functional outcome.
- Older age and larger tear size are associated with retear.
- Repair techniques that approximate the rotator cuff footprint may enhance healing potential.
- No consensus exists in the literature as to the optimal treatment of partial-thickness rotator cuff tears.
- Treatment for partial-thickness rotator cuff tears should take into account the patient's age and activity level as well as the amount of tendon involvement.

Introduction

Rotator cuff tears are increasingly common in the mature athlete.[1-3] Prevalence reported in the literature ranges from 22% of patients older than 65 years[1] to 54% of those older than 60.[3] Although a tear can be asymptomatic,[3] shoulder scores tend to be be worse in patients with tears.[1] Furthermore, there is a risk of tear progression and the development of symptoms over time.[4] Yamanaka and Matsumoto[5] followed 40 patients with an average age of 61 years with articular-side partial rotator cuff tears as diagnosed by arthrography and found that 11 progressed to full-thickness tears at a mean of 412 days after the initial arthrography. Progression to full-thickness tears was associated with increasing age.[5] In a study by Yamaguchi et al,[4] 23 of 45 previously asymptomatic rotator cuff tears as diagnosed by ultrasonography became symptomatic over a mean of 2.8 years, and 9 of these patients had tear progression.

Partial Tears

Partial tears of the supraspinatus have been categorized by Fukuda et al[6] into bursal-side, intratendinous, and joint-side tears. Ellman[7] further classified partial-thickness tears into three groups based on the depth of the tear: articular surface tears, extending to a depth less than 3 mm; bursal surface tears, extending 3 to 6 mm deep or less than 50% of the thickness of the tendon; and interstital tears, extending more than 6 mm deep or involving more than 50% of the thickness of the tendon.

Arthroscopy is often used as the gold standard for assessing the extent of the rotator cuff tear.[8]

Treatment Options

Treatment of partial-thickness rotator cuff tears is controversial, with many opinions but few objective data. Possible treatment options include arthroscopic débridement (with or without subacromial decompression), repair in situ, completion of the tear and repair, and treating only associated pathologies, such as a superior labrum anterior-to-posterior (SLAP) lesion or capsular laxity.

Débridement of partial rotator cuff tears, with or without subacromial decompression, is one treatment option. Andrews et al[9] recommended arthroscopic débridement in a young, athletic patient population; the authors believed this helped to "initiate a healing response." However, at a mean 3-year follow-up, Oglivie-Harris and Wiley[10] found that only half of their patients who underwent an arthroscopic débridement had successful results. They theorized that intra-articular débridement did not remove the extra-articular impingement that led to the tear.[10] Fukuda et al[2] described partial-thickness bursal-side tears as originating from a watershed area in the supraspinatus tendon that corresponded to impingement from the anterior margin of the acromion.

Several authors have reported on their results with subacromial decompression. Esch et al[11] reported an 82% satisfaction rate at 1 year in patients who had an arthroscopic subacromial decompression for a partial rotator cuff tear. Gartsman[12] retrospectively reviewed his experience with treating patients with a partial rotator cuff tear who had a minimum 2-year follow-up. He found a 93% success rate in patients who had an arthroscopic subacromial decompression and tendon débridement for a partial tear.[12] Tear length ranged from 0.3 to 3 cm, with an average of 1.1 × 1.6 cm. Patients who were receiving workers' compensation had only a 58% satisfactory result.

Not all authors have had success with débridement and acromioplasty alone. Weber[8] retrospectively reviewed his results with arthroscopic débridement and acromioplasty versus arthroscopic acromioplasty and open repair of tears greater than 50% of the thickness of the tendon. None of the patients in the repair group had symptoms of a retear, and there were no reoperations. However, six patients in the arthroscopic group underwent reoperation, with no evidence of healing in three and propagation of the tear in three. This led the author to conclude that acromioplasty alone did not prevent further tearing. Progression of tears also has been seen after an arthroscopic subacromial decompression and débridement. Kartus et al[13] found on postoperative ultrasonography that 9 of 26 tears progressed to full-thickness tears. Good results with completion of the tear and repair have also been reported. Kamath et al[14] reviewed their results with arthroscopic completion of the tear and suture anchor repair of a high-grade (>50% thickness) tear of the supraspinatus. Ultrasonography was performed at a minimum of 6 months after surgery, and healing was demonstrated in 37 of 42 patients. The mean age of the patients with the healed repair was significantly less than the age of the patients with the recurrent defect (51.8 years versus 62.8 years). Although older patients have a lower rate of healing of a repaired rotator cuff tear, a repair may convert the tear from a symptomatic to an asymptomatic tear.[15]

In situ repair of tears greater than 50% of the thickness of the tendon has been advocated by some authors for restoring the medial row while preserving the lateral row to better approximate the supraspinatus footprint and to restore the correct muscle-tendon length/tension relationship.[16,17] Furthermore, a biomechanical study by Mazzocca et al[18] demonstrated significantly higher articular tendon strain in tears greater than 50%. This strain was decreased to close to the intact state with in situ repair. Gonzalez-Lomas et al[19] argued that débridement of remaining cuff may actually lead to resection of healthy tissue that is detrimental, and they advocated in situ repair. They performed a cadaveric study in which they compared in situ transtendon repairs with completion of the tear and repair of a 50% partial articular-side supraspinatus tear. They found significantly less gap formation and higher load to ultimate failure with the in situ repair. The authors theorized that preservation of tendon and preserving the lateral footprint may help with more even distribution of loads across the repair site. A significant improvement in functional outcome scores was reported at a minimum 2-year follow-up in patients who had undergone arthroscopic transtendon repair of a partial articular-side supraspinatus tear.[20]

Authors' Preference

Indications for débridement include young, athletic patients; patients with instability or internal impingement; a treatable labral lesion (especially a SLAP lesion); and involvement of less than 75% of the tendon. If more than 75% of the tendon is involved or there is a large intratendinous extension, in situ repair is considered, but caution is exercised to avoid overtightening.

Indications for arthroscopic débridement and subacromial decompression include older patients with degenerative disease; acromial changes; bursal findings at arthroscopy; involvement of the nondominant arm; and involvement of less than 25% to 50% of the tendon.

Indications for repair include involvement of more than 25% to 50% of the tendon, significant delamination or complexity of the tear, involvement of the dominant arm, and high demand or activity level. Currently, we prefer to complete and repair degenerative tears in older patients rather than undertake in situ repair.

Open Versus Arthroscopic Rotator Cuff Repair

The integrity of the repaired cuff has been found to be critical to functional outcome.[21-23] Reported rates of intact cuff repairs as seen on postoperative MRI or ultrasonography range from 63%[24] to 80%.[23] Harryman et al[22] found that only 68 of 105 (65%) of the rotator cuffs they repaired using an open technique remained intact as seen on ultrasonography at a mean of 5 years (range, 2 to 11 years) postoperatively. Patients who had intact repairs at follow-up had better function with regard to activities of daily living, as well as range of motion and strength, than patients with retears. Gazielly et al[21] reported 76% of cuffs repaired by an open technique to be intact, as evaluated by ultrasonography, at a minimum of 2 years postoperatively. Better Constant score, mobility, and strength were correlated with an intact repair. Thomazeau et al[23] had a 20% retear rate seen on MRI at a mean follow-up of 21.1 months. Worse flexion strength and poorer Constant scores were correlated with retear. Size of the

postoperative tear as seen on MRI, as well as postoperative fatty degeneration of the infraspinatus and subscapularis, also have been found to correlate with clinical outcome.[25]

Retears after arthroscopic repair also have been reported and appear to be associated with size of the initial tear. Galatz et al[26] evaluated 18 patients at minimum 12-month follow-up after arthroscopic repair of tears larger than 2 cm and reported recurrent tears in 17. Boileau et al[27] reported on their results with arthroscopic repair of supraspinatus tears and found that 46 of 65 patients had an intact cuff at follow-up imaging (MRI or CT arthrogram) performed at a minimum of 6 months after surgery. Patients older than 65 years also had a significantly lower rate of healing ($P = 0.001$). The authors also found a lower rate of healing with initial tear extension to the infraspinatus and subscapularis ($P = 0.02$). Bishop et al[28] also found that tears larger than 3 cm repaired with an open technique had a significantly higher intact rate than tears repaired using an arthroscopic technique (62% versus 24%; $P < 0.036$). However, no significant difference was found in overall retear rate between the two groups. Morse et al[29] performed a meta-analysis of level I to III evidence studies on arthroscopic versus mini-open rotator cuff repair. Of the five studies that met the inclusion criteria, there was no difference in functional outcome scores or complications between the two groups. However, no postoperative imaging studies were performed in any of the selected studies.

Strategies to Improve Tendon Healing

Whether an open or arthroscopic technique is used, the repair should have high initial fixation strength, allowing minimal gap formation and maintaining mechanical stability until solid healing.[30]

Single-Row, Double-Row, and Transosseous-Equivalent Repair

Using a three-dimensional digitizer in cadaveric shoulders, Apreleva et al[31] demonstrated that the supraspinatus footprint is only partially restored by single row techniques. The double-row technique, using a medial row of anchors placed at the articular margin and a lateral row placed in the greater tuberosity, has been described by several authors to better restore the footprint of the supraspinatus than single-row repair.[32-36] Biomechanically, better initial strength and stiffness,[37,38] as well as decreased gap formation and strain, have been found with the double-row repair versus the single-row repair.[37] A higher time-zero ultimate tensile load for double-row fixation, versus three different single-row techniques, has also been found in cadaveric specimins.[39]

Failure rates for the arthroscopic double-row technique have ranged from 5% to 60% and appear to depend on tear size.[40] Smaller tears have been found to have a higher postoperative intact rate than larger tears.[40-42] Huijsmans et al[42] reported an overall intact repair rate of 83% (174 of 210), with better results in small tears (88%; 14 of 16) and medium tears (93%; 113 of 121) versus large tears (78%; 32 of 41) or massive tears (47%; 15 of 32). Sugaya et al[40] also found a lower retear rate on MRI for small to medium tears (5%) versus large and massive tears (40%). Lafosse et al[41] had no retears in the small cuff tears but reported structural failure in 12 of 69 large and massive tears. Clinically, smaller tears achieved greater mean strength than the large and massive tears at final follow-up.

Both double-row and transosseous-equivalent techniques have been found to have greater contact area than the single-row technique in a cadaveric model.[43] Park et al[44] demonstrated that the transosseous-equivalent technique has greater pressurized contact area and mean pressure between the supraspinatus tendon and its footprint than the double-row technique. Furthermore, the transosseous-equivalent technique has a higher mean ultimate load to failure versus the double-row technique, although no significant difference was seen for gap formation or stiffness.[45] In their cadaveric study, Busfield et al[46] found that the addition of knots in the medial row of a transosseous-equivalent repair decreased gap formation and improved ultimate load more than when medial row knots were not used.

Despite the biomechanical advantages of double- versus single-row repair, clinical studies have demonstrated no significant difference in healing or functional outcome between single- and double-row repairs.[47-50] Charousset et al[51] found no significant difference in integrity of repair between tears repaired with single- or double-row technique, but they did find significantly better anatomic healing with the double-row repair. There was also no difference in Constant score at final follow-up between the groups.[51] Franceschi et al[47] conducted a randomized controlled trial comparing single- versus double-row repair and found no statistically significant difference in healing as assessed by magnetic resonance arthrography. Furthermore, there was no difference in University of California at Los Angeles (UCLA) score or range of motion at final follow-up of 2 years.[47] A randomized controlled trial performed by Burks et al[48] found no difference on MRI in terms of footprint coverage, tendon thickness, or tendon signal. The authors also found no difference in outcome as measured by UCLA, Constant, Western Ontario Rotator Cuff Index (WORC), single assessment numeric evaluation (SANE), and American Shoulder and Elbow Surgeons (ASES) scores or range of motion and internal or external rotation strength.[48] Grasso et al[49] also found no difference in Disabilities of the Arm, Shoulder, and Hand (DASH) score, DASH work score, Constant score, or muscle strength at a mean follow-up of 24.8 months in their randomized controlled trial. However, no postoperative imaging was obtained. Park et al[50] found no significant difference in functional outcome as measured by the ASES and Constant scores when comparing results of single- and double-row repairs. When results were stratified by tear size, however, functional outcome scores were significantly improved in patients with a large to massive tears (>3 cm) who had had a double-row rather than a single-row repair. The authors recommended using a double-row repair for large to massive tears to enhance healing potential. MRI performed at a minimum of 1 year postoperatively demonstrated intact repairs in 22 of 25 patients in whom arthroscopic transosseous-equivalent suture-bridge technique was used.[52] The authors did not find a correlation with tear size; however, this was most likely due to the small sample size.

Authors' Preference

Our preference is to perform transosseous-equivalent suture bridge technique rotator cuff repairs arthroscopically for all primary tears except some traumatic tears in which the subscapularis is adhered to the axillary nerve. Arthroscopic repair is also used for revision cases, where

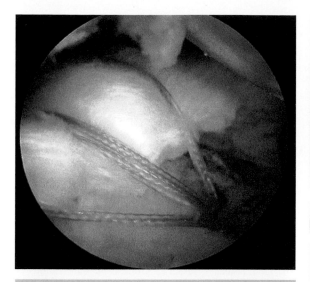

Figure 1 Arthroscopic view of transosseous-equivalent rotator cuff repair. (Reproduced with permission from Lutton DM, Parsons BO, Flatow EL: Arthroscopic rotator cuff techniques: Single-row, double-row, and the transosseous equivalent. *Curr Orthop Pract* 2009;20(4):349-354.)

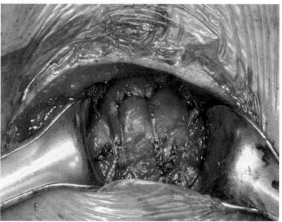

Figure 2 Intraoperative photograph shows a completed mini-open rotator cuff repair, transosseous-equivalent technique. (Reproduced with permission from Lutton DM, Parsons BO, Flatow EL: Arthroscopic rotator cuff techniques: Single-row, double-row, and the transosseous equivalent. *Curr Orthop Pract* 2009; 20(4):349-354.)

there may be stiffness or impingement but good tissue is still present, and for elderly patients with massive tears. A transosseous-equivalent technique is used when possible (**Figure 1**). A double-row technique is occasionally used with tissue that is of poor quality, and a single-row technique is occasionally used with very retracted cuffs, to prevent overtensioning. Open repairs are reserved for some traumatic subscapularis tears that are adhered to the axillary nerve, as well as revision cases in which a graft or tendon transfer is considered (**Figure 2**). Open repair is also used in patients who have coexisting arthritis if possible arthroplasty is anticipated.

Parsons et al[53] reviewed their results with 56 arthroscopic rotator cuff repairs that were treated postoperatively in a sling for 6 weeks. At 6 weeks, 10 of 43 patients were "stiff" (forward elevation <100° and external rotation <30°), and 33 were "non-stiff." At 1 year postoperatively, there was no significant difference in forward elevation or external rotation between the groups. Both groups also had significant improvement in ASES and Constant scores. When repair integrity was assessed using MRI at 1 year, there was an overall 44% intact rate. However, when the groups were separated into "stiff" or "non-stiff," the "stiff" group had a 70% intact rate, and the "non-stiff" group had a 36% intact rate ($P = 0.079$). Postoperatively, patients with small to medium tears (1 to 2 cm with good tissue) are kept in a sling for 6 weeks and allowed to perform gentle external rotation. Patients with massive tears are restricted from range of motion for 6 weeks. Overhead exercises, such as with the pulley, are also prohibited in the first 6 weeks. For golfers, limited putting is allowed at 8 to 10 weeks, chipping and putting at 3 months, gradual start to drives at 4 to 5 months, and playing 18 holes is allowed at 5 to 6 months. Tennis is permitted at 4 to 5 months for light hitting, and full return to the game is allowed at 6 months. Few studies have examined return to sports after rotator cuff repair in mature athletes. Vives et al[54] found that 23 of 29 golfers (mean age, 60 years) who underwent open or mini-open rotator cuff repair were able to return to their presymptomatic competitive level without pain. Sonnery-Cottet et al[55] found that 80% of their middle-aged patients (mean age, 51 years) who underwent an open rotator cuff repair were able to play tennis at a mean 9.8 months after surgery.

References

1. Fehringer EV, Sun J, VanOeveren LS, Keller BK, Matsen FA III: Full-thickness rotator cuff tear prevalence and correlation with function and co-morbidities in patients sixty-five years and older. *J Shoulder Elbow Surg* 2008;17(6):881-885.

2. Fukuda H, Hamada K, Yamanaka K: Pathology and pathogenesis of bursal-side rotator cuff tears viewed from en bloc histologic sections. *Clin Orthop Relat Res* 1990;(254):75-80.

3. Sher JS, Uribe JW, Posada A, Murphy BJ, Zlatkin MB: Abnormal findings on magnetic resonance images of asymptomatic shoulders. *J Bone Joint Surg Am* 1995; 77(1):10-15.

4. Yamaguchi K, Tetro AM, Blam O, Evanoff BA, Teefey SA, Middleton WD: Natural history of asymptomatic rotator cuff tears: A longitudinal analysis of asymptomatic tears detected sonographically. *J Shoulder Elbow Surg* 2001;10(3):199-203.

5. Yamanaka K, Matsumoto T: The joint side tear of the rotator cuff: A followup study by arthrography. *Clin Orthop Relat Res* 1994;(304):68-73.

6. Fukuda H, Mikasa M, Yamanaka K: Incomplete thickness rotator cuff tears diagnosed by subacromial bursography. *Clin Orthop Relat Res* 1987;(223):51-58.

7. Ellman H: Diagnosis and treatment of incomplete rotator cuff tears. *Clin Orthop Relat Res* 1990;(254): 64-74.

8. Weber SC: Arthroscopic debridement and acromioplasty versus mini-open repair in the treatment of significant partial-thickness rotator cuff tears. *Arthroscopy* 1999;15(2):126-131.

9. Andrews JR, Broussard TS, Carson WG: Arthroscopy of the shoulder in the management of partial tears of the rotator cuff: A preliminary report. *Arthroscopy* 1985;1(2):117-122.

10. Ogilvie-Harris DJ, Wiley AM: Arthroscopic surgery of the shoulder: A general appraisal. *J Bone Joint Surg Br* 1986;68(2):201-207.

11. Esch JC, Ozerkis LR, Helgager JA, Kane N, Lilliott N: Arthroscopic subacromial decompression: Results according to the degree of rotator cuff tear. *Arthroscopy* 1988;4(4):241-249.

12. Gartsman GM: Arthroscopic acromioplasty for lesions of the rotator cuff. *J Bone Joint Surg Am* 1990;72(2): 169-180.

13. Kartus J, Kartus C, Rostgård-Christensen L, Sernert N, Read J, Perko M: Long-term clinical and ultrasound evaluation after arthroscopic acromioplasty in patients with partial rotator cuff tears. *Arthroscopy* 2006; 22(1):44-49.

14. Kamath G, Galatz LM, Keener JD, Teefey S, Middleton W, Yamaguchi K: Tendon integrity and functional outcome after arthroscopic repair of high-grade partial-thickness supraspinatus tears. *J Bone Joint Surg Am* 2009;91(5):1055-1062.

15. Chafik D, Yamaguchi K: Outcomes after rotator cuff repair: Does healing matter? *Semin Arthroplasty* 2009; 20(2):116-121.

16. Ide J, Maeda S, Takagi K: Arthroscopic transtendon repair of partial-thickness articular-side tears of the rotator cuff: Anatomical and clinical study. *Am J Sports Med* 2005;33(11):1672-1679.

17. Lo IK, Burkhart SS: Transtendon arthroscopic repair of partial-thickness, articular surface tears of the rotator cuff. *Arthroscopy* 2004;20(2):214-220.

18. Mazzocca AD, Rincon LM, O'Connor RW, et al: Intra-articular partial-thickness rotator cuff tears: Analysis of injured and repaired strain behavior. *Am J Sports Med* 2008;36(1):110-116.

19. Gonzalez-Lomas G, Kippe MA, Brown GD, et al: In situ transtendon repair outperforms tear completion and repair for partial articular-sided supraspinatus tendon tears. *J Shoulder Elbow Surg* 2008;17(5): 722-728.

20. Castagna A, Delle Rose G, Conti M, Snyder SJ, Borroni M, Garofalo R: Predictive factors of subtle residual shoulder symptoms after transtendinous arthroscopic cuff repair: A clinical study. *Am J Sports Med* 2009;37(1):103-108.

21. Gazielly DF, Gleyze P, Montagnon C: Functional and anatomical results after rotator cuff repair. *Clin Orthop Relat Res* 1994;(304):43-53.

22. Harryman DT II, Mack LA, Wang KY, Jackins SE, Richardson ML, Matsen FA III: Repairs of the rotator cuff: Correlation of functional results with integrity of the cuff. *J Bone Joint Surg Am* 1991;73(7):982-989.

23. Thomazeau H, Boukobza E, Morcet N, Chaperon J, Langlais F: Prediction of rotator cuff repair results by magnetic resonance imaging. *Clin Orthop Relat Res* 1997;(344):275-283.

24. Gerber C, Fuchs B, Hodler J: The results of repair of massive tears of the rotator cuff. *J Bone Joint Surg Am* 2000;82(4):505-515.

25. Jost B, Pfirrmann CW, Gerber C, Switzerland Z: Clinical outcome after structural failure of rotator cuff repairs. *J Bone Joint Surg Am* 2000;82(3):304-314.

26. Galatz LM, Ball CM, Teefey SA, Middleton WD, Yamaguchi K: The outcome and repair integrity of completely arthroscopically repaired large and massive rotator cuff tears. *J Bone Joint Surg Am* 2004; 86-A(2):219-224.

27. Boileau P, Brassart N, Watkinson DJ, Carles M, Hatzidakis AM, Krishnan SG: Arthroscopic repair of full-thickness tears of the supraspinatus: Does the tendon really heal? *J Bone Joint Surg Am* 2005;87(6): 1229-1240.

28. Bishop J, Klepps S, Lo IK, Bird J, Gladstone JN, Flatow EL: Cuff integrity after arthroscopic versus open rotator cuff repair: A prospective study. *J Shoulder Elbow Surg* 2006;15(3):290-299.

29. Morse K, Davis AD, Afra R, Kaye EK, Schepsis A, Voloshin I: Arthroscopic versus mini-open rotator cuff repair: A comprehensive review and meta-analysis. *Am J Sports Med* 2008;36(9):1824-1828.

30. Gerber C, Schneeberger AG, Beck M, Schlegel U: Mechanical strength of repairs of the rotator cuff. *J Bone Joint Surg Br* 1994;76(3):371-380.

31. Apreleva M, Ozbaydar M, Fitzgibbons PG, Warner JJ: Rotator cuff tears: The effect of the reconstruction method on three-dimensional repair site area. *Arthroscopy* 2002;18(5):519-526.

32. Brady PC, Arrigoni P, Burkhart SS: Evaluation of residual rotator cuff defects after in vivo single- versus double-row rotator cuff repairs. *Arthroscopy* 2006; 22(10):1070-1075.

33. Fealy S, Kingham TP, Altchek DW: Mini-open rotator cuff repair using a two-row fixation technique: outcomes analysis in patients with small, moderate, and large rotator cuff tears. *Arthroscopy* 2002;18(6): 665-670.

34. Lo IK, Burkhart SS: Double-row arthroscopic rotator cuff repair: Re-establishing the footprint of the rotator cuff. *Arthroscopy* 2003;19(9):1035-1042.

35. Mazzocca AD, Millett PJ, Guanche CA, Santangelo SA, Arciero RA: Arthroscopic single-row versus double-row suture anchor rotator cuff repair. *Am J Sports Med* 2005;33(12):1861-1868.

36. Meier SW, Meier JD: Rotator cuff repair: The effect of double-row fixation on three-dimensional repair site. *J Shoulder Elbow Surg* 2006;15(6):691-696.

37. Kim DH, Elattrache NS, Tibone JE, et al: Biomechanical comparison of a single-row versus double-row suture anchor technique for rotator cuff repair. *Am J Sports Med* 2006;34(3):407-414.

38. Meier SW, Meier JD: The effect of double-row fixation on initial repair strength in rotator cuff repair: A biomechanical study. *Arthroscopy* 2006;22(11):1168-1173.

39. Ma CB, Comerford L, Wilson J, Puttlitz CM: Biomechanical evaluation of arthroscopic rotator cuff repairs: Double-row compared with single-row fixation. *J Bone Joint Surg Am* 2006;88(2):403-410.

40. Sugaya H, Maeda K, Matsuki K, Moriishi J: Repair integrity and functional outcome after arthroscopic double-row rotator cuff repair: A prospective outcome study. *J Bone Joint Surg Am* 2007;89(5):953-960.

41. Lafosse L, Brozska R, Toussaint B, Gobezie R: The outcome and structural integrity of arthroscopic rotator cuff repair with use of the double-row suture anchor technique. *J Bone Joint Surg Am* 2007;89(7):1533-1541.

42. Huijsmans PE, Pritchard MP, Berghs BM, van Rooyen KS, Wallace AL, de Beer JF: Arthroscopic rotator cuff repair with double-row fixation. *J Bone Joint Surg Am* 2007;89(6):1248-1257.

43. Tuoheti Y, Itoi E, Yamamoto N, et al: Contact area, contact pressure, and pressure patterns of the tendon-bone interface after rotator cuff repair. *Am J Sports Med* 2005;33(12):1869-1874.

44. Park MC, ElAttrache NS, Tibone JE, Ahmad CS, Jun BJ, Lee TQ: Part I: Footprint contact characteristics for a transosseous-equivalent rotator cuff repair technique compared with a double-row repair technique. *J Shoulder Elbow Surg* 2007;16(4):461-468.

45. Park MC, Tibone JE, ElAttrache NS, Ahmad CS, Jun BJ, Lee TQ: Part II: Biomechanical assessment for a footprint-restoring transosseous-equivalent rotator cuff repair technique compared with a double-row repair technique. *J Shoulder Elbow Surg* 2007;16(4):469-476.

46. Busfield BT, Glousman RE, McGarry MH, Tibone JE, Lee TQ: A biomechanical comparison of 2 technical variations of double-row rotator cuff fixation: The importance of medial row knots. *Am J Sports Med* 2008;36(5):901-906.

47. Franceschi F, Ruzzini L, Longo UG, et al: Equivalent clinical results of arthroscopic single-row and double-row suture anchor repair for rotator cuff tears: A randomized controlled trial. *Am J Sports Med* 2007; 35(8):1254-1260.

48. Burks RT, Crim J, Brown N, Fink B, Greis PE: A prospective randomized clinical trial comparing arthroscopic single- and double-row rotator cuff repair: Magnetic resonance imaging and early clinical evaluation. *Am J Sports Med* 2009;37(4):674-682.

49. Grasso A, Milano G, Salvatore M, Falcone G, Deriu L, Fabbriciani C: Single-row versus double-row arthroscopic rotator cuff repair: A prospective randomized clinical study. *Arthroscopy* 2009;25(1):4-12.

50. Park JY, Lhee SH, Choi JH, Park HK, Yu JW, Seo JB: Comparison of the clinical outcomes of single- and double-row repairs in rotator cuff tears. *Am J Sports Med* 2008;36(7):1310-1316.

51. Charousset C, Grimberg J, Duranthon LD, Bellaiche L, Petrover D: Can a double-row anchorage technique improve tendon healing in arthroscopic rotator cuff repair? A prospective, nonrandomized, comparative study of double-row and single-row anchorage techniques with computed tomographic arthrography tendon healing assessment. *Am J Sports Med* 2007; 35(8):1247-1253.

52. Frank JB, ElAttrache NS, Dines JS, Blackburn A, Crues J, Tibone JE: Repair site integrity after arthroscopic transosseous-equivalent suture-bridge rotator cuff repair. *Am J Sports Med* 2008;36(8):1496-1503.

53. Parsons BO, Gruson KI, Chen DD, Harrison AK, Gladstone J, Flatow EL: Does slower rehabilitation after arthroscopic rotator cuff repair lead to long-term stiffness? *J Shoulder Elbow Surg* 2010;19(7):1034-1039.

54. Vives MJ, Miller LS, Rubenstein DL, Taliwal RV, Becker CE: Repair of rotator cuff tears in golfers. *Arthroscopy* 2001;17(2):165-172.

55. Sonnery-Cottet B, Edwards TB, Noel E, Walch G: Rotator cuff tears in middle-aged tennis players: Results of surgical treatment. *Am J Sports Med* 2002;30(4): 558-564.

Chapter 21

Massive Rotator Cuff Tears: Options Other Than Repair

Gregory Stranges, MD
Richard J. Hawkins, MD

Key Points

- Massive irreparable rotator cuff tears in the active baby boomer population are challenging to treat because of the high activity levels and functional demands of these patients.
- In the case of irreparable tears, the most appropriate treatment option depends on the patient's level of pain, functional status, and desire to return to sports or vigorous activities.
- Biceps tenotomy and rotator cuff débridement is often effective for pain relief in the patient with preserved active range of motion.
- Partial repair, tendon transfers, or biologic augmentation may be considered in the high-demand boomer population, although return of strength and function may be difficult to predict.
- Reverse shoulder arthroplasty (RSA) may provide predictable return of active elevation, but it must be used with caution in the high-demand baby boomer because of the potential complications and lack of understanding of the stresses it can withstand.

Introduction

Rotator cuff tears are a common musculoskeletal disorder in the baby boomer age group. The prevalence of rotator cuff tears in asymptomatic shoulders has been found to be 23% to 34%.[1] The frequency increases with age, from approximately 13% to 28% in the fifth and sixth decades of life to 31% to 51% in individuals older than 70 years.[2] It is not known what proportion of these tears are irreparable.[3] Massive rotator cuff tears can unfortunately occur even in the mature athlete. It is often surprising that some patients can continue to function well in overhead activi-ties despite the presence of a massive rotator cuff tear. However, patients who do develop pain and/or functional deficits present a unique challenge in that many of them desire a treatment plan that allows them to maintain or return to an active lifestyle.

The ability to identify tears that are massive or irreparable is critical in choosing an appropriate treatment plan. Attempted repair of tears that are too large or have poor prognostic features may not provide a satisfactory outcome for the mature athlete who would like to remain active postoperatively. In these cases, other

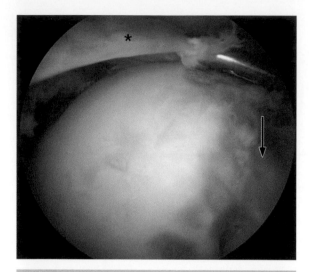

Figure 1 Arthroscopic view of a massive irreparable rotator cuff tear. The tendon (asterisk) is not reducible to the tuberosity footprint (arrow) despite traction sutures.

surgical options may be better suited to the patient's expectations. Unfortunately, this is not always a clear distinction, and the decision must be based on a combination of factors found in the history, physical examination, and diagnostic imaging.

Classification and Definition of Massive Rotator Cuff Tears

Various classification systems have been proposed to help guide the treatment of rotator cuff tears. DeOrio and Cofield[4] classified rotator cuff tears based on size, according to the length of the greatest diameter of the tear in either the coronal or sagittal plane. Tears were categorized as small (≤1 cm), medium (1 to 3 cm), large (3 to 5 cm), and massive (>5 cm). This remains the most widely accepted classification system.

Harryman et al[5] classified rotator cuff tears according to the number of tendons involved: type 0 (intact cuff), type 1A (partial-thickness defect of one tendon [supraspinatus]), type 1B (full-thickness defect of one tendon [supraspinatus]), type 2 (full-thickness defect involving two tendons [supraspinatus and infraspinatus]), and type 3 (full-thickness defect involving three tendons [supraspinatus, infraspinatus, and subscapularis]). The authors further grouped the surgical types

into small (types 1A and 1B) and large (types 2 and 3) and found that repairs of large tears had a substantially higher rate of recurrent defects in the rotator cuff tendon on follow-up. The development of ultrasonographic imaging of the rotator cuff provided the ability to classify tears with this system preoperatively.

Perhaps the most simple classification scheme was proposed by Gerber et al,[6] who typed tears as repairable or irreparable (unable to reinsert tendon to its insertion despite abduction of arm to 60°) (**Figure 1**). Of course, this system relies on intraoperative evaluation to categorize the tear and does not provide any guidance in surgical decision making. Gerber et al[7] also proposed that massive tears be defined as those that involve the detachment of at least two entire tendons, which may be more useful for preoperative staging based on the results of diagnostic imaging.

Massive rotator cuff tears can go on to develop rotator cuff tear arthropathy. This has been estimated to occur in only 4% of untreated rotator cuff tears and is therefore relatively uncommon in active baby boomers.[8] As described by Neer et al,[8] upward migration of the humeral head with pseudoarticulation against the undersurface of the acromion and acromioclavicular (AC) joint was found to produce characteristic radiographic findings. These include instability of the glenohumeral joint with proximal migration of the humerus, collapse of the superior humeral head, and erosion of the glenoid, acromion, and acromioclavicular joint[8] (**Figure 2**). Osteophyte formation, although common in primary osteoarthritis, is not routinely observed in cuff tear arthropathy.

It is evident that no single classification system can consistently predict the repairability of a rotator cuff tear for every specific instance. However, the systems outlined above identify important characteristics of the tear such as size or number of involved tendons that improve the surgeon's ability to predict whether a rotator cuff tear can be repaired. This may aid in selection of a treatment plan that includes alternate surgical options if an attempted repair is likely to be unsuccessful.

Historical Perspective

Surgical repair of massive rotator cuff tears has shown variable success in previous literature. Early reports of open repair demonstrated successful outcomes in only 50% to 60% of cases.[9] Later reports of both open and

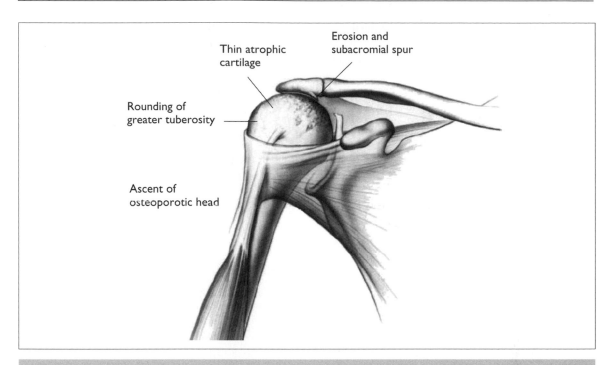

Figure 2 Anatomic illustration shows characteristic features of rotator cuff tear arthropathy as originally described by Neer et al. Later stage of involvement exhibits segmental collapse of the humeral head. (Reproduced with permission from Neer CS, Craig EV, Fukuda H: Cuff-tear arthropathy. *J Bone Joint Surg Am* 1983;65(9): 1232-1244.)

arthroscopic repair showed higher rates of pain relief but less success with restoration of full strength and functional status in these shoulders.[7,9-12] Based on preoperative clinical and MRI findings, there is a subset of tears that may be deemed irreparable or may have a poor chance for success even if the tendon can be surgically reapproximated.[7,13,14]

Using ultrasonography, Harryman et al[5] evaluated the integrity of 105 open repairs of large rotator cuff tears at an average of 5 years postoperatively. The authors compared motion, strength, and functional data for each patient. Shoulders with an intact rotator cuff tendon at follow-up were most likely to have a successful outcome. Recurrent defects were found in more than 50% of larger tears (two- and three-tendon involvement), and although the size of these residual defects correlated with increasing loss of function, these patients were still satisfied with their repair.

In 1995, Rockwood et al[15] reported on the results of open subacromial decompression and débridement of 53 massive rotator cuff tears. Satisfactory results were obtained in 83% of the shoulders, but weakness or absence of anterior deltoid function as a result of the open surgery was found to increase the likelihood of a poor outcome. Ellman et al[16] found that rotator cuff tears treated with arthroscopic decompression and débridement only demonstrated postoperative relief of pain that was size-dependent. Gartsman[17] found that results of arthroscopic decompression and débridement were poor in patients with full-thickness rotator cuff defects compared with those who had partial-thickness tears or isolated subacromial impingement. He later published results from 33 irreparable tears showing improvement in satisfaction, pain, and activities of daily living, but he conceded that these results were still inferior to repair of the rotator cuff.[18]

Finally, in 2004, Galatz et al[19] reported on results of arthroscopic repair of a series of 18 mostly large rotator cuff tears followed for a minimum of 2 years. Seventeen of 18 were found to have a recurrent defect in the repaired tendon, with most defects measured as the same size as the tear before repair. Interestingly, all patients in the study were satisfied with their surgery with improvements in pain, strength, range of motion, and outcome scores. The clinical improvement, however, deteriorated with time between the 1-year and 2-year follow-up.

In summary, large and massive rotator cuff tears occur even in the boomer population. Repair of these tears can be challenging, and these repairs may fail more often than we would like. Early studies do not specifically address the mature athlete patient group. However, they do provide guidance on surgical options in rotator cuff tears and insight into the outcomes when repair is not possible or has failed.

Evaluation

For massive rotator cuff tears, the separate elements of the clinical evaluation are equally crucial for proper decision making. The patient history is usually adequate to establish the diagnosis and, in combination with the physical examination, suggest the severity or size of the tear. Diagnostic imaging serves to confirm the diagnosis, identify the morphologic qualities of the tear, and identify any concomitant pathology. Combined with patient factors such as functional demands, general health, and treatment expectations, this information can help guide the clinician and patient toward the most appropriate treatment pathway.

Patient History

The presenting symptom in tears of the rotator cuff is generally a combination of pain and weakness. As demonstrated by Gerber et al,[20] after hypertonic saline injections into the subacromial space, pain from this location is typically localized to the lateral acromion and lateral deltoid to its insertion on the upper arm. Less frequently, it may occur more anterior, more posterior, or even distal to the elbow, which may cloud the diagnosis made on history. Any description of pain in an alternate distribution may suggest associated pathology, such as involvement of the long head of the biceps or the AC joint. Of course, any radiation of pain below the elbow or into the hand should spur further questioning about neck pain and sensory changes that may suggest cervical radiculopathy.

Rotator cuff tears are often a chronic degenerative process, but they also can be secondary to a traumatic injury. It is important to establish the acuity and mechanism of injury to identify massive tears that may be amenable to early repair. The typical symptom is chronic, progressive symptoms in the absence of trauma. However, the active mature athlete may also describe a dramatic loss of motion and strength after a traction injury or glenohumeral dislocation while participating in sporting activities. In this setting, the surgeon should be highly suspicious of acute massive rotator cuff tear but might also consider the presence of an associated neurologic injury as a result of the initial trauma.

Physical Examination

Certain findings on physical examination may indicate the presence of a massive, irreparable rotator cuff tear. Inspection of the posterior shoulder may reveal atrophy of the posterosuperior rotator cuff musculature. Infraspinatus atrophy is easier to detect because of its superficial location relative to the supraspinatus, which lies deep to the trapezius muscle. Inspection from the front may show an asymmetric proximal contour to the biceps muscle belly, which is exacerbated with biceps contraction and is more obvious in thin patients. This "Popeye deformity" indicates rupture of the long head of the biceps tendon and is frequently associated with large full-thickness rotator cuff tears.

Range-of-motion testing frequently yields clues that a suspected rotator cuff tear may be massive or irreparable. Significant limitation of active forward elevation in the setting of normal or near-normal passive elevation usually indicates significant rotator cuff dysfunction such as with a massive tear. Inability to actively elevate more than 20° manifests as a shoulder shrug, or pseudoparalysis, which is virtually pathognomonic for a massive rotator cuff tear. In the extreme situation, loss of constraint provided by the coracoacromial arch may allow anterosuperior escape of the humeral head, which may be visible or palpable as the patient contracts the deltoid when attempting to elevate the arm. External rotation should also be carefully evaluated, as an increase in passive external rotation on the symptomatic side may indicate complete rupture of the subscapularis.[21]

Strength testing is extremely important in trying to define the size and repairability of a rotator cuff tear. Strength test results can be difficult to interpret when the examination elicits significant pain. In these instances, it is more accurate to repeat this portion of the examination after subacromial injection of local anesthetic to eliminate the inhibitory effects of pain. Although active range of motion may be maintained in some massive tears, patients will usually exhibit weakness of the involved muscles to resistance testing. Profound weakness to external rotation indicates extension of the cuff tear posteriorly to involve the infraspinatus and possibly the teres minor tendon. The external rotation lag sign and hornblower sign may be seen in these cases.[22] Internal rotation weakness and positive lift-off and belly press signs indicate an anterosuperior tear pattern with subscapularis involvement.[23] Weakness of both external and internal rotation is indicative of a 3-tendon tear.

A complete shoulder examination should be performed to detect associated pathology. Palpation of the AC joint may expose concomitant symptomatic degenerative arthritis at this site. Further provocative testing would include the cross-body adduction test and O'Brien active compression test, which was originally described as a way to distinguish between the deep pain of superior labrum anterior-to-posterior (SLAP) tears and the superior pain of the AC joint.[24] Pain originating from the long head of the biceps tendon is elicited by direct palpation of the bicipital groove and a positive Speed test. Subacromial impingement produces pain with Neer and Hawkins impingement testing.[25] Differential injections of local anesthetic into the subacromial space, AC joint, or bicipital groove are a useful diagnostic aid to help confirm the presence or absence of these concurrent conditions.[21]

Diagnostic Imaging

Radiography

Initial evaluation of suspected massive rotator cuff tears includes plain radiography. Three views are usually adequate in the setting of massive cuff tears. Additional views may be required if associated pathology such as AC joint arthritis is suspected. A true AP Grashey view of the glenohumeral joint is used to evaluate humeral head height, flattening of the greater tuberosity second-

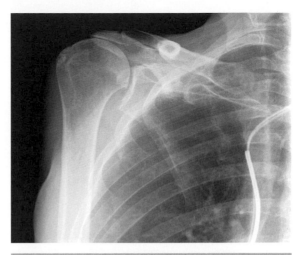

Figure 3   AP radiograph of a shoulder with a massive rotator cuff tear displays proximal migration of the humeral head and narrowed acromiohumeral distance.

ary to subacromial impingement, and degenerative changes secondary to rotator cuff arthropathy. Superior migration of the humerus resulting in an acromiohumeral distance of less than 5 mm is suggestive of a massive rotator cuff tear[26,27] (**Figure 3**), but not all irreparable cuff tears have a high-riding humeral head. The axillary view may demonstrate glenohumeral joint space narrowing and allows visualization of the AC joint or an os acromiale if present. Acromial morphology is best viewed on the supraspinatus outlet view and may demonstrate any anterior spurs located superior to the rotator cuff tear.

Ultrasonography

Ultrasonography has been shown to be a very accurate modality for visualizing the rotator cuff tendon and detecting full-thickness tears.[28,29] Many studies have shown it to be as accurate as MRI in detecting both partial- and full-thickness tears.[29-31] Ultrasonography is noninvasive and cost effective and can be performed easily in the ambulatory setting. It is helpful not only for diagnosis but also for follow-up evaluation, and it allows easy imaging of both shoulders. However, the accuracy of ultrasonography is operator dependent, and it has limited ability to detect intra-articular pathology,

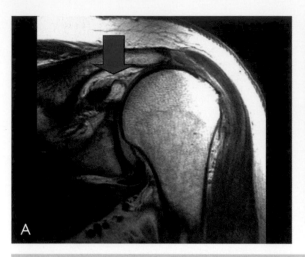
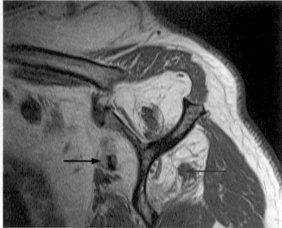

Figure 4 T1-weighted MRIs of a massive rotator cuff tear. **A,** Coronal plane view demonstrates retraction of the supraspinatus tendon to the level of the glenoid (arrow). **B,** Sagittal plane image demonstrates atrophy and fatty infiltration of the supraspinatus (asterisk), infraspinatus (red arrow), and subscapularis (black arrow) muscles.

which decreases its utility compared with other imaging methods.[32,33]

Magnetic Resonance Imaging

MRI is most commonly used to image the soft-tissue structures of the shoulder. It is extremely accurate in detecting tears of the rotator cuff. A recent meta-analysis of 65 previous studies showed an overall sensitivity of 92.1% and specificity of 92.9% for full-thickness cuff tears.[34] Detection of partial-thickness tears is less reliable, with a sensitivity of 63.6% and specificity of 91.7%. Interestingly, ultrasonography was found to be just as accurate for both groups, and magnetic resonance arthrography was more sensitive and specific for both full-thickness tears (sensitivity, 95.4%; specificity, 98.9%) and partial-thickness tears (sensitivity, 85.9%; specificity, 96.0%).

MRI is able to provide more information regarding the characteristics of the tear. It can quantify the size of the tear in the anterior-posterior direction and the retraction medial-laterally (**Figure 4,** *A*). Atrophy or fatty infiltration of the involved muscle belly can be evaluated on sagittal plane images of the supraspinatus and infraspinatus fossae (**Figure 4,** *B*). Because the presence of these factors has been shown to correlate with poor outcomes and function after rotator cuff repair, it is important to request that imaging include more medial cuts, as standard MRI protocols of the shoulder may fail to visualize this vitally important region.[7,13,14,35] Muscle atrophy is evaluated on the most lateral sagittal image in which the scapular spine is still in contact with the scapular body. It may be calculated by the occupation ratio as described by Thomazeau et al.[36] Alternatively, atrophy may be evaluated by the tangent sign,[37] which is positive if the supraspinatus muscle belly does not cross a line connecting the superior borders of the coracoid and the scapular spine (**Figure 5**). Fatty infiltration is routinely classified by the grading system of Goutallier et al[13] (**Table 1**). This was originally described for evaluation on CT images, but has also been shown to be reproducible when assessed by MRI.[38]

MRI is also valuable in detecting associated pathology. The AC joint, articular cartilage defects, and labral pathology all may be visualized better with MRI than with ultrasonography.[33] The presence of the long head of the biceps tendon in the bicipital groove and abnormalities of its intra-articular portion also may be seen. This information is particularly useful for preoperative planning and counseling the patient with regard to the expected intraoperative findings and their impact on

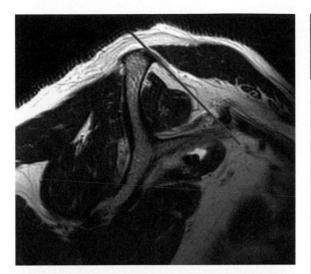

Figure 5 Sagittal plane T1-weighted MRI shows mild atrophy of the supraspinatus muscle (asterisk) and a positive tangent sign. The tangent between the scapular spine and the coracoid is indicated by the red line.

Table 1: Goutallier Classification of Fatty Muscle Degeneration in Rotator Cuff Ruptures

Stage	Fatty Infiltration
0	None
1	Fatty streaks within muscle
2	Muscle > fat
3	Muscle = fat
4	Fat > muscle

Adapted with permission from Goutallier D, Postel JM, Bernageau J, Lavau L, Voisin MC: Fatty muscle degeneration in cuff ruptures: Pre-and postoperative evaluation by CT scan. *Clin Orthop Relat Res* 1994;(304):78-83.

postoperative outcomes and rehabilitation. Disadvantages of MRI include the relative cost, contraindications such as incompatible medical implants, and difficulties with imaging claustrophobic patients.[32]

Computed Tomography

CT arthrography of the shoulder may be an effective tool to visualize the rotator cuff when MRI is not possible. Shorter imaging times make it effective in claustrophobic patients, and metallic hardware around the shoulder does not impact the final images to the same extent as with MRI.[39] This modality is as effective as MRI in detecting tears of the rotator cuff, and in some European centers, it is the preferred method of advanced imaging of the shoulder.[40] CT arthrography should therefore be considered in patients who cannot undergo MRI.

Treatment

The surgeon must combine information gleaned from the patient history, clinical examination, and imaging to select the most appropriate treatment path. First, the clinician must establish whether the patient's chief symptom is pain, loss of motion or loss of strength, or a combination. Second, the patient's functional goals should be confirmed, as lower functioning individuals may desire only pain relief, whereas active baby boomers may wish to return to more strenuous activities, including sports. Next, clinical examination findings such as pseudoparalysis and lag signs should be combined with information about tear size and tissue quality on imaging to predict repairability of the tear. Proper counseling is essential to explain that even successful repair of a tear with poor prognostic features such as fatty infiltration and atrophy may not produce satisfactory functional results. In addition, some massive tears with significant preoperative weakness or pseudoparalysis may not allow return to high-demand activities regardless of the treatment method selected. Although repair of a rotator cuff tear is the goal in the boomer population, patients must be informed that large and massive tears may fail even if repaired.

Nonsurgical Treatment

Common nonsurgical treatment modalities used in rotator cuff tears include physical therapy, nonsteroidal anti-inflammatory medications, and corticosteroid injections. Numerous studies have reported good success rates for nonsurgical treatment of full-thickness

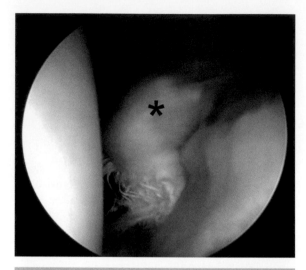

Figure 6 Arthroscopic view shows fraying and near-complete rupture of the biceps tendon (asterisk), a common source of pain associated with rotator cuff tears.

Surgical Treatment

Arthroscopic Débridement

Débridement of irreparable rotator cuff tears, both open and arthroscopic, has been shown to be an effective treatment option for certain patient groups. Decompression of the subacromial space and débridement of painful tear edges and bursa is performed to relieve pain, but because the tear itself is not addressed, functional improvement is less predictable. A better term for decompression might be "smoothing" of a bone spur. Because of concerns about removing the fulcrum around which the deltoid functions, a complete subacromial decompression with acromioplasty may be contraindicated in the setting of a massive rotator cuff tear. Rather, a limited decompression with excision of the bone spur but preservation of the anterior fibers of the coracoacromial ligament may be valuable to preserve the coracoacromial arch.

As discussed previously, historical literature has shown open surgical débridement to improve patient satisfaction, pain, and function in massive tears.[15,18] As shoulder arthroscopy has become more common, recent literature has focused on results of arthroscopic débridement of massive tears. Generally, these studies have reported reliable pain relief but marginal improvement in function.[47-53] Therefore, débridement and decompression of irreparable rotator cuff tears is best suited as a pain-relief procedure in patients with low functional demands. As improvement may not occur or may be short-lived, it may not allow the active middle-aged athlete to return to strenuous activities or sports that depend on the affected extremity. An appropriate preoperative discussion of this is essential to establish realistic expectations.

Biceps Tenotomy

The biceps tendon has been established as a common source of pain in the painful shoulder with rotator cuff pathology,[54-56] and changes in the tendon are frequently associated with rotator cuff tears[57,58] (**Figure 6**). Kempf et al[59] reported in 1999 that tenotomy of the long head of the biceps tendon produced beneficial effects both when combined with acromioplasty and as an isolated procedure in the treatment of full-thickness rotator cuff tears. The positive effects of biceps tenot-

tears,[41-44] with results commonly diminishing as duration of symptoms increase.[42,45] Few authors, however, have looked at nonsurgical treatment specifically for massive irreparable cuff tears. Short-term improvements have been shown after 12 weeks of a specific exercise therapy protocol.[46] More recently, Zingg et al[27] reported successful outcomes for function (Constant score 83% of age- and sex-matched normal shoulders) and pain (mean of 11.5 points on visual analog scale where 15 = no pain) in 19 patients with massive rotator cuff tears over a mean follow-up of 4 years. However, active range of motion did not improve, and tear size, fatty infiltration, atrophy, and degenerative changes all progressed.[27] Of the original nonsurgical group, 18% eventually underwent surgery for increasing pain or dysfunction. These results suggest that nonsurgical treatment would be most suitable for patients with minimal painful symptoms and low functional demands. This contrasts with the baby boomer population, in whom return to sports such as golf and tennis is often the goal. In these cases, pain relief is an essential consideration in treatment of a large of massive tear, but functional performance may be more important.

omy were magnified in the presence of a massive irreparable tear.

Walch et al[60] demonstrated an 87% satisfaction rate and improvement in shoulder outcome scores after biceps tenotomy in 307 patients with irreparable cuff tears. Despite the possible role of the biceps as a secondary humeral head depressor, the acromiohumeral distance was found to decrease by only 1.3 mm over the mean follow-up of 57 months. Klinger et al[50] also demonstrated that biceps tenotomy in the setting of massive cuff tears did not result in significant proximal humeral migration.

Boileau et al[61] later reported the results of 72 isolated arthroscopic biceps tenotomies or tenodeses for irreparable tears: 78% of patients were satisfied with the procedure, the average Constant score increased by 20 points, and the acromiohumeral distance did not decrease significantly. However, although some patients with loss of active elevation secondary to pain did regain the ability to elevate overhead, patients with true pseudoparalysis did not regain active elevation postoperatively. No difference was seen between the tenotomy and tenodesis groups, in keeping with Gill et al,[55] who reported significant pain relief and improved functional outcomes after 30 arthroscopic tenotomies for various biceps pathologies. Tenotomy may have the advantage of shorter recovery time and fewer complications at the expense of cosmetic deformity and possible cramping with repeated supination stresses. However, when compared retrospectively, no statistical difference was found between the two procedures for anterior shoulder pain, muscle cramping, or cosmetic deformity.[62] On the basis of these studies, biceps tenotomy or tenodesis can be recommended as an effective procedure for patients with massive rotator cuff tears with a chief symptom of pain. However, it cannot be expected to improve active motion or function and therefore should be considered in patients who have maintained satisfactory preoperative active motion despite the rotator cuff deficiency, or whose motion is limited due to pain.

Partial Repair

Burkhart[63] proposed that partial repairs of massive rotator cuff tears can be helpful to reduce pain and improve function when complete repair is not possible. The first step in a partial repair of a U-shaped tear consists of side-to-side sutures of the tendon from me-dial to lateral until the anterior and posterior limbs can no longer be approximated. Next, the anterior and posterior margins of the remaining defect are repaired from tendon to bone with suture anchors.[64]

The general principle behind this concept is that the impact of a residual defect in the superior cuff is minimized when the posterior or anterior component of the rotator cuff tear is repaired. This restores the "transverse force couple" and balances the forces exerted by the cuff on both the anterior and posterior aspects of the glenohumeral joint[64] (**Figure 7**). The effect of balancing these forces is to maintain the humeral head centered in the glenoid, providing a stable fulcrum for the deltoid to act on when elevating the humerus. The margin convergence portion of the repair also reduces strain along the entire free margin of the tendon, protecting the tendon-to-bone portion of the posterior or anterior repair.[65,66] However, one must keep in mind that the forces that caused the large or massive tear in the first place may result in a recurrence of the tear.

In 14 patients followed an average of 20.8 months after partial repair of a massive rotator cuff tear, Burkhart et al[63] reported impressive improvements in active elevation (90.8°), strength (2.3 grades on 0 to 5 scale), functional outcomes (University of California at Los Angeles [UCLA] score increase from 9.8 to 27.6), and satisfaction (13 of 14). The results of a more recent study by Duralde and Bair[67] were not as dramatic, but significant improvements were demonstrated in active elevation (40°), and the ability to elevate to 135° overhead was restored in 8 of 24 patients; 15 patients did gain one grade of strength, and no patients lost strength. Finally, results were judged as excellent or good in 16 patients and as fair or poor in 8 patients.[67] These studies suggest that in active patients with massive rotator cuff tears, a partial repair may be effective in restoring function and possibly allow a return to athletic activities. However, because the deforming forces remain in place on the residual defect to perpetuate the tear, the duration of these beneficial effects is still unclear.

Tendon Transfers

Although not usually considered in elderly patients with rotator cuff tears, tendon transfers may be an option in baby boomers with high functional demands

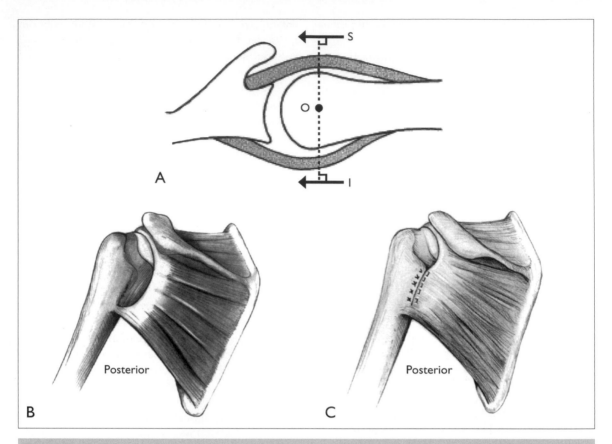

Figure 7   A, Transverse force couples are balanced when the infraspinatus and subscapularis tendons are intact and functional. S = subscapularis, O = center of rotation, I = infraspinatus. **B,** Massive posterosuperior cuff tear with infraspinatus deficiency. **C,** Partial repair of rotator cuff with restoration of the infraspinatus portion of the transverse force couple. (Panel A is adapted with permission from Burkhart SS: Reconciling the paradox of rotator cuff repair versus debridement: A unified biomechanical rationale for the treatment of rotator cuff tears. *Arthroscopy* 1994;10(1):4-19. Panels B and C are reproduced with permission from Burkhart SS, Nottage WM, Ogilvie-Harris DJ, Kohn HS, Pachelli A: Partial repair of irreparable rotator cuff tears. *Arthroscopy* 1994;10(4):363-370.)

for work or recreational activities. Ideally, the chief symptom should be weakness rather than pain. Tendon transfers may improve strength and function both actively, through force exerted on the humerus in the direction of muscle contraction, and passively, by acting as a humeral head depressor to keep the head centered in the glenoid as a pivot for the deltoid to function.[6,68]

The anatomic pattern of a rotator cuff deficiency dictates the specific transfers that may be useful (**Table 2**). Posterosuperior rotator cuff deficiency secondary to a massive tear involving the supraspinatus, infraspinatus, and teres minor is the most common pattern.

Latissimus dorsi transfers are the most frequent choice to address these tears. Anterosuperior tears involving the supraspinatus and subscapularis tendons are most often addressed with pectoralis major transfers. Tendon transfers may be considered as primary treatment for an irreparable tear or as salvage treatment for a previous failed repair. Potential candidates for tendon transfer include relatively young high-demand patients with mild to moderate weakness, such as may be seen in the active baby boomer. A tendon transfer should not be expected to restore elevation in a patient with severe weakness or pseudoparalysis.[68]

Latissimus dorsi tendon transfer for massive postero-superior rotator cuff tears involves mobilization and release of the latissimus tendon from its proximal humeral insertion through a posterior incision. The tendon is then rerouted to a superior shoulder incision and is inserted onto the humeral head via transosseous sutures.[6] Gerber[69] originally published early follow-up data on 16 latissimus transfers at an average of 33 months postoperatively. He found satisfactory pain relief on exertion in 13 patients, a mean increase in flexion of 52°, and age- and sex-adjusted shoulder function scores of 73% of normal.[69] Longer term results reviewing 69 latissimus transfers at an average 53-month follow-up were recently published by Gerber et al.[70] Significant improvements in functional outcome scores and pain were demonstrated, but radiographic arthritic changes did advance slightly.[70] An increase of 19° of flexion was also shown, which was somewhat diminished from the earlier short-term results. Both studies demonstrated clearly inferior results for the subset of patients who also had poor subscapularis function preoperatively. Miniaci and MacLeod[71] published 2- to 5-year results showing significant improvements in pain and function for 14 of 17 patients who underwent salvage latissimus transfer for failed previous rotator cuff repairs. However, Warner and Parsons[72] later showed worse overall outcomes for latissimus transfers performed as salvage versus primary procedures.

Recently, latissimus dorsi and teres major transfers have been combined with reverse shoulder arthroplasty (RSA) through the deltopectoral approach to improve postoperative external rotation. Gains of up to 34° and improvements in both activities of daily living and functional outcomes have been reported with this procedure.[73,74] These results suggest that this transfer should also be considered in the athletic boomer patient with a rotator cuff tear who desires a gain in active external rotation.[75,76]

Pectoralis major tendon transfers are most commonly used for irreparable anterosuperior rotator cuff defects.[77] Wirth and Rockwood[78] originally described transfer of the superior portion of the tendon to the inferior greater tuberosity lateral to the bicipital groove. Since then, other modifications have been described, including subcoracoid transfers deep to the conjoined tendon to more accurately replicate the vector of pull

Table 2: Historical Tendon Transfer Options for Rotator Cuff Deficits

Tear Pattern	Tendon Transfers
Posterosuperior (infraspinatus deficit)	Latissimus, teres major, deltoid flap, trapezius, subscapularis
Anterosuperior (subscapularis deficit)	Pectoralis major, teres major, trapezius

for the subscapularis.[79-82] Resch et al[79] reported excellent or good results in 9 of 12 subcoracoid pectoralis transfers, with significant reductions in pain and improved subjective function and outcome scores. Galatz et al[83] also reported improved pain and function, with satisfactory results in 11 of 14 pectoralis transfers. Although forward elevation was improved postoperatively, average flexion was still only 60.8°, and only three patients were able to elevate above the horizontal plane. More recently, Elhassan et al[84] reported on pectoralis major transfers for various causes of subscapularis insufficiency. In their subgroup consisting of patients with massive rotator cuff tears, they noted an improvement in Constant score from 28.7 to 52.3.

Published results for the various tendon transfers for irreparable rotator cuff tears consistently show improvements in both pain and function. However, these are complex surgical procedures with significant associated morbidity and complex rehabilitation requirements. Despite this, the overall magnitude of functional improvements is guarded, which underscores the importance of careful patient selection when considering this treatment option in the mature athlete.

Biologic Augmentation

Because of limited functional improvement and high rates of recurrent defects, the management of massive rotator cuff tears in mature, active individuals is challenging. Often the repaired tissue is of poor quality, with little biologic chance of healing. In an effort to improve rotator cuff tendon healing rates, tissue engineering has been used to produce various biologic patch grafts to augment the repair (**Figure 8**). These grafts may be xenograft tissue, such as bovine dermis or por-

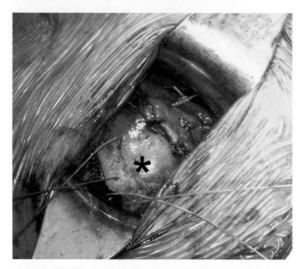

Figure 8 Intraoperative photograph shows biologic augmentation of a rotator cuff defect with a tissue patch graft (asterisk).

cine small intestinal submucosa (SIS), or allograft derived from human dermis.[85] The biologic graft tissue provides a favorable environment for the host healing response, acting as an extracellular matrix scaffold for the host fibroblasts to infiltrate during the reparative process.[86] Cross-linking of the tissue slows its reabsorption once implanted and may strengthen the tissue.[87] In addition, the graft is rendered acellular to minimize any host immune response against the foreign tissue.[88]

Animal studies have shown promising results for biologic augmentation of rotator cuff repair. Dejardin et al[89] tested SIS patches in canine rotator cuff tears and showed excellent integration to surrounding tissues with failure load similar to a reimplanted tendon group. In sheep rotator cuff repairs, Schlegel et al[90] showed no difference in load to failure in tendons augmented with an SIS patch versus nonaugmented repairs, but they did find a significant increase in stiffness of the augmented repair. A recent study in rat rotator cuff repairs showed a higher force to failure in a group augmented with human dermal matrix compared with an unrepaired defect group, but still lower than that of an intact tendon control.[88]

Few human studies have evaluated biologic graft augmentation, and these do not match the promising results from the animal studies. Sclamberg et al[91] noted retears in 10 of 11 large and massive cuff repairs augmented with an SIS patch at 6-month MRI follow-up. Both Ianotti et al,[86] in 2006, and Walton et al,[92] in 2007, found no clinical benefit and high rates of retears in porcine SIS-augmented rotator cuff repairs. Badhe et al[93] later published more encouraging 3- to 5-year follow-up data, showing high patient satisfaction, functional improvement, and intact tendons in eight of ten extensive cuff tear repairs augmented with porcine dermal xenograft tissue. The study included no comparison with a control group, however, so it is not possible to draw conclusions on the relative benefit of the graft versus that of the surgical repair. Because the basic science data show the potential benefit for biologic augmentation of rotator cuff repairs, it may be an option in the mature athletic patient with an irreparable tear. However, as there are presently no human data that can show any benefit, it is difficult to recommend this treatment over the other options at this time.

Arthroplasty

Although traditionally reserved for elderly, lower demand patients, various forms of shoulder arthroplasty may be considered in certain active baby boomer–age patients. Familiarity with the various indications, contraindications, and potential pitfalls is essential when considering these options for the younger patient with higher functional demands.

Total Shoulder Arthroplasty

In primary glenohumeral arthritis, total shoulder arthroplasty has been shown to be superior to hemiarthroplasty for pain relief, function, and patient satisfaction.[94,95] However, because of the "rocking horse" effect, with proximal migration of the humerus and consequent repetitive edge loading on the superior margin of the glenoid component, high rates of glenoid loosening and prosthetic failure have been shown with total shoulder arthroplasty in the setting of rotator cuff deficiency.[96-98] For this reason, glenoid resurfacing should not be performed for cuff tear arthropathy.

Hemiarthroplasty

Historically, shoulder arthroplasty has been performed chiefly for pain relief in rotator cuff tear arthropathy, with a "limited goals" approach to functional improvement.[8,99,100] Multiple authors have demonstrated reliable reduction in painful symptoms with standard hemiarthroplasty.[101-104] However, changes in range of motion and function have been less consistent in previous published reports, with various factors being associated with poor results. Williams and Rockwood[101] reported on the results of hemiarthroplasty in 21 cuff-deficient shoulders and described satisfactory results in 18 and a mean 50° increase in flexion. However, five patients were unable to flex to 90°, and overall results were inferior to hemiarthroplasties with intact rotator cuffs.

Field et al[102] reported 10 successful outcomes in 16 hemiarthroplasties for rotator cuff arthropathy. Poor results were more likely in patients with previous acromioplasty and disruption of the coracoacromial arch, which occurred in 4 of the 6 unsuccessful results. Sanchez-Sotelo et al[103] also noted a high rate of unsatisfactory results and anterosuperior instability in patients who underwent hemiarthroplasty after a previous acromioplasty. In 34 hemiarthroplasties for rotator cuff deficiencies, Goldberg et al[104] reported 26 satisfactory results and an average increase in elevation from 78° to 111°. Patients who could elevate 90° or more preoperatively were more likely to have improved pain and function and a satisfactory outcome.

When contained by the coracoacromial arch, superior migration of the proximal humerus often leads to femoralization of the humeral head and acetabularization of the acromion.[8] A hemiarthroplasty prosthesis with an extended coverage head has been developed for these patients.[100] Visotsky et al[105] reported significant decreases in pain, increased American Shoulder and Elbow Surgeons (ASES) scores, and an average improvement in forward flexion from 56° to 116° with the use of a cuff tear arthropathy prosthesis. The authors recommended that this prosthesis not be used in cases of loss of the coracoacromial arch and anterosuperior escape of the humeral head.

Reverse Total Shoulder Arthroplasty

Results of conventional shoulder arthroplasty or hemiarthroplasty in the setting of rotator cuff deficiency are less than satisfactory, especially with regard to active motion and function. The biomechanical rationale for use of the reverse ball-and-socket shoulder prosthesis is to convert the shear forces applied by the deltoid to compressive forces, allowing active glenohumeral motion that does not rely on the rotator cuff musculature.[98,106] This prosthesis was initially introduced by Grammont and Baulot[107] and consists of a convex surface applied to the glenoid to articulate with a concave shell placed on the proximal humerus[108] (**Figure 9**).

RSA has been studied for painful rotator cuff arthropathy. In a study by Boileau et al[109] of outcomes for various surgical indications, a subgroup of 21 patients with cuff tear arthropathy were found to exhibit significant improvements in satisfaction, outcome scores, and forward elevation (from 53° preoperatively to 123° postoperatively). Complications occurred in 4 of the 21 patients in this group. Frankle et al[110] reported significant improvements in pain scores and outcome measures and a 50° increase in average forward flexion in 60 patients treated with RSA for rotator cuff deficiency with arthritis. In this study, 8 glenoid baseplate failures were observed. A later study with authors in common did not show any baseplate failures at 2-year follow-up of a prosthetic design with improved baseplate fixation,[111] highlighting the importance of proper technique and the high potential complication rate with this technique.

The results of RSA have also been shown for massive irreparable rotator cuff tears without arthritic changes in the glenohumeral joint. Wall et al[112] published the outcomes of 191 reverse prostheses at an average follow-up of 39.9 months postoperatively. These were performed for various indications, including massive cuff tears both with and without arthritis, revision arthroplasties, posttraumatic arthritis, rheumatoid disease, and acute fractures. In terms of function, pain, and motion, the subgroup of 41 RSAs performed for massive cuff tears without arthritis were shown to have an average postoperative forward elevation of 143° and equal functional outcomes to both the cuff tear arthropathy and primary arthritis with cuff tear groups. These three groups were shown to have superior results compared to those performed for the other etiologies. Boileau et al[113] recently showed that RSA after failed rotator cuff surgery is more successful in pseudoparalytic shoulders than in painful shoulders with good

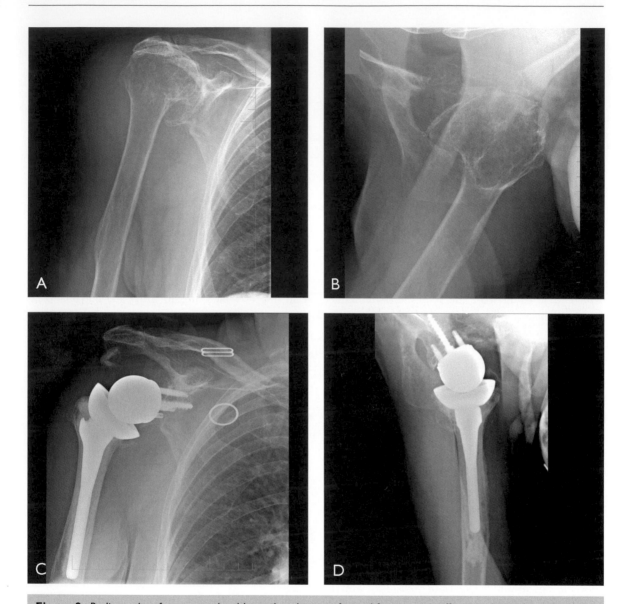

Figure 9 Radiographs of a reverse shoulder arthroplasty performed for rotator cuff tear arthropathy. Preoperative AP (**A**) and axillary (**B**) radiographs. Postoperative AP (**C**) and axillary (**D**) radiographs. An acromial fracture is present on the postoperative radiographs.

motion. However, results were still inferior to those for primary RSA.

Although short-term results for RSA are very encouraging, long-term data are presently sparse. Guery et al[114] published the survivorship results on 80 RSAs at a mean of 5 to 6 years (range, 5 to 10 years) postopera-

tively. Arthroplasties performed for cuff tear arthropathy demonstrated an overall survival rate of 95% at 10 years. However, despite viability of the implant, both pain and function significantly deteriorated after 6 years. By 10 years, only 46 shoulders had satisfactory functional scores and only 49 had a pain score below the desired score. These results mirrored those of an earlier study by Sirveaux et al,[115] which also showed significant decreases in survivorship and function after 7 years. These data represent the early generations of RSA implants and may not be representative of the survivorship of newer designs. Nevertheless, it may be of concern when considering RSA in the mature active patient with an irreparable rotator cuff tear.

In recent years, RSA has become more commonly used for treatment of cuff tear arthropathy, and the indications have expanded to include massive cuff tear with pseudoparalysis in the absence of arthritis.[106] The complication rate, however, has been shown to be higher than that of conventional shoulder arthroplasty. Major complications include hematoma formation, infection, glenoid loosening, scapular notching, dislocation, and acromial fracture.[108] Prosthetic design and surgical techniques are constantly evolving and improving, which may reduce the frequency of these in the future. Because of the present high complication rate and lack of long-term longevity data, strict patient selection is critical when considering this option. However, even in the baby boomer population, RSA is sometimes the only viable option. We have performed RSA in mature athletes, and some were able to return to activities such as tennis or golf, although because of a lack of long-term follow-up data, we do not know how such return to activities will affect survivorship of the implant.

Summary

Massive rotator cuff tears present a challenge to the orthopaedic surgeon because of the variability in pain, range of motion, strength, and function with which such patients may present. Treatment becomes more complex in the mature active patient because of their higher functional goals and expectations. It is critically important to evaluate for elements of repairability to better select the appropriate treatment choice and properly inform the patient about the likelihood of success. Historical features such as the acuity and mechanism of onset and reports of pain or weakness are important to clarify. Poor prognostic features for repairability on the physical examination include pseudoparalysis and lag signs. Radiographic studies that exhibit diminished acromiohumeral distance and significant tendon retrac-

tion, atrophy, and fatty infiltration of the rotator cuff are concerning features that may indicate worse outcomes with attempted repair.

When the rotator cuff tear is felt to be irreparable, treatment options should be based on the clinical symptoms, function, and expectations of the patient. A painful shoulder with acceptable active motion is often improved with a biceps tenotomy combined with débridement and careful acromial smoothing with presentation of the coracoacromial ligament. This approach is not as successful if there is associated glenohumeral arthritis. Biceps release should also be considered in a shoulder with poor motion if it is suspected that the limitation in motion is secondary to pain. A diagnostic subacromial local anesthetic injection is useful in determining whether active motion is improved with relief of pain. If the limited motion is not due to pain but rather to cuff weakness, a biceps tenotomy would not be expected to improve active range of motion or function.

In an active patient with limited active range of motion and function secondary to an irreparable massive rotator cuff tear, treatment options include partial repair, tendon transfers, and biologic augmentation of the rotator cuff. Improvement in function and outcomes for each of these choices may be unpredictable but would be compatible with heavier demands and activities postoperatively. RSA may be more predictable in restoring motion in massive rotator cuff tears, but it is usually reserved for the patient with glenohumeral arthritis or lower postoperative functional demands on the shoulder. In certain active mature patients, RSA may be the only reliable option to return active elevation and function, but it should used with caution because of the potential complications.

References

1. Sher JS, Uribe JW, Posada A, Murphy BJ, Zlatkin MB: Abnormal findings on magnetic resonance images of asymptomatic shoulders. *J Bone Joint Surg Am* 1995; 77(1):10-15.

2. Tempelhof S, Rupp S, Seil R: Age-related prevalence of rotator cuff tears in asymptomatic shoulders. *J Shoulder Elbow Surg* 1999;8(4):296-299.

3. Dines DM, Moynihan DP, Dines JS, McCann P: Irreparable rotator cuff tears: what to do and when to

do it; the surgeon's dilemma. *J Bone Joint Surg Am* 2006;88(10):2294-2302.

4. DeOrio JK, Cofield RH: Results of a second attempt at surgical repair of a failed initial rotator-cuff repair. *J Bone Joint Surg Am* 1984;66(4):563-567.

5. Harryman DT II, Mack LA, Wang KY, Jackins SE, Richardson ML, Matsen FA III: Repairs of the rotator cuff: Correlation of functional results with integrity of the cuff. *J Bone Joint Surg Am* 1991;73(7):982-989.

6. Gerber C, Vinh TS, Hertel R, Hess CW: Latissimus dorsi transfer for the treatment of massive tears of the rotator cuff: A preliminary report. *Clin Orthop Relat Res* 1988;(232):51-61.

7. Gerber C, Fuchs B, Hodler J: The results of repair of massive tears of the rotator cuff. *J Bone Joint Surg Am* 2000;82(4):505-515.

8. Neer CS II, Craig EV, Fukuda H: Cuff-tear arthropathy. *J Bone Joint Surg Am* 1983;65(9):1232-1244.

9. Green A: Chronic massive rotator cuff tears: Evaluation and management. *J Am Acad Orthop Surg* 2003;11(5): 321-331.

10. Hawkins RJ, Misamore GW, Hobeika PE: Surgery for full-thickness rotator-cuff tears. *J Bone Joint Surg Am* 1985;67(9):1349-1355.

11. Burkhart SS, Barth JR, Richards DP, Zlatkin MB, Larsen M: Arthroscopic repair of massive rotator cuff tears with stage 3 and 4 fatty degeneration. *Arthroscopy* 2007;23(4):347-354.

12. Wolf BR, Dunn WR, Wright RW: Indications for repair of full-thickness rotator cuff tears. *Am J Sports Med* 2007;35(6):1007-1016.

13. Goutallier D, Postel JM, Bernageau J, Lavau L, Voisin MC: Fatty muscle degeneration in cuff ruptures: Pre- and postoperative evaluation by CT scan. *Clin Orthop Relat Res* 1994;(304):78-83.

14. Gladstone JN, Bishop JY, Lo IK, Flatow EL: Fatty infiltration and atrophy of the rotator cuff do not improve after rotator cuff repair and correlate with poor functional outcome. *Am J Sports Med* 2007;35(5): 719-728.

15. Rockwood CA Jr, Williams GR Jr, Burkhead WZ Jr: Débridement of degenerative, irreparable lesions of the rotator cuff. *J Bone Joint Surg Am* 1995;77(6):857-866.

16. Ellman H, Kay SP, Wirth M: Arthroscopic treatment of full-thickness rotator cuff tears: 2- to 7-year follow-up study. *Arthroscopy* 1993;9(2):195-200.

17. Gartsman GM: Arthroscopic acromioplasty for lesions of the rotator cuff. *J Bone Joint Surg Am* 1990;72(2): 169-180.

18. Gartsman GM: Massive, irreparable tears of the rotator cuff: Results of operative debridement and subacromial decompression. *J Bone Joint Surg Am* 1997;79(5):715-721.

19. Galatz LM, Ball CM, Teefey SA, Middleton WD, Yamaguchi K: The outcome and repair integrity of completely arthroscopically repaired large and massive rotator cuff tears. *J Bone Joint Surg Am* 2004;86(2): 219-224.

20. Gerber C, Galantay RV, Hersche O: The pattern of pain produced by irritation of the acromioclavicular joint and the subacromial space. *J Shoulder Elbow Surg* 1998;7(4):352-355.

21. Deutsch A, Ramsey ML, Iannotti JP: Diagnosis, patient selection and clinical decision making, in Iannotti JP, Williams GR, eds: *Disorders of the Shoulder: Diagnosis & Management*, ed 2. Philadelphia, PA, Lippincott Williams & Wilkins, 2006, pp 40-41.

22. Walch G, Boulahia A, Calderone S, Robinson AH: The 'dropping' and 'hornblower's' signs in evaluation of rotator-cuff tears. *J Bone Joint Surg Br* 1998;80(4): 624-628.

23. Tokish JM, Decker MJ, Ellis HB, Torry MR, Hawkins RJ: The belly-press test for the physical examination of the subscapularis muscle: Electromyographic validation and comparison to the lift-off test. *J Shoulder Elbow Surg* 2003;12(5):427-430.

24. O'Brien SJ, Pagnani MJ, Fealy S, McGlynn SR, Wilson JB: The active compression test: A new and effective test for diagnosing labral tears and acromioclavicular joint abnormality. *Am J Sports Med* 1998;26(5): 610-613.

25. Tennent TD, Beach WR, Meyers JF: A review of the special tests associated with shoulder examination: Part I. The rotator cuff tests. *Am J Sports Med* 2003;31(1): 154-160.

26. Weiner DS, Macnab I: Superior migration of the humeral head: A radiological aid in the diagnosis of tears of the rotator cuff. *J Bone Joint Surg Br* 1970; 52(3):524-527.

27. Zingg PO, Jost B, Sukthankar A, Buhler M, Pfirrmann CW, Gerber C: Clinical and structural outcomes of nonoperative management of massive rotator cuff tears. *J Bone Joint Surg Am* 2007;89(9):1928-1934.

28. Al-Shawi A, Badge R, Bunker T: The detection of full thickness rotator cuff tears using ultrasound. *J Bone Joint Surg Br* 2008;90(7):889-892.

29. Kelly AM, Fessell D: Ultrasound compared with magnetic resonance imaging for the diagnosis of rotator cuff tears: A critically appraised topic. *Semin Roentgenol* 2009;44(3):196-200.

30. Kang CH, Kim SS, Kim JH, et al: Supraspinatus tendon tears: Comparison of 3D US and MR arthrography with surgical correlation. *Skeletal Radiol* 2009;38(11):1063-1069.

31. Vlychou M, Dailiana Z, Fotiadou A, Papanagiotou M, Fezoulidis IV, Malizos K: Symptomatic partial rotator cuff tears: Diagnostic performance of ultrasound and magnetic resonance imaging with surgical correlation. *Acta Radiol* 2009;50(1):101-105.

32. Shahabpour M, Kichouh M, Laridon E, Gielen JL, De Mey J: The effectiveness of diagnostic imaging methods for the assessment of soft tissue and articular disorders of the shoulder and elbow. *Eur J Radiol* 2008;65(2):194-200.

33. Rutten MJ, Spaargaren GJ, van Loon T, de Waal Malefijt MC, Kiemeney LA, Jager GJ: Detection of rotator cuff tears: The value of MRI following ultrasound. *Eur Radiol* 2010;20(2):450-457.

34. de Jesus JO, Parker L, Frangos AJ, Nazarian LN: Accuracy of MRI, MR arthrography, and ultrasound in the diagnosis of rotator cuff tears: A meta-analysis. *AJR Am J Roentgenol* 2009;192(6):1701-1707.

35. Gerber C, Schneeberger AG, Hoppeler H, Meyer DC: Correlation of atrophy and fatty infiltration on strength and integrity of rotator cuff repairs: A study in thirteen patients. *J Shoulder Elbow Surg* 2007;16(6):691-696.

36. Thomazeau H, Boukobza E, Morcet N, Chaperon J, Langlais F: Prediction of rotator cuff repair results by magnetic resonance imaging. *Clin Orthop Relat Res* 1997;(344):275-283.

37. Zanetti M, Gerber C, Hodler J: Quantitative assessment of the muscles of the rotator cuff with magnetic resonance imaging. *Invest Radiol* 1998;33(3):163-170.

38. Fuchs B, Weishaupt D, Zanetti M, Hodler J, Gerber C: Fatty degeneration of the muscles of the rotator cuff. Assessment by computed tomography versus magnetic resonance imaging. *J Shoulder Elbow Surg* 1999;8(6):599-605.

39. Lecouvet FE, Simoni P, Koutaïssoff S, Vande Berg BC, Malghem J, Dubuc JE: Multidetector spiral CT arthrography of the shoulder: Clinical applications and limits, with MR arthrography and arthroscopic correlations. *Eur J Radiol* 2008;68(1):120-136.

40. Woertler K: Multimodality imaging of the postoperative shoulder. *Eur Radiol* 2007;17(12):3038-3055.

41. Blair B, Rokito AS, Cuomo F, Jarolem K, Zuckerman JD: Efficacy of injections of corticosteroids for subacromial impingement syndrome. *J Bone Joint Surg Am* 1996;78(11):1685-1689.

42. Bokor DJ, Hawkins RJ, Huckell GH, Angelo RL, Schickendantz MS: Results of nonoperative management of full-thickness tears of the rotator cuff. *Clin Orthop Relat Res* 1993;(294):103-110.

43. Goldberg BA, Nowinski RJ, Matsen FA III: Outcome of nonoperative management of full-thickness rotator cuff tears. *Clin Orthop Relat Res* 2001;(382):99-107.

44. Maman E, Harris C, White L, Tomlinson G, Shashank M, Boynton E: Outcome of nonoperative treatment of symptomatic rotator cuff tears monitored by magnetic resonance imaging. *J Bone Joint Surg Am* 2009;91(8):1898-1906.

45. Bartolozzi A, Andreychik D, Ahmad S: Determinants of outcome in the treatment of rotator cuff disease. *Clin Orthop Relat Res* 1994;(308):90-97.

46. Ainsworth R: Physiotherapy rehabilitation in patients with massive, irreparable rotator cuff tears. *Musculoskeletal Care* 2006;4(3):140-151.

47. Zvijac JE, Levy HJ, Lemak LJ: Arthroscopic subacromial decompression in the treatment of full thickness rotator cuff tears: A 3- to 6-year follow-up. *Arthroscopy* 1994;10(5):518-523.

48. Scheibel M, Lichtenberg S, Habermeyer P: Reversed arthroscopic subacromial decompression for massive rotator cuff tears. *J Shoulder Elbow Surg* 2004;13(3):272-278.

49. Klinger HM, Steckel H, Ernstberger T, Baums MH: Arthroscopic debridement of massive rotator cuff tears: Negative prognostic factors. *Arch Orthop Trauma Surg* 2005;125(4):261-266.

50. Klinger HM, Spahn G, Baums MH, Steckel H: Arthroscopic debridement of irreparable massive rotator cuff tears—a comparison of debridement alone and combined procedure with biceps tenotomy. *Acta Chir Belg* 2005;105(3):297-301.

51. Liem D, Lengers N, Dedy N, Poetzl W, Steinbeck J, Marquardt B: Arthroscopic debridement of massive irreparable rotator cuff tears. *Arthroscopy* 2008;24(7): 743-748.

52. Elhassan B, Endres NK, Higgins LD, Warner JJ: Massive irreparable tendon tears of the rotator cuff: Salvage options. *Instr Course Lect* 2008;57:153-166.

53. Angelo RL: The arthroscopic management of large to massive rotator cuff tears. *Tech Shoulder Elbow Surg* 2008;9(4):226-236.

54. Hitchcock HH, Bechtol CO: Painful shoulder: Observations on the role of the tendon of the long head of the biceps brachii in its causation. *J Bone Joint Surg Am* 1948;30A(2):263-273.

55. Gill TJ, McIrvin E, Mair SD, Hawkins RJ: Results of biceps tenotomy for treatment of pathology of the long head of the biceps brachii. *J Shoulder Elbow Surg* 2001;10(3):247-249.

56. Szabó I, Boileau P, Walch G: The proximal biceps as a pain generator and results of tenotomy. *Sports Med Arthrosc* 2008;16(3):180-186.

57. Neer CS II: Anterior acromioplasty for the chronic impingement syndrome in the shoulder: A preliminary report. *J Bone Joint Surg Am* 1972;54(1):41-50.

58. Murthi AM, Vosburgh CL, Neviaser TJ: The incidence of pathologic changes of the long head of the biceps tendon. *J Shoulder Elbow Surg* 2000;9(5):382-385.

59. Kempf JF, Gleyze P, Bonnomet F, et al: A multicenter study of 210 rotator cuff tears treated by arthroscopic acromioplasty. *Arthroscopy* 1999;15(1):56-66.

60. Walch G, Edwards TB, Boulahia A, Nové-Josserand L, Neyton L, Szabo I: Arthroscopic tenotomy of the long head of the biceps in the treatment of rotator cuff tears: Clinical and radiographic results of 307 cases. *J Shoulder Elbow Surg* 2005;14(3):238-246.

61. Boileau P, Baqué F, Valerio L, Ahrens P, Chuinard C, Trojani C: Isolated arthroscopic biceps tenotomy or tenodesis improves symptoms in patients with massive irreparable rotator cuff tears. *J Bone Joint Surg Am* 2007;89(4):747-757.

62. Osbahr DC, Diamond AB, Speer KP: The cosmetic appearance of the biceps muscle after long-head tenotomy versus tenodesis. *Arthroscopy* 2002;18(5): 483-487.

63. Burkhart SS, Nottage WM, Ogilvie-Harris DJ, Kohn HS, Pachelli A: Partial repair of irreparable rotator cuff tears. *Arthroscopy* 1994;10(4):363-370.

64. Burkhart SS: Partial repair of massive rotator cuff tears: The evolution of a concept. *Orthop Clin North Am* 1997;28(1):125-132.

65. Burkhart SS, Athanasiou KA, Wirth MA: Margin convergence: A method of reducing strain in massive rotator cuff tears. *Arthroscopy* 1996;12(3):335-338.

66. Burkhart SS: The principle of margin convergence in rotator cuff repair as a means of strain reduction at the tear margin. *Ann Biomed Eng* 2004;32(1):166-170.

67. Duralde XA, Bair B: Massive rotator cuff tears: The result of partial rotator cuff repair. *J Shoulder Elbow Surg* 2005;14(2):121-127.

68. Iannotti JP, Hennigan S, Herzog R, et al: Latissimus dorsi tendon transfer for irreparable posterosuperior rotator cuff tears: Factors affecting outcome. *J Bone Joint Surg Am* 2006;88(2):342-348.

69. Gerber C: Latissimus dorsi transfer for the treatment of irreparable tears of the rotator cuff. *Clin Orthop Relat Res* 1992;(275):152-160.

70. Gerber C, Maquieira G, Espinosa N: Latissimus dorsi transfer for the treatment of irreparable rotator cuff tears. *J Bone Joint Surg Am* 2006;88(1):113-120.

71. Miniaci A, MacLeod M: Transfer of the latissimus dorsi muscle after failed repair of a massive tear of the rotator cuff: A two to five-year review. *J Bone Joint Surg Am* 1999;81(8):1120-1127.

72. Warner JJ, Parsons IM IV : Latissimus dorsi tendon transfer: A comparative analysis of primary and salvage reconstruction of massive, irreparable rotator cuff tears. *J Shoulder Elbow Surg* 2001;10(6):514-521.

73. Boileau P, Rumian AP, Zumstein MA: Reversed shoulder arthroplasty with modified L'Episcopo for combined loss of active elevation and external rotation. *J Shoulder Elbow Surg* 2010;19(2, Suppl)20-30.

74. Gerber C, Pennington SD, Lingenfelter EJ, Sukthankar A: Reverse Delta-III total shoulder replacement combined with latissimus dorsi transfer: A preliminary report. *J Bone Joint Surg Am* 2007;89(5):940-947.

75. Gerhardt C, Lehmann L, Lichtenberg S, Magosch P, Habermeyer P: Modified L'Episcopo tendon transfers for irreparable rotator cuff tears: 5-year follow-up. *Clin Orthop Relat Res* 2010;468(6):1572-1577.

76. Boileau P, Chuinard C, Roussanne Y, Neyton L, Trojani C: Modified latissimus dorsi and teres major transfer through a single delto-pectoral approach for external rotation deficit of the shoulder: As an isolated procedure or with a reverse arthroplasty. *J Shoulder Elbow Surg* 2007;16(6):671-682.

77. Neri BR, Chan KW, Kwon YW: Management of massive and irreparable rotator cuff tears. *J Shoulder Elbow Surg* 2009;18(5):808-818.

78. Wirth MA, Rockwood CA Jr: Operative treatment of irreparable rupture of the subscapularis. *J Bone Joint Surg Am* 1997;79(5):722-731.

79. Resch H, Povacz P, Ritter E, Matschi W: Transfer of the pectoralis major muscle for the treatment of irreparable rupture of the subscapularis tendon. *J Bone Joint Surg Am* 2000;82(3):372-382.

80. Klepps SJ, Goldfarb C, Flatow E, Galatz LM, Yamaguchi K: Anatomic evaluation of the subcoracoid pectoralis major transfer in human cadavers. *J Shoulder Elbow Surg* 2001;10(5):453-459.

81. Klepps S, Galatz L, Yamaguchi K: Subcoracoid pectoralis major transfer: A salvage procedure for irreparable subscapularis deficiency. *Tech Shoulder Elbow Surg* 2001;2(2):85-91.

82. Gerber A, Clavert P, Millett PJ, Holovacs TF, Warner JJ: Split pectoralis major and teres major tendon transfers for reconstruction of irreparable tears of the subscapularis. *Tech Shoulder Elbow Surg* 2004;5(1): 5-12.

83. Galatz LM, Connor PM, Calfee RP, Hsu JC, Yamaguchi K: Pectoralis major transfer for anterior-superior subluxation in massive rotator cuff insufficiency. *J Shoulder Elbow Surg* 2003;12(1):1-5.

84. Elhassan B, Ozbaydar M, Massimini D, Diller D, Higgins L, Warner JJ: Transfer of pectoralis major for the treatment of irreparable tears of subscapularis: does it work? *J Bone Joint Surg Br* 2008;90(8):1059-1065.

85. Iannotti JP, Codsi MJ, Lafosse L, Flatow EL: Management of rotator cuff disease: Intact and repairable cuff, in Iannotti JP, Williams GR, eds: *Disorders of the Shoulder: Diagnosis & Management*, ed 2. Philadelphia, PA, Lippincott Williams & Wilkins, 2006, pp 80-82.

86. Iannotti JP, Codsi MJ, Kwon YW, Derwin K, Ciccone J, Brems JJ: Porcine small intestine submucosa augmentation of surgical repair of chronic two-tendon rotator cuff tears: A randomized, controlled trial. *J Bone Joint Surg Am* 2006;88(6):1238-1244.

87. Coons DA, Alan Barber F: Tendon graft substitutes-rotator cuff patches. *Sports Med Arthrosc* 2006;14(3): 185-190.

88. Ide J, Kikukawa K, Hirose J, Iyama K, Sakamoto H, Mizuta H: Reconstruction of large rotator-cuff tears with acellular dermal matrix grafts in rats. *J Shoulder Elbow Surg* 2009;18(2):288-295.

89. Dejardin LM, Arnoczky SP, Ewers BJ, Haut RC, Clarke RB: Tissue-engineered rotator cuff tendon using porcine small intestine submucosa: Histologic and mechanical evaluation in dogs. *Am J Sports Med* 2001;29(2):175-184.

90. Schlegel TF, Hawkins RJ, Lewis CW, Motta T, Turner AS: The effects of augmentation with Swine small intestine submucosa on tendon healing under tension: Histologic and mechanical evaluations in sheep. *Am J Sports Med* 2006;34(2):275-280.

91. Sclamberg SG, Tibone JE, Itamura JM, Kasraeian S: Six-month magnetic resonance imaging follow-up of large and massive rotator cuff repairs reinforced with porcine small intestinal submucosa. *J Shoulder Elbow Surg* 2004;13(5):538-541.

92. Walton JR, Bowman NK, Khatib Y, Linklater J, Murrell GA: Restore orthobiologic implant: Not recommended for augmentation of rotator cuff repairs. *J Bone Joint Surg Am* 2007;89(4):786-791.

93. Badhe SP, Lawrence TM, Smith FD, Lunn PG: An assessment of porcine dermal xenograft as an augmentation graft in the treatment of extensive rotator cuff tears. *J Shoulder Elbow Surg* 2008; 17(1, Suppl)35S-39S.

94. Gartsman GM, Roddey TS, Hammerman SM: Shoulder arthroplasty with or without resurfacing of the glenoid in patients who have osteoarthritis. *J Bone Joint Surg Am* 2000;82(1):26-34.

95. Radnay CS, Setter KJ, Chambers L, Levine WN, Bigliani LU, Ahmad CS: Total shoulder replacement compared with humeral head replacement for the treatment of primary glenohumeral osteoarthritis: A systematic review. *J Shoulder Elbow Surg* 2007;16(4): 396-402.

96. Franklin JL, Barrett WP, Jackins SE, Matsen FA III: Glenoid loosening in total shoulder arthroplasty: Association with rotator cuff deficiency. *J Arthroplasty* 1988;3(1):39-46.

97. Hawkins RJ, Bell RH, Jallay B: Total shoulder arthroplasty. *Clin Orthop Relat Res* 1989;(242): 188-194.

98. Werner CM, Steinmann PA, Gilbart M, Gerber C: Treatment of painful pseudoparesis due to irreparable rotator cuff dysfunction with the Delta III reverse ball-and-socket total shoulder prosthesis. *J Bone Joint Surg Am* 2005;87(7):1476-1486.

99. Neer CS II, Watson KC, Stanton FJ: Recent experience in total shoulder replacement. *J Bone Joint Surg Am* 1982;64(3):319-337.

100. Wiater JM, Fabing MH: Shoulder arthroplasty: prosthetic options and indications. *J Am Acad Orthop Surg* 2009;17(7):415-425.

101. Williams GR Jr, Rockwood CA Jr: Hemiarthroplasty in rotator cuff-deficient shoulders. *J Shoulder Elbow Surg* 1996;5(5):362-367.

102. Field LD, Dines DM, Zabinski SJ, Warren RF: Hemiarthroplasty of the shoulder for rotator cuff arthropathy. *J Shoulder Elbow Surg* 1997;6(1):18-23.

103. Sanchez-Sotelo J, Cofield RH, Rowland CM: Shoulder hemiarthroplasty for glenohumeral arthritis associated with severe rotator cuff deficiency. *J Bone Joint Surg Am* 2001;83-A(12):1814-1822.

104. Goldberg SS, Bell JE, Kim HJ, Bak SF, Levine WN, Bigliani LU: Hemiarthroplasty for the rotator cuff-deficient shoulder. *J Bone Joint Surg Am* 2008;90(3):554-559.

105. Visotsky JL, Basamania C, Seebauer L, Rockwood CA, Jensen KL: Cuff tear arthropathy: Pathogenesis, classification, and algorithm for treatment. *J Bone Joint Surg Am* 2004;86-A(2, Suppl 2)35-40.

106. Gerber C, Pennington SD, Nyffeler RW: Reverse total shoulder arthroplasty. *J Am Acad Orthop Surg* 2009; 17(5):284-295.

107. Grammont PM, Baulot E: Delta shoulder prosthesis for rotator cuff rupture. *Orthopedics* 1993;16(1):65-68.

108. Matsen FA III, Boileau P, Walch G, Gerber C, Bicknell RT: The reverse total shoulder arthroplasty. *J Bone Joint Surg Am* 2007;89(3):660-667.

109. Boileau P, Watkinson D, Hatzidakis AM, Hovorka I: Neer Award 2005: The Grammont reverse shoulder prosthesis. Results in cuff tear arthritis, fracture sequelae, and revision arthroplasty. *J Shoulder Elbow Surg* 2006;15(5):527-540.

110. Frankle M, Siegal S, Pupello D, Saleem A, Mighell M, Vasey M: The Reverse Shoulder Prosthesis for glenohumeral arthritis associated with severe rotator cuff deficiency: A minimum two-year follow-up study of sixty patients. *J Bone Joint Surg Am* 2005;87(8):1697-1705.

111. Cuff D, Pupello D, Virani N, Levy J, Frankle M: Reverse shoulder arthroplasty for the treatment of rotator cuff deficiency. *J Bone Joint Surg Am* 2008; 90(6):1244-1251.

112. Wall B, Nové-Josserand L, O'Connor DP, Edwards TB, Walch G: Reverse total shoulder arthroplasty: A review of results according to etiology. *J Bone Joint Surg Am* 2007;89(7):1476-1485.

113. Boileau P, Gonzalez JF, Chuinard C, Bicknell R, Walch G: Reverse total shoulder arthroplasty after failed rotator cuff surgery. *J Shoulder Elbow Surg* 2009;18(4):600-606.

114. Guery J, Favard L, Sirveaux F, Oudet D, Mole D, Walch G: Reverse total shoulder arthroplasty: Survivorship analysis of eighty replacements followed for five to ten years. *J Bone Joint Surg Am* 2006;88(8):1742-1747.

115. Sirveaux F, Favard L, Oudet D, Huquet D, Walch G, Molé D: Grammont inverted total shoulder arthroplasty in the treatment of glenohumeral osteoarthritis with massive rupture of the cuff: Results of a multicentre study of 80 shoulders. *J Bone Joint Surg Br* 2004;86(3):388-395.

Chapter 22

Proximal Humerus Fractures

Gita Pillai, MD
Bradford Parsons, MD
Evan L. Flatow, MD

Key Points

- Proximal humerus fractures are common, and most are amenable to nonsurgical treatment.
- Surgical treatment of proximal humerus fractures has evolved considerably, and many options are now available.
- Percutaneous treatments offer a minimally invasive approach, which minimizes scarring and optimizes outcome.
- Locking plate technology has allowed many fractures that previously would have required arthroplasty to be treated successfully with open reduction and internal fixation (ORIF).
- Hemiarthroplasty and reverse total shoulder arthroplasty are indicated in select comminuted fractures in the elderly.

Introduction

Proximal humerus fractures are common, accounting for 5% of all fractures, and are especially prevalent in the aging population.[1,2] In people older than 65 years, proximal humerus fractures are the third most common fracture, following hip and distal radius fractures. Although most proximal humerus fractures are nondisplaced and therefore amenable to nonsurgical treatment, displaced fractures in active patients often warrant surgical management. Recent advances have given surgeons multiple options in the surgical treatment of proximal humerus fractures, including percutaneous pinning, open reduction and internal fixation (ORIF) with anatomically contoured locking or nonlocking plates, and hemiarthroplasty. With the evolution in management of these fractures toward less invasive techniques, improved fixation implants, and soft-tissue–sparing procedures, many patients can successfully return to pre-injury activities, including sports, following fracture management.

Fracture Classification and Pathoanatomy

Displaced proximal humerus fractures are classified based on fracture anatomy. As classically delineated by Neer[3] in his four-part fracture classification, the proximal humerus is divided into the following segments: the anatomic head, the greater and lesser tuberosities, and the shaft/surgical neck. Most two-part fractures involve displaced surgical neck or greater tuberosity fractures. Three-part fractures commonly involve the humeral head, greater tu-

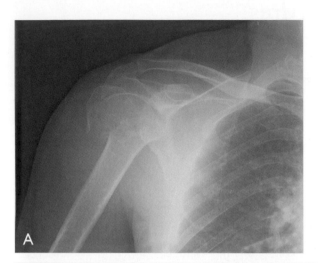
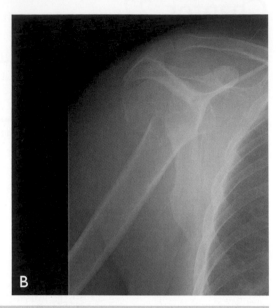

Figure 1   AP (**A**) and scapular Y (**B**) views of a four-part valgus-impacted fracture.

berosity, and shaft as fragments, with the lesser tuberosity remaining attached to the humeral head. Classic four-part fractures involve displacement of all components of the proximal humerus from the shaft and each other. Fractures also may be associated with glenohumeral joint dislocation, increasing the severity of soft-tissue injury. Fragment displacement and pathoanatomy is most influenced by the pull of the rotator cuff on the tuberosities, often leading to alteration of the normal version (three-part fractures) or inclination of the proximal humerus. As severity of displacement and number of fracture fragments increases, so does the likelihood of disruption of the vascularity of the humeral head, increasing the possibility of osteonecrosis. Recently, a variation of the classic four-part fracture pattern has been described, termed the "four-part valgus-impacted fracture," in which the humeral head falls into valgus displacement with disruption of the tuberosities[4] (**Figure 1**). This fracture has been associated with a lower incidence of osteonecrosis than the classic four-part fracture because the medial soft-tissue sleeve is intact and the blood supply to the articular surface is preserved. Thus these fractures often may be managed with ORIF as opposed to hemiarthroplasty, the classic treatment for displaced four-part fractures.

Treatment Decision Making

Age, bone quality, fracture pattern, humeral head vascularity, and timing of surgery are all important factors when deciding upon a treatment course, whether nonsurgical or surgical. Smith et al[5] found that osteoporotic fractures, which are common in elderly patients, were associated with a higher rate of complications, even in the face of improved fixation implants such as locking plates. Similarly, younger patients (<70 years) were found to have superior outcomes compared with patients older than 70 years in the same series.[5]

When considering humeral head–preserving techniques versus replacement, fracture pattern and humeral head viability are critical to decision making. Fractures with extensive disruption of the proximal humerus, such as four-part fractures or fracture-dislocations, have been associated with a relatively high rate of osteonecrosis, leading many surgeons to advocate hemiarthroplasty for these fractures. More recently, radiographic parameters examining fracture involvement of the humeral calcar have been described. Humeral head ischemia was found to correlate with fractures that involve and separate the anatomic neck. Radiographic findings of such fractures include mini-

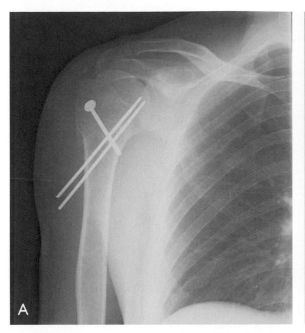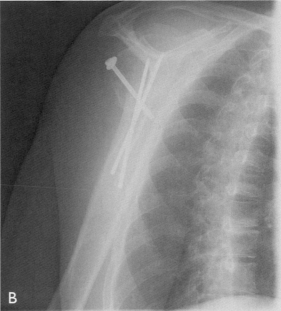

Figure 2   AP (**A**) and scapular Y (**B**) views of percutaneous pinning of a four-part valgus-impacted fracture.

mal metaphyseal fracture extension attached to the humeral head (<8 mm) and greater than 2-mm disruption of the medial humeral calcar. The presence of both radiographic findings was found to yield a 97% positive predictive value for later humeral head ischemia.[6]

Timing of surgery is also important. Most fractures are amenable to surgical treatment within the first 2 weeks following injury. When considering percutaneous pinning as a treatment option, however, early management is critical to success. Delays of even 1 week can lead to fragment scarring and early soft callus formation, making percutaneous reduction of fragments more difficult or impossible. Fractures treated with conventional ORIF or arthroplasty have been found to have inferior results when delayed 4 weeks or more from injury.[7,8]

Nonsurgical Management

Most proximal humerus fractures are either nondisplaced or minimally displaced and can be treated nonsurgically. Minimally displaced or nondisplaced two- and three-part fractures are initially immobilized in a sling for 2 to 3 weeks, depending on fracture stability.

Fluoroscopic or physical examination assessment of fracture stability may allow early (around 2 weeks) gentle passive motion if stability is confirmed. Active motion is usually allowed at 4 weeks, once callus is evident. Function is related to initial fracture displacement as well as final fracture union.[9]

Surgical Management

Displaced fractures are typically indicated for surgical treatment, as functional outcome may be compromised following nonsurgical treatment. Options for surgical management include percutaneous reduction and fixation (pinning), formal ORIF, or hemiarthroplasty reconstruction. Choice of treatment is dependent upon multiple factors, such as fracture pattern, bone quality, and timing of surgery, as discussed above.

Percutaneous Pinning

Recently, many authors have described successful results of percutaneous treatment of two-part, select three-part, and valgus-impacted four-part fractures (**Figure 2**). Keener et al[10] reported on a series of 36 patients with two-, three-, and four-part fractures treated

Table 1: Results of Percutaneous Pinning of Proximal Humerus Fractures

Study	Patient Age (Years)	Mean Follow-up (Months)	No. of Patients
Jaberg et al (1992)[11]	63	36	48
Resch et al (1997)[12]	54	24	27
Chen et al (1998)[14]	43	21	19
Soete et al (1999)[13]	68	45	31
Herscovici et al (2000)[15]	54	40	41
Fenichel et al (2006)[16]	50	30	50
Keener et al (2007)[10]	61	35	36

ASES = American Shoulder and Elbow Surgeons.

with percutaneous pinning with a minimum follow-up of 1 year; final average American Shoulder and Elbow Surgeons (ASES) and Constant scores were 83.4 and 73.9, respectively. Similarly, Jaberg et al[11] reported on a series of 48 patients with two-, three-, and four-part proximal humerus fractures treated with percutaneous pinning. They reported good or excellent results using the Saillant scale in 71% of patients and a low rate of complications, including osteonecrosis. Other series have reported similar outcomes[12-16] (**Table 1**).

Although percutaneous techniques are attractive from the standpoint of minimal soft-tissue disruption and scarring, they are not appropriate for all fractures. Further, percutaneous pinning of proximal humerus fractures requires a learning curve and is technically demanding, especially when malrotation of fragments is apparent, such as in three-part fractures.

Contraindications to percutaneous pinning include severely osteoporotic bone, as this may lead to hardware failure or migration; comminuted fractures involving the greater tuberosity such that the tuberosity cannot be adequately fixed with cannulated screws; and metaphyseal comminution of the medial calcar. In the latter scenario, the head fragment is often displaced in varus malangulation because of the loss of the calcar buttress (**Figure 3**). Percutaneous pins may not adequately stabilize such a fracture pattern, and the fracture is at risk for redisplacing into varus; as such, these fractures often require formal ORIF with plate constructs.

Following percutaneous fixation, patients are immobilized in a sling for 3 to 4 weeks. Typically at 4 weeks, pin fixation is removed and the patient begins a range-of-motion protocol. Early problems with pin-tract infection and wound problems have led most surgeons to advocate cutting percutaneously placed pins beneath the skin with a plan for staged removal at 3 to 4 weeks, as skin integrity and fracture healing allow.

Open Reduction and Internal Fixation

Historically, ORIF of proximal humeral fractures has used a variety of fixation methods, including sutures, plates, and intramedullary devices, with mixed outcomes.[9,17-19] In elderly patients with osteoporotic bone, suture or tension band constructs have often been used, as the rotator cuff attachment offers superior fixation compared with conventional plate options in osteoporotic bone.[20] However, with the advent of locking plate technology and the development of anatomic contoured proximal humeral locking plate options, the role of plate fixation of these fractures has evolved and undergone a resurgence. Recent biomechanical studies have demonstrated superior stiffness, torsional resistance, ultimate load, and displacement characteristics of locking plates compared with conventional buttress

Table 1: (*continued*)

No. of Two-part Fractures	No. of Three-part Fractures	No. of Four-part Fractures	Results
32	8	5	Saillant: 70% good
0	9	18	Constant: 3-part, 85.4; 4-part, 82.5
13	6	0	Neer: 84% good to excellent
7	20	4	Constant: 80; 5 osteonecrosis (3 were displaced 4-part fractures)
21	16	4	Modified ASES: 2-part, 78; 3-part, 70; 4-part, 37
24	26	0	Constant: 81
11	9	16 valgus	ASES: 83.4 Constant: 73.9

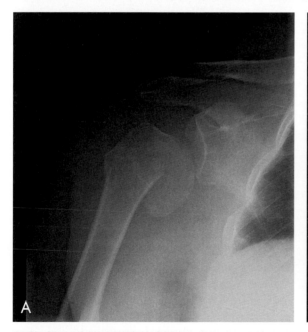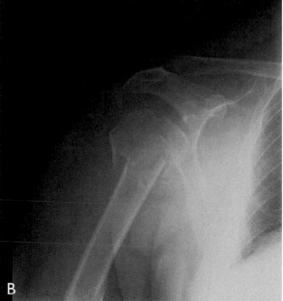

Figure 3   Grashey (**A**) and AP (**B**) views of a proximal humerus fracture with varus angulation and metaphyseal comminution of the medial calcar.

plate, blade plate, or T-plate fixation in the proximal humerus.[21-23]

Although locking plates offer improved fixation in osteoporotic bone, they are not a panacea, and anatomic reduction and adequate osseous fixation is still critical. In addition, most conventional locking plate implants offer the ability to reinforce fixation by allowing sutures from the rotator cuff to be incorporated into the plate fixation, yielding a "belt-and-suspenders" construct that should be routinely used. In addition to

Table 2: Results of Open Reduction and Internal Fixation of Proximal Humerus Fractures

Study	No. of Fractures	Mean Age (Years)	Mean Follow-up (Months)	No. of Two-part Fractures
Wijgman et al (2002)[24]	50	48	120	0
Robinson et al (2003)[17]	25	67	12	0
Fankhauser et al (2005)[18]	29	64	12	5
Plecko and Kraus (2005)[19]	36	57.5	31	8

DASH = Disabilities of the Arm, Shoulder, and Hand.

concerns over adequate fixation with historical plating techniques and implants, many early series examining nonlocking plate fixation reported an unsatisfactory level of osteonecrosis, which is often thought to be a consequence of soft-tissue stripping. Studies performed on the newer locking plates have reported a lower incidence of symptomatic osteonecrosis.[18,19] One risk unique to locking plates is that if the head collapses from osteonecrosis, the screw, because it is "locked" into the plate, does not slide but remains prominent, thus damaging the glenoid and requiring removal. Removable percutaneous pins may therefore be preferable when the risk of osteonecrosis is high.

Currently, only a few studies have reported on long-term outcomes using locking plate technology. Two recent series have found good outcomes with the use of proximal humeral locking plates for two-, three-, and select four-part fractures[18,19] (**Table 2**). Complications surrounding plate fixation remain, mostly associated with inadequate reduction, tuberosity malpositioning, articular surface malrotation (version), or failure to reestablish appropriate neck-shaft angulation.[24] One anatomic series examined the likelihood of screw penetration into the articular surface and found that posterosuperior screws are most likely to encroach on the joint. Careful assessment of screw lengths and orienta-

tion is critical, and fluoroscopic assessment in multiple planes (axillary, AP, and lateral) can be helpful in identifying screws that penetrate the humeral articular surface.[25] Dynamic, or "live," fluoroscopy with range of motion of the shoulder in all planes once fixation is complete also may be useful in identifying potentially prominent screws.

Postoperative rehabilitation is guided by fracture fixation and stability, with most patients starting an early passive motion protocol within 1 week of surgery. Active motion typically occurs at 4 to 6 weeks, followed by later strengthening.

Hemiarthroplasty

Primary arthroplasty for fracture is undertaken when the humeral head is at high risk for osteonecrosis or when stable fracture fixation seems unlikely with ORIF. The risk of osteonecrosis is particularly likely after head-splitting fractures, classic four-part fractures with displacement of the anatomic neck from the medial calcar, or in four-part fracture-dislocations. As such, hemiarthroplasty is indicated for these situations as well as for some three-part fractures in patients with osteoporotic bone (**Figure 4**).

Hemiarthroplasty generally provides good pain relief, but patient outcomes and postoperative range of

Table 2: (*continued*)

No. of Three-part Fractures	No. of Four-part Fractures	Implant and Approach	Results
40	20	Deltopectoral T-plates Cerclage wires	Constant: excellent, 30%; good, 57%; poor, 13%
5	20	Deltoid split Small-fragment plates/screws	Constant: 80 DASH: 22
15	9	Deltopectoral AO locking plates	Constant: 74.6
9	19	Deltopectoral AO locking plates	Constant: 63

motion have been variable[7,26-30] (**Table 3**). Although variability in study parameters makes full comparison of series difficult, most series report a mean elevation of 100°, with some patients achieving greater motion; however, many series report inferior motion.[7,27-29] Critical to success are tuberosity healing and restoration of normal anatomy, such as humeral height and tuberosity-head and tuberosity-tuberosity relationships. Often, a full-length radiograph of the contralateral humerus is useful to define the normal anatomic relationships, such as calcar and/or humeral head height and neck-shaft angle.[29,31-33] In a large multicenter study, the average Constant score was 49 points in patients with nonunited tuberosities, 53 points in those healed in an incorrect position, and 64 points in those healed anatomically.[28] Recently, newer prosthetic designs with dedicated fracture stems and bony ingrowth capabilities have improved radiographic and functional outcomes.[34]

Timing of surgical intervention does affect outcomes following hemiarthroplasty for fracture. The optimal timing in regard to ease of the procedure is generally in the acute period. Recent studies have shown better results for acute reconstructions versus late reconstructions.[7,8] One study, however, found no difference in outcomes between early (<30 days) and late (>30 days) reconstruction.[26]

Postoperative rehabilitation is guided by tuberosity fixation and bone quality. Secure fixation of the tuberosities to the implant, shaft, and each other allows early passive motion and may optimize the outcome. However, concerns over tuberosity nonunion and resorption, especially in elderly patients, even when the tuberosity is appropriately positioned and securely fixed, have led some surgeons to decelerate rehabilitation following hemiarthroplasty management of proximal humerus fractures in an effort to improve tuberosity healing.

Reverse Total Shoulder Arthroplasty

Recently, reverse total shoulder arthroplasty has been considered as a primary option for severe proximal humerus fractures in elderly, low-demand patients. This is generally not a viable option for an athlete.

Summary

The treatment approach in the mature athlete with a proximal humerus fracture is predicated on bone quality, age, and fracture pattern with resultant risk for osteonecrosis. In general, fracture patterns likely to develop osteonecrosis are best treated with hemiarthroplasty. With the recent advances in locking plate technology, however, many comminuted three- and four-part fractures that were traditionally managed with

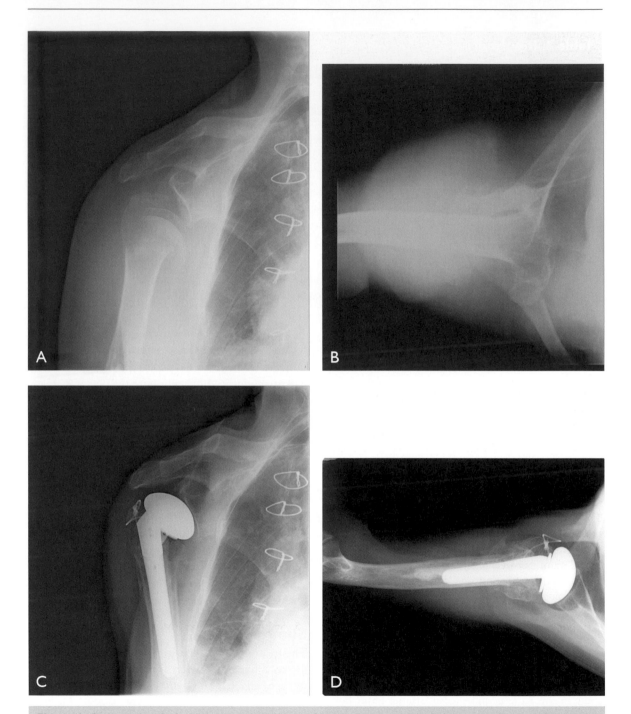

Figure 4   Radiographs of a four-part proximal humerus fracture with head split. Preoperative Grashey (**A**) and axillary (**B**) views. Grashey (**C**) and axillary (**D**) views obtained after hemiarthroplasty.

Table 3: Results of Hemiarthoplasty for Proximal Humerus Fractures

Study	No. of Fractures	Mean Age (Years)	Mean Follow-up (Months)	Results
Prakash et al (2002)[26]	15	69	33	Subjective outcome: 93% good
Boileau et al (2002)[29]	66	66	27	Constant: 56
Mighell et al (2003)[7]	72	66	36	ASES: 76.6 SST: 7.5
Robinson et al (2003)[30]	138	69	12	Constant: 64
Christoforakis et al (2004)[27]	26	65	49.6	Constant: 70.4
Kralinger et al (2004)[28]	167	70	29	Constant: 55

ASES = American Shoulder and Elbow Surgeons, SST = simple shoulder test.

hemiarthroplasty may now be amenable to fixation. Further, refinement of technique and use of less invasive soft-tissue–sparing procedures, such as percutaneous pinning of select fractures, offer the possibility of decreased scarring and improved function, potentially enabling mature athletes to return to their sport.

Four-part proximal humeral fractures in very osteopenic bone, head-splitting fractures, and fracture-dislocations are still most commonly managed by hemiarthroplasty, even in the mature athlete. Performing a hemiarthroplasty in an active patient requires realistic expectations postoperatively. Historically, mean range of motion is elevation to shoulder level, although greater range of motion has been reported recently with newer prosthetic designs and tuberosity fixation methods.

With the advent of newer techniques such as percutaneous pinning, improved implants such as low-profile locking plates, and dedicated fracture stems for hemiarthroplasty, surgeons have the ability to optimally manage displaced fractures in all patients, including the mature athlete. These recent advances in fixation capabilities and surgical technique afford multiple options to the surgeon and patients and may be critical in returning the mature athlete to sports participation.

References

1. Lind T, Krøner K, Jensen J: The epidemiology of fractures of the proximal humerus. *Arch Orthop Trauma Surg* 1989;108(5):285-287.

2. Palvanen M, Kannus P, Niemi S, Parkkari J: Update in the epidemiology of proximal humeral fractures. *Clin Orthop Relat Res* 2006;442:87-92.

3. Neer CS II: Displaced proximal humeral fractures: I. Classification and evaluation. *J Bone Joint Surg Am* 1970;52(6):1077-1089.

4. Jakob RP, Miniaci A, Anson PS, Jaberg H, Osterwalder A, Ganz R: Four-part valgus impacted fractures of the proximal humerus. *J Bone Joint Surg Br* 1991;73(2): 295-298.

5. Smith AM, Mardones RM, Sperling JW, Cofield RH: Early complications of operatively treated proximal humeral fractures. *J Shoulder Elbow Surg* 2007;16(1): 14-24.

6. Hertel R, Hempfing A, Stiehler M, Leunig M: Predictors of humeral head ischemia after intracapsular fracture of the proximal humerus. *J Shoulder Elbow Surg* 2004;13(4):427-433.

7. Mighell MA, Kolm GP, Collinge CA, Frankle MA: Outcomes of hemiarthroplasty for fractures of the

proximal humerus. *J Shoulder Elbow Surg* 2003; 12(6):569-577.

8. Becker R, Pap G, Machner A, Neumann WH: Strength and motion after hemiarthoplasty in displaced four-fragment fracture of the proximal humerus: 27 patients followed for 1-6 years. *Acta Orthop Scand* 2002; 73(1):44-49.

9. Koval KJ, Gallagher MA, Marsicano JG, Cuomo F, McShinawy A, Zuckerman JD: Functional outcome after minimally displaced fractures of the proximal part of the humerus. *J Bone Joint Surg Am* 1997;79(2): 203-207.

10. Keener JD, Parsons BO, Flatow EL, Rogers K, Williams GR, Galatz LM: Outcomes after percutaneous reduction and fixation of proximal humeral fractures. *J Shoulder Elbow Surg* 2007; 16(3):330-338.

11. Jaberg H, Warner JJ, Jakob RP: Percutaneous stabilization of unstable fractures of the humerus. *J Bone Joint Surg Am* 1992;74(4):508-515.

12. Resch H, Povacz P, Fröhlich R, Wambacher M: Percutaneous fixation of three- and four-part fractures of the proximal humerus. *J Bone Joint Surg Br* 1997; 79(2):295-300.

13. Soete PJ, Clayson PE, Costenoble VH: Transitory percutaneous pinning in fractures of the proximal humerus. *J Shoulder Elbow Surg* 1999;8(6):569-573.

14. Chen CY, Chao EK, Tu YK, Ueng SW, Shih CH: Closed management and percutaneous fixation of unstable proximal humerus fractures. *J Trauma* 1998;45(6):1039-1045.

15. Herscovici D Jr, Saunders DT, Johnson MP, Sanders R, DiPasquale T: Percutaneous fixation of proximal humeral fractures. *Clin Orthop Relat Res* 2000; (375):97-104.

16. Fenichel I, Oran A, Burstein G, Perry Pritsch M: Percutaneous pinning using threaded pins as a treatment option for unstable two- and three-part fractures of the proximal humerus: A retrospective study. *Int Orthop* 2006;30(3):153-157.

17. Robinson CM, Page RS: Severely impacted valgus proximal humeral fractures: Results of operative treatment. *J Bone Joint Surg Am* 2003;85(9):1647-1655.

18. Fankhauser F, Boldin C, Schippinger G, Haunschmid C, Szyszkowitz R: A new locking plate for unstable

fractures of the proximal humerus. *Clin Orthop Relat Res* 2005;(430):176-181.

19. Plecko M, Kraus A: Internal fixation of proximal humerus fractures using the locking proximal humerus plate. *Oper Orthop Traumatol* 2005;17(1):25-50.

20. Banco SP, Andrisani D, Ramsey M, Frieman B, Fenlin JM Jr: The parachute technique: Valgus impaction osteotomy for two-part fractures of the surgical neck of the humerus. *J Bone Joint Surg Am* 2001; 83-A Suppl 2(Pt 1):38-42.

21. Siffri PC, Peindl RD, Coley ER, Norton J, Connor PM, Kellam JF: Biomechanical analysis of blade plate versus locking plate fixation for a proximal humerus fracture: Comparison using cadaveric and synthetic humeri. *J Orthop Trauma* 2006;20(8):547-554.

22. Walsh S, Reindl R, Harvey E, Berry G, Beckman L, Steffen T: Biomechanical comparison of a unique locking plate versus a standard plate for internal fixation of proximal humerus fractures in a cadaveric model. *Clin Biomech (Bristol, Avon)* 2006;21(10):1027-1031.

23. Weinstein DM, Bratton DR, Ciccone WJ II, Elias JJ: Locking plates improve torsional resistance in the stabilization of three-part proximal humeral fractures. *J Shoulder Elbow Surg* 2006;15(2):239-243.

24. Wijgman AJ, Roolker W, Patt TW, Raaymakers EL, Marti RK: Open reduction and internal fixation of three and four-part fractures of the proximal part of the humerus. *J Bone Joint Surg Am* 2002;84(11):1919-1925.

25. Klepps SJ, Miller SL, Lin J, Gladstone J, Flatow EL: Determination of radiographic guidelines for percutaneous fixation of proximal humerus fractures using a cadaveric model. *Orthopedics* 2007;30(8): 636-641.

26. Prakash U, McGurty DW, Dent JA: Hemiarthroplasty for severe fractures of the proximal humerus. *J Shoulder Elbow Surg* 2002;11(5):428-430.

27. Christoforakis JJ, Kontakis GM, Katonis PG, Stergiopoulos K, Hadjipavlou AG: Shoulder hemiarthroplasty in the management of humeral head fractures. *Acta Orthop Belg* 2004;70(3):214-218.

28. Kralinger F, Schwaiger R, Wambacher M, et al: Outcome after primary hemiarthroplasty for fracture of the head of the humerus: A retrospective multicentre study of 167 patients. *J Bone Joint Surg Br* 2004; 86(2):217-219.

29. Boileau P, Krishnan SG, Tinsi L, Walch G, Coste JS, Molé D: Tuberosity malposition and migration: reasons for poor outcomes after hemiarthroplasty for displaced fractures of the proximal humerus. *J Shoulder Elbow Surg* 2002;11(5):401-412.

30. Robinson CM, Page RS, Hill RM, Sanders DL, Court-Brown CM, Wakefield AE: Primary hemiarthroplasty for treatment of proximal humeral fractures. *J Bone Joint Surg Am* 2003;85(7):1215-1223.

31. Frankle MA, Greenwald DP, Markee BA, Ondrovic LE, Lee WE III: Biomechanical effects of malposition of tuberosity fragments on the humeral prosthetic reconstruction for four-part proximal humerus fractures. *J Shoulder Elbow Surg* 2001;10(4):321-326.

32. Murachovsky J, Ikemoto RY, Nascimento LG, Fujiki EN, Milani C, Warner JJ: Pectoralis major tendon reference (PMT): A new method for accurate restoration of humeral length with hemiarthroplasty for fracture. *J Shoulder Elbow Surg* 2006;15(6):675-678.

33. Balg F, Boulianne M, Boileau P: Bicipital groove orientation: Considerations for the retroversion of a prosthesis in fractures of the proximal humerus. *J Shoulder Elbow Surg* 2006;15(2):195-198.

34. Krishnan SG, Bennion PW, Reineck JR, Burkhead WZ: Hemiarthroplasty for proximal humeral fracture: Restoration of the Gothic arch. *Orthop Clin North Am* 2008;39(4):441-450.

Chapter 23
Elbow Disorders and Upper Arm Injuries

Brett Franklin, MD
Michael J. Kissenberth, MD

Key Points
- Overuse injuries resulting in tendon disorders around the elbow are common conditions seen in mature athletes.
- Most chronic tendon injuries can be managed successfully with nonsurgical measures, and those that fail can be handled successfully with either open or arthroscopic techniques.
- Symptomatic elbow osteoarthritis (OA) that fails nonsurgical management can usually be successfully managed with either open or arthroscopic débridement with capsular resections/releases.
- Newer biologic modalities to treat elbow disorders in the mature athlete are still under investigation.

Introduction

Elbow pain is common in the mature athlete and can originate from acute traumatic injuries, chronic and overuse injuries, or OA. With the increased level of athletic participation in the older population, these injuries are becoming more and more prevalent. This chapter will cover the most common age-related elbow injuries in the mature athlete, including medial and lateral epicondylitis, biceps and triceps tendon injuries, OA and stiffness, and ulnar nerve neuropathy.

Lateral Epicondylitis

Lateral epicondylitis was first described by Runge[1] in 1873. In 1882, in a letter published in *The Lancet*, Henry J. Morris used the term "lawn tennis arm" because of the condition's association with the sport. Since the original identification and description of this entity, understanding of its pathophysiology has expanded dramatically. This has in turn led to more effective nonsurgical and surgical treatment modalities.

Epidemiology

Lateral epicondylitis ("tennis elbow") occurs across a wide age range, with most patients presenting in the fourth to fifth decade of life.[2] The prevalence appears to be equal in males and females. Approximately 75% of cases occur in the dominant arm.[3] Numerous sports and occupational activities have been associated with lateral epicondylitis. The common factor in all cases of lateral epicondylitis appears to be repetitive overuse secondary to sport, occupation, or daily activities. Nirschl and Ashman[4] described the following etiologic factors as most likely to be associated with elbow overuse injury: patient older than 35 years of age; high activity level in either sport or occupation, with a frequency of 3 times per week or greater and a duration of 30 minutes or more per session; and demanding activity technique. Haahr and Andersen[5] identified the following additional risk factors: nonneutral postures of the hand and arms, use of heavy hand tools, and repetitive significant strain while performing activities. Shiri et al[6] evaluated 4,783 subjects in Finland and found a prevalence of 1.3% among those aged 30 to 64 years, with the highest prevalence in subjects aged 45 to 54 years. The authors identified smoking, obesity, repetitive movements, and forceful activities as the most common associated risk factors.

With regard to sport, a direct correlation has been found between tennis playing time and the risk of developing symptomatic lateral epicondylitis, with a 2 to 3.5 times greater risk in club players with more than 2 hours of racket time per week versus those with less than 2 hours.[3] Age is also a predictive risk factor, with players older than 40 years of age having a two- to fourfold greater incidence than players younger than 40 years.[3]

Several factors in tennis have been implicated with regard to increased risk of developing symptomatic lateral epicondylitis. These include the greater forces generated during ball strike secondary to the greater ball momentum created by harder court surfaces, improper grip size and racket weight for an individual player, excessively high string tension, and improper swing mechanics.[7] Using electromyography (EMG) and cinematographic analysis, Kelley et al[8] demonstrated increased extensor carpi radialis brevis (ECRB) activity and altered swing mechanics in symptomatic tennis players versus control subjects. Poor one-handed backhand technique is also thought to be a factor leading to lateral epicondylitis.

Pathophysiology

Originally, epicondylitis was thought to represent an inflammatory condition; the term *tendinitis* is perhaps a misnomer. Tendinopathy is a more appropriate term to describe the histopathologic changes seen in epicondylitis, as histopathologic studies have not confirmed the presence of acute inflammatory cells at the site of injury.[9,10] More recent evidence has suggested that the process represents a repetitive pattern of micro tears and failed healing attempts at the site of injury.[11] Histologic studies have identified a fibroblastic and vascular response, which has been termed "angiofibroblastic tendinosis" to distinguish this degenerative process from a true inflammatory process.[11] This distinction is important in understanding the correct etiology and treatment of the problem.

The ECRB is considered the most common site of histopathologic change. Nirschl and Pettrone[2] evaluated 88 cases of surgically treated lateral epicondylitis and demonstrated the origin of the ECRB as being the primary area involved in 97% of cases, with 35% of cases demonstrating gross tendon rupture. Degenerative tendinosis has also been described in the extensor digitorum communis (EDC) in 35% to 50% of cases.[2,4] The extensor carpi radialis longus origin has been implicated as well, but to a much lesser extent than the ECRB and EDC.

Diagnosis and Evaluation

Lateral epicondylitis has a common presentation of insidious onset of pain that originates over the lateral elbow and radiates down the dorsal forearm along the course of the common wrist extensors. The pain is typically sharp and associated with activities that involve repetitive motion and active wrist extension. Patients will often report the inability to hold items such as a gallon of milk or a cup of coffee.

Physical examination typically reveals tenderness to palpation over the common extensor origin, with the point of maximal tenderness lying just anterior and distal to the lateral epicondyle over the origin of the ECRB and EDC muscles (**Figure 1,** *A*). Provocative tests, including manual resisted wrist and finger extension with the elbow extended, will reproduce the patient's symptoms (**Figure 1,** *B*). Elbow motion is usually well preserved. Weakness is noticed at the wrist with extension and grip strength testing. Dorf et al[12] demonstrated that grip strength was diminished by 50% and 69% on the affected side versus the unaffected side in elbow extension and flexion, respectively. The authors suggested that evaluating grip strength is a useful objective tool in the diagnosis of lateral epicondylitis.

A thorough history and physical examination is warranted in the evaluation of lateral epicondylitis to rule

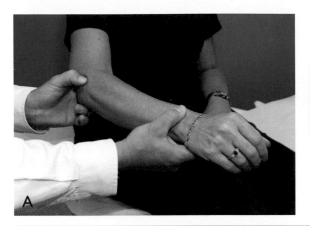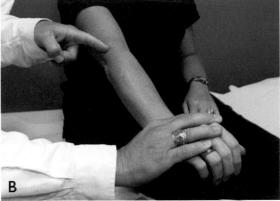

Figure 1 Photographs show physical examination for lateral epicondylitis. **A,** The examiner is palpating the area near the extensor carpi radialis brevis (ECRB) origin, which is commonly the area of maximal tenderness in lateral epicondylitis. The area is usually just distal and anterior to the lateral epicondyle. **B,** Test for lateral epicondylitis. Pain is elicited at the area of maximal tenderness with elbow extension and resisted wrist extension.

out common conditions with similar presentations. Degenerative cervical disk disease with radiculopathy, radial tunnel syndrome, intra-articular pathology including articular cartilage and synovial disease, and posterolateral elbow instability all should be included in the differential diagnosis. Additionally, some patients may have increased tenderness to palpation along the lateral synovial plica; this area of tenderness is posterior to the "typical" area of tenderness with lateral epicondylitis. Many patients also will report pain that radiates dorsally into the common extensor origin.

Although radiographs are often normal, Nirschl and Ashman[4] found a 20% incidence of calcification within the extensor origin at the lateral epicondyle; however, this did not correlate with prognosis. MRI has been shown to be effective in the preoperative evaluation of lateral epicondylitis, with imaging studies revealing edema, thickening, and degeneration within the ECRB origin; these have subsequently correlated with intraoperative and histopathologic findings.[13] However, MRI findings must be viewed in light of the patient's history and physical examination, as positive MRI findings are seen in 14% to 54% of asymptomatic individuals.[14] Ultrasonography is an additional noninvasive method of evaluating lateral epicondylitis. Intrasubstance tears, peritendinous fluid, and thickening of the common extensor origin are seen on ultrasonograms in symptomatic individuals.[15] As with all ultrasonographic techniques, the sensitivity and specificity is user- and interpreter-dependent.

Treatment

Multiple treatment modalities, both surgical and nonsurgical, have been used for lateral epicondylitis, but no clear consensus exists as to which is the most effective. Regardless of the treatment, symptoms improve in most patients by 1 year, and only 4% to 11% of those who seek medical treatment require subsequent surgery.[14] Smidt et al[16] determined that long duration of symptoms, concomitant neck pain, and severe pain at initial presentation were associated with poorer outcomes at 12 months in those patients managed nonsurgically. Haahr and Andersen[5] found poor improvement in patients involved in manual labor involving a high level of physical strain, dominant-side involvement, and high baseline pain levels. Nirschl and Ashman[4] described an ordered treatment algorithm that is designed to work with and enhance the natural biology of the healing response. Their approach begins with relief of pain and control of inflammation and hemorrhage, followed by promotion of tissue healing, general fitness, control of force loads, and finally removal of pathologic tissue surgically if necessary.[4]

Nonsurgical Management

Nonsurgical management consists of rest, activity modifications, nonsteroidal anti-inflammatory drugs (NSAIDs), counterforce bracing, physical therapy, various types of injections, and noninvasive modalities. NSAIDs are one of the most common modalities implemented in the treatment of lateral epicondylitis. Their effectiveness is thought to be secondary to their effect on adjacent synovitis and inflammation in surrounding muscle and connective tissue. The utility of both oral and topical NSAIDs has been both supported and refuted in the literature. With regard to particular NSAIDs, the only study to date comparing various NSAIDs head to head is that of Stull and Jokl,[17] who found no difference between diflunisal and naproxen.

Corticosteroid injections have been implemented and studied extensively in the management of lateral epicondylitis. Randomized trials have shown that local corticosteroid injections result in improved pain, satisfaction, and outcome measures in patients versus other modalities in the short term (<6 weeks).[18,19] Longer term studies, however, have failed to demonstrate lasting impact beyond 6 weeks. Possible complications associated with corticosteroid injections include skin discoloration, subcutaneous fat necrosis, and, rarely, tendon atrophy and rupture. Botulinum toxin and autologous blood injections have received attention in the treatment of lateral epicondylitis. Autologous platelet-rich plasma (PRP), thought to produce a local healing response, has generated much interest recently in the treatment of chronic tendinopathies. The indications for PRP use have outpaced strong evidence-based research, but many studies are under way. Mishra and Pavelko[20] prospectively evaluated the use of PRP in lateral epicondylitis and demonstrated improvement in their small sample size. A summary of recent studies investigating NSAIDs, corticosteroid injections, botulinum injections, autologous blood injection, and PRP is included in **Table 1**.[18,20-28]

Extracorporeal shockwave therapy has been used in the treatment of lateral epicondylitis. It is thought to exert its effect through stimulation of local healing response and possible inhibition of pain receptors. Buchbinder et al[29] performed a systematic review of the literature on this treatment for lateral epicondylitis and found it provided little or no benefit.

Physical therapy protocols along with various orthoses also are often used in the management of lateral epicondylitis. Most include various stretches, including wrist flexion with the elbow in full extension. In a recent randomized controlled trial, isokinetic eccentric strengthening was compared with traditional strengthening rehabilitation and was found to be more effective with regard to pain control, elimination of strength deficits, improved tendon quality as determined by MRI, and improvement in patient disability status.[30] In a 2002 Cochrane Database review, Struijs et al[31] evaluated the effectiveness of orthotic devices used for lateral epicondylitis and were unable to substantiate significant benefits from the use of common orthoses such as cock-up wrist splints and counterforce braces.

Surgical Management

Surgical management is reserved for patients whose symptoms have not responded fully to a prolonged course of nonsurgical treatment. According to one study, only 5% of patients in general practice and 25% in a referral practice required surgery.[11] Surgery has traditionally consisted of open or percutaneous techniques with either release of the common extensor tendon or débridement of pathologic degenerative tissue within the ECRB or EDC. Arthroscopic techniques have been developed with similar success and a quicker recovery. Baker and Baker[32] have demonstrated very successful arthroscopic management of lateral epicondylitis with long-term results. One of the benefits of arthroscopy is the ability to fully evaluate the elbow joint. During arthroscopy, tendinosis in the extensor tendons is easily visualized (**Figure 2,** *A*). Once visualized, the pathologic tissue can then be easily removed (**Figure 2,** *B*). A summary of recent studies evaluating the surgical management of lateral epicondylitis is included in **Table 2**.[33-35]

Complications of lateral elbow surgery have been reported and well described. With both open and arthroscopic procedures, excessive débridement can lead to iatrogenic posterolateral rotary instability. Keeping the area of débridement anterior to the midline of the lateral epicondyle minimizes the risk of iatrogenic damage to the lateral stabilizing structures.[36] Additional complications reported have included neuroma of the posterior cutaneous nerve of the forearm and heterotopic ossification of the lateral elbow.[36,37]

Table 1: Nonsurgical Management of Lateral Epicondylitis

Authors	Study Design	Treatment	Results
Labele et al[21]	Multicenter PRCT	Diclofenac vs placebo	Diclofenac > placebo for pain relief Function/grip equal
Hay et al[18]	Multicenter PRCT	Corticosteroid + naproxen vs placebo	No difference
Green et al[22]	Systematic review 14 RCTs	Topical NSAIDs vs placebo	Topical NSAIDs provided better pain control and patient satisfaction
Smidt et al[23]	Systematic review 13 RCTs	Corticosteroid vs placebo, local anesthetics	Improved pain, grip strength, patient satisfaction short term (≤6 weeks) with corticosteroid injection
Hayton et al[24]	DBRCT	Botulinum toxin vs placebo	No difference in grip strength, pain, patient satisfaction
Wong et al[25]	DBRCT	Botulinum toxin vs placebo	Improved pain scores with botulinum up to 18 weeks Some digit paresis
Placzek et al[26]	DBRCT	Botulinum toxin vs placebo	Improved pain scores with botulinum up to 18 weeks Some digit paresis
Edwards and Calandruccio[27]	RCT	Autologous blood	Improved pain relief and return to activity (maximal effect delayed 3-6 weeks) No controls
Connell et al[28]	RCT	Autologous blood	Improved pain relief and return to activity (maximal effect delayed 3-6 weeks) No controls
Mishra and Pavelko[20]	Cohort Level 2	PRP injection in 15 patients	Improved pain with PRP, but small sample size

PRCT = prospective randomized controlled trial, NSAIDs = nonsteroidal anti-inflammatory drugs, RCT = randomized controlled trial; DBRCT = double-blind RCT; PRP = platelet-rich plasma.

Medial Epicondylitis

Epidemiology

As with *lateral epicondylitis,* the term *medial epicondylitis* is a misnomer because few, if any, inflammatory cells are found within the common flexor-pronator origin in symptomatic patients. Lateral epicondylitis occurs 7 to 20 times more frequently than medial epicondylitis.[38]

Patient demographics are similar, with individuals in the fourth to fifth decades of life being most commonly affected and males and females being affected equally. Although it is commonly referred to as "golfer's elbow," medial epicondylitis is seen in any sport or occupational activity in which the elbow is subjected to repetitive valgus stress, or with repetitive overuse of the flexor-pronator muscles.

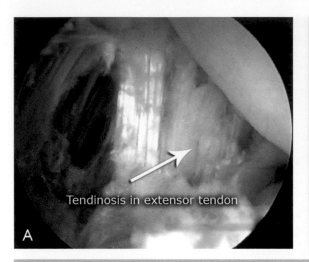
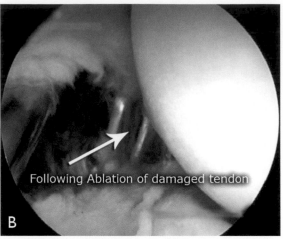

Tendinosis in extensor tendon

A

Following Ablation of damaged tendon

B

Figure 2   Arthroscopic views of an elbow with lateral epicondylitis. **A,** View from the proximal medial portal demonstrates ECRB tendinosis. **B,** View from the proximal medial portal after removal of pathologic tissue.

Table 2: Surgical Management of Lateral Epicondylitis

Authors	Study Design	Treatment	Results
Szabo et al[33]	Retrospective review	Open vs arthroscopic vs percutaneous débridement	Improvement in all groups, but no significant difference at 2-year follow-up
Dunkow et al[34]	RCT	Percutaneous vs open	Improved DASH scores and earlier return to work in percutaneous group
Lo et al[35]	Systematic review	Open vs arthroscopic vs percutaneous débridement	No difference in long-term outcome Earlier return to work with arthroscopic and percutaneous techniques
Baker and Baker[32]	Retrospective review Case series	Arthroscopic	87% satisfied with arthroscopic treatment at mean follow-up of 130 months

RCT = randomized controlled trial, DASH = Disabilities of the Arm, Shoulder, and Hand.

Diagnosis

Medial epicondylitis usually presents as medial elbow pain that is worse with activities involving wrist flexion and forearm pronation such as gripping, throwing, and batting. Strength, range of motion, and sensation are typically normal; however, symptoms of ulnar nerve irritation have been identified in 23% to 60% of pa-tients in some series which, if unrecognized, may result in treatment failure.[4,39,40] Physical examination reveals tenderness distal and lateral to the medial epicondyle directly over the pronator teres and flexor carpi radialis (**Figure 3**). Pain is typically reproduced with resisted wrist flexion and forearm pronation. Pienimäki et al[41] found that patients with medial epicondylitis showed a

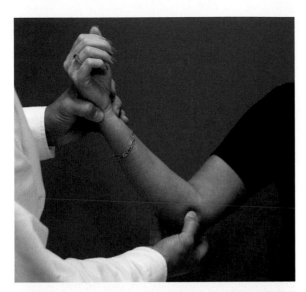

Figure 3   Photograph shows an examiner palpating the area over the flexor-pronator mass, which is commonly tender in medial epicondylitis.

lower level of impairment with regard to pain and muscle function than did patients with lateral epicondylitis. A careful assessment of medial elbow stability to valgus stress should be performed to evaluate for ulnar collateral ligament laxity, which can coexist. Plain radiographs are typically normal; however, throwing athletes may show calcification of the ulnar collateral ligament or medial traction spurs at the flexor-pronator mass origin. MRI will show the typical changes consistent with tendinosis but is not usually required to make the diagnosis.

Treatment

As with lateral epicondylitis, the mainstay of treatment of medial epicondylitis is nonsurgical management consisting of rest, activity modification, NSAIDs, physical rehabilitation, counterforce bracing, corticosteroid injections, and a gradual return to 'activities. Multiple authors have demonstrated successful outcomes with a nonsurgical approach.[38] Stahl and Kaufman[42] evaluated the effectiveness of steroid injections in treating medial epicondylitis in a prospective, randomized fashion and found they provided short-term (<6 weeks) benefit compared to therapy alone, but they failed to show any advantage at 3 months and 1 year.

Surgical intervention is warranted in patients with chronic medial epicondylitis that has not responded adequately to nonsurgical management. The same principles of surgical management that apply to lateral epicondylitis also apply to medial epicondylitis, with the goal being débridement of abnormal, degenerative tissue and reapproximation of healthy tissues. The surgical treatment of medial epicondylitis has not been as successful as that for lateral epicondylitis. One explanation for this is likely the coexistence of ulnar nerve neuropathy in patients with medial epicondylitis that is not discovered preoperatively or addressed intraoperatively. Kurvers and Verhaar[43] retrospectively evaluated their results of surgical treatment of medial epicondylitis and found a success rate of 68% in patients with isolated tendinosis, versus 12% in patients with coexisting ulnar neuritis. Similarly, Gabel and Morrey[44] found 96% good or excellent results in patients with isolated medial epicondylitis, versus 40% good or excellent results in patients with moderate to severe ulnar neuropathy. Arthroscopic approaches to medial epicondylitis are being developed, but there currently are no reports of the safety or effectiveness of these techniques.[45]

Distal Biceps Ruptures

Epidemiology

Injuries to the distal biceps tendon and its insertion are relatively uncommon, with an incidence of 1.2 per 100,000 patients; however, when they do occur, they result in significant disability.[46] According to the literature, the average age of rupture is 45 to 50 years, and ruptures are more common in men, in the dominant arm, in those who smoke, and in patients who body build or use anabolic steroids.[46-48] It is estimated that distal tendon ruptures represent approximately 3% of all biceps tendon injuries. They typically occur as a single traumatic event involving a sudden eccentric contraction without preceding symptomatology.[47]

Pathophysiology

Multiple mechanisms have been proposed for biceps tendon ruptures. No clear consensus on the exact etiology has emerged, suggesting it is most likely multifactorial in nature. Several authors have proposed that an irregularity of the radial tuberosity or anatomic variants such as bony prominences may be a source of mechanical irritation to the tendon.[49,50] Other authors have suggested that the tendon is weakened secondary to intrasubstance degeneration as revealed in histopathologic specimens showing mucoid degeneration.[51] Seiler et al[52] suggested a vascular cause, reporting a zone of relative hypovascularity approximately 2 cm proximal to the tendon insertion that may lead to attritional degeneration. A combination of local tendon pathology and biomechanical factors seems to be the most likely etiology of tendon failure.

Diagnosis and Evaluation

Patients typically present with a history of sudden anterior elbow pain and possibly a "pop" following an eccentric contraction of the elbow. Along with the sudden pain, they experience immediate weakness of both elbow flexion and supination that often improves as the pain subsides. Patients may notice a marked deformity of the anterior arm as the biceps retracts proximally, resulting in the so-called "Popeye" deformity. After the acute phase of pain, swelling, and weakness subsides, patients often report a dull ache and cramping with physical activities.

Physical examination immediately after injury will reveal swelling and tenderness in the antecubital fossa. Acutely, it is sometimes difficult to assess for a palpable defect secondary to pain and swelling. As the injury becomes more subacute to chronic, examination often reveals an appreciable defect when the bicipital aponeurosis (lacertus fibrosus) is involved in the injury. If no defect is appreciated and the mechanism and history are consistent with distal biceps injury, then a partial tear or an intact lacertus should be suspected. The hook test described by O'Driscoll et al[53] is a helpful diagnostic tool to aid in the diagnosis of distal biceps ruptures. The hook test is performed as follows: The patient is asked to actively supinate the elbow while it is at 90° of flexion. The examiner attempts to hook his or her index finger under the biceps from the lateral side. If the examiner is unable to hook a cordlike structure, it is likely that the biceps has been avulsed from the radial tuberosity. Once the pain subsides, physical examination typically reveals normal motion with notable deficits in supination and elbow flexion strength compared to the contralateral side.

Patient history and physical examination are often all that is necessary to confirm the diagnosis. Plain radiographs are often of little benefit; however, they may reveal an avulsion of the distal insertion or irregularity of the bicipital tuberosity.[54] MRI and ultrasonography are useful adjuncts in chronic or difficult cases in which the history and mechanism are not well known. MRI can be very useful to distinguish between partial and complete ruptures and also to visualize the amount of retraction of the torn tendon.[55]

Treatment

Treatment of distal biceps tendon injuries is based on the timing from injury, the integrity of the tendon, and the patient's expectations and demands. Acute injuries are arbitrarily defined as those occurring within 4 weeks of presentation; chronic injuries are defined as those more than 4 weeks old. Tears can be categorized as partial or complete, with reports of partial tears being much less common than complete tears.[55] Another important factor in determining treatment is the integrity of the bicipital aponeurosis. When it is intact, in theory, proximal migration of the distal tendon and muscle belly may be limited and direct repair may be possible even in the chronic setting.[56] In cases of complete rupture, tendon reattachment should be performed in an expedient fashion once swelling subsides. Chronic cases may require extensive approaches to retrieve the distal biceps tendon and release adhesions. When chronic retraction results in an inability to bring the tendon to the bicipital tuberosity without undue tension, an interpositional graft may be necessary.

Surgical management has become the standard of care for complete distal biceps tendon ruptures and for partial ruptures that fail to improve completely with nonsurgical care. Although early studies showed normal function and early return to work with nonsurgical treatment, numerous studies have since demonstrated that anatomic repair results in improved strength and function.[57-59] The current recommendation is that nonsurgical management of complete tendon ruptures should be reserved for elderly patients or those who have a sedentary lifestyle or are not medically fit for surgery. It is crucial to emphasize to these patients that chronic pain and weakness of elbow flexion and supination may occur.

Multiple techniques have been developed for the repair of distal biceps tendon ruptures. These have been grouped into techniques involving two incisions and those performed through a single incision. Early techniques involved an extensile anterior approach with direct reinsertion or reattachment of the avulsed tendon to the tuberosity or the brachialis. This resulted in numerous reports of radial nerve injury. To avoid risk to the nerve during exposure, Boyd and Anderson[60] developed a two-incision technique in 1961 in which they used a secondary posterolateral incision to eliminate the need for extensive dissection in the antecubital fossa. Although this technique did lower the risk of neurovascular injury, the outcomes of repair were complicated by the development of radioulnar synostosis and heterotopic ossification in some cases.[61] To diminish the subperiosteal dissection that was thought to contribute to the ossification seen in the Boyd-Anderson technique, Morrey et al[62] modified the posterolateral approach to a muscle-splitting technique through the common extensor tendons. This technique has been validated by multiple authors with regard to restoration of strength and motion and return to activities including sport.[47,58,63,64]

More recently, there has been a renewed interest in single-incision techniques secondary to the advent of new technologies for tendon fixation, including suture anchors, interference screws, and cortical button techniques. The technique for a single incision is similar to the two-incision technique with regard to tendon retrieval and preparation. After the tendon and tuberosity have been visualized and prepared, the tendon is secured using one of several methods. Suture anchors may be placed directly into the tendon attachment site; these are preferred by many surgeons because they are easy to use, the products are familiar, and outcomes are reliably good to excellent.[65,66] Mazzocca et al[67,68] has recently described two techniques using an interference screw. One uses an interference screw in isolation. The other incorporates a cortical button device on the opposite cortex in addition to the interference screw. In an application first described by Bain et al,[69] Greenberg et al[70] evaluated the use of an EndoButton (Smith & Nephew, Andover, MA) in isolation with regard to both clinical and biomechanical results and showed excellent results, with a higher pull-out strength than bone tunnels or suture anchors. Repair of the distal biceps using the EndoButton and endoscopic visualization has even been reported.[71]

Complications have been reported for both the single- and two-incision techniques. As mentioned previously, the main concern with the two-incision technique is the risk of heterotopic ossification and possible radioulnar synostosis, but this complication has also been reported in single-incision techniques using an EndoButton.[72] Both techniques put the anterior neurovascular structures at risk, and there are multiple reports of injury using either technique. The lateral antebrachial cutaneous nerve and the posterior interosseous nerve are the two structures most commonly involved.[48] Fortunately, these injuries are usually traction-related and transient in nature and may be minimized by meticulous attention to technique and forearm position during surgery.

Excellent outcomes can be achieved with either single- or two-incision techniques, with most studies showing little functional difference between the two. **Table 3** summarizes several recent comparative articles.[73-75]

Postoperatively, patients are typically immobilized for a short period to allow skin healing. Traditionally, patients were immobilized for prolonged periods to allow soft-tissue healing to the tuberosity. With the advent of more secure fixation techniques, however, postoperative protocols allowing early protected range of motion have been shown to be safe and effective.[76]

Triceps Ruptures

Epidemiology

Injuries to the distal triceps are extremely uncommon and may be the rarest of all tendon injuries about the elbow, representing fewer than 1% of problems reported in the literature. In a retrospective study looking over a 20-year period at a major referral center, only 22 patients with 23 injuries were identified who required surgical treatment of a distal triceps rupture.[77] In this same study, 10 of the 23 triceps ruptures were initially misdiagnosed, likely secondary to the infrequency with which this injury is seen. This injury occurs more often in males than in females, at a ratio of approximately 2:1.[78,79] Although these injuries have been reported across all ages, patients in the largest study group to date

Table 3: Surgical Management of Distal Biceps Ruptures

Authors	Study Design	Treatment	Results
El-Hawary et al[73]	Prospective cohort 19 patients	Single vs two incisions	Earlier recovery and lower complication rate with two incisions
Johnson et al[74]	Retrospective review 26 patients	Single vs two incisions	95% satisfaction both groups Slightly improved strength and endurance with two incisions but not statistically significant
Chaven et al[75]	Systematic review Level IV	Single vs two incisions	Increased unsatisfactory results with two-incision technique Loss of rotation motion and strength

had an average age of 47 years at the time of injury.[77] Most injuries occur in otherwise healthy patients; however, associations have been found with anabolic steroid use, renal osteodystrophy, and metabolic bone disease.[54]

Diagnosis and Evaluation

Tendon disruption typically occurs at the tendo-osseous junction as a result of a sudden eccentric contraction, most commonly associated with trauma such as a fall on an outstretched hand. Acutely, physical examination reveals posterior elbow pain, swelling, triceps weakness, and a palpable defect in some cases. As mentioned previously, because of the rarity of this injury, the diagnosis is often missed at initial presentation, leading to a delay in surgical treatment.[80,81] Radiographs will occasionally show intratendinous calcification or possibly a bony "fleck sign," which can be seen with tendinous avulsions. Plain radiographs can also rule out associated injuries such as radial head fractures that have been associated with triceps tendon avulsions.[82] In difficult cases or where partial versus complete tearing cannot be differentiated, MRI can be confirmatory.

Treatment

As with complete biceps tendon ruptures, the current recommendation for most complete acute triceps ruptures is acute surgical repair; for chronic injuries, repair is recommended versus reconstruction. Nonsurgical management is reserved for patients with partial ruptures who have maintained most of their extension strength and for those patients with complete ruptures who are not medically fit for surgery.

Multiple techniques have been described in the literature for acute repair and chronic reconstruction. In patients with a significant bony avulsion, fixation of the bone fragment and attached tendon is recommended.[83] When the tendo-osseous attachment is disrupted, primary attachment through drill holes placed in the olecranon is recommended.[77,78] Unlike biceps tendon avulsions, in which retraction is common in the chronic setting, retraction is typically not found in triceps ruptures, so these often can be repaired as primary or acute injuries.[54] For chronic cases with significant tendon retraction, reconstructive techniques using allograft, autograft, and local muscle and fascial augmentation have been described.[77,78] Postoperatively, the elbow is typically immobilized in midflexion for 2 to 4 weeks, with gradual progression from passive to active motion over a 4- to 6-week period.

Elbow Osteoarthritis
Epidemiology

Although not directly related to sports activity in the mature athlete, primary OA of the elbow can have detrimental effects on performance secondary to pain and stiffness. Elbow OA affects less than 2% of the population. It is more common in men (4:1 ratio of males to females), presents at an average age of 50 years, and has been associated with a history of strenuous work, heavy lifting, and hand dominance.[84,85] Unlike other joints, the elbow affected by primary OA demonstrates relative maintenance of the articular surfaces and joint space. Elbow OA is better characterized by hypertrophic osteophyte formation, capsular contracture, and degeneration primarily found within the radiocapitellar joint laterally that may or may not progress medially.[86,87] Secondary elbow OA has multiple causes, including, but not limited to, trauma, rheumatoid arthritis, osteochondritis dissecans, and synovial chondromatosis. Primary elbow OA and posterior impingement are discussed here.

Diagnosis and Evaluation

Primary elbow OA typically presents in an insidious manner, with patients reporting pain and stiffness with a loss of terminal extension. Up to 50% of patients have mechanical symptoms such as painful catching or locking secondary to loose osteochondral fragments.[88,89] The arc of motion is invariably affected, with mechanical blocks at the extremes of motion secondary to hypertrophic osteophyte formation at the anterior coracoid process and the posterior olecranon fossa, as well as capsular contractures.[88,90]

Physical examination can reveal crepitus, pain at the extremes of motion, and effusion. A thorough neurovascular examination, especially of the ulnar nerve, is important, as ulnar neuropathy has been found in up to 55% of patients presenting for ulnohumeral arthroplasty.[89,90]

The radiographic workup should include standard AP, lateral, and oblique views, which will often reveal loose bodies; osteophyte formation, most commonly at the coronoid process and olecranon fossa; and relative preservation of the ulnohumeral joint space.[91] In more advanced cases, radiocapitellar changes may be identified as well.[88,92] CT may serve as a useful adjunctive study in preoperative planning because it can further localize and define the presence of loose bodies and osteophytes in areas not well visualized by plain radiographs, such as the coronoid fossa, olecranon fossa, and medial gutter.

Treatment

Nonsurgical management of elbow OA consists of medical treatment, including NSAIDs and occasional intra-articular corticosteroid injections, activity modification, and physical therapy. Viscosupplementation with sodium hyaluronan has been found to be effective in the short term (<3 months); however, further studies are needed to determine its role in elbow OA, and it should be noted that viscosupplementation is not currently approved by the US Food and Drug Administration (FDA) for use in elbow OA.[93] Although activity modification may eliminate symptoms in most patients, this is difficult to maintain in the active lifestyle of the mature athlete. Formal physical therapy is not typically required, although a home exercise program focusing on maintenance of range of motion and strength is recommended.

Surgical management is indicated for patients in whom a course of nonsurgical management has failed and in whom disability has adversely affected quality of life from a work or sport perspective. Multiple surgical options exist, which can be broadly categorized into joint-preserving and joint-resurfacing procedures. Joint-preserving treatment options include open joint débridement and ulnohumeral arthroplasty and arthroscopic joint débridement with capsular release. Joint-resurfacing options include interposition arthroplasty and replacement arthroplasty. Because activity restrictions are required after joint resurfacing procedures, this chapter focuses on joint-preserving procedures, which allow mature athletes to return to participation in sports.

Open Joint Débridement and Ulnohumeral Arthroplasty

Open joint débridement and ulnohumeral arthroplasty is indicated for young, active patients whose primary symptom is loss of motion and impingement pain at the extremes of motion. Multiple approaches have been described to address both the capsular pathology and osteophyte formation. Some authors advocate a medial or lateral incision to address the anterior pathology; however, a second incision is often needed to gain access to the posterior and opposite side of the joint.[90,92] Others have suggested a single posterior approach with the development of medial and lateral musculocutane-

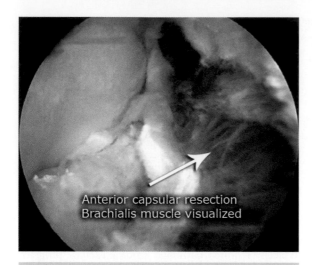

Figure 4   Arthroscopic view of the anterior compartment of an elbow with OA after removal of osteophytes and anterior capsular resection.

ous flaps and an anterior capsulotomy.[88,89] The Outerbridge-Kashiwagi procedure is another surgical option in which a posterior approach is used along with trephination of the olecranon and coronoid fossa to gain access to the anterior osteophytes.[94] Regardless of approach, multiple studies have proven that good to excellent results can be achieved with these techniques. Antuña et al[89] achieved good to excellent results in 74% of their patients followed for a mean of 6.7 years and were able to improve the average arc of motion from 79° to 101°. Phillips et al[95] reported 85% good to excellent results as determined by Disabilities of the Arm, Shoulder and Hand (DASH) scores at a mean 6.3 years of follow-up. Although clinical success has been documented by these and other studies, radiographic signs of recurrence have been found in 50% to 100% of patients followed for 10 years or more.[92,95] The clinical significance of these radiographic findings is unknown, with most patients reporting continued improvements in pain and function despite recurrence of flexion contractures and osteophyte formation.[96]

Arthroscopic Osteocapsular Arthroplasty

The surgical indications for and goals of arthroscopic management of primary elbow OA are identical to those for open procedures. The technique of elbow arthroscopy and portal placement has been well described by multiple authors, but it remains a very technically demanding procedure requiring experience in advanced arthroscopic techniques. An arthroscopic approach has several advantages over open procedures, including improved visualization of the entire joint surface, less soft-tissue trauma, decreased postoperative pain, and potentially faster recovery.[97] In spite of clinical success with arthroscopic techniques, complications remain, with injuries to radial, median, and ulnar nerves all having been reported.[98,99]

Arthroscopic débridement for the osteoarthritic elbow should address all offending pathology, including capsular contractures, osteophyte formation, and loose bodies. In patients with a prominent flexion contracture, the procedure should begin within the anterior compartment, with removal of osteophytes and anterior capsular resection[97] (**Figure 4**). The median nerve is the structure at greatest risk, but the risk of injury can be diminished with the use of retractors placed through accessory portals.[37] Simultaneously, the olecranon and olecranon fossa should be assessed for osteophyte formation, and these should be removed as needed. The ulnar nerve should be protected during posterior and posteriomedial procedures with retractors placed via accessory portals.[37] Upon completion of the procedure, final range of motion should be assessed intraoperatively, and a thorough neurovascular examination should be performed in the recovery area. Postoperatively, maintenance of range of motion and adequate pain control are extremely important for clinical success. Several authors advocate the use of continuous passive motion or even static or dynamic splints in addition to an aggressive physical therapy protocol to maintain range of motion.[97,100]

Multiple authors have shown favorable outcomes with arthroscopic osteocapsular arthroplasty. **Table 4** provides a summary of their results.[101-104]

In patients in whom open and arthroscopic treatment for OA of the elbow is unsuccessful, either interpositional arthroplasty or total elbow arthroplasty (TEA) may be considered. When considering these options in the active, mature athlete, the indications to perform these procedures should be carefully scrutinized. The results for interpositional arthroplasty have shown some success in posttraumatic OA, but they are

Table 4: Arthroscopic Management of Elbow Osteoarthritis

Authors	Study Design	Treatment	Results
Savoie et al[101]	Case series 24 patients	Arthroscopic modification of the Outerbridge-Kashiwagi technique	92% good to excellent results 81° improvement in arc of motion
Kim and Shin[102]	Case series 63 patients	Arthroscopic débridement	92% success rate Improved ROM: 79° preoperatively, 121° postoperatively
Adams et al[103]	Retrospective review 41 patients	Arthroscopic osteophyte resection and capsular release	81% good to excellent results Improved pain, motion, and functional scores (MEPS 67.5 preoperatively, 84.4 postoperatively)
Cohen et al[104]	Nonrandomized trial 44 patients	Open vs arthroscopic débridement and capsular release	No significant difference between groups

ROM = range of motion, MEPS = Mayo Elbow Performance Score.

less predictable in primary OA. TEA can provide dramatic pain relief and improved function, but it may result in early loosening and excess wear in the more active patient.[105]

Ulnar Nerve Neuropathy

Ulnar nerve neuropathy is the second most common nerve compression syndrome in the upper extremity, after carpal tunnel syndrome. The ulnar nerve is the most commonly involved nerve around the elbow. Cubital tunnel syndrome is commonly seen in association with other conditions about the elbow, especially medial epicondylitis and elbow OA, and it is important to recognize the presence of this pathology as it can affect the overall outcome when treating these other conditions. A complete review of the pathology and treatment of ulnar nerve compression is beyond the scope of this chapter; however, a few details with regard to the diagnosis and management of ulnar nerve neuropathy in the mature athlete deserve mention.

Diagnosis and Evaluation

The workup for ulnar nerve compression at the elbow begins with a thorough history and physical examination. Patients typically present with reports of either medial elbow pain or parasthesias involving the small finger and ulnar half of the ring finger. Patients often report nocturnal pain and paresthesias. They may also report weakness with grip or hand function secondary to hand intrinsic involvement. A careful evaluation should be performed to rule out other pathologies that may mimic ulnar nerve neuropathy, such as cervical radiculopathy (C8-T1), brachial plexopathy, thoracic outlet syndrome, or ulnar nerve entrapment distally at the wrist. Examination of the extremity should include inspection for nerve subluxation with elbow range of motion. A Tinel sign and an elbow flexion test reproducing the symptoms should be performed as part of the physical examination. A complete sensory examination should be performed distally to include slowly adapting fibers (static two-point discrimination and Semmes-Weinstein monofilament test), quickly adapting fibers (moving two-point discrimination and vibratory testing), and nerve density tests (static and moving two-point discrimination).[106] A complete motor examination should be performed, as well as testing for ulnarly innervated extrinsic (flexor digitorum profundus to the ring and little fingers) and intrinsic musculature. Although ulnar nerve compression is primarily diagnosed through history and physical examination, electrodiagnostic studies can be confirmatory. In cases of compression neuropathy, the studies will show increased distal latency times and decreased conduction velocity across the cubital tunnel.

Treatment

Nonsurgical management is indicated for patients with mild or moderate symptoms and no signs of distal atrophy. Options include NSAIDs, protective padding, ergonomic changes in the home and work environment, and night splinting to limit elbow flexion. Surgical intervention is warranted if symptoms do not respond adequately to nonsurgical management and for patients in whom EMG indicates muscle wasting or signs of significant compression. Multiple techniques have been described to surgically manage cubital tunnel syndrome, including in situ decompression, medial epicondylectomy, and subcutaneous or submuscular transposition. All of the techniques have advantages and disadvantages and have been supported in the literature, with no clear distinction as to which is most effective. Several studies have compared in situ decompression with transposition techniques and recommended simple decompression because it offers similar results, is less technically demanding, and has fewer complications.[107-109] Regardless of the technique used, a key principle is to achieve complete decompression at all potential sites of entrapment or pressure, making sure the nerve is tension free and glides freely throughout the arc of elbow motion.

Summary

Elbow disorders affecting the mature athlete are most often the result of tendon and articular surface degeneration from repetitive use. Most chronic conditions can be managed effectively with a nonsurgical program including rehabilitation, activity modification, and medical treatments. Newer biologic treatment modalities are currently under investigation and will hopefully prove to be beneficial. Lateral epicondylitis and mild OA are very common chronic conditions in the mature athlete. Surgical management with open and arthroscopic techniques is effective in restoring function and mobility to the elbow.

References

1. Runge F: Zur Genese und Behandlung des Schreibekrampfes. *Berlin Klin Wochenschr* 1873;10:245-248.

2. Nirschl RP, Pettrone FA: Tennis elbow: The surgical treatment of lateral epicondylitis. *J Bone Joint Surg Am* 1979;61(6A):832-839.

3. Gruchow HW, Pelletier D: An epidemiologic study of tennis elbow: Incidence, recurrence, and effectiveness of prevention strategies. *Am J Sports Med* 1979;7(4):234-238.

4. Nirschl RP, Ashman ES: Elbow tendinopathy: Tennis elbow. *Clin Sports Med* 2003;22(4):813-836.

5. Haahr JP, Andersen JH: Physical and psychosocial risk factors for lateral epicondylitis: A population based case-referent study. *Occup Environ Med* 2003;60(5):322-329.

6. Shiri R, Viikari-Juntura E, Varonen H, Heliövaara M: Prevalence and determinants of lateral and medial epicondylitis: A population study. *Am J Epidemiol* 2006;164(11):1065-1074.

7. Jobe FW, Ciccotti MG: Lateral and medial epicondylitis of the elbow. *J Am Acad Orthop Surg* 1994;2(1):1-8.

8. Kelley JD, Lombardo SJ, Pink M, Perry J, Giangarra CE: Electromyographic and cinematographic analysis of elbow function in tennis players with lateral epicondylitis. *Am J Sports Med* 1994;22(3):359-363.

9. Jozsa LG, Kannus P: Overuse injuries of tendons, in Jozsa LG, Kannus P, eds: *Human Tendons: Anatomy, Physiology, and Pathology*. Champaign, IL, Human Kinetics, 1997, pp 164-253.

10. Regan W, Wold LE, Coonrad R, Morrey BF: Microscopic histopathology of chronic refractory lateral epicondylitis. *Am J Sports Med* 1992;20(6):746-749.

11. Kraushaar BS, Nirschl RP: Tendinosis of the elbow (tennis elbow): Clinical features and findings of histological, immunohistochemical, and electron microscopy studies. *J Bone Joint Surg Am* 1999;81(2):259-278.

12. Dorf ER, Chhabra AB, Golish SR, McGinty JL, Pannunzio ME: Effect of elbow position on grip strength in the evaluation of lateral epicondylitis. *J Hand Surg Am* 2007;32(6):882-886.

13. Potter HG, Hannafin JA, Morwessel RM, DiCarlo EF, O'Brien SJ, Altchek DW: Lateral epicondylitis:

Correlation of MR imaging, surgical, and histopathologic findings. *Radiology* 1995;196(1):43-46.

14. Calfee RP, Patel A, DaSilva MF, Akelman E: Management of lateral epicondylitis: Current concepts. *J Am Acad Orthop Surg* 2008;16(1):19-29.

15. Connell D, Burke F, Coombes P, et al: Sonographic examination of lateral epicondylitits. *ARJ Am J Roentgenol* 2001;176(3):777-782.

16. Smidt N, Lewis M, van der Windt DA, Hay EM, Bouter LM, Croft P: Lateral epicondylitis in general practice: Course and prognostic indicators of outcome. *J Rheumatol* 2006;33(10):2053-2059.

17. Stull PA, Jokl P: Comparison of diflunisal and naproxen in the treatment of tennis elbow. *Clin Ther* 1986;9(Suppl C):62-66.

18. Hay EM, Paterson SM, Lewis M, Hosie G, Croft P: Pragmatic randomised controlled trial of local corticosteroid injection and naproxen for treatment of lateral epicondylitis of elbow in primary care. *BMJ* 1999;319(7215):964-968.

19. Smidt N, van der Windt DA, Assendelft WJ, Devillé WL, Korthals-de Bos IB, Bouter LM: Corticosteroid injections, physiotherapy, or a wait-and-see policy for lateral epicondylitis: A randomised controlled trial. *Lancet* 2002;359(9307):657-662.

20. Mishra A, Pavelko T: Treatment of chronic elbow tendinosis with buffered platelet-rich plasma. *Am J Sports Med* 2006;34(11):1774-1778.

21. Labelle H, Guibert R, The University of Montreal Orthopaedic Research Group: Efficacy of diclofenac in lateral epicondylitis of the elbow also treated with immobilization. *Arch Fam Med* 1997;6(3):257-262.

22. Green S, Buchbinder R, Barnsley L, et al: Non-steroidal anti-inflammatory drugs (NSAIDs) for treating lateral elbow pain in adults. *Cochrane Database Syst Rev* 2002;(2):CD003686.

23. Smidt N, Assendelft WJ, van der Windt DA, Hay EM, Buchbinder R, Bouter LM: Corticosteroid injections for lateral epicondylitis: A systematic review. *Pain* 2002;96(1-2):23-40.

24. Hayton MJ, Santini AJ, Hughes PJ, Frostick SP, Trail IA, Stanley JK: Botulinum toxin injection in the treatment of tennis elbow: A double-blind, randomized, controlled, pilot study. *J Bone Joint Surg Am* 2005;87(3):503-507.

25. Wong SM, Hui AC, Tong PY, Poon DW, Yu E, Wong LK: Treatment of lateral epicondylitis with

botulinum toxin: A randomized, double-blind, placebo-controlled trial. *Ann Intern Med* 2005;143(11):793-797.

26. Placzek R, Drescher W, Deuretzbacher G, Hempfing A, Meiss AL: Treatment of chronic radial epicondylitis with botulinum toxin A: A double-blind, placebo-controlled, randomized multicenter study. *J Bone Joint Surg Am* 2007;89(2):255-260.

27. Edwards SG, Calandruccio JH: Autologus blood injections for refractory lateral epicondylitis. *J Hand Surg Am* 2003;28(2):272-278.

28. Connell DA, Ali KE, Ahmad M, Lambert S, Corbett S, Curtis M: Ultrasound-guided autologous blood injection for tennis elbow. *Skeletal Radiol* 2006;35(6):371-377.

29. Buchbinder R, Green SE, Youd JM, Assendelft WJ, Barnsley L, Smidt N: Systematic review of the efficacy and safety of shock wave therapy for lateral elbow pain. *J Rheumatol* 2006;33(7):1351-1363.

30. Croisier JL, Foidart-Dessalle M, Tinant F, Crielaard JM, Forthomme B: An isokinetic eccentric programme for the management of chronic lateral epicondylar tendinopathy. *Br J Sports Med* 2007;41(4):269-275.

31. Struijs PA, Smidt N, Arola H, van Dijk CN, Buchbinder R, Assendelft WJ: Orthotic devices for tennis elbow: A systematic review. *Br J Gen Pract* 2001;51(472):924-929.

32. Baker CL Jr, Baker CL III: Long-term follow-up of arthroscopic treatment of lateral epicondylitis. *Am J Sports Med* 2008;36(2):254-260.

33. Szabo SJ, Savoie FH III, Field LD, Ramsey JR, Hosemann CD: Tendinosis of the extensor carpi radialis brevis: An evaluation of three methods of operative treatment. *J Shoulder Elbow Surg* 2006;15(6):721-727.

34. Dunkow PD, Jatti M, Muddu BN: A comparison of open and percutaneous techniques in the surgical treatment of tennis elbow. *J Bone Joint Surg Br* 2004;86(5):701-704.

35. Lo MY, Safran MR: Surgical treatment of lateral epicondylitis: A systematic review. *Clin Orthop Relat Res* 2007;463:98-106.

36. Sodha S, Nagda SH, Sennett DJ: Heterotopic ossification in a throwing athlete after elbow arthroscopy. *Arthroscopy* 2006;22(7):802, e1-e3.

37. Kelly EW, Morrey BF, O'Driscoll SW: Complications of elbow arthroscopy. *J Bone Joint Surg Am* 2001; 83(1):25-34.

38. Leach RE, Miller JK: Lateral and medial epicondylitis of the elbow. *Clin Sports Med* 1987;6(2):259-272.

39. Nirschl RP: Sports and overuse injuries to the elbow: Muscle and tendon trauma, in Morrey BF, ed: *The Elbow and Its Disorders*, ed 2. Philadelphia, PA, WB Saunders, 1985, pp 537-552.

40. Vangsness CT Jr, Jobe FW: Surgical treatment of medial epicondylitis: Results in 35 elbows. *J Bone Joint Surg Br* 1991;73(3):409-411.

41. Pienimäki TT, Siira PT, Vanharanta H: Chronic medial and lateral epicondylitis: A comparison of pain, disability, and function. *Arch Phys Med Rehabil* 2002; 83(3):317-321.

42. Stahl S, Kaufman T: The efficacy of an injection of steroids for medial epicondylitis: A prospective study of sixty elbows. *J Bone Joint Surg Am* 1997;79(11):1648-1652.

43. Kurvers H, Verhaar J: The results of operative treatment of medial epicondylitis. *J Bone Joint Surg Am* 1995;77(9):1374-1379.

44. Gabel GT, Morrey BF: Operative treatment of medical epicondylitis: Influence of concomitant ulnar neuropathy at the elbow. *J Bone Joint Surg Am* 1995; 77(7):1065-1069.

45. Porcellini G, Paladini P, Campi F, Merolla G: Arthroscopic neurolysis of the ulnar nerve at the elbow. *Chir Organi Mov* 2005;90(2):191-200.

46. Safran MR, Graham SM: Distal biceps tendon ruptures: incidence, demographics, and the effect of smoking. *Clin Orthop Relat Res* 2002;(404): 275-283.

47. D'Alessandro DF, Shields CL Jr, Tibone JE, Chandler RW: Repair of distal biceps tendon ruptures in athletes. *Am J Sports Med* 1993;21(1):114-119.

48. Mazzocca AD, Spang JT, Arciero RA: Distal biceps rupture. *Orthop Clin North Am* 2008;39(2):237-249.

49. Morrey BF: Injuries of the flexors of the elbow: Biceps in tendon injury, in Morrey BF, ed: *The Elbow and Its Disorders*, ed 3. Philadelphia, PA, WB Saunders, 2000, pp 468-478.

50. Davis WM, Yassine Z: An etiological factor in tear of the distal tendon of the biceps brachii; report of two cases. *J Bone Joint Surg Am* 1956;38-A(6):1365-1368.

51. Kannus P, Józsa L: Histopathological changes preceding spontaneous rupture of a tendon: A controlled study of 891 patients. *J Bone Joint Surg Am* 1991;73(10):1507-1525.

52. Seiler JG III, Parker LM, Chamberland PD, Sherbourne GM, Carpenter WA: The distal biceps tendon: Two potential mechanisms involved in its rupture: arterial supply and mechanical impingement. *J Shoulder Elbow Surg* 1995;4(3):149-156.

53. O'Driscoll SW, Goncalves LB, Dietz P: The hook test for distal biceps tendon avulsion. *Am J Sports Med* 2007;35(11):1865-1869.

54. Vidal AF, Drakos MC, Allen AA: Biceps tendon and triceps tendon injuries. *Clin Sports Med* 2004;23(4): 707-722.

55. Rokito AS, McLaughlin JA, Gallagher MA, Zuckerman JD: Partial rupture of the distal biceps tendon. *J Shoulder Elbow Surg* 1996;5(1):73-75.

56. Aldridge JW, Bruno RJ, Strauch RJ, Rosenwasser MP: Management of acute and chronic biceps tendon rupture. *Hand Clin* 2000;16(3):497-503.

57. Pearl ML, Bessos K, Wong K: Strength deficits related to distal biceps tendon rupture and repair: A case report. *Am J Sports Med* 1998;26(2):295-296.

58. Baker BE, Bierwagen D: Rupture of the distal tendon of the biceps brachii: Operative versus non-operative treatment. *J Bone Joint Surg Am* 1985;67(3):414-417.

59. Bell RH, Wiley WB, Noble JS, Kuczynski DJ: Repair of distal biceps brachii tendon ruptures. *J Shoulder Elbow Surg* 2000;9(3):223-226.

60. Boyd HB, Anderson LB: A method for reinsertion of the distal biceps brachii tendon. *J Bone Joint Surg Am* 1961;43:1041-1043.

61. Failla JM, Amadio PC, Morrey BF, Beckenbaugh RD: Proximal radioulnar synostosis after repair of distal biceps brachii rupture by the two-incision technique: Report of four cases. *Clin Orthop Relat Res* 1990;(253): 133-136.

62. Morrey BF, Askew LJ, An KN, Dobyns JH: Rupture of the distal tendon of the biceps brachii: A biomechanical study. *J Bone Joint Surg Am* 1985;67(3):418-421.

63. Karunakar MA, Cha P, Stern PJ: Distal biceps ruptures: A followup of Boyd and Anderson repair. *Clin Orthop Relat Res* 1999;(363):100-107.

64. Davison BL, Engber WD, Tigert LJ: Long term evaluation of repaired distal biceps brachii tendon ruptures. *Clin Orthop Relat Res* 1996;(333):186-191.

65. Sotereanos DG, Pierce TD, Varitimidis SE: A simplified method for repair of distal biceps tendon ruptures. *J Shoulder Elbow Surg* 2000;9(3):227-233.

66. Lintner S, Fischer T: Repair of the distal biceps tendon using suture anchors and an anterior approach. *Clin Orthop Relat Res* 1996;(322):116-119.

67. Mazzocca AD, Alberta FG, ElAttrache NS, Romeo AA: Single incision technique using an interference screw for the repair of distal biceps tendon ruptures. *Oper Tech Sports Med* 2003;11(1):36-41.

68. Mazzocca AD, Bicos J, Arciero RA, et al: Repair of distal biceps tendon ruptures using a combined anatomic interference screw and cortical button. *Tech Shoulder Elbow Surg* 2005;6(2):108-115.

69. Bain GI, Prem H, Heptinstall RJ, Verhellen R, Paix D: Repair of distal biceps tendon rupture: A new technique using the Endobutton. *J Shoulder Elbow Surg* 2000;9(2):120-126.

70. Greenberg JA, Fernandez JJ, Wang T, Turner C: EndoButton-assisted repair of distal biceps tendon ruptures. *J Shoulder Elbow Surg* 2003;12(5):484-490.

71. Sharma S, MacKay G: Endoscopic repair of distal biceps tendon using an EndoButton. *Arthroscopy* 2005;21(7):897.

72. Agrawal V, Stinson MJ: Case report: Heterotopic ossification after repair of distal biceps tendon rupture utilizing a single-incision Endobutton technique. *J Shoulder Elbow Surg* 2005;14(1):107-109.

73. El-Hawary R, Macdermid JC, Faber KJ, Patterson SD, King GJ: Distal biceps tendon repair: Comparison of surgical techniques. *J Hand Surg Am* 2003;28(3):496-502.

74. Johnson TS, Johnson DC, Shindle MK, et al: One-versus two-incision technique for distal biceps tendon repair. *HSS J* 2008;4(2):117-122.

75. Chavan PR, Duquin TR, Bisson LJ: Repair of the ruptured distal biceps tendon: A systematic review. *Am J Sports Med* 2008;36(8):1618-1624.

76. Cheung EV, Lazarus M, Taranta M: Immediate range of motion after distal biceps tendon repair. *J Shoulder Elbow Surg* 2005;14(5):516-518.

77. van Riet RP, Morrey BF, Ho E, O'Driscoll SW: Surgical treatment of distal triceps ruptures. *J Bone Joint Surg Am* 2003;85(10):1961-1967.

78. Morrey BF: Rupture of the triceps tendon, in Morrey BF, ed: *The Elbow and Its Disorders*, ed 3. Philadelphia, PA, WB Saunders Co, 2000, pp 479-484.

79. Strauch RJ: Biceps and triceps injuries of the elbow. *Orthop Clin North Am* 1999;30(1):95-107.

80. Pantazopoulos T, Exarchou E, Stavrou Z, Hartofilakidis-Garofalidis G: Avulsion of the triceps tendon. *J Trauma* 1975;15(9):827-829.

81. Tarsney FF: Rupture and avulsion of the triceps. *Clin Orthop Relat Res* 1972;83:177-183.

82. Levy M, Fishel RE, Stern GM: Triceps tendon avulsion with or without fracture of the radial head—a rare injury? *J Trauma* 1978;18(9):677-679.

83. Viegas SF: Avulsion of the triceps tendon. *Orthop Rev* 1990;19(6):533-536.

84. Ortner DJ: Description and classification of degenerative bone changes in the distal joint surfaces of the humerus. *Am J Phys Anthropol* 1968;28(2):139-155.

85. Stanley D: Prevalence and etiology of symptomatic elbow osteoarthritis. *J Shoulder Elbow Surg* 1994;3:386-389.

86. Goodfellow JW, Bullough PG: The pattern of ageing of the articular cartilage of the elbow joint. *J Bone Joint Surg Br* 1967;49(1):175-181.

87. Murato H, Ikuta Y, Murakami T: Anatomic investigation of the elbow joint with specific reference to the aging of the articular cartilage. *J Shoulder Elbow Surg* 1993;2:175-181.

88. Morrey BF: Primary degenerative arthritis of the elbow: Treatment by ulnohumeral arthroplasty. *J Bone Joint Surg Br* 1992;74(3):409-413.

89. Antuña SA, Morrey BF, Adams RA, O'Driscoll SW: Ulnohumeral arthroplasty for primary degenerative arthritis of the elbow: Long-term outcome and complications. *J Bone Joint Surg Am* 2002;84-A(12):2168-2173.

90. Oka Y: Debridement arthroplasty for osteoarthrosis of the elbow: 50 patients followed mean 5 years. *Acta Orthop Scand* 2000;71(2):185-190.

91. Minami M: Roentgenological studies of osteoarthritis of the elbow joint [in Japanese]. *Nippon Seikeigeka Gakkai Zasshi* 1977;51:1223-1236.

92. Wada T, Isogai S, Ishii S, Yamashita T: Débridement arthroplasty for primary osteoarthritis of the elbow. *J Bone Joint Surg Am* 2004;86-A(2):233-241.

93. van Brakel RW, Eygendaal D: Intra-articular injection of hyaluronic acid is not effective for the treatment of post-traumatic osteoarthritis of the elbow. *Arthroscopy* 2006;22(11):1199-1203.

94. Kashiwagi D: Intra-articular changes of the osteoarthritic elbow, especially about the fossa olecranon. *Jpn Orthop Assn* 1978;52:1367-1382.

95. Phillips NJ, Ali A, Stanley D: Treatment of primary degenerative arthritis of the elbow by ulnohumeral arthroplasty: A long-term follow-up. *J Bone Joint Surg Br* 2003;85(3):347-350.

96. Gramstad GD, Galatz LM: Management of elbow osteoarthritis. *J Bone Joint Surg Am* 2006;88(2):421-430.

97. Steinmann SP, King GJ, Savoie FH III, American Academy of Orthopaedic Surgeons: Arthroscopic treatment of the arthritic elbow. *J Bone Joint Surg Am* 2005;87(9):2114-2121.

98. Haapaniemi T, Berggren M, Adolfsson L: Complete transection of the median and radial nerves during arthroscopic release of post-traumatic elbow contracture. *Arthroscopy* 1999;15(7):784-787.

99. Hahn M, Grossman JA: Ulnar nerve laceration as a result of elbow arthroscopy. *J Hand Surg Br* 1998;23(1):109.

100. Cheung EV, Adams R, Morrey BF: Primary osteoarthritis of the elbow: Current treatment options. *J Am Acad Orthop Surg* 2008;16(2):77-87.

101. Savoie FH III, Nunley PD, Field LD: Arthroscopic management of the arthritic elbow: Indications, technique, and results. *J Shoulder Elbow Surg* 1999;8(3):214-219.

102. Kim SJ, Shin SJ: Arthroscopic treatment for limitation of motion of the elbow. *Clin Orthop Relat Res* 2000;(375):140-148.

103. Adams JE, Wolff LH III, Merten SM, Steinmann SP: Osteoarthritis of the elbow: Results of arthroscopic osteophyte resection and capsulectomy. *J Shoulder Elbow Surg* 2008;17(1):126-131.

104. Cohen AP, Redden JF, Stanley D: Treatment of osteoarthritis of the elbow: A comparison of open and arthroscopic debridement. *Arthroscopy* 2000;16(7):701-706.

105. Kozak TK, Adams RA, Morrey BF: Total elbow arthroplasty in primary osteoarthritis of the elbow. *J Arthroplasty* 1998;13(7):837-842.

106. Elhassan B, Steinmann SP: Entrapment neuropathy of the ulnar nerve. *J Am Acad Orthop Surg* 2007;15(11):672-681.

107. Bartels RH, Verhagen WI, van der Wilt GJ, Meulstee J, van Rossum LG, Grotenhuis JA: Prospective randomized controlled study comparing simple decompression versus anterior subcutaneous transposition for idiopathic neuropathy of the ulnar nerve at the elbow: Part 1. *Neurosurgery* 2005;56(3):522-530.

108. Nabhan A, Ahlhelm F, Kelm J, Reith W, Schwerdtfeger K, Steudel WI: Simple decompression or subcutaneous anterior transposition of the ulnar nerve for cubital tunnel syndrome. *J Hand Surg Br* 2005;30(5):521-524.

109. Biggs M, Curtis JA: Randomized, prospective study comparing ulnar neurolysis in situ with submuscular transposition. *Neurosurgery* 2006;58(2):296-304.

Chapter 24

Hand and Wrist

Ky Kobayashi, MD
William Hallier, MD

Key Points

- Management of hand and wrist injuries in the growing population of mature athletes can be a challenge and requires a good assessment of sport-specific athletic demands and the degree of impairment incurred by the athlete.
- Common conditions (arthritis, tendinitis, fractures, and neuropathy) occurring in the mature athlete often blur the line between acute injury, overuse, and normal degenerative change.
- Nonsurgical management may be all that is required for the athlete to continue performing well and without symptoms; however, more definitive procedures such as arthroplasty, arthroscopy, and internal fixation are sometimes necessary to alleviate pain and preserve athletic function.

Introduction

Management of hand and wrist injuries in the mature athlete can be challenging and requires a thorough assessment of sport-specific athletic demands and the degree of impairment incurred by the athlete. Nonsurgical management consisting of splints, medications, and hand therapy is beneficial in most cases; however, more definitive procedures are sometimes necessary to alleviate pain and preserve athletic function. This chapter covers common conditions and injuries sustained by athletes in their fourth to sixth decades of life who compete in racquet sports, golf, cycling, and rowing. Many of these conditions can present as a result of participation in a variety of sports, occupational pursuits, and as a normal consequence of aging.

Conditions occurring in the mature athlete often blur the line between acute injury, overuse, and normal degenerative change. Management almost always requires a thoughtful blending of treatment modalities used in the young athlete with those typically reserved for aging patients.

Wrist Arthritis

Arthritis of the hand and wrist is a common condition frequently encountered by surgeons treating mature athletes. Multiple factors play a role in the etiology of hand and wrist arthritis, and it can be related to post-traumatic conditions such as fractures or intercarpal instability. One of the more common causes of wrist arthritis as described by Watson and Ballet[1] is scapholunate advanced collapse (SLAC), which is a progressive

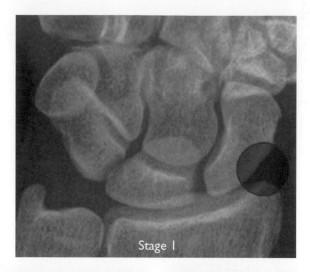

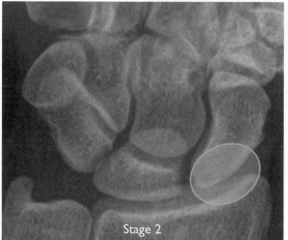

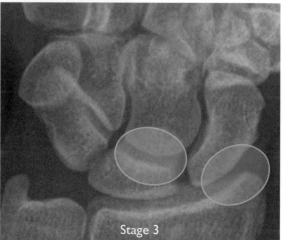

Figure 1   Stages of SLAC wrist degeneration follow a progressive arthritic pattern of degenerative arthritis that starts at the radial styloid (stage 1), involves the entire radioscaphoid articulation (stage 2), and advances to the midcarpal joint (stage 3). (Reproduced with permission from Watson HK, Ballet FL: The SLAC wrist: Scapholunate advanced collapse pattern of degenerative arthritis. *J Hand Surg Am* 1984;9(3):358-365.)

arthritic condition related to scapholunate ligament tears and abnormal loading of the radioscaphoid joint. More than 70% of arthritic wrists demonstrate evidence of SLAC wrist degeneration, with scapholunate ligament injury being the most common and scaphoid nonunion advanced collapse (SNAC) being the second most common.[1-3] Disruption of the ligamentous support of the proximal pole of the scaphoid results in dorsal intercalated segment instability (DISI). This al-

lows abnormal motion and loading stresses across the radioscaphoid joint of the wrist and accelerates degenerative changes. SLAC wrist degeneration progresses from the distal radioscaphoid joint to the midcarpal joint[1] (**Figure 1**).

Patients typically present with dorsal wrist pain and limited painful motion. History may reveal several years of wrist discomfort that has progressively worsened. Radiographs may reveal progression in a classic degen-

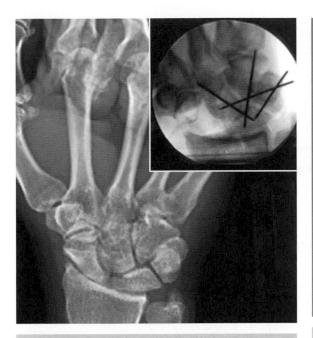

Figure 2   PA radiograph of the wrist of a 50-year-old racquetball player with a stage 3 SLAC wrist after scaphoid excision and four-corner fusion.

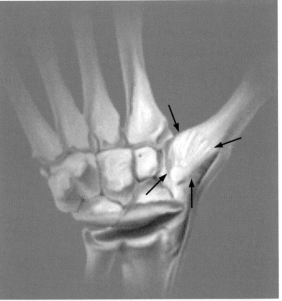

Figure 3   Thumb CMC joint anatomy. (Adapted with permission from Chiavaras MM, Harish S, Oomen G, Popowich T, Wainman B, Bain JR: Sonography of the anterior oblique ligament of the trapeziometacarpal joint: A study of cadavers and asymptomatic volunteers. *Am J Roentgenol* 2010;195(6):W428-434.)

erative pattern. Surgery should be considered only when nonsurgical measures, including activity modification, immobilization, medications, therapy, and steroid injections, have failed. Surgical treatment should be carefully discussed with the mature athlete, especially considering that approximately 50% of motion can be lost with a limited arthrodesis or with a proximal row carpectomy[4-6] (**Figure 2**). Pain reduction and motion preservation should be the goal of any planned intervention and should be considered in the context of the athlete's specific sport. Some SLAC changes may be treated by arthroscopic radial styloidectomy; however, these results may be variable and are indicated only for early stages of degeneration involving the distal radial styloid.[7] Although reports comparing limited arthrodesis and proximal row carpectomy have demonstrated similar subjective and objective outcomes, we tend to favor limited arthrodesis (scaphoidectomy, neutral carpal alignment, and four-corner fusion) for active, higher demand patients.[4-6]

Thumb Carpometacarpal Joint Arthritis

Thumb carpometacarpal (CMC) joint arthritis, also called first CMC joint arthritis or basal joint arthritis, is one of the most common arthritic conditions affecting the mature athlete. The basal joint of the thumb is a semiconstrained joint with three axes of motion and is primarily supported by ligamentous constraints[8] (**Figure 3**). The combination of this inherent mobility and its prominent role in pinch and grip predispose the thumb CMC joint to degeneration that is related to dysfunction of the palmar oblique ligament, which normally prevents dorsal subluxation of the metacarpal on the trapezium.[8]

   With thumb CMC joint arthritis, patients generally report pain localized at the thumb base that is aggravated by grip-intensive sports such as tennis, golf, and rowing.[9] Examination of the thumb CMC joint may

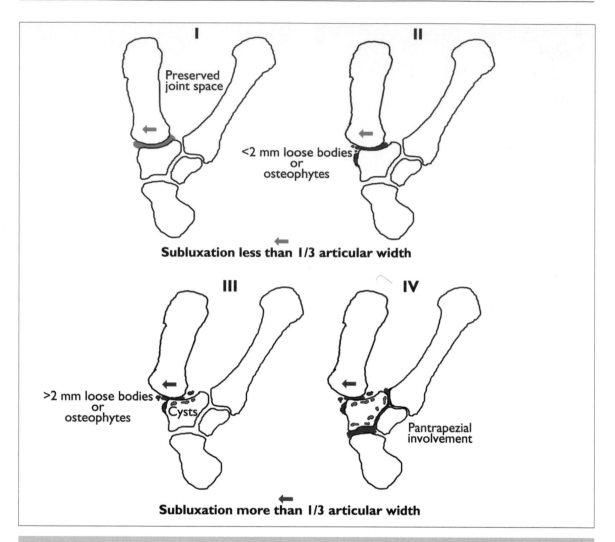

Figure 4 Eaton classification of thumb CMC arthritis. In stage I CMC arthritis, the joint space is maintained or slightly widened secondary to synovitis or joint effusion. Stage II changes include slight joint space narrowing, minimal dorsoradial subluxation, and sclerosis. Stage III is characterized by more arthritic changes. Stage IV disease reveals more extensive pantrapezial arthritic changes. (Adapted from Barron OA, Glickel SZ, Eaton RG: Basal joint arthroplasty of the thumb. J Am Acad Orthop Surg 2000;8(5):314-323.)

reveal a dorsally subluxated metacarpal base with pain and swelling. Provocative testing by axially loading the trapeziometacarpal joint combined with small-arc rotation of the thumb CMC joint (grind test) also elicits discomfort in symptomatic patients.

The Eaton classification, which is the most common radiographic assessment of thumb CMC arthritis, defines stages ranging from early degenerative changes to pantrapezial arthritis and subluxation of the thumb CMC joint[10] (**Figure 4**). Although the Eaton classification is useful in documentating the progress of CMC arthritis, it is less reliable in predicting progression or in correlating the degree of symptoms in any given athlete.[8]

Nonsurgical management of thumb CMC arthritis has had limited study but can be effective early in the

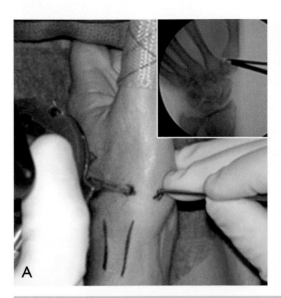
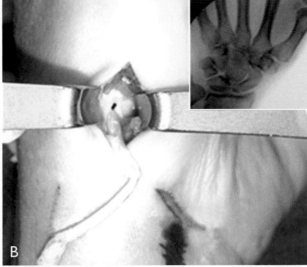

Figure 5   Intraoperative photographs show an arthroscopic partial trapezium resection (**A**) and tendon interposition with palmaris longus autograft (**B**). (Photographs courtesy of Roderick J. Bruno, MD, Exeter, NH.)

course of the disease or in the less symptomatic patient. Splinting, injections, and rest may be all that is required for the athlete to continue performing well and without symptoms.[8] Surgical treatment options for CMC arthritis can be divided into early joint-preserving procedures and those reserved for late disease. Although only case series reports for early stages of CMC joint arthritis are available for review, good results have been reported with arthroscopy (débridement, synovectomy, and thermal shrinkage), volar ligament reconstruction, and metacarpal extension osteotomy.[11] As disease and symptoms progress, surgery is generally aimed at resecting the diseased trapezium partially or completely. This can be accomplished with or without ligament stabilization and with or without spacer interposition[8,11] (**Figure 5**). Interposition of a spacer in the setting of either partial or complete trapeziectomy has been accomplished most commonly by the well-accepted ligament "anchovy" procedure.[8] Randomized prospective studies comparing different techniques described for management of late disease show little difference in outcomes, calling into question whether one surgical option is clearly superior to another.[11] Although there may be some debate on the best surgical option for advanced CMC joint arthritis, CMC joint arthroplasty

will benefit patients in whom nonsurgical treatment has failed.

Proximal Interphalangeal Joint Arthritis

Proximal interphalangeal (PIP) joint disability of the hand can occur secondary to traumatic and nontraumatic arthritis. Advanced disease affecting the ulnar digits impairs grip strength, whereas index finger involvement results in decreased pinch strength. Loss of key pinch and grip strength can result in loss of function and performance in racquet sports and golf. If nonsurgical management consisting of activity modification, hand therapy, and medication fails to relieve significant PIP joint discomfort, surgical intervention may be warranted. Arthrodesis of the PIP joint is acceptable; however, arthroplasty is preferred when feasible, to preserve motion. Arthroplasty techniques include fibrous interposition, volar plate advancement, hinge implants, and semiconstrained prostheses.[12] The best candidate for PIP arthroplasty is the athlete with a painful PIP joint secondary to degenerative or posttraumatic arthritis in one of the ulnar three digits, who has near full extension and 30° to 40° of flexion. When good bone stock,

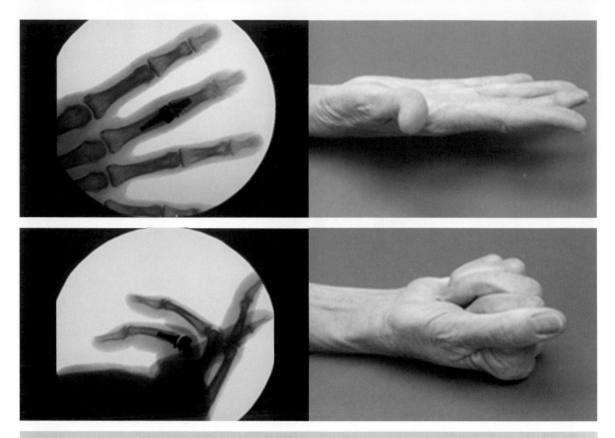

Figure 6   Radiographs and clinical photographs of the hand of a 58-year-old equestrian after PIP joint arthroplasty show the hand in extension (top) and flexion (bottom).

minimal deformity, and a preserved extensor and flexor mechanism are present, the prognosis for eliminating pain and improving motion is good.[13] PIP joint arthrodesis is recommended for the index finger because flexion is not as crucial, strong pinch is necessary, and lateral deviation after PIP joint arthroplasty may occur. Silicone PIP joint arthroplasties demonstrated an average range of motion of 45° to 60°, with approximately 70% of patients obtaining more than 40° of motion.[14] Improved results are obtained in patients with degenerative and posttraumatic arthritis. Although very little information is available for semiconstrained surface replacement arthroplasty, short-term follow-up is encouraging.[13,15]

Johnstone[15] reported on 20 surface replacement arthroplasty PIP joint implants (CoCr/polyethylene) primarily used for osteoarthritis and posttraumatic arthri-

tis. Average follow-up time was 14.6 months, with all patients noting pain reduction and 90% of that subset reporting excellent pain relief. No patient lost motion, and 70% of patients demonstrated an average arc of motion of 73°. Poor results were associated with high levels of early postoperative pain and poor compliance with hand therapy. Although very little information is available for semiconstrained surface replacement arthroplasty, short-term follow-up is encouraging[13] (**Figure 6**).

Distal Radius Fractures

Distal radius fractures are common injuries in the mature athlete. The severity of these fractures can be sport-specific, with high-energy trauma seen in contact sports and biking and low-energy trauma seen in racquet

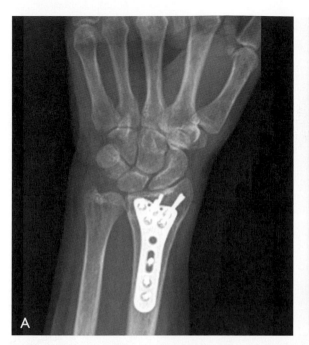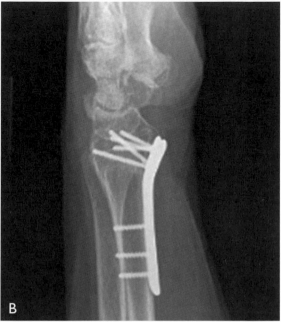

Figure 7   PA (**A**) and lateral (**B**) radiographs obtained after ORIF of a distal radius intra-articular fracture.

sports, particularly in patients with diminished bone density secondary to osteoporosis or osteomalacia. Athletes may present with pain, swelling, and bruising about the wrist. Radiographs should include at least three views of the wrist (AP, lateral, and oblique) to determine displacement, shortening, or intra-articular involvement. CT may be necessary to better visualize intra-articular fracture patterns. MRI also may be appropriate to evaluate associated intrinsic ligament injuries of the proximal carpal row and triangular fibrocartilage complex (TFCC). The goal of treatment is to restore normal alignment of the distal radius; this can be accomplished with various techniques and devices. Casting of stable distal radius fractures with close follow-up is the treatment of choice. Distal radius fractures with more than 5 mm of shortening, more than 20° of dorsal tilt, and more than 2 mm of intra-articular step-off should be reduced and stabilized with internal or external fixation.[16] Open reduction and internal fixation (ORIF) has gained popularity with the use of volar locking plates and fragment-specific fixation (**Figure 7**). Short-term follow-up has demonstrated improved motion and increased grip strength; however,

long-term follow-up demonstrates little difference in clinical outcomes. Rozental et al[17] demonstrated better functional results in the early postoperative period in association with ORIF and suggests considering this form of treatment for patients requiring a faster return to function after injury. Rehabilitation and return to sport requires careful monitoring and judgment. Internal fixation may allow early motion; however, return to play should be based on sport and position played.

Hook of Hamate Fractures

Although hook of hamate fractures represent only 2% of all carpal fractures, they are frequently seen in certain sports such as golf, baseball, and hockey.[18,19] Hook of hamate fractures are thought to be caused by a direct blow such as experienced when grounding a golf club or checking a swing in baseball. Because these injuries may be difficult to diagnose, they must be suspected when an athlete who competes in racquet or club sports presents with ulnar-side wrist pain. Examination findings may demonstrate pain over the hook of the hamate and pain with resisted flexion of the ring and small

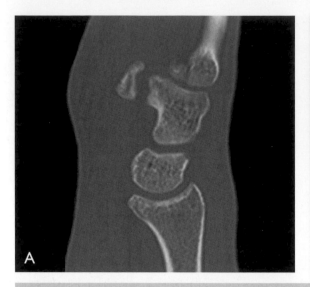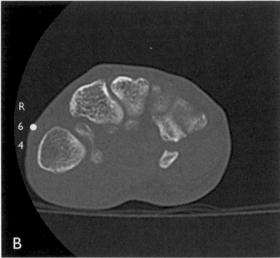

Figure 8   Sagittal CT scan of the wrist (**A**) and axial CT scan through the distal row of the carpus (**B**) reveal a fracture through the hook of hamate.

fingers. In chronic cases, ulnar nerve dysfunction at the wrist may be detected. Radiographic visualization of a fracture of the hook of the hamate can be difficult even with oblique and carpal tunnel views. CT is the image modality of choice when a fracture of the hook of the hamate is suspected[18] (**Figure 8**).

Treatment of hook of hamate fractures begins with cast immobilization; however, nonunion often occurs because of multiple intrinsic forces on the hamate hook fragment. ORIF has had variable results, and excision of the hamate hook is the usual treatment of choice.[18,20]

Scaphoid Fractures

The scaphoid is the most commonly and problematically injured carpal bone; scaphoid fractures constitute approximately 75% of all carpal fractures.[18] The mechanism of injury is usually a fall on an outstretched hand that results in hyperextension of the wrist. These injuries are often misdiagnosed as sprains, and treatment is often delayed. This may result in a decreased rate of healing; the increased time to healing presents a serious problem for the competitive athlete.[16]

The athlete with a scaphoid fracture presents with tenderness and pain over the radial aspect of the wrist

(anatomic snuffbox and scaphoid tubercle). Multiple radiographs, including ulnar-deviated PA views, should be obtained; however, initial radiographs may not show fracture. Treatment of athletes typically requires immediate diagnosis and can be best visualized with MRI. MRI is sensitive in demonstrating the presence or absence of a scaphoid fracture and facilitates decision making regarding safe return to sport.[16,18,21]

Treatment of scaphoid fractures in athletes requires careful discussion with the athlete regarding the potential for nonunion and malunion. Treatment of acute, stable, nondisplaced scaphoid fractures in casts results in healing rates higher than 90% at 2 to 3 months.[18] A variety of cast types (long arm versus short arm) have been used; however, no data conclusively support one particular type of cast.[22] Surgical treatment of nondisplaced scaphoid waist fractures is somewhat controversial; however, internal fixation is becoming more accepted for the athlete who desires earlier use of the hand and less time in a cast.[18,23,24] Unstable fractures, including those with more than 1 mm of displacement and associated carpal instability, require reduction and stabilization.[16] Unprotected return to sport should be

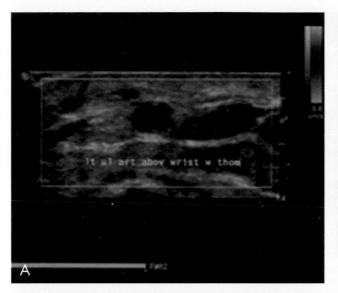 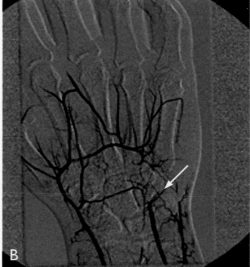

Figure 9   Duplex ultrasonogram (**A**) and angiogram (**B**) demonstrate ulnar artery thrombosis (arrow).

allowed only when full healing of the scaphoid has been established by both clinical and radiographic evaluation. The best imaging modality for assessing scaphoid healing is CT; complete healing can be difficult to assess by radiographs alone.[16,23,24]

Hypothenar Hammer Syndrome

Hypothenar hammer syndrome (HHS) is a vascular phenomenon that typically results from repetitive blunt trauma to the hypothenar aspect of the hand where the relatively unprotected ulnar artery remains superficial as it exits the Guyon canal. Although HHS has classically been described in the dominant hand of middle-aged male workers who habitually use the ulnar palm as a tool to hammer objects, it also has been reported in athletes participating in a variety of sports, including baseball, golf, tennis, biking, and weight lifting. The pathophysiology of HHS is related to trauma to the ulnar artery as it travels around the hook of the hamate, with the hook acting as an "anvil" upon which the artery may be impacted.[25-27] HSS symptoms occur secondarily as a result of thrombosis with or without embolic events. Ischemia in the ulnar digits of the hand associated with cold sensitivity, paresthesias, and pain are common findings. Other findings may include a fracture of the hook of the hamate and ulnar tunnel syndrome. The Allen test[25,26] is clinically useful to evaluate the patency of the ulnar artery and superficial palmar arch. Imaging may be accomplished with ultrasonography; however, angiography is the accepted standard for definitively establishing the diagnosis of HHS and localizing the site of occlusion or aneurysm[25,26] (**Figure 9**).

Nonsurgical treatment is aimed at avoiding repetitive insults in episodically symptomatic patients. Calcium channel blockers and oral sympatholytics have been shown to be equally effective in this subset of patients.[25] Surgery is the only treatment that will prevent recurrence of emboli and decompresses the adjacent neurologic structures. Surgical options include ligation of the ulnar artery if a complete radial arch exists. Excision of the damaged artery and reconstruction with an interposition vein graft is more common[25-27] (**Figure 10**). Because a subset of the population appears to be inherently susceptible to developing HHS, prevention is accomplished by ensuring that athletes wear proper protective equipment and are taught proper grip techniques.

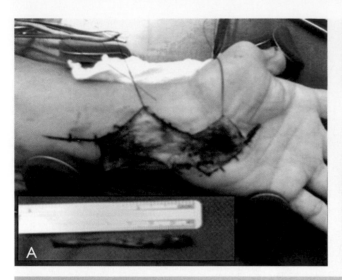
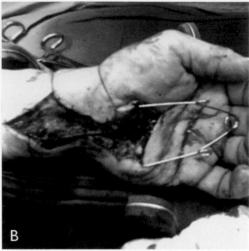

Figure 10   Intraoperative photographs show resection of a thrombosed ulnar artery (**A**) and reconstruction with vein graft (**B**).

Ulnar Collateral Ligament Injuries of the Thumb Metacarpophalangeal Joint

Thumb injuries involving the ulnar collateral ligament (UCL) commonly affect mature athletes involved in contact sports, cycling, and snow skiing. Athletes typically describe a hyperabduction injury to the thumb metacarpophalangeal (MCP) joint after a fall or pole injury while skiing. Pain and swelling on the ulnar aspect of the thumb MCP joint are typically observed on physical examination. Instability testing in full extension and 30° of flexion will demonstrate more than 30° of deformity or more than 15° of side-to-side difference, representing a complete tear.[28] More than 80% of patients with a complete tear will have a Stener lesion[16] (**Figure 11**). Stener lesions occur when the UCL detaches and becomes incarcerated proximal to the adductor aponeurosis. Examination may reveal a palpable lump, but this may be difficult to discern if significant swelling is present. Imaging studies, including MRI and ultrasonography, can be useful tools when diagnosis is difficult. Treatment is dictated by clinical and radiographic findings. Stener lesions are best repaired early, within 2 to 3 weeks, because long-term outcome can be poor with surgical delay.[18] Sprains, partial thickness tears, or nondisplaced complete tears may be treated with a short-arm thumb spica cast or splint for 6 weeks. Casting followed by splinting and taping will allow most athletes a safe return to their sport.

de Quervain Syndrome

de Quervain syndrome is the most common tendon disorder of the wrist. It is characterized by tenosynovitis of the first dorsal compartment (abductor pollicis longus [APL] and extensor pollicis brevis [EPB]).[29] de Quervain syndrome is common in the mature athlete and results from repetitive wrist motion seen in racquet sports, golf, and fly fishing.[30] Friction is thought to cause the thickening and degeneration; this may be related to anatomic variations such as additional tendon slips and septa within the first dorsal compartment. Examination reveals radial-side wrist pain over the first dorsal compartment and a positive Finkelstein test.[30] The Finkelstein test is performed by grasping the patient's thumb and ulnarly deviating the wrist through traction on the thumb. Nonsurgical management is usually very effective, and more than 80% of patients may experience resolution with steroid injections, rest, and immobilization.[18] Surgical treatment is aimed at

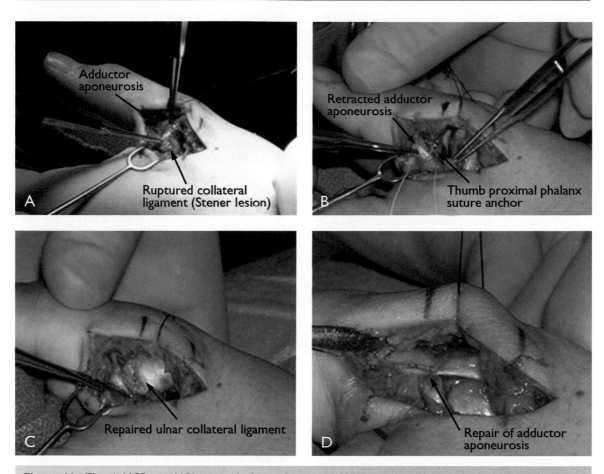

Figure 11   Thumb MCP joint UCL repair. **A,** Stener lesion with UCL incarcerated proximal to the adductor aponeurosis. **B,** The adductor aponeurosis is retracted, and a suture anchor is placed. **C,** The repaired UCL. **D,** The repaired adductor aponeurosis.

releasing the first dorsal compartment by incising the dorsal aspect or the retinaculum in line with the APL and EPB tendons, leaving the volar portion of the retinaculum to prevent subluxation of the tendons. Care must be taken to ensure release of common septa between the APL and EPB, and superficial radial nerve injury must be avoided. Surgery is supplemented by a thumb spica splint postoperatively until suture removal. Cure rates approach 90% with surgery.[31] Satisfaction is generally very high with surgery and is increased in patients who have symptoms for longer periods before resorting to surgery than for those who undergo surgery shortly after the onset of symptoms.[31]

Resuming normal activity after the removal of the splint, if one is used, is sufficient to return the patient to full function once symptoms have abated.

TFCC Injuries

TFCC injuries are common in athletes and may result from repetitive trauma seen in racquet sports or falls onto an extended pronated wrist. The TFCC is generally regarded as an important stabilizer of the distal radioulnar joint and a load absorber of the wrist.[18,32] Palmer et al[33-35] have demonstrated that axial load transmission across the TFCC and ulna is approximately 20% and increases with positive ulnar variance. Ulnar-side wrist pain associated with TFCC tears may be vague and associated with clicks and pops with wrist motion, particularly circumduction. Examination may reveal pain in the fovea of the wrist between the extensor carpi ulnaris and flexor carpi ulnaris distal to the ulnar head. Pain may be reproduced with resisted supination or pronation. Imaging studies, including a PA zero rotation view, a clenched-fist pronation PA view, and contralateral views, will assess ulnar variance and may impact treatment decisions when ulnocarpal abutment is suspected.[36] MRI has significant false-negative rates because of granulation of peripheral tears, making the test more useful for central tears.[18,32] Treatment of high-level athletes may require early arthroscopic evaluation of the wrist if symptoms persist after a trial of nonsurgical treatment; this offers the advantage of being both diagnostic and therapeutic.[18,32]

TFCC tears are classified as either traumatic or degenerative according to Palmer.[37] Traumatic tears are generally amenable to arthroscopic débridement (central tears) or repair (peripheral tears) if neutral or negative ulnar variance and no evidence of chondral changes are present to suggest ulnocarpal abutment syndrome. Arthroscopic central débridement is associated with 90% good to excellent results and allows early return to activity in 1 to 2 months.[18,38] Peripheral repairs are protected in a cast for at least 6 weeks followed by therapy and strengthening. Return to sport occurs in 3 to 4 months with 90% good to excellent results.[18,39]

Degenerative tears of the TFCC, which are common in the mature athlete, need to be assessed carefully. Positive ulnar variance as well as associated injuries on the ulnar aspect of the wrist, including chondral injuries and lunotriquetral ligament injuries, may necessitate shortening of the ulna by a wafer resection (<3 mm positive ulnar variance) or formal ulnar shortening osteotomy.[32,40] The failure rate following arthroscopic débridement of degenerative central tears is not encouraging. Hulsizer et al[41] noted poor results in 13 of 97 patients after simple débridement. After ulnar shortening osteotomy was performed on those 13 patients, 12 reported complete relief of pain. Minami et al[42,43] noted poor results after débridement of degenerative tears and reported significant improvement in a follow-up study after ulnar shortening osteotomy for

positive ulnar variance in 23 of 25 patients. Tomaino et al[44] evaluated 12 patients after combined TFCC débridement and Feldon wafer resection and noted relief of symptoms in all patients.

Treating the mature athlete with TFCC injuries can be challenging. Careful attention to associated injuries and ulnar variance will help guide treatment and the postoperative regimen to ensure timely return to athletic competition.

Carpal Tunnel Syndrome

Median nerve compression at the wrist is the most common neuropathy of the upper extremity and is exacerbated by extreme wrist positions (as in cycling) or repetitive forceful use of the hand (as in rowing). Clinical findings include pain and paresthesias on the palmar-radial aspect of the hand associated with dropping objects and decreased strength. Pain typically occurs with activity and at night. Diagnosis of carpal tunnel syndrome (CTS) is best accomplished by using a variety of tests, including the carpal tunnel compression test and nerve studies. Hand symptom diagrams, on which a patient shades in symptomatic areas on a pictorial representation of a hand, also can be useful to the examining surgeon.[45] Documentation of severity should be tested by two-point discrimination as well as grip strength. Nonsurgical treatment consists of splinting, anti-inflammatory medications, and medical management of underlying systemic diseases (eg, hypothyroidism, diabetes) associated with CTS. Steroid injections are effective in 80% of patients; however, only 22% of patients will be symptom free at 1 year.[46] Patients with mild symptoms of less than 1 year duration who are treated with a combination of splints and steroids are most likely to benefit from nonsurgical management. Surgical treatment is indicated when nonsurgical management fails. Controversy exists regarding the benefits of open versus endoscopic release.[45] Many argue that open procedures afford better visualization of the nerve and less chance of nerve injury. Others feel that endoscopic release can provide symptomatic relief and early return to normal activities.[45]

Summary

The mature athlete can present an interesting clinical challenge because of the overlap between injury, degenerative changes, and susceptibility to overuse phenomena from repetitive activities experienced during either recreation or work-related activity. Most of the entities described in this chapter are found in all age groups, but the treatment may be different in a mature athlete because of overlapping degenerative changes, physical limitations, or sport-specific considerations in the individual. Thoughtful consideration of all of these factors will lead to a more satisfactory outcome for the mature athlete, including the goal of a safe and expedient return to sports activities.

References

1. Watson HK, Ballet FL: The SLAC wrist: Scapholunate advanced collapse pattern of degenerative arthritis. *J Hand Surg Am* 1984;9(3):358-365.

2. Mastella DJ, Ashmead D, Watson HK: Scapholunate advanced collapse wrist arthritis. *Tech Orthop* 2009; 24(1):13-18.

3. Ruby LK, Leslie BM: Wrist arthritis associated with scaphoid nonunion. *Hand Clin* 1987;3(4):529-539.

4. Tomaino MM, Delsignore J, Burton RI: Long-term results following proximal row carpectomy. *J Hand Surg Am* 1994;19(4):694-703.

5. Dacho AK, Baumeister S, Germann G, Sauerbier M: Comparison of proximal row carpectomy and midcarpal arthrodesis for the treatment of scaphoid nonunion advanced collapse (SNAC-wrist) and scapholunate advanced collapse (SLAC-wrist) in stage II. *J Plast Reconstr Aesthet Surg* 2008;61(10):1210-1218.

6. Cohen MS, Kozin SH: Degenerative arthritis of the wrist: Proximal row carpectomy versus scaphoid excision and four-corner arthrodesis. *J Hand Surg Am* 2001;26(1):94-104.

7. Yao J, Osterman AL: Arthroscopic techniques for wrist arthritis (radial styloidectomy and proximal pole hamate excisions). *Hand Clin* 2005;21(3):519-526.

8. Van Heest AE, Kallemeier P: Thumb carpal metacarpal arthritis. *J Am Acad Orthop Surg* 2008;16(3):140-151.

9. Forthman CL: Management of advanced trapeziometacarpal arthrosis. *J Hand Surg Am* 2009; 34(2):331-334.

10. Eaton RG, Glickel SZ: Trapeziometacarpal osteoarthritis: Staging as a rationale for treatment. *Hand Clin* 1987;3(4):455-471.

11. Shuler MS, Luria S, Trumble TE: Basal joint arthritis of the thumb. *J Am Acad Orthop Surg* 2008;16(7): 418-423.

12. Murray PM: Prosthetic replacement of the proximal interphalangeal joint. *Hand Clin* 2006;22(2):201-206.

13. Kobayashi K, Terrono AL: Proximal interphalangeal joint arthroplasty of the hand. *J Am Soc Surg Hand* 2003;3(4):219-226.

14. Iselin F, Conti E, Perrotte R, Stephan E: Long-term results of proximal interphalangeal resection-arthroplasty using the Swanson silastic implant. *Ann Chir Main Memb Super* 1995;14(3):126-133.

15. Johnstone BR: Proximal interphalangeal joint surface replacement arthroplasty. *Hand Surg* 2001;6(1):1-11.

16. Morgan WJ, Slowman LS: Acute hand and wrist injuries in athletes: Evaluation and management. *J Am Acad Orthop Surg* 2001;9(6):389-400.

17. Rozental TD, Blazar PE, Franko OI, Chacko AT, Earp BE, Day CS: Functional outcomes for unstable distal radial fractures treated with open reduction and internal fixation or closed reduction and percutaneous fixation: A prospective randomized trial. *J Bone Joint Surg Am* 2009;91(8):1837-1846.

18. Rettig AC: Athletic injuries of the wrist and hand: Part I. Traumatic injuries of the wrist. *Am J Sports Med* 2003;31(6):1038-1048.

19. Geissler WB: Carpal fractures in athletes. *Clin Sports Med* 2001;20(1):167-188.

20. Parker RD, Berkowitz MS, Brahms MA, Bohl WR: Hook of the hamate fractures in athletes. *Am J Sports Med* 1986;14(6):517-523.

21. Beeres FJ, Rhemrev SJ, den Hollander P, et al: Early magnetic resonance imaging compared with bone scintigraphy in suspected scaphoid fractures. *J Bone Joint Surg Br* 2008;90(9):1205-1209.

22. Ring D, Jupiter JB, Herndon JH: Acute fractures of the scaphoid. *J Am Acad Orthop Surg* 2000;8(4):225-231.

23. Ram AN, Chung KC: Evidence-based management of acute nondisplaced scaphoid waist fractures. *J Hand Surg Am* 2009;34(4):735-738.

24. Grewal R, King GJ: An evidence-based approach to the management of acute scaphoid fractures. *J Hand Surg Am* 2009;34(4):732-734.

25. Ablett CT, Hackett LA: Hypothenar hammer syndrome: Case reports and brief review. *Clin Med Res* 2008;6(1):3-8.

26. Stuart JJ, Joe KJ, Kobayashi KM: Surgical management of ulnar artery thrombosis: Poster presentation. *Society of Military Orthopaedic Surgeons.* 2007.

27. Wong GB, Whetzel TP: Hypothenar hammer syndrome–Review and case report. *Vasc Surg* 2001;35(2):163-166.

28. Heyman P: Injuries to the ulnar collateral ligament of the thumb metacarpophalangeal joint. *J Am Acad Orthop Surg* 1997;5(4):224-229.

29. Ranney D, Wells R, Moore A: Upper limb musculoskeletal disorders in highly repetitive industries: Precise anatomical physical findings. *Ergonomics* 1995; 38(7):1408-1423.

30. Moore JS: De Quervain's tenosynovitis: Stenosing tenosynovitis of the first dorsal compartment. *J Occup Environ Med* 1997;39(10):990-1002.

31. Ta KT, Eidelman D, Thomson JG: Patient satisfaction and outcomes of surgery for de Quervain's tenosynovitis. *J Hand Surg Am* 1999;24(5):1071-1077.

32. Papapetropoulos PA, Ruch DS: Repair of arthroscopic triangular fibrocartilage complex tears in athletes. *Hand Clin* 2009;25(3):389-394.

33. Palmer AK, Glisson RR, Werner FW: Ulnar variance determination. *J Hand Surg Am* 1982;7(4):376-379.

34. Palmer AK, Glisson RR, Werner FW: Relationship between ulnar variance and triangular fibrocartilage complex thickness. *J Hand Surg Am* 1984;9(5): 681-682.

35. Werner FW, Glisson RR, Murphy DJ, Palmer AK: Force transmission through the distal radioulnar carpal joint: Effect of ulnar lengthening and shortening. *Handchir Mikrochir Plast Chir* 1986;18(5):304-308.

36. Tomaino MM: The importance of the pronated grip x-ray view in evaluating ulnar variance. *J Hand Surg Am* 2000;25(2):352-357.

37. Palmer AK: Triangular fibrocartilage complex lesions: A classification. *J Hand Surg Am* 1989;14(4):594-606.

38. Bednar JM, Osterman AL: The role of arthroscopy in the treatment of traumatic triangular fibrocartilage injuries. *Hand Clin* 1994;10(4):605-614.

39. Corso SJ, Savoie FH, Geissler WB, Whipple TL, Jiminez W, Jenkins N: Arthroscopic repair of peripheral avulsions of the triangular fibrocartilage complex of the wrist: A multicenter study. *Arthroscopy* 1997;13(1):78-84.

40. Feldon P, Terrono AL, Belsky MR: Wafer distal ulna resection for triangular fibrocartilage tears and/or ulna impaction syndrome. *J Hand Surg Am* 1992;17(4): 731-737.

41. Hulsizer D, Weiss AP, Akelman E: Ulna-shortening osteotomy after failed arthroscopic debridement of the triangular fibrocartilage complex. *J Hand Surg Am* 1997;22(4):694-698.

42. Minami A, Ishikawa J, Suenaga N, Kasashima T: Clinical results of treatment of triangular fibrocartilage complex tears by arthroscopic debridement. *J Hand Surg Am* 1996;21(3):406-411.

43. Minami A, Kato H: Ulnar shortening for triangular fibrocartilage complex tears associated with ulnar positive variance. *J Hand Surg Am* 1998;23(5):904-908.

44. Tomaino MM, Weiser RW: Combined arthroscopic TFCC debridement and wafer resection of the distal ulna in wrists with triangular fibrocartilage complex tears and positive ulnar variance. *J Hand Surg Am* 2001;26(6):1047-1052.

45. Bonauto DK, Silverstein BA, Fan ZJ, Smith CK, Wilcox DN: Evaluation of a symptom diagram for identifying carpal tunnel sydrome. *Occup Med (Lond)* 2008;58(8):561-566.

46. Szabo RM, Steinberg DR: Nerve entrapment syndromes in the wrist. *J Am Acad Orthop Surg* 1994;2(2):115-123.

SECTION 4

LOWER EXTREMITY AND SPINE

Nicholas A. DiNubile, MD
Section Editor

Chapter 25

Hip Arthroscopy in the Mature Athlete

Marc J. Philippon, MD
Bruno G. Schröder e Souza, MD
Karen K. Briggs, MPH

Key Points

- Sports training improves functional status, health, and quality of life in older adults.
- Sports and recreational activities are risk factors for knee and hip osteoarthritis, which is directly correlated to the intensity and duration of the exposure.
- Until recently, options for treating patients with hip pain without significant osteoarthritic changes were limited. Many patients were told to stop their activities, take prescription medications, and wait until their joints had enough degeneration to be treated with replacement.
- Hip arthroscopy has been shown to effectively improve symptoms, regardless of age, in patients with hip joint pathology and with a preoperative joint space of at least 2 mm.
- Studies are being conducted to assess whether hip arthroscopy will be able to stop or delay the progress of degenerative changes related to subtle bone deformities that are associated with intra-articular lesions (eg, labral tears and chondral damage), such as in femoroacetabular impingement (FAI).

Introduction

Current knowledge indicates that the process of maturing is accompanied by age-related declines in health that include decreased energy expenditure at rest and during exercise, and increased body fat with accompanying dyslipidemia and reduced insulin sensitivity. Quality of life is also affected by reduced strength and endurance and increased difficulty in being physically active.[1] Many of these effects have been shown to be reversible with adequate resistance training and participation in sports activity.[1]

Both the knee and the hip joint are especially prone to developing degenerative changes related to osteoarthritis with age.[2] That tendency can be increased by participation in sports and recreational activities. Direct correlation between the intensity and duration of exposure and the development of osteoarthritis has been reported, although this risk seems to be lower than that associated with a history of trauma or obesity. Exercises directed to pursue health improvement have been found to have a beneficial effect on symptoms and function of patients with degenerative articular changes.[2]

As the population ages and still wishes to remain active,[3] the number of patients with prearthritic hip symptoms seeking nonarthroplasty solutions has increased. Many of these patients are no longer willing to accept the traditional treatments that are commonly offered: decrease in level of activity, symptomatic medication, and other nonsurgical measures. They should be advised of the risks and benefits of their participation in physical activities[2] and be made aware of the new concepts in the pathomechanics of joint degeneration,[4,5] as well as the current options to treat this condition.[6-10]

Hip arthroscopy has been shown to be an effective means of treating many intra-articular conditions of the hip.[11-13] For conditions that do not improve with nonsurgical treatment, arthroscopy is considered an excellent option because it bears relatively low morbidity and is associated with a relatively short recovery time.[6,10-12] Few age-related contraindications to hip arthroscopy exist, but the presence of established osteoarthritis, especially with a joint space of less than 2 mm, has been shown to correlate with worse outcomes.[6] In these patients, prosthetic replacement should strongly be considered.

The Aging Hip

Aging is a natural phenomenon that results in complex changes in multiple physiologic systems, including a decline in organ functions and tissue properties, which are usually accompanied by a lowered threshold for lesions and limited function. The musculoskeletal system is often a mirror of these changes with age, and the hip, as a major joint, is an excellent example of the changes related to senescence.[13] The age-related changes in the hip joint increase the risk for injury and degenerative joint disease. The mature athlete should be aware of this risk as well as the benefits of exercising.[2] Patient education on the limitations imposed by aging can be an important ally in the prevention of serious lesions and progression of osteoarthritis.

In the femur and acetabulum, the most notable transformation is the loss of bone mass and quality of bone.[14] Osteoporosis increases the risk for fractures, even in minor trauma such as that experienced by participants in noncontact sports. Moreover, mature athletes, especially those involved in endurance sports, also carry an increased risk of stress fractures,[15] as such activities may compound the effects of bone fatigue and insufficiency.

The articular cartilage matrix demonstrates decreased concentration of proteoglycan, decreased water content, and increased joint loading with diminished fluid flux with age.[16] In addition, the response to hormones is decreased, leading to higher susceptibility to injuries and degenerative risk, as well as a predominance of catabolic metabolism, which predisposes to osteoarthritis. Early detection of chondral lesions and correction of predisposing factors may play a role in improving patients' prognosis. The labrum is also affected by aging, and the decrease in its mechanical and physical properties may lead to increased forces on the articular cartilage and make anticipated repairs more difficult.

The strength, water content, and metabolic activity of the joint capsule and ligaments decreases over time. Additionally, the concentration of cross-links between collagen fibers increases, causing an increase in the stiffness of these structures. Limitations in joint range of motion and a predisposition to lesions in more extreme positions may result.[13]

As tendons become drier and stiffer as a result of biochemical changes in composition and organization related to age, their ability to handle imposed stress decreases.[13] Moreover, a limited potential to heal has been observed. Because of that, periarticular lesions are especially prevalent in older athletes, and recurrent symptoms are not uncommon.[17] Surgical intervention may be necessary to treat degenerative tendon tears.

The skeletal muscle loses type II fibers, strength, mass, and elasticity with age.[18] Moreover, there is a trend to rapid deterioration of strength and endurance related to immobility that is usually difficult to regain. This reinforces the need for early mobilization and muscle conditioning immediately after surgery in this population.

Evaluation
Differential Diagnosis
Hip or groin pain is frequently related to injuries of the hip joint and the surrounding structures, although other conditions in the differential diagnosis should be considered as well[7,9,17,19-22] (**Table 1**).

In mature athletes presenting with peripheral arthropathy, it is mandatory to investigate autoimmune arthritis, crystal-induced arthritis, Lyme disease, and pigmented villonodular synovitis. Musculoskeletal soft-tissue disorders (eg, bursitis, tendinopathies, enthesitis) are a frequent cause of pain and disability in both competitive and recreational athletes and are related to acute injuries or overuse, especially in elderly populations.[19]

History

The first step in the diagnosis of patients with hip pain is to obtain a detailed history.[22] Physical examination should determine whether the pain has an intra- or extra-articular source. Signs of instability and impingement can be inferred from physical examination.[23,24]

Patients with femoroacetabular impingement (FAI) often present with discomfort in the groin.[23] The onset of symptoms may be insidious or related to a new sports activity. A history of pain related to activities that demand excessive hip flexion under load, such as squatting and leg-press exercises, is common.[23,24] Although FAI is usually due to abnormal morphology of the hip, it may occur in normal hips with increased range of movement.[25] Women often present with intermittent pain due to excessive hip flexion, with pincer deformity a common finding. In many cases, patients take part in sports activities or have occupations in which some discomfort is an accepted part of the activity. For this reason, delayed diagnosis is not uncommon. Some patients with marked acetabular retroversion, when asked to sit on the floor, may be more comfortable with their hips flexed, abducted, and externally rotated. Some describe a dislike of sitting in a chair with their legs crossed, especially with the symptomatic leg crossed over the other.[26] Intolerance to long periods of sitting in a low chair is very common. In more dramatic cases, hip flexion may be limited to as little as 90°, progressing to a full range of motion only when the hip is able to move simultaneously into external rotation and abduction, known as the Drehmann sign.[27-29] In these cases, contact of the femoral neck with the edge of the acetabulum on maximum flexion necessitates contouring the femoral neck to avoid contact in full range of motion. The limb tends to lie at rest in an externally rotated position

of the hip, and the range of external rotation, especially in the 90° flexed position, is more generous than usual, often exceeding 60°. The range of internal rotation may be limited proportionally.

The onset of symptoms may also be related to a traumatic event,[12] usually acute chondral or labral dam-

Table 1: Differential Diagnoses of Hip Pain

Extra-articular

Pubalgia ("sports hernia")

Hernias (inguinal hernia, femoral hernia)

Abdominal conditions (eg, diverticular disease, urinary tract conditions, endometriosis, tumors)

Nerve compression (lumbar disk herniation, piriformis syndrome, meralgia paresthetica)

Adenopathy (sexually transmitted disease, acute or chronic infection in the lower limb)

Tendinitis and bursitis (snapping hip, iliopsoas, rectus femoris)

Lateral trochanteric pain syndrome

Intra-articular

Stress fracture (femoral neck and acetabulum)

Inflammatory diseases (eg, rheumatoid arthritis, ankylosing spondylitis, psoriasis)

Deposit diseases (gout, chondrocalcinosis)

Metabolic diseases (osteomalacia, Otto pelvis, Paget disease)

Infectious diseases (pyoarthrosis, articular tuberculosis)

Mechanical disorders (loose bodies, femoroacetabular impingement, hip dysplasia and instability)

Tumors (eg, osteoid osteoma, osteochondromas, chondroblastoma)

Traumatic disorders (eg, hip pointer, labral tear, ligament teres tear, acetabular fracture)

Miscellaneous (eg, osteonecrosis, transient osteoporosis, synovial chondromatosis)

age. The patient may report an acute episode of pain, with limping and sometimes blocking. When the pain eventually subsides, instability symptoms (such as popping) and position/activity-related pain become the main problems reported by patients.[23,24]

Mechanical symptoms (such as blocking, popping, and catching) and limitation of sports and activities of daily living may be present and usually indicate intra-articular soft-tissue damage such as labral tears, loose bodies, or ligamentum teres lesions.[9] Degenerative signs may predominate after a prolonged time without treatment and may include global limitation of motion.[29]

Physical Examination

Physical examination has been reported to have high sensitivity for the diagnosis of labral tears.[30] A systematic clinical evaluation should be able to raise suspicion for this condition.[23,24,30] When findings are positive or inconclusive, complementary examinations should be conducted to determine the exact source of pain and to help formulate a treatment strategy. When labral pathology is suspected, the physician should always keep in mind that this condition rarely occurs in isolation; therefore, the etiology of the labral dysfunction must be sought.[4]

Physical examination should include a general health examination. The patient's morphology, gait, and posture should be assessed. Shortening of the stance phase or shortening of the length of the stride on the affected side should be noted. During the examination, pelvic obliquity, limb-length inequality, muscle contractures, and scoliosis should be identified.[22,23]

The hip joint is palpated to determine locations of tenderness, delineate the integrity of muscular structures surrounding the hip, and locate areas of atrophy. Tenderness upon palpation should raise suspicion of an extra-articular condition, such as greater trochanteric pain syndrome. This condition usually affects older patients who present with localized pain over the greater trochanter and the insertion of the gluteus medius tendons.[22] A snapping iliopsoas tendon also should be considered. This is assessed by moving the hip from flexion, abduction, and external rotation to extension, adduction, and internal rotation. A palpable or audible

pop in the inguinal region may indicate snapping hip syndrome, but it does not rule out the possibility of a labral tear.[17,31]

Hip range of motion is evaluated and compared with the contralateral hip. Not uncommonly, a patient will have bilateral hip symptoms. Decreased range of motion in flexion and internal rotation is an expected finding for impingement, but it may be subtle.[32] Lack of internal rotation of the flexed hip correlates strongly with decreased space between the acetabular rim and the femoral head-neck junction on MRI.[33,34] Limited abduction and pain may be present in cases of lateral impingement. Global decrease in the range of motion is more common in osteoarthritis.[29] Excessive range of motion raises suspicion of hip instability.[9,22]

Painful hip flexion, adduction, and internal rotation (impingement test)[32] may suggest the presence of intra-articular pathology, most commonly a labral tear. The sensitivity of this test for labral tears was reported to vary from 95% to 100%.[30] A positive apprehension sign (discomfort and a subluxation sensation during passive extension and external rotation of the hip) should raise suspicion for hip instability. Pain during the apprehension test may also be present in cases of posteroinferior impingement.[9] Pain during the log-roll test suggests intra-articular pathology. Excessive external rotation and a soft end point compared with the asymptomatic side during this test is another sign of instability. The traction test with the leg extended may cause apprehension or, less frequently, reproduce an audible or palpable popping reported by the patient in cases of instability. The FABER (flexion, abduction, and external rotation) test is used to identify hip and sacroiliac pain. More recently, we have been using the FABER distance test to identify FAI and labral tears. Increases in the distance between the lateral femoral epicondyle and the examination table during that test were found to correlate with an increased α angle on radiographs.[6] Other elements of the physical examination include the Ober test, a resisted leg raise in the supine position, and forced internal rotation while applying an axial load. The final elements of the examination are motor strength testing and a neurovascular examination.[9,17,22,23]

Imaging

Imaging is often useful to determine morphologic aspects of the hip that might explain signs of dysplasia or impingement. Intra-articular lesions such labral tears, chondral damage, cysts, and ligamentum teres lesions may be confirmed with magnetic resonance arthrograms. Imaging is also useful to assess the stage of joint degeneration and identify nonmechanical causes for symptoms, such as tumors, metabolic disorders, stress fractures, and osteonecrosis.[33,34]

Plain radiographic assessment is the first step in assessing possible morphologic causes of pain. At least three orthogonal radiographic views are necessary to evaluate the presence of altered morphology[28] (**Table 2**).

An AP pelvic radiograph should be obtained in all patients to compare the affected side with the contralateral hip. The direction and position of the x-ray beam influences the interpretation of all the radiographic signs. Pelvic positioning must be considered when interpreting the radiographic signs associated with pincer impingement. With the coccyx and symphysis pubis aligned, the pelvis should be in neutral flexion/extension, which means that the distance between the top of the pubic symphysis and the sacrococcygeal junction should be 32 mm for men and 47 mm for women.[28] Images obtained with the patient in a position that increases the pubic symphysis–sacrococcygeal junction distance will overemphasize signs of impingement, whereas a position that decreases the distance may result in underdetection of impingement. The AP pelvic radiograph is the most valuable study for confirming retroversion or coxa profunda in a patient suspected of having pincer-type impingement.[26] The presence of one of the following three findings indicates a retroverted acetabulum: the crossover sign,[35] the posterior wall sign,[26] or the ischial sign.[36] Coxa profunda is recognized on the AP pelvic radiograph when the medial wall of the acetabulum lies on or medial to the ilioischial line. Protrusio acetabulum, which represents the more severe form of coxa profunda, is diagnosed when the femoral head crosses the ilioischial line. Hip dysplasia and proximal femur deformities also can be observed on this view.[28]

A frog-lateral view of the proximal femur is essential for the diagnosis of cam impingement, which is characterized by asphericity of the femoral head.[32] This abnormality typically occurs in the anterolateral portion of the head-neck junction, so it may not be seen on an AP pelvic radiograph or a simple lateral radiograph of the hip. A cross-table lateral view (with the hip in 10° of internal rotation) or a Dunn view (an AP radiograph of the hip in neutral rotation, 20° of abduction, and 90° of flexion) is required. Most studies have considered an α angle greater than 50° to be diagnostic for the abnormality.[6,28,37] In addition, a head-neck offset ratio less than 0.15 on the cross-table lateral radiograph has been reported to have a sensitivity of 68% and specificity of 82% for the diagnosis of cam impingement. The offset ratio is measured by dividing the anterior offset by the femoral head diameter.[28] The anterior offset is the distance between two parallel lines, one adjacent to the anterior aspect of the neck and the other touching the most anterior part of the femoral head and both parallel to the femoral neck axis. In a comparison of four different lateral radiographic views used to detect femoral head asphericity, Meyer et al[38] found that the modified Dunn view (an AP radiograph of the hip in neutral rotation, 20° of abduction, and 45° of flexion) was the most sensitive and the cross-table lateral view and the standard Dunn view were satisfactory.

In some cases, signs of dysplasia can be observed only on the false profile view of the pelvis, described by Lequesne and de Sèze.[39] The vertical-center-anterior (VCA) angle is calculated from the radiographic view. The patient stands at a 65° angle to the x-ray beam, with the foot on the affected side parallel to the x-ray cassette and the focal distance set to 1 m. The tip of the greater trochanter forms the horizontal center, and the vertical center is midway between the symphysis pubis and the anterior superior iliac spine. A vertical line through the center of the femoral head subtends the VCA angle by connecting with a second line through the center of the hip and the foremost aspect of the acetabulum. A VCA angle of 25° is generally regarded as normal, 25° to 20° is considered borderline, and less than 20° is considered pathologic, although more recent studies suggest that a VCA angle 17° or greater can be regarded as normal.[40]

Whether additional imaging studies are indicated depends on the conditions suspected. MRI studies have low sensitivity for intra-articular pathology but are of great value when extra-articular conditions are sus-

Table 2: Radiographic Evaluation of the Hip

Factor	Criterion for Dysplasia
Acetabular inclination	Tonnis angle[a] >10°
Hip center	Lateralized[b]
Congruency[c]	Incongruence (divergent)
Shenton's line[d]	Superior migration of the femur
CE angle[e]	<20°
Extrusion index[f]	>20%

Factor	Criterion for Femoroacetabular Impingement
Acetabular retroversion	Crossover sign[g] positive
α angle[h]	>50°
Pistol grip deformity	Present
Ischial spine sign[i]	Positive
Posterior wall sign[j]	Positive
Acetabular inclination	Tonnis angle < 0°
CE angle[e]	> 39°
Acetabular depth	Coxa profunda[k]/acetabulum protrusio[l]
Congruency[c]	Incongruence (convergent)

[a]Angle subtended by the horizontal line of the pelvis and another running through the most inferior point of the sclerotic acetabular sourcil to the lateral margin of the acetabular sourcil on the AP radiograph.

[b]The hip center is considered lateralized if the medial aspect of the femoral head is greater than 10 mm from the ilioischial line.

[c]Incongruence is defined as nonparallel contours of the femoral head and acetabulum. It is considered divergent if the articular distance is increased laterally and decreased medially. It is considered convergent if the articular distance is increased medially and decreased laterally.

[d]Line formed by the inferior margin of the femoral neck and the superior border of the obturator foramen.

[e]Center-edge (CE) angle is subtended by a perpendicular line to the horizontal plane of the pelvis passing through the center of the femoral head and another connecting the acetabular border to this point.

[f]The extrusion index is obtained by dividing the distance of the femoral head not covered by the acetabulum by the greater horizontal diameter of the femoral head.

[g]Crossover sign: The hip is considered retroverted if the anterior wall crosses the posterior wall of the acetabulum before reaching the lateral edge of the sourcil.

[h]The α angle is subtended by a line drawn in the center of the femoral neck and another that connects the center of the femoral neck and the point at which the head loses its sphericity anteriorly. This angle is measured in the lateral view.

[i]Ischial spine sign: The ischial spine projects into the pelvic cavity on AP pelvic radiograph.

[j]Posterior wall sign: The center of the femoral head lies lateral to the posterior wall.

[k]Coxa profunda: The floor of the fossa acetabuli touches or is medial to the ilioischial line.

[l]Acetabulum protrusio: The medial edge of the femoral head is medial to the ilioischial line.

pected. CT and magnetic resonance arthrography with gadolinium contrast are useful for confirming impingement deformity, identifying associated pathologic changes, and facilitating surgical planning.[33,34,41,42] CT scans provide three-dimensional surface renderings of hip morphology and aid in determining the area of bone resection when surgery is being considered. For patients who cannot undergo magnetic resonance arthrography, contrast-enhanced CT has shown similar sensitivity and specificity.[43] Magnetic resonance arthrography with gadolinium contrast can demonstrate abnormalities of the acetabular rim such as labral tears, paralabral cysts, and cartilage delamination.[41] Magnetic resonance arthrography has been reported to have from 63% to 100% sensitivity[34,42] and from 0% to 94% specificity for labral tears. MRI is also useful for distinguishing dysplasia from impingement. With impingement, the labrum may be normal in size or small, whereas a hypertrophied labrum is associated with a dysplastic acetabulum.[37,44] Fibrocystic changes at the femoral head-neck junction (also known as synovial herniation pits, or Pitt's pits),[45] which are often visible on plain radiographs but are more easily seen on CT or MRI scans, have been reported to be 91% specific and to have a positive predictive value of 71% for the diagnosis of FAI.[37]

Nonsurgical Management

Patients who wish to delay arthroscopy begin general exercises that can be tolerated without pain. It is important that they avoid pushing the hip to extremes of motion that engage the bony impingement. Following a 3-month rehabilitation program, patients return for surgical evaluation. We discourage patients with labral tears or chondral defects from delaying surgery too long, as research has shown that results are less satisfactory when patients delay surgery for more than 1 year. It is also important to determine if the pain the patient is experiencing is the same pain that brought the patient to the clinic. This can be accomplished by performing an injection of a local anesthetic and a corticosteroid in the office. After sterile preparation, an 18-gauge spinal needle is placed within the hip capsule, and the anesthetic/steroid mixture is administered. After approximately 5 minutes, the physical examination tests are repeated and any improvement in symptoms is noted. This test is typically diagnostic. The injection can also be used therapeutically during the time the patient is awaiting surgical intervention.

Indications for Hip Arthroscopy
Femoroacetabular Impingement

FAI is a condition in which subtle abnormal bone morphology of the proximal femur and/or the acetabulum causes a bony conflict within the hip joint in a normal range of motion.[32] Types of FAI are pincer impingement, cam impingement, and combined pincer and cam impingement. In pincer impingement, an abutment of the femoral neck against a retroverted or deep acetabulum causes compression of the hip labrum and subluxation of the joint with a typically posteromedial contrecoup chondral lesion.[26,32] In cam impingement, an osseous bump located in the femoral head-neck junction is forced into the joint, most commonly in a flexed and adducted position with internal rotation, causing displacement of the labrum with eventual labral tear and detachment of the acetabular cartilage due to increased load, friction, and shear forces.[32,37,46]

The natural history of FAI is not yet completely understood, although strong anatomic, biomechanical, and epidemiologic evidence links FAI to the development of osteoarthritis.[5,28,46] In a radiographic study, Bardakos and Villar[47] found that approximately one third of patients with signs of FAI also had signs of progressive joint degeneration at 10-year follow-up. The only predictors for osteoarthritis progression in that study were the modified anatomic proximal femoral angle and the posterior wall sign.

Arthroscopic treatment of FAI includes resection of bone deformities (rim trimming and femoral neck osteoplasty) and correction of intra-articular lesions (usually labral repair and ligamentum teres débridement)[6,8,9,35] (**Figure 1**). The procedure is indicated in a patient who has intra-articular symptoms that do not improve after 3 to 6 months of nonsurgical treatment, as well as radiographic and clinical signs of FAI. In the mature population, caution must be exercised not to exaggerate the bone resection of the femoral neck.[6] Resection of more than 30% of the femoral neck has been recognized as a risk factor for fractures in experimental studies.[48] In the elderly population, especially

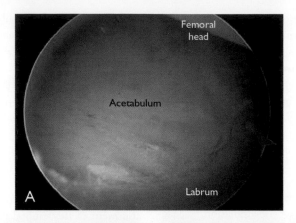

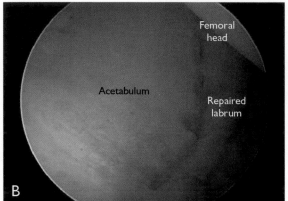

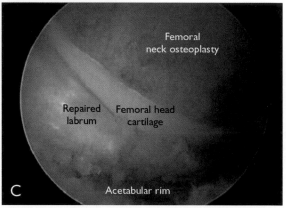

Figure 1 Arthroscopic views of the knee in a 55-year-old patient with femoroacetabular impingement (FAI). **A,** Before repair, signs of labral degeneration were present: detachment, fraying, and yellowish color. **B,** Selective labral débridement and repair with anchors was performed, along with acetabular rim trimming and femoral neck osteoplasty. **C,** Dynamic examination demonstrates repaired labrum providing seal with the femoral head.

those at higher risk for osteoporosis, the resection must be limited to the amount required for impingement-free movement, and the contours of the osteoplasty should be smooth so that stress risers are not created. Femoral neck fractures have been reported following FAI treatment, and some authors recommend the use of crutches for a limited time after surgery, especially in higher risk patients in whom the resection was large.[6,15,35]

Early treatment of FAI is advised, as longer duration of symptoms has been found to correlate with more severe intra-articular damage, including grade IV chondral lesions and more complex labral tears.[6,46] Grade IV chondral lesions are even more challenging in older patients, particularly if microfracture is indicated in patients who may have weak bone due to osteoporosis. Moreover, older patients may have difficulties with the non–weight-bearing period of 8 weeks required when microfracture is performed. This difficulty with non-weight bearing can be related to joint stiffness, decrease in bone mass, decrease in muscle strength, and overload of other joints due to age.[13,16] Complex labral tears also have been found in patients who were symptomatic for a long period of time.[6,49] In these patients, labral repair may not be an option; however, labral débridement or reconstruction may be a viable choice.[6,23,50] Patient satisfaction after labral reconstruction was found to be greater in younger patients; however, age is not a contraindication for the procedure, especially in more active patients and those presenting with some degree of hip instability.[50] Unfortunately, more severe intra-articular lesions are often found in that population, and special attention to a rehabilitation program, including continuous passive motion and muscle strengthening, is paramount to optimize results.

Labral Tears

Labral lesions were divided by Lage et al[51] into four categories based on etiology: traumatic, congenital, degenerative, and idiopathic. Based on novel knowledge of the etiology of labral pathology,[4] we modified the classification proposed by Lage et al.[51] We currently consider labral pathology to be secondary to morphologic alterations, functional alterations, trauma, or degenerative articular changes.[22] **Table 3** describes common causes and aspects of labral pathology.

Labral tears are believed to contribute to early development of osteoarthritis.[11,25,52] Correct diagnosis is essential for the proper treatment of labral lesions. Patients with isolated labral lesions may benefit from partial débridement or labral repair. When indicated, labral repair has shown to provide better results than débridement.[6,53,54] In the great majority of cases, concomitant pathologies are present and need to be addressed to lower the risk of treatment failure.[25] By not recognizing hip impingement or dysplasia, the potential exists to impede improvement or worsen the condition. Any additional intra-articular lesions that are present, such as chondral defects, ligament teres lesions, and loose bodies, should be adequately treated. In most cases, an arthroscopic approach is able to correct both the labral condition and its underlying cause. Open procedures are reserved for cases of dysplasia without arthritis and cases of extremely abnormal bone morphology.

Hip Instability

Nonsurgical treatment is usually unsuccessful in the resolution of symptoms of hip instability.[55] However, identification and correction of provocative postures and movements, as well as local or global muscle weakness, may play a decisive adjunctive role in whether the treatment succeeds in allowing the patient to return to sports and/or activities of daily living. Surgical treatment must be directed to solve the underlying cause of the instability.[9] This is not always easy, especially in cases associated with systemic diseases. We seek to anatomically restore faulty stabilizing structures either by repair or reconstruction.[9] The technique for hip arthroscopy used by the senior author (M.J.P.) has been described in detail. Labral tears should be repaired whenever possible, and débridement should be limited. In cases of complex tears, labral reconstruction with iliotibial band autograft may be an attractive alternative to extensive débridement.[50]

Capsular laxity should be recognized and treated in all patients with instability. The capsule is probed in the regions of the iliofemoral and ischiofemoral ligaments, and areas of redundancy are noted. A flexible monopolar radiofrequency probe is used for thermal capsulorrhaphy. Temperature and power settings are closely monitored to keep them precisely at 67°C and 40 W. The probe is moved across the redundant tissue, with minimal contact, in a striped pattern.[9] To encourage healing in the treated tissue, sufficient healthy tissue should be left between the stripes. As the probe is moved across the tissue, the color and shrinkage of the capsular tissue is monitored visually. Overheating of the tissue must be avoided by monitoring the probe temperatures and avoiding excessive heating time in a single region of the capsule. Following focal thermal capsulorrhaphy, capsular plication may be performed as needed to further reduce capsular volume. Sutures are placed through the tissue and tied to reduce capsule volume. Plication sutures are placed between the lateral arm of the iliofemoral ligament and the ischiofemoral ligament.[9] In cases that demand larger capsulotomies (eg, FAI treatment), care is taken not to violate the iliofemoral ligament in its whole extension, and attentive capsular closure or plication is performed at the end of the procedure to avoid iatrogenic instability.

Ligamentum Teres Lesions

Arthroscopic débridement and thermal shrinkage are the treatments of choice for ligamentum teres lesions. Such lesions may be highly symptomatic and are not always detected with imaging.[56] The integrity of the ligamentum is assessed by rotating the limb internally, when the ligamentum is loose, and then externally, with the ligamentum taut. Débridement of frayed, loose

Table 3: Common Causes of Labral Pathology

Type	Base condition	Labral Morphology	Labral Lesion	Common Location[a]
Morphologic alterations	Femoroacetabular impingement			
	Cam	Normal	Labral tear (usually base detachment in the watershed zone associated with chondral lesion)	Mean: 12.8 o'clock (range, 7-3 o'clock; SD = 1.6 h)
	Pincer	Hypotrophic	Labral degeneration (bruising, fraying, with eventual cysts and ossification)	Mean: 12.5 o'clock (range, 6-5 o'clock; SD = 2.7 h)
	Mixed type	Normal/hypotrophic areas	Labral tear associated with degeneration signs	Same as pincer
	Dysplasia	Hypertrophic	Myxoid degeneration and/or detachment from the osseous rim	Anterosuperior
Functional alterations	Instability	Normal	Labral tear (usually base detachment in the watershed zone)	Anterior
	Iliopsoas impingement	Normal	Inflammation, labral tear, or mucoid degeneration Scarring to the anterior capsule	3 o'clock
Trauma	Traumatic	Normal	Variable	Anterior
Degeneration	Hip degenerative disease	Hypotrophic	Labral degeneration (yellow color, bruising, fraying, with eventual cysts and ossification)	Global

[a]All positions are normalized for the right hip.

fibers of partially ruptured ligaments and of the stump in completely ruptured ligaments usually relieves mechanical symptoms.[56] Curved-blade shavers and flexible radiofrequency ablation probes can be used to assess the lesion, and rotation of the limb helps to expose the structure for the arthroscopic approach (**Figure 2**).

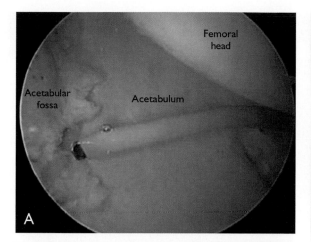

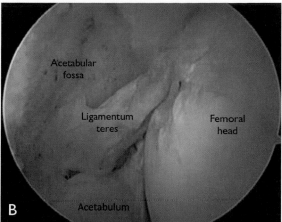

Figure 2 Arthroscopic views show a flexible radiofrequency device used to approach the acetabular fossa (**A**) and treat ligamentum teres pathology (**B**).

Thermal shrinkage is especially useful in patients with partial ruptures and signs of instability. Shrinkage should be performed with the hip in neutral rotation and should should be done conservatively, as excessive shrinkage may lead to restricted external rotation of the hip. The senior author has performed reconstruction of the ligamentum teres using an autograft of fascia lata as a salvage procedure for patients with complete tears of the ligament and extremely symptomatic instability.

Chondral Lesions

Diffuse chondral lesions are more common in elderly populations. This condition is difficult to treat but may respond relatively well when the contributing factor for the persistent damage is removed. Common instances are removal of loose bodies and treatment of a labral tear or impingement.[8] The success of such treatment has been shown to correlate with adequate joint space as seen on preoperative radiographs. A joint space less than 2 mm on any part of the weight-bearing surface was correlated with worse outcomes after hip arthroscopy.[6] Chondroplasty using thermal devices may be used to treat cartilage fraying.[12]

Localized chondral injuries are usually related to trauma or FAI. A direct correlation exists between the α angle and the presence of large grade IV chondral lesions.[46] Débridement of chondral flaps is usually very effective in resolving pain and mechanical symptoms.

Peripheral acetabular lesions often disappear after rim trimming is completed. For the other grade IV lesions, microfracture has been proven to be effective on both the acetabulum and femoral head[6,49,57] (**Figure 3**).

Loose Bodies

Removal of loose bodies is probably one of the most well-defined indications for hip arthroscopy. Synovial chondromatosis, long-standing chondral lesions, and trauma are common sources of loose bodies. Mechanical symptoms usually predominate. Symptomatic relief is often immediate after surgery. The prognosis depends on the etiology and the amount of intra-articular damage diagnosed at the time of surgery.

Internal Snapping Hip

The three types of coxa saltans, or snapping hip, are (1) intra-articular snapping caused by several conditions, including loose bodies and labral pathology; (2) internal snapping caused by the iliopsoas tendon moving over a bony prominence; and (3) external snapping from the iliotibial band or gluteus maximus tendon snapping over the greater trochanter.[17,31,58,59] Internal snapping of the iliopsoas tendon over the iliopectineal eminence, femoral head, or lesser trochanter may or may not be painful. Pain or discomfort associated with internal snapping is an indication of associated iliopsoas tendinitis, either as a result of acute inflammation or

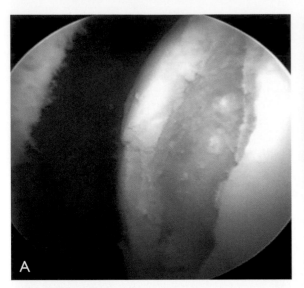 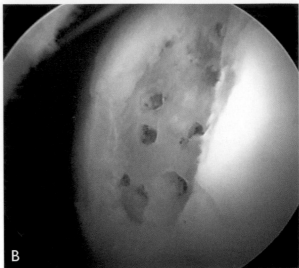

Figure 3 Arthroscopic views show a chondral defect on the femoral head. **A,** The defect following preparation for microfracture. **B,** The defect following microfracture. Note the blood and marrow elements coming from the holes.

more chronic degeneration and tendinopathy.[58,59] Initial management of painful iliopsoas tendinitis consists of nonsteroidal anti-inflammatory drugs and physical therapy.[21,59-61] If pain persists, an ultrasound-guided injection of lidocaine and corticosteroid can provide relief and predict the response to surgical release.[29,60] For patients who have recurrent pain after local injection, arthroscopic release at the musculotendinous junction or near the tendon insertion on the lesser trochanter has been described, and good results have been reported.[58-61]

Ilizaliturri et al[60] reported on six patients (seven hips) who underwent endoscopic release of the iliopsoas tendon using the Sampson technique (extra-articular, next to the insertion) and experienced complete relief of symptoms. The authors noted significant loss of flexor strength that improved after 8 weeks. Flanum et al[59] also noted postoperative weakness. They also reported recurrent ischial bursitis and sacroiliac joint pain as complications of the altered gait pattern caused by the complete release of the iliopsoas tendon at its insertion on the lesser trochanter.

Our current approach involves tenotomy of the iliopsoas tendon by an intra-articular approach.[62] In this approach, the tendon is visualized through an anterior capsulotomy during arthroscopy. Some muscle tissue usually is attached to the tendon at this point. We selectively divide the tendinous portion using an arthroscopic blade or radiofrequency device, leaving the muscle intact. For that reason, the tenotomy can be considered complete but some continuity between the muscle and its insertion is maintained. This often prevents postoperative weakness; however, the incidence of undercorrection or recurrence is expected to be greater.

Ilizaliturri et al[63] reported no difference between the two approaches in a randomized controlled trial. Regardless of the technique, care should be taken to avoid surgical violation of the iliopsoas tendon, which carries a risk of heterotopic ossification. Prophylaxis is recommended even with endoscopic methods.[63]

Lateral Trochanteric Syndrome

Mature athletes are especially susceptible to lateral hip pain. Hip abductor tendinopathy is a frequent cause of greater trochanteric pain syndrome; many cases diagnosed as bursitis are probably more related to tendon lesions.[20,64] The hip abductor muscles can be thought of as analogous to the rotator cuff of the shoulder.[65-67]

LaBan et al[68] described a case of complete detachment of those muscles from the trochanter, which was referred to as the "bald trochanter." The authors suggested that symptomatic patients who had no improvement from nonsurgical measures should undergo MRI. Patients with lesions found on MRI that do not respond to nonsurgical treatment have demonstrated good results when treated surgically.[68]

Hip arthroscopy is often performed to rule out and treat concomitant intra-articular problems. The hip is abducted to 15° and the subcutaneous plane is dissected just above the fascia lata. A cruciform incision is then made just above the greater trochanter, to decompress the underlying tissue. All of the redundant bursa is débrided. The insertions of the gluteus medius and minimus tendons are identified, and the tear/detachment is exposed. Débridement of scar tissue over the trochanter is performed so that bleeding bone is exposed at the original footprints of the tendons in preparation for reinsertion. Large metallic anchors are placed on those locations at a minimum angle of 45° to the force vector of the tendinous insertions (to minimize risk of avulsion). Mattress sutures are used to reattach the conjoined tendon to its original site.

Outcomes

Few studies have reported outcomes following hip arthroscopy in the mature population. In one study, predictors of worse outcomes in patients with FAI and chondral/labral dysfunction included joint space narrowing of 2 mm of more, low preoperative modified Harris hip score, concomitant grade IV lesions of the acetabulum and femoral head requiring microfracture (kissing lesions), and labral débridement (instead of labral repair). Although age was significantly associated with worse outcomes, that relationship may have been caused by the presence of degenerative changes in older patients. In fact, when multivariate analysis was conducted, functional outcomes were not associated with age but with joint space, preoperative functional score, and labral treatment.[6] In a 10-year follow-up study, Byrd and Jones[69] also found that that when patients presenting with signs of osteoarthritis were excluded, the outcomes in the older group were similar to those found in younger populations.

Summary

As the population ages, many people want to remain active, but the number of people seeking treatment for prearthritic hip symptoms has increased. Abnormal bone morphology or FAI can progress to early osteoarthritis. If FAI and the associated chondrolabral lesion are identified and treated, older patients can get back to activity. By maintaining good exercise regimens that minimize extreme hip flexion, the athlete may prevent further chondrolabral damage in the hip. The goal of hip arthroscopy in the mature athlete is to repair damaged tissue and improve the joint environment by removing areas of conflict. This treatment will protect the repaired areas and prevent continued damage to the joint. Although no evidence exists that this treatment will prevent osteoarthritis, early clinical data suggest that by resolving the bony impingement, prevention of further labral and chondral damage is possible.

References

1. Hunter GR, McCarthy JP, Bamman MM: Effects of resistance training on older adults. *Sports Med* 2004; 34(5):329-348.

2. Vignon E, Valat JP, Rossignol M, et al: Osteoarthritis of the knee and hip and activity: A systematic international review and synthesis (OASIS). *Joint Bone Spine* 2006;73(4):442-455.

3. Vandervoort AA: Potential benefits of warm-up for neuromuscular performance of older athletes. *Exerc Sport Sci Rev* 2009;37(2):60-65.

4. Wenger DE, Kendell KR, Miner MR, Trousdale RT: Acetabular labral tears rarely occur in the absence of bony abnormalities. *Clin Orthop Relat Res* 2004;(426): 145-150.

5. Ganz R, Leunig M, Leunig-Ganz K, Harris WH: The etiology of osteoarthritis of the hip: An integrated mechanical concept. *Clin Orthop Relat Res* 2008; 466(2):264-272.

6. Philippon MJ, Briggs KK, Yen YM, Kuppersmith DA: Outcomes following hip arthroscopy for femoroacetabular impingement with associated chondrolabral dysfunction: Minimum two-year follow-up. *J Bone Joint Surg Br* 2009;91(1):16-23.

7. Philippon MJ, Stubbs AJ, Schenker ML, Maxwell RB, Ganz R, Leunig M: Arthroscopic management of femoroacetabular impingement: Osteoplasty technique

and literature review. *Am J Sports Med* 2007;35(9): 1571-1580.

8. Philippon MJ, Schenker ML: A new method for acetabular rim trimming and labral repair. *Clin Sports Med* 2006;25(2):293-297.

9. Philippon MJ: New frontiers in hip arthroscopy: The role of arthroscopic hip labral repair and capsulorrhaphy in the treatment of hip disorders. *Instr Course Lect* 2006;55:309-316.

10. Byrd JW: The role of hip arthroscopy in the athletic hip. *Clin Sports Med* 2006;25(2):255-278.

11. McCarthy J, Barsoum W, Puri L, Lee JA, Murphy S, Cooke P: The role of hip arthroscopy in the elite athlete. *Clin Orthop Relat Res* 2003;(406):71-74.

12. Philippon MJ, Kuppersmith DA, Wolff AB, Briggs KK: Arthroscopic findings following traumatic hip dislocation in 14 professional athletes. *Arthroscopy* 2009;25(2):169-174.

13. Singh H: Senescent changes in the human musculoskeletal system, in Speer KP, ed: *Injury Prevention and Rehabilitation for Active Older Adults.* Champaign, IL, Human Kinetics, 2005, pp 3-17.

14. Lane JM, Russell L, Khan SN: Osteoporosis. *Clin Orthop Relat Res* 2000;(372):139-150.

15. Egol KA, Koval KJ, Kummer F, Frankel VH: Stress fractures of the femoral neck. *Clin Orthop Relat Res* 1998;(348):72-78.

16. Buckwalter JA, Woo SL, Goldberg VM, et al: Soft-tissue aging and musculoskeletal function. *J Bone Joint Surg Am* 1993;75(10):1533-1548.

17. Tibor LM, Sekiya JK: Differential diagnosis of pain around the hip joint. *Arthroscopy* 2008;24(12):1407-1421.

18. Luff AR: Age-associated changes in the innervation of muscle fibers and changes in the mechanical properties of motor units. *Ann N Y Acad Sci* 1998;854:92-101.

19. Jennings F, Lambert E, Fredericson M: Rheumatic diseases presenting as sports-related injuries. *Sports Med* 2008;38(11):917-930.

20. American Academy of Orthopaedic Surgeons: Hip pain may be torn tendon, not bursitis. *Acad News* February 15, 1997. www2.aaos.org/aaos/archives/acadnews/97news/gluteus1. Accessed July 15, 2011.

21. Little TL, Mansoor J: Low back pain associated with internal snapping hip syndrome in a competitive cyclist. *Br J Sports Med* 2008;42(4):308-309.

22. Philippon MJ, Schröder e Souza BG: Identifying labral tears in daily practice. *Sports Med Update* 2009;2:3-6.

23. Philippon MJ, Maxwell RB, Johnston TL, Schenker M, Briggs KK: Clinical presentation of femoroacetabular impingement. *Knee Surg Sports Traumatol Arthrosc* 2007;15(8):1041-1047.

24. Burnett RS, Della Rocca GJ, Prather H, Curry M, Maloney WJ, Clohisy JC: Clinical presentation of patients with tears of the acetabular labrum. *J Bone Joint Surg Am* 2006;88(7):1448-1457.

25. Beaulé PE, O'Neill M, Rakhra K: Acetabular labral tears. *J Bone Joint Surg Am* 2009;91(3):701-710.

26. Reynolds D, Lucas J, Klaue K: Retroversion of the acetabulum: A cause of hip pain. *J Bone Joint Surg Br* 1999;81(2):281-288.

27. Drehmann F: Drehmann's sign: A clinical examination method in epiphysiolysis (slipping of the upper femoral epiphysis). Description of signs, aetiopathogenetic considerations, clinical experience (author's transl). *Z Orthop Ihre Grenzgeb* 1979;117(3):333-344.

28. Tannast M, Siebenrock KA, Anderson SE: Femoroacetabular impingement: Radiographic diagnosis—what the radiologist should know. *AJR Am J Roentgenol* 2007;188(6):1540-1552.

29. Maheshwari AV, Malik A, Dorr LD: Impingement of the native hip joint. *J Bone Joint Surg Am* 2007;89(11): 2508-2518.

30. Leibold MR, Huijbregts PA, Jensen R: Concurrent criterion-related validity of physical examination tests for hip labral lesions: A systematic review. *J Man Manip Ther* 2008;16(2):E24-E41.

31. Winston P, Awan R, Cassidy JD, Bleakney RK: Clinical examination and ultrasound of self-reported snapping hip syndrome in elite ballet dancers. *Am J Sports Med* 2007;35(1):118-126.

32. Ganz R, Parvizi J, Beck M, Leunig M, Nötzli H, Siebenrock KA: Femoroacetabular impingement: A cause for osteoarthritis of the hip. *Clin Orthop Relat Res* 2003;(417):112-120.

33. Leunig M, Podeszwa D, Beck M, Werlen S, Ganz R: Magnetic resonance arthrography of labral disorders in hips with dysplasia and impingement. *Clin Orthop Relat Res* 2004;(418):74-80.

34. Leunig M, Werlen S, Ungersböck A, Ito K, Ganz R: Evaluation of the acetabular labrum by MR arthrography. *J Bone Joint Surg Br* 1997;79(2):230-234.

35. Sampson TG: Arthroscopic treatment of femoroacetabular impingement. *Am J Orthop (Belle Mead NJ)* 2008;37(12):608-612.

36. Kalberer F, Sierra RJ, Madan SS, Ganz R, Leunig M: Ischial spine projection into the pelvis: A new sign for acetabular retroversion. *Clin Orthop Relat Res* 2008; 466(3):677-683.

37. Nötzli HP, Wyss TF, Stoecklin CH, Schmid MR, Treiber K, Hodler J: The contour of the femoral head-neck junction as a predictor for the risk of anterior impingement. *J Bone Joint Surg Br* 2002;84(4): 556-560.

38. Meyer DC, Beck M, Ellis T, Ganz R, Leunig M: Comparison of six radiographic projections to assess femoral head/neck asphericity. *Clin Orthop Relat Res* 2006;445:181-185.

39. Lequesne M, de Sèze: False profile of the pelvis: A new radiographic incidence for the study of the hip. Its use in dysplasias and different coxopathies. *Rev Rhum Mal Osteoartic* 1961;28:643-652.

40. Crockarell JR Jr, Trousdale RT, Guyton JL: The anterior centre-edge angle: A cadaver study. *J Bone Joint Surg Br* 2000;82(4):532-534.

41. Fadul DA, Carrino JA: Imaging of femoroacetabular impingement. *J Bone Joint Surg Am* 2009;91(Suppl 1): 138-143.

42. Chan YS, Lien LC, Hsu HL, et al: Evaluating hip labral tears using magnetic resonance arthrography: A prospective study comparing hip arthroscopy and magnetic resonance arthrography diagnosis. *Arthroscopy* 2005;21(10):1250.

43. Yamamoto Y, Tonotsuka H, Ueda T, Hamada Y: Usefulness of radial contrast-enhanced computed tomography for the diagnosis of acetabular labrum injury. *Arthroscopy* 2007;23(12):1290-1294.

44. Klaue K, Durnin CW, Ganz R: The acetabular rim syndrome: A clinical presentation of dysplasia of the hip. *J Bone Joint Surg Br* 1991;73(3):423-429.

45. Pitt MJ, Graham AR, Shipman JH, Birkby W: Herniation pit of the femoral neck. *AJR Am J Roentgenol* 1982;138(6):1115-1121.

46. Johnston TL, Schenker ML, Briggs KK, Philippon MJ: Relationship between offset angle alpha and hip chondral injury in femoroacetabular impingement. *Arthroscopy* 2008;24(6):669-675.

47. Bardakos NV, Villar RN: Predictors of progression of osteoarthritis in femoroacetabular impingement: A radiological study with a minimum of ten years follow-up. *J Bone Joint Surg Br* 2009;91(2):162-169.

48. Mardones RM, Gonzalez C, Chen Q, Zobitz M, Kaufman KR, Trousdale RT: Surgical treatment of femoroacetabular impingement: Evaluation of the effect of the size of the resection. *J Bone Joint Surg Am* 2005; 87(2):273-279.

49. Philippon MJ, Schenker ML, Briggs KK, Kuppersmith DA, Maxwell RB, Stubbs AJ: Revision hip arthroscopy. *Am J Sports Med* 2007;35(11):1918-1921.

50. Philippon MJ, Schröder e Souza BG, Briggs KK: Arthroskopische Rekonstruktion des Labrum acetabulare mit einem autologen Tractus-iliotibialis-Transplantat. *Arthroskopie* 2009;22(4):306-311.

51. Lage LA, Patel JV, Villar RN: The acetabular labral tear: An arthroscopic classification. *Arthroscopy* 1996;12(3):269-272.

52. McCarthy JC: The diagnosis and treatment of labral and chondral injuries. *Instr Course Lect* 2004;53: 573-577.

53. Larson CM, Giveans MR: Arthroscopic debridement versus refixation of the acetabular labrum associated with femoroacetabular impingement. *Arthroscopy* 2009;25(4):369-376.

54. Espinosa N, Rothenfluh DA, Beck M, Ganz R, Leunig M: Treatment of femoro-acetabular impingement: Preliminary results of labral refixation. *J Bone Joint Surg Am* 2006;88(5):925-935.

55. Bellabarba C, Sheinkop MB, Kuo KN: Idiopathic hip instability: An unrecognized cause of coxa saltans in the adult. *Clin Orthop Relat Res* 1998;(355):261-271.

56. Byrd JW, Jones KS: Traumatic rupture of the ligamentum teres as a source of hip pain. *Arthroscopy* 2004;20(4):385-391.

57. Lienert JJ, Rodkey WG, Steadman JR Jr, Philippon MJ, Sekiya JK: Microfracture techniques in hip arthroscopy. *Oper Tech Orthop* 2005;15:267-272.

58. Blankenbaker DG, De Smet AA, Keene JS: Sonography of the iliopsoas tendon and injection of the iliopsoas bursa for diagnosis and management of the painful snapping hip. *Skeletal Radiol* 2006;35(8):565-571.

59. Flanum ME, Keene JS, Blankenbaker DG, Desmet AA: Arthroscopic treatment of the painful "internal" snapping hip: Results of a new endoscopic technique and imaging protocol. *Am J Sports Med* 2007;35(5): 770-779.

60. Ilizaliturri VM Jr , Villalobos FE Jr , Chaidez PA, Valero FS, Aguilera JM: Internal snapping hip syndrome: treatment by endoscopic release of the iliopsoas tendon. *Arthroscopy* 2005;21(11):1375-1380.

61. Hölmich P: Long-standing groin pain in sportspeople falls into three primary patterns, a "clinical entity" approach: A prospective study of 207 patients. *Br J Sports Med* 2007;41(4):247-252.

62. Wettstein M, Jung J, Dienst M: Arthroscopic psoas tenotomy. *Arthroscopy* 2006;22(8):907, e1-e4.

63. Ilizaliturri VM Jr, Chaidez C, Villegas P, Briseño A, Camacho-Galindo J: Prospective randomized study of 2 different techniques for endoscopic iliopsoas tendon release in the treatment of internal snapping hip syndrome. *Arthroscopy* 2009;25(2):159-163.

64. Kingzett-Taylor A, Tirman PF, Feller J, et al: Tendinosis and tears of gluteus medius and minimus muscles as a cause of hip pain: MR imaging findings. *AJR Am J Roentgenol* 1999;173(4):1123-1126.

65. Bunker TD, Esler CN, Leach WJ: Rotator-cuff tear of the hip. *J Bone Joint Surg Br* 1997;79(4):618-620.

66. Kagan A: Five cases of disruptions of the abductor mechanism of the hip. *Orthop Trans* 1996;20:329.

67. Kagan A II: Rotator cuff tears of the hip. *Clin Orthop Relat Res* 1999;(368):135-140.

68. LaBan MM, Weir SK, Taylor RS: 'Bald trochanter' spontaneous rupture of the conjoined tendons of the gluteus medius and minimus presenting as a trochanteric bursitis. *Am J Phys Med Rehabil* 2004; 83(10):806-809.

69. Byrd JW, Jones KS: Hip arthroscopy for labral pathology: Prospective analysis with 10-year follow-up. *Arthroscopy* 2009;25(4):365-368.

Chapter 26

Total Hip Arthroplasty and Total Knee Arthroplasty

Matthew J. Kraay, MS, MD
Victor M. Goldberg, MD

Key Points

- The over-65 age group is the fastest growing segment of the US population.
- Demand for total joint arthroplasty is expected to increase dramatically by the year 2030.
- The baby boomer generation has high lifestyle and activity expectations following total joint arthroplasty.
- Improvements in implant design and surgical techniques allow patients to return to reasonably active lifestyles following total joint arthroplasty.
- Current total joint implants and techniques provide the patient with a durable and potentially lifelong solution for end-stage arthritis.

Introduction and Demographics

"Seniors," defined as those older than 65 years, represent the fastest growing segment of the US population. Based on data from the Centers for Disease Control in 2005, nearly one in three adults in the United States is affected with arthritis, and arthritis and other rheumatic conditions are the leading cause of disability in Americans. Healthcare expenses for the treatment of arthritis and other related chronic joint disorders in the United States are estimated at more than $116 billion annually. In the over-65 age group, nearly 50% have at least one joint significantly affected with osteoarthritis. At the same time, this senior segment of the population is healthier and more active and has higher expectations for an active lifestyle than did prior members of this demographic group. As the US population ages, the impact of these chronic joint disorders on society will continue to increase steadily.

In 2005, approximately 428,000 total knee arthroplasties (TKAs) and more than 209,000 total hip arthroplastics (THAs) were performed in the United States, numbers that appear to be increasing steadily. By 2030, the number of joint replacements performed in the United States is expected to increase to an incredible 3.5 million TKAs and 500,000 THAs.[1]

Since the introduction of modern total joint arthroplasty nearly 4 de-

Table 1: Mean Maximum Resultant Forces for Activities 2 Months After Total Hip Arthroplasty

Activity	Maximum Resultant Force (× body weight)
Straight-leg raise	1.8
Getting out of bed	1.4
Single-leg stance	2.1
Walking with cane	2.6
Unassisted walking	2.5
Fast walking	3.6
Running	4.5

Adapted with permission from Davy DT, Kotzar GM, Brown RH, et al: Telemetric force measurements across the hip after total hip arthroplasty. *J Bone Joint Surg Am* 1988;70(1):45-50.

cades ago, improvements in implant design, implant materials, and surgical techniques have resulted in dramatic improvements in the clinical outcomes and durability of both TKA and THA. Long-term follow-up studies suggest that more than 90% of cemented condylar TKAs and cemented or uncemented THAs can be expected to survive 15 to 20 years.[2,3]

Although the pain relief and long-term clinical survival of these procedures are excellent, today's typical TKA and THA patients are frequently not satisfied with the activity and lifestyle limitations historically recommended following these procedures. Many of these patients have unusually high expectations with regard to their ability to return to "normal" activities following total joint arthroplasty, including rigorous athletic activities such as downhill skiing, singles tennis, weight lifting, and even running. Patient-perceived stiffness and persistent pain following these procedures have been suggested as important reasons why some of these high expectations are not met.

The mechanical and functional limitations of modern joint arthroplasty devices are real, and most joint arthroplasty surgeons have concerns about patients' un-

realistic expectations to return to extremely high levels of activity and participation in certain sports following THA and TKA. Both the hip and knee can be subjected to extremely high joint reactive forces that can exceed 8 to 10 times body weight in association with some of these activities (**Table 1**). Despite improvements in implant materials and designs, premature failure due to polyethylene wear, osteolysis, and mechanical loosening is a significant concern in the patient who expects to return to these joint-overloading activities following TKA or THA. Dislocation is one of the most common reasons for revision following THA, and certain activities that can result in the hip being put into extremes of position clearly predispose to this complication.

Although high-impact and certain joint-overloading activities are a concern, appropriate exercise following THA and TKA has numerous benefits for the aging patient. Weight-bearing and light resistive exercise helps to maintain bone health by minimizing osteoporosis and maintaining muscle strength and coordination. The aerobic effects of an appropriate exercise program are important in weight control, cardiovascular fitness, and even psychologic health. Joint arthroplasty has been shown to have beneficial effects on maximum oxygen consumption, workload, and exercise duration.[4] Activity recommendations for joint arthroplasty patients clearly need to be carefully formulated and take all the above factors into consideration.

Several issues must be raised when discussing total joint arthroplasty with patients who want to continue in active sports. The optimum surgical and postoperative treatment plan for the active baby boomer patient requiring THA or TKA should take into consideration the patient's preoperative activities and postoperative expectations as well as available implant technology. Although the surgical approach and individualized treatment plan may enhance a rapid return to preoperative activities, the possibility of premature implant failure and bearing surface wear and considerations about the type of fixation used are important issues to discuss with the patient preoperatively.

THA in Baby Boomers

The most common causes of failure of contemporary THA are dislocation, infection, loosening, and wear (and associated osteolysis). The annualized linear wear rate of THAs performed with conventional polyethylene has been shown to be an important determinant of the need for eventual revision.[5] Development of osteolysis appears to be somewhat dose-dependent and is considerably more likely to occur when annualized linear wear exceeds what has been termed the osteolysis threshold of 0.1 mm/y.[6] Schmalzried and Huk[7] demonstrated that wear correlates directly with activity following THA. We reviewed the postoperative activity levels in 78 THA patients younger than 55 years of age at the time of surgery followed for 10 years at our institution (VM Goldberg, unpublished data, 2009). Fifty-two of these patients were very active, and 50 of these 52 returned to sports. Half of these patients were able to return to their preoperative sport; the other half had to return to a sport of lesser intensity. Failure rate due to osteolysis was 3.5% at 10 years after surgery; however, only one revision was performed.

Implant fixation in elderly patients appears to be durable regardless of the method of fixation. In younger patients, however, who are typically more active, uncemented fixation appears to be more durable[8] (**Table 2**). In addition to activity-related concerns, the recent trend toward the use of "less invasive" surgical approaches has resulted in a significant increase in the use of uncemented THA regardless of patient age.

As most patients age, alterations in the endosteal geometry of the proximal femur and overall deterioration in bone quality can adversely affect the degree of initial implant stability required to obtain satisfactory uncemented implant fixation. Age-related increases in the diameter of the medullary canal typically warrant the use of larger diameter uncemented stems, which predispose to stress shielding and undesirable stress-induced remodeling of the proximal femur. Traditionally, this concern has been managed by use of a cemented femoral component, which, because of the mechanical properties of polymethyl methacrylate, has a composite stiffness closer to that of a normal femur than does a large-diameter, canal-filling, distally fixed uncemented femoral component. Several attempts have been made to develop an isoelastic uncemented femoral component out of polymeric materials that have mechanical properties closer to that of the native femur than the traditional femoral components made of the standard implant alloys (ie, CoCrMo [cobalt chrome]

or TiAlV [titanium]). The only currently available femoral component of this type is the EPOCH (extensively porous coated hip) stem (Zimmer, Warsaw, IN). This implant uses a central structural core of CoCrMo with a molded polyaryletherketone (PAEK) filler and a surrounding fixation surface of titanium fiber metal (**Figure 1**). Early to intermediate-term results indicate that stress shielding and adverse bone remodeling are minimized with this novel design[9,10] (**Figure 2**).

Strategies to minimize wear have been a major focus of research in THA during the last 15 years. Radiation sterilization of the ultra-high-molecular-weight polyethylene (UHMWPE) liner in an oxygen environment has been shown to lead to oxidative degradation of the UHMWPE with dramatic reduction in the mechanical and wear properties of this widely used implant material due to subsurface delamination and cracking.[11,12] Irradiation sterilization of UHMWPE in an oxygen-free, inert environment and introduction of barrier packaging have been shown to significantly decrease these oxidation-related effects on mechanical properties.[13] Despite many improvements in material quality, manufacturing, and sterilization, conventional polyethylene does not appear to be the optimal bearing surface for THA in the younger and more active patient of today. Within the last 8 to 10 years, new alternative bearing materials have been introduced in the hopes of reducing wear and eliminating osteolysis in THA. Based on hip wear–simulator evaluation, all of these alternative bearing materials appear to have substantially better wear properties than conventional UHMWPE. However, each of these new alternative bearing materials also seems to carry some unique concerns.[14]

Cross-linked UHMWPE (XLPE) is currently the most widely used alternative bearing material for THA. Although the wear properties of XLPE are significantly better than those of conventional polyethylene, the fracture toughness and fatigue properties of this relatively brittle polymeric material are a concern.[11] Certain implant design features and technical factors that result in localized stress concentrations and edge-loading conditions have been implicated as risk factors for rare reported cases of implant fracture. Although the relative bioreactivity of wear debris generated by XLPE bearing surfaces in comparison with conventional polyethylene and the other alternative bearing surfaces is

Table 2: Total Hip Arthroplasty Survival by Patient Age, Type of Stem, and Type of Fixation[a]

Stem Groups by Age Group	No. of Primary Operations	Mean Follow-up (Years)	No. at Risk at 10 Years	10-Year Survival[b]
55-64 years				
Uncemented straight	4,261	6.0	859	98 (98-99)
Uncemented fit and fill	2,875	7.1	978	96 (95-97)
Composite-beam cemented	3,705	10.2	1,876	87 (85-88)
Loaded taper cemented	1,821	5.6	332	92 (90-94)
Subtotal	12,662			
65-74 years				
Uncemented straight	2,494	5.3	372	98 (97-99)
Uncemented fit and fill	2,257	5.7	447	97 (95-98)
Composite-beam cemented	12,878	8.6	5,420	92 (91-93)
Loaded taper cemented	6,663	4.7	665	95 (93-96)
Subtotal	24,292			
≥75 years				
Uncemented straight	390	4.9	45	99 (97-100)
Uncemented fit and fill	611	4.4	50	99 (99-100)
Composite-beam cemented	8,288	6.6	2,116	96 (96-97)
Loaded taper cemented	4,725	3.9	254	98 (97-99)
Subtotal	14,014			
All (≥55 years)				
Uncemented straight	7,145	5.7	1,276	98 (98-99)
Uncemented fit and fill	5,743	6.3	1,474	97 (96-97)
Composite-beam cemented	24,871	8.2	9,412	92 (92-92)
Loaded taper cemented	13,209	4.6	1,250	95 (94-95)
Total	50,968			

[a]The end point was defined as revision because of aseptic loosening of the stem.

[b]Ten-, 15-, and 20-year survival rates were obtained from the Kaplan-Meier analysis. The values are given as the mean percentage, with 95% confidence interval in parentheses.

[c]The risk ratio is from the Cox regression analysis (other stem groups were compared with the loaded-taper cemented stems; adjustment was made for age and sex). The 95% confidence interval is given in parentheses.

[d]The difference was not significant.

NR = not reported.

Adapted with permission from Mäkelä KT, Eskelinen A, Pulkkinen P, Paavolainen P, Remes V: Total hip arthroplasty for primary osteoarthritis in patients fifty-five years of age or older: An analysis of the Finnish arthroplasty registry. *J Bone Joint Surg Am* 2008;90(10):2160-2170.

Table 2: *(continued)*

No. at Risk at 15 Years	15-Year Survival[b]	No. at Risk at 20 Years	20-Year Survival[b]	Adjusted Risk Ratio for Revision[c]	P Value
49	91 (86-95)	NR	NR	0.27 (0.20-0.38)	<0.001
108	90 (85-94)	1	NR	0.39 (0.29-0.53)	<0.001
977	76 (74-78)	357	70 (67-72)	1.40 (1.12-1.76)	0.003
104	77 (72-83)	37	66 (57-74)	1.0	NR
25	98 (97-99)	NR	NR	0.31 (0.20-0.50)	<0.001
36	92 (86-98)	NR	NR	0.50 (0.34-0.74)	<0.001
1897	87 (86-88)	378	84 (82-85)	1.60 (1.33-1.93)	<0.001
156	89 (86-92)	26	82 (76-89)	1.0	NR
1	NR	NR	NR	0.84 (0.26-2.76)	0.78[d]
1	NR	NR	NR	0.40 (0.10-1.69)	0.21[d]
423	95 (93-95)	37	95 (93-96)	2.01 (1.37-2.94)	<0.001
18	NR	NR	NR	1.0	NR
75	93 (90-96)	NR	NR	0.28 (0.22-0.36)	<0.001
145	91 (87-94)	1	NR	0.41 (0.33-0.52)	<0.001
3297	85 (85-87)	771	82 (80-83)	1.55 (1.35-1.77)	<0.001
277	85 (84-89)	63	77 (71-82)	1.0	NR

still unknown, at 8 to 10 years after their introduction, osteolysis appeared to be extremely rare with XLPE bearings.

Metal-on-metal (MOM) alternative bearings are, at least theoretically, an appealing option for THA. In addition to having an extremely low volumetric wear rate in THA wear simulators, MOM THA makes possible the use of a large femoral head that closely resembles the diameter of the patient's own femoral head. The increased range of motion and reduction of dislocation afforded by a large femoral head prosthesis is especially appealing in the athletically active patient following THA. The large-diameter MOM head concept also has revived interest in femoral head resurfacing arthroplasty of the hip, which proponents advocate as a "conservative" approach to THA that is especially appealing for the young, active patient with arthritis of the hip. Two randomized clinical trials of MOM surface replacement arthroplasty versus large-head MOM THA have failed to show any difference between the two groups in Western Ontario and McMaster Universities Osteoarthritis Index (WOMAC) function score,

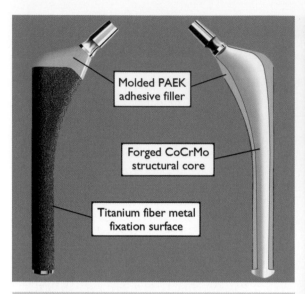

Figure 1 Frontal (left) and cut-away cross-sectional (right) views of the EPOCH composite hip stem demonstrate its composite structure. PAEK = polyaryletherketone. (Courtesy of Zimmer, Warsaw, IN.)

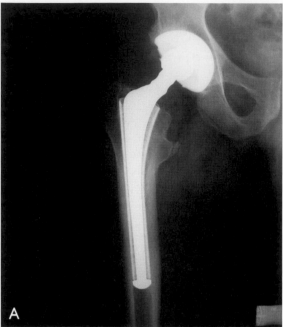

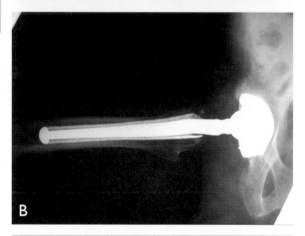

Figure 2 Radiographs of the hip of an active patient who underwent THA with an EPOCH stem. AP (**A**) and lateral (**B**) radiographs at 8-year follow-up demonstrate preservation of bone density.

University of California at Los Angeles (UCLA) activity score, or pain score at 1 or 2 years.[15] Serum cobalt and chromium levels were increased in both the THA and resurfacing groups compared with baseline levels. Theoretical concerns about excess cobalt and chromium metal ion release from these MOM bearings include local tissue toxicity, renal damage, chromosomal damage, and the potential for malignant cellular transformation. Although the MOM alternative might seem to be a preferred bearing surface for THA, long-term concerns about systemic effects of wear debris from MOM THA and increasing reports of local toxicity associated with these devices (aseptic lymphocytic vasculitis-associated lesions [ALVAL])[16,17] and local pseudotumors around these implants[18] have resulted in recent moderation of their clinical use. Suboptimal component positioning that results in edge loading and excessive wear and implant design have been demonstrated to contribute to increased metal ion levels and development of pseudotumors in MOM THAs.[19,20] Several authors have suggested, however, that pseudotumor-like reactions can occur in patients with low wear who have a hypersensitivity reaction to metal

ions.[21,22] Glyn-Jones et al[23] reported a 1.8% incidence of revision for pseudotumor in a group of 1,224 surface replacements. Although the rate of revision for men was 0.5%, the incidence of revision for pseudotumors was 6% for women older than 40 years and 13% for women younger than 40 years. Patients with small femoral head size also appeared to be at increased risk of revision for pseudotumor.

Ceramic-on-ceramic bearings have the lowest wear rate of any of the alternative bearing surfaces currently available. In addition, wear debris from ceramic bearings appears to be very bioinert and well tolerated in the body. Although historically ceramic femoral head components have been associated with an unacceptable rate of breakage and catastrophic failure, improvements in ceramic implant manufacturing techniques have reduced the incidence of fracture to as low as 1 in 25,000 for BIOLOX (CeramTec AG, Plochingen, Germany) alumina femoral heads. These materials are extremely brittle and subject to several unique types of damage, however, including chipping and "stripe wear," under eccentric and impact-loading conditions. Chipping can occur during insertion of the ceramic liner into the metal shell at the time of surgery if the components are not perfectly aligned or postoperatively if there is neck-on-liner impingement. "Stripe wear" appears to be due to repetitive separation and impact loading of the ceramic femoral head against the acetabular liner during the gait cycle or impingement of the ceramic components against the metal portions of the stem or cup.[14] Microscopic damage to the highly polished ceramic-on-ceramic articulation can result in squeaking due to impaired fluid-film lubrication of the ceramic surfaces.[24] Not only is this a considerable annoyance for the patient, but the long-term consequences of this damage to the bearing surface and alteration of the normal lubrication mechanism of the ceramic-on-ceramic bearing raises concerns about long-term in vivo performance and durability.

TKA in Baby Boomers

The most common causes of failure of contemporary TKA are aseptic loosening, wear and associated osteolysis, instability and malalignment, infection, and extensor mechanism complications. Excessive mechanical overloading has been associated with failure following TKA, as with THA. Diduch et al[25] reported a 94% rate of survival of the femoral and tibial components and a 90% rate of survival of the femoral, tibial, and patellar components at 18-year follow-up in a group of active patients. Mont et al[26] reviewed the outcomes of TKA in two matched groups of patients. One group returned to

moderate-impact sports after surgery, and the other returned to low-impact sports. No differences in radiographic or clinical outcome were seen in the two groups, and no revisions had been performed in either group at a mean follow-up of 7 years. Lavernia et al[27] analyzed wear in 28 retrieved components and found significant correlations between damage due to creep and deformation and UCLA activity score. Analysis of patients from the Swedish Knee Registry by Knutson et al[28] revealed that the 10-year revision rate was three times higher for younger, more active patients. Rand et al[29] reported the overall outcome of more than 10,000 TKAs done at the Mayo Clinic. Survival at 10 years was 94% for patients older than 75 years, 88% for patients between 56 and 70 years, and only 77% for patients younger than 55 years.

Posterior cruciate–retaining TKAs in 104 patients followed for a minimum of 10 years were reviewed with regard to return to activities (VM Goldberg, unpublished data, 2009). The patients were younger than 60 years at the time of surgery. Of the 60 patients who were very active in sports according to Mont's criteria, 55 returned to their sport after TKA. Before and after surgery, Knee Society knee scores and function scores were comparable in patients whether they participated in sports or not. No revisions were performed in either group, and no radiographic evidence of osteolysis was seen.

Unicompartmental knee arthroplasty (UKA), done through a minimally invasive surgical (MIS) approach, has seen increased use as an alternative to TKA or osteotomy in the patient with isolated unicompartmental arthritis. Advantages of MIS UKA include reduced hospital length of stay, recovery, and rehabilitation; a more "conservative" procedure with the potential for later conversion to a TKA; a more predictable outcome than a proximal tibial osteotomy; and reported 10-year survival rates greater than 95%.[30] Although the 10-year results of UKA appear comparable to those of TKA, the longer term outcomes are unknown. Disadvantages of UKA include the potential for degeneration of the unresurfaced compartments and possibly inferior fixation in comparison to TKA, both of which may result in the need for conversion to a TKA. Patient selection for UKA is critical because pain relief is disappointing in patients with significant involvement in the other com-

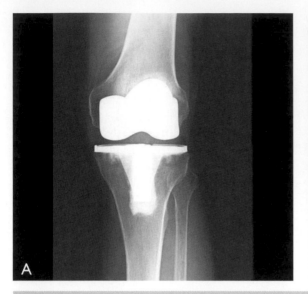
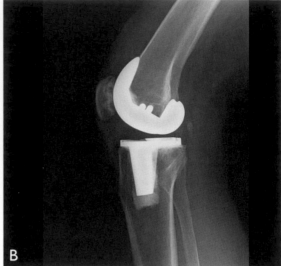

Figure 3   AP (**A**) and lateral (**B**) radiographs of an active 59-year-old man with a high-flexion knee. The patient obtained more than 155° of knee flexion postoperatively and returned to unlimited walking, biking, and squash.

partments of the knee. In certain active patients with predominantly unicompartmental knee arthritis yet with limited patellofemoral degenerative changes and symptoms, a UKA can be offered as the "first stage" of a TKA. The risk of revision of a UKA appears to be higher in patients younger than 65 years. Conversion of a painful or failed UKA to a TKA can give clinical outcomes that are comparable to a primary TKA if major bone deficiency is not present. These significant bone deficiencies are typically the result of an excessive initial tibial resection, an insufficiency fracture of the resurfaced tibial plateau, or subsidence of a loose tibial component.

Increased functional demands in the active knee arthroplasty patient who wants to return to athletic activities have stimulated interest in "high-flexion" knee designs and strategies to minimize wear in TKA (**Figure 3,** *A* and *B*). Although these high-flexion implants are designed to allow for knee flexion of up to 155°, patient selection, surgical technique, and postoperative rehabilitation are other important determinants of range of motion following TKA. Essential features of high-flexion designs include maintenance of sufficient contact area over the full range of motion to minimize

contact stresses, promotion of femoral rollback, minimization of patellar tendon and posterior cruciate ligament impingement, optimization of tibiofemoral rotation, and posterior cruciate ligament tensioning and balancing. Long-term follow-up studies are lacking, but early results do not demonstrate any functional differences between these implants and similar non–high-flexion components.[31-33]

Wear reduction in TKA has focused on mobile-bearing designs and use of XLPE. Fixed-bearing TKA designs, in which all motion occurs at one surface only (ie, between the femoral component and the polyethylene articular surface), must be of a relatively nonconforming geometry to prevent kinematic conflict and to allow physiologic range of motion following surgery. The mobile-bearing concept, however, allows for motion to occur at the polyethylene bearing surfaces in contact with both the femoral component and the tibial tray. Unlike fixed-bearing designs, this results in two contact surfaces of high conformity and low polyethylene contact stresses. Although the mobile-bearing concept appears to have a theoretical advantage over fixed-bearing designs with regard to wear, no conclusive clinical data exist to support the superiority of mobile-bearing over fixed-bearing TKA. McEwen et al[34] reported that in young, active patients, the wear rate appears to be higher with fixed-bearing TKA versus mobile-bearing TKA. The consensus of current data, however, suggests that mobile-bearing TKA offers no advantage in terms of function or failure rate in comparison with current fixed-bearing TKA designs.

Conventional UHMWPE has performed well in TKA. Elimination of calcium stearate, incorporation of net shape-molding manufacturing techniques, sterilization by irradiation in an oxygen-free environment, and barrier packaging have resulted in a bearing surface material that combines strength, toughness, wear resistance, and stable material properties. Irradiation-induced cross-linking of polyethylene has been shown to improve wear and delamination resistance in TKA simulators, and XLPE has recently been introduced for use in TKA. Because fracture toughness and fatigue are more of a concern in TKA than in THA, XLPEs used in TKA are treated with a reduced amount of irradiation to better maintain their mechanical properties and simultaneously provide a modest improvement in wear properties over conventional UHMWPE. Femoral components made of oxidized zirconium have been shown to reduce polyethylene wear in TKA simulators and may result in reduction of polyethylene wear in TKA.[35]

Summary

In summary, the function and durability of THA and TKA have improved substantially, and patients undergoing these procedures can expect many years of active use from their total joint arthroplasty. Although high-impact and certain joint-overloading activities are a concern, appropriate exercise following THA and TKA has numerous benefits for the aging patient and should be encouraged. Success of THA and TKA depends on numerous factors, including patient selection, implant design, surgical technique, and postoperative rehabilitation. Recent improvements in bearing surfaces for THA and TKA hold the promise of total joint arthroplasties with even more durability.

References

1. Kurtz S, Ong K, Lau E, Mowat F, Halpern M: Projections of primary and revision hip and knee arthroplasty in the United States from 2005 to 2030. *J Bone Joint Surg Am* 2007;89(4):780-785.

2. Joshi AB, Markovic L, Gill G: Knee arthroplasty in octogenarians: Results at 10 years. *J Arthroplasty* 2003;18(3):295-298.

3. Ma HM, Lu YC, Ho FY, Huang CH: Long-term results of total condylar knee arthroplasty. *J Arthroplasty* 2005;20(5):580-584.

4. Ries MD, Philbin EF, Groff GD, Sheesley KA, Richman JA, Lynch F Jr: Improvement in cardiovascular fitness after total knee arthroplasty. *J Bone Joint Surg Am* 1996;78(11):1696-1701.

5. McAuley JP, Szuszczewicz ES, Young A, Engh CA Sr: Total hip arthroplasty in patients 50 years and younger. *Clin Orthop Relat Res* 2004;(418):119-125.

6. Dowd JE, Sychterz CJ, Young AM, Engh CA: Characterization of long-term femoral-head-penetration rates: Association with and prediction of osteolysis. *J Bone Joint Surg Am* 2000;82-A(8):1102-1107.

7. Schmalzried TP, Huk OL: Patient factors and wear in total hip arthroplasty. *Clin Orthop Relat Res* 2004;(418):94-97.

8. Mäkelä KT, Eskelinen A, Pulkkinen P, Paavolainen P, Remes V: Total hip arthroplasty for primary osteoarthritis in patients fifty-five years of age or older: An analysis of the Finnish arthroplasty registry. *J Bone Joint Surg Am* 2008;90(10):2160-2170.

9. Glassman AH, Crowninshield RD, Schenck R, Herberts P: A low stiffness composite biologically fixed prosthesis. *Clin Orthop Relat Res* 2001;(393):128-136.

10. Akhavan S, Matthiesen MM, Schulte L, et al: Clinical and histologic results related to a low-modulus composite total hip replacement stem. *J Bone Joint Surg Am* 2006;88(6):1308-1314.

11. Rimnac CM, Pruitt L: Implant Wear Symposium 2007 Engineering Work Group: How do material properties influence wear and fracture mechanisms? *J Am Acad Orthop Surg* 2008;16(Suppl 1):S94-S100.

12. Kurtz SM, Rimnac CM, Hozack WJ, et al: In vivo degradation of polyethylene liners after gamma sterilization in air. *J Bone Joint Surg Am* 2005;87(4):815-823.

13. Crowninshield RD, Muratoglu OK: Implant Wear Symposium 2007 Engineering Work Group: How have new sterilization techniques and new forms of polyethylene influenced wear in total joint replacement? *J Am Acad Orthop Surg* 2008;16(Suppl 1): S80-S85.

14. Clarke IC, Manley MT: Implant Wear Symposium 2007 Engineering Work Group: How do alternative bearing surfaces influence wear behavior? *J Am Acad Orthop Surg* 2008;16(Suppl 1):S86-S93.

15. Lavigne M, Therrien M, Nantel J, Roy A, Prince F, Vendittoli P: RCT comparing clinical outcome and gait characteristics after large head THA and hip resurfacing, Paper 318. *AAOS Annual Meeting Proceedings*. Rosemont, IL, American Academy of Orthopaedic Surgeons, 2009, vol 10, p 457.

16. Garbuz DS, Tanzer M, Greidanus NV, Masri BA, Duncan CP: The John Charnley Award: Metal-on-metal hip resurfacing versus large-diameter head metal-on-metal total hip arthroplasty. A randomized clinical trial. *Clin Orthop Relat Res* 2010;468(2):318-325.

17. Davies AP, Willert HG, Campbell PA, Learmonth ID, Case CP: An unusual lymphocytic perivascular infiltration in tissues around contemporary metal-on-metal joint replacements. *J Bone Joint Surg Am* 2005; 87(1):18-27.

18. Willert HG, Buchhorn GH, Fayyazi A, et al: Metal-on-metal bearings and hypersensitivity in patients with artificial hip joints: A clinical and histomorphological study. *J Bone Joint Surg Am* 2005;87(1):28-36.

19. De Haan R, Pattyn C, Gill HS, Murray DW, Campbell PA, De Smet K: Correlation between inclination of the acetabular component and metal ion levels in metal-on-metal hip resurfacing replacement. *J Bone Joint Surg Br* 2008;90(10):1291-1297.

20. Langton DJ, Jameson SS, Joyce TJ, Hallab NJ, Natu S, Nargol AV: Early failure of metal-on-metal bearings in hip resurfacing and large-diameter total hip replacement: A consequence of excess wear. *J Bone Joint Surg Br* 2010;92(1):38-46.

21. Pandit H, Glyn-Jones S, McLardy-Smith P, et al: Pseudotumours associated with metal-on-metal hip resurfacings. *J Bone Joint Surg Br* 2008;90(7):847-851.

22. Campbell P, Ebramzadeh E, Nelson S, Takamura K, De Smet K, Amstutz HC: Histological features of pseudotumor-like tissues from metal-on-metal hips. *Clin Orthop Relat Res* 2010;468(9):2321-2327.

23. Glyn-Jones S, Pandit H, Kwon YM, Doll H, Gill HS, Murray DW: Risk factors for inflammatory pseudotumour formation following hip resurfacing. *J Bone Joint Surg Br* 2009;91(12):1566-1574.

24. Jacobs CA, Greenwald AS, Anderson PA, Kraay MJ, Mihalko WM: Squeaky hips make media, medical noise. *AAOS NOW* Oct 2008. Available at http://www.aaos.org/news/aaosnow/oct08/clinical1.asp. Accessed July 12, 2010.

25. Diduch DR, Insall JN, Scott WN, Scuderi GR, Font-Rodriguez D: Total knee replacement in young, active patients: Long-term follow-up and functional outcome. *J Bone Joint Surg Am* 1997;79(4):575-582.

26. Mont MA, Marker DR, Seyler TM, Gordon N, Hungerford DS, Jones LC: Knee arthroplasties have similar results in high- and low-activity patients. *Clin Orthop Relat Res* 2007;460:165-173.

27. Lavernia CJ, Sierra RJ, Hungerford DS, Krackow K: Activity level and wear in total knee arthroplasty: A study of autopsy retrieved specimens. *J Arthroplasty* 2001;16(4):446-453.

28. Knutson K, Lewold S, Robertsson O, Lidgren L: The Swedish knee arthroplasty register: A nation-wide study of 30,003 knees 1976-1992. *Acta Orthop Scand* 1994; 65(4):375-386.

29. Rand JA, Trousdale RT, Ilstrup DM, Harmsen WS: Factors affecting the durability of primary total knee prostheses. *J Bone Joint Surg Am* 2003;85-A(2): 259-265.

30. Berger RA, Meneghini RM, Jacobs JJ, et al: Results of unicompartmental knee arthroplasty at a minimum of ten years of follow-up. *J Bone Joint Surg Am* 2005; 87(5):999-1006.

31. Chaudhary R, Beaupré LA, Johnston DW: Knee range of motion during the first two years after use of posterior cruciate-stabilizing or posterior cruciate-retaining total knee prostheses: A randomized clinical trial. *J Bone Joint Surg Am* 2008;90(12):2579-2586.

32. Kim YH, Choi Y, Kwon OR, Kim JS: Functional outcome and range of motion of high-flexion posterior cruciate-retaining and high-flexion posterior cruciate-substituting total knee prostheses: A prospective, randomized study. *J Bone Joint Surg Am* 2009;91(4): 753-760.

33. Kim YH, Choi Y, Kim JS: Range of motion of standard and high-flexion posterior cruciate-retaining total knee prostheses a prospective randomized study. *J Bone Joint Surg Am* 2009;91(8):1874-1881.

34. McEwen HM, Barnett PI, Bell CJ, et al: The influence of design, materials and kinematics on the in vitro wear of total knee replacements. *J Biomech* 2005;38(2):357-365.

35. Laskin RS: An oxidized Zr ceramic surfaced femoral component for total knee arthroplasty. *Clin Orthop Relat Res* 2003;(416):191-196.

Chapter 27

Athletic Activity After Arthroplasty

Joshua Baumfeld, MD
Michael Thompson, MD
William L. Healy, MD

Key Points

- Total joint arthroplasty has been shown to improve general and cardiovascular health and may benefit mental health as well.
- Demand for joint arthroplasty is projected to increase in the first 3 decades of the 21st century.
- Patient expectations are changing, and many patients choose to undergo joint arthroplasty to continue to participate in athletic activity.
- The orthopaedic literature regarding athletic activity after joint arthroplasty is limited to retrospective studies with short-term or midterm follow-up and must be interpreted with caution.
- In general, consensus opinion suggests patients may participate in low-impact activity and should avoid high-impact sports following joint arthroplasty.
- Expert opinion exists for athletic activity following total hip, knee, and shoulder arthroplasty, which can help guide surgeons when discussing patient expectations and limitations for postoperative activity.

Introduction

The number of arthroplasties in the United States has increased significantly in recent years. One report estimates that in 2008, more than 400,000 primary total hip arthroplasties (THAs) and more than 500,000 primary total knee arthroplasties (TKAs) were performed in the United States.[1] Kurtz et al[2] have estimated 170% growth in primary THAs and 670% growth in primary TKAs by the year 2030. Historically, joint arthroplasty operations were performed for control of pain. During the last decade, patient expectations have expanded, and many pa-

tients choose to undergo joint arthroplasty to improve function and return to high-demand sports.[3] Mancuso et al[4] have shown that patients undergoing joint arthroplasty have multiple expectations, including relief of symptoms, improvement in physical function, and improvement in psychosocial well-being. Although patients may choose to undergo a joint arthroplasty operation to participate in sports, it has been difficult for orthopaedic surgeons to provide an evidence-based answer to a patient who asks, "What can I do after my joint replacement?"

General Health Benefits

Osteoarthrosis is associated with pain that may lead to deconditioning and a decrease in cardiovascular status. Regular exercise reduces anxiety, depression, and mortality, and it improves cardiovascular and bone health.[5,6] Regular exercise also can be beneficial for patients with obesity, high blood pressure, coronary disease, diabetes, osteoporosis, and low back pain.[7] Ries et al[8] have demonstrated an overall health benefit associated with increased activity following TKA. They followed two groups of patients with knee osteoarthritis, one of which underwent TKA. After 2 years, there was a significant improvement in maximum oxygen consumption compared with the nonarthroplasty group. They also showed improvement in Arthritis Impact Measurement Scales for mobility, walking, and bending as well as performing household tasks. They noted that resuming routine walking activities after TKA improved cardiovascular fitness.

Röder et al[9] evaluated over 12,000 patients undergoing THA for preoperative and postoperative pain, mobility, and motion. They showed a significant increase in the percentage of patients who were able to ambulate more than 60 minutes following joint arthroplasty. This indicates that joint arthroplasty can have a beneficial impact on general health and cardiovascular health.

Contrary to common belief, however, patients are still at risk of gaining weight following TKA. Zeni and Snyder-Mackler[10] compared patients who had undergone TKA with an age-matched control group and found that 66% of the surgical group gained weight over a 2-year follow-up period. The authors noted that it is important to encourage TKA patients to take advantage of their functional gain.

Effect of Activity on Bearing Surface Wear and Implant Survivorship

The orthopaedic literature is not clear as to the long-term effects of activity on survival rates of joint implants. Chandler et al[11] demonstrated that an increased level of activity was associated with premature loosening in 67% of patients with cemented THAs. Dorr et al[12] showed increased failure rates with increased activity in a population younger than 45 years at the time of

their index cemented THA. Kilgus et al[13] divided active patients with cemented THAs into a high-impact group (tennis, jogging, horseback riding, racquetball, backpacking, and other sports as well heavy labor) and a low-impact group. The high-impact group had a 28% revision rate versus a 6% revision rate in the low-impact population. Kilgus et al also demonstrated that older patients, including those over 70, have a higher rate of failure with increased activity. Mintz et al[14] reported that younger, active patients had an increased rate of component failure with the porous-coated anatomic TKA using predominantly uncemented fixation.

Charnley and Halley[15] demonstrated that THA patients with cemented fixation and 22-mm femoral heads had 5 to 10 times normal bearing surface wear using conventional (ie, non–cross-linked) ultra-high–molecular-weight polyethylene (UHMWPE). Schmalzried et al[16] have shown that more than 500,000 submicron-size conventional polyethylene particles can be released with every step taken following THA. These small polyethylene particles have been implicated in osteolysis, which can lead to aseptic loosening of joint implants. In another study, Schmalzried et al[17] reported that wear is a function of use, not necessarily time. They studied 37 THAs and showed a positive correlation with higher walking speeds and wear. Maloney et al[18] demonstrated that polyethylene wear and osteolysis about the pelvis was correlated with wear rate and patient age. They noted that patients under 50 years of age had increased wear rates and an associated increased risk of osteolysis with conventional polyethylene. Lavernia et al[19] evaluated retrieved polyethylene inserts after TKA at a mean of 74 months after implantation and noted a positive correlation between wear rate and activity level and length of implantation.

In sharp contrast, other investigators have shown no difference in revision rates among patients who participate in athletic activity. Diduch et al[20] examined TKA patients younger than 55 years with mean 8-year follow-up and noted excellent Knee Society and functional scores; at 18-year follow-up the survival rate was 87%. They reported that some of these patients played high-impact sports such as tennis. Gschwend et al[21] examined 2 groups of 50 patients with 5- to 10-year follow-up. One group regularly participated in alpine or cross-country skiing; the second group did not participate in any winter sports. At 5 years, there were no signs of loosening in the active group, but 5 of the 60 implants in the less active group showed loosening. At 10 years, there was a higher average rate of wear in the active group (2.1 mm versus 1.5 mm). The authors concluded that there was no evidence that alpine or cross-country skiing had a negative effect on the acetabular or femoral components in THA. They recommended avoiding short-radius turns on steep slopes and moguls.

Mont et al[22] evaluated active and inactive patients who were younger than 50 years of age at the time of TKA with a follow-up of 7 years. The authors noted no difference in rates of revision or implant failure. They also studied tennis players following THA and TKA. They noted a 5% revision rate with midterm follow-up after THA,[3] and similar findings were shown after TKA. At approximately 9-year follow-up, Kim et al[23] reported no cases of loosening in active patients younger than 50 years. Jones et al[24] evaluated 26 patients who underwent revision TKA and 26 who did not in a matched control study. Using telephone interviews regarding athletic activity, the authors concluded that physical activity did not appear to be a risk factor for revision in TKA.

Total Hip Arthroplasty

THA has been shown to improve activity for patients with osteoarthritis. Chatterji et al[25] surveyed patients before and after THA and reported that more patients participated in sports postoperatively. Patients indicated that they felt there was a beneficial effect on their performance following THA. However, they noted that the number of sporting activities decreased. Activities such as exercise walking and water aerobics increased, but more demanding sports activities such as golf, tennis, and jogging decreased. The conclusions of this study were that patients adopted lower impact activity following THA, and that the total number of patients performing a sport increased postoperatively, but the total amount of sports played decreased.

Mont et al[3] evaluated tennis players following THA. The study involved sending questionnaires to United States Tennis Association (USTA) members. Mean patient age at the time of the index surgery was 58 years. Patients were asked their surgeon's preference as to whether they should continue to play tennis following arthroplasty; the responses indicated that 14% of surgeons approved of singles, 34% approved of doubles only, and 52% opposed tennis completely. Despite this, 21% of patients chose to have THA surgery specifically to continue playing tennis: 36% to play and for pain relief, and 43% to play and improve their range of motion. A 5% revision rate was noted. Patients returned to play at an average of 6.7 months, and they returned to nearly the same level of play as preoperatively. They played an average of three times per week, similar to their premorbid rate. Patients noted increased mobility but decreased court speed. In addition, 9% had activity-related groin pain, and 16% had some pain and stiffness. This study shows that patients can successfully return to tennis at a high level. However, there was significant selection bias in the study, as all of the players surveyed had remained active USTA members after THA.

Mallon et al[26] showed that golfers at both the professional and amateur levels can return to their sport after THA. The mean age at the time of THA was 58 to 59 years, with a mean follow-up period of 4 to 5 years. Most patients returned to golf 3 to 4 months after their THA, and 92% reported no pain with playing. There was a 9% revision rate, and one patient sustained an open periprosthetic fracture after a slip and fall while playing. Hip Society members were polled; although none considered golf contraindicated after THA, 69% encouraged the use of a cart. Some respondents advised patients who had an uncemented hip prosthesis to decrease their golfing activity during the first 6 to 8 months postoperatively.

Participation in mountain sports is also possible after THA. Peters[27] reported on mountain sports such as 6- to 7-hour mountain walks, trekking, and high-altitude activities following THA. Patients who wish to participate in these activities following THA should have significant preoperative experience. The author felt that it is important that the patient has regained proprioception, balance, and strength and be in excellent physical condition in order to successfully return to mountain sports.

Sechriest et al[28] reviewed 34 patients following THA with a mean follow-up of 6.3 years and a mean age of 42 years at the time of surgery. They found that patients' perception of activity did not correlate with wear and gait cycles per year and noted that young patients with THA might not be as active as the patients themselves perceived. The authors found that linear polyethylene wear rates did not exceed those seen in patients who are older. They also noted that advanced age and obesity correlated negatively with postoperative walking activity. Also, patients with systemic polyarticular disease were less active after THA than were THA patients with local hip disease such as osteonecrosis and dysplasia.

Many of the studies evaluating activity following THA were performed with conventional polyethylene and older-generation implants. Current trends in joint arthroplasty include the use of alternative bearing surfaces such as highly cross-linked polyethylene (HXLPE), ceramics, and metal-on-metal. Potential advantages of these bearing surfaces include decreased wear rates, decreased osteolysis, and lower rates of aseptic loosening. Most of the studies documenting high failure rates of THA in young, active patients have examined patients treated with metal or conventional polyethylene bearing surfaces. More recent data, such as the reviews of the Finnish Arthroplasty Register by Eskelinen et al,[29,30] demonstrate that second-generation uncemented femoral stems have greater than 90% survival rates at 10 years. In their review of 2,000 tapered titanium porous plasma–sprayed femoral components, Lombardi et al[31] showed a 99% stem survival rate at 10, 15, and 20 years. In a study with minimum follow-up of 13 years with a porous-coated uncemented femoral stem in young patients, Davies et al[32] found no stem failures or evidence of loosening. Similarly, Healy et al[33] showed a 99.8% survivorship at 9-year follow-up with an uncemented, flat, tapered-wedge femoral stem design.

Wear-related osteolysis is the major cause of arthroplasty failure, so some surgeons restrict athletic activity and avoid operating on younger, more active patients. With increasing demand for joint arthroplasty, as well as increasing desire to continue or resume athletic activity, emphasis has been placed on providing more durable joint implants. Recent studies evaluating HXLPE in vivo have demonstrated significant improvements in wear rates. In a double-blinded, randomized controlled trial of conventional UHMWPE versus HXLPE over 2 years, HXLPE had a wear rate 40% lower than that of conventional UHMWPE.[34] Another study reported a 72% reduction in wear at 5 years.[35] More recently, McCalden et al[36] reported a 95% reduction of wear at a mean of 6 years. The increased wear resistance of HXLPE may be associated with decreased fatigue crack resistance, as demonstrated by Bradford et al.[37] This is of particular concern in cups that are positioned in excessive inclination or have faulty locking mechanisms.

In addition to HXLPE, other alternative bearing surfaces have been developed in an effort to reduce osteolysis. These bearings have theoretical promise, but each has demonstrated potential drawbacks. Ceramic-on-ceramic bearing surfaces have low wear rates, but they have demonstrated "squeaking," and these components require smaller heads by design limitation, which may lead to instability. Additionally, there are reports of ceramic fracture, with rates from 0.02% to as high as 5% with older ceramics.[38] Metal-on-metal articulations have low wear rates, may reduce osteolysis, and can be used with large, stable femoral heads. A unique issue with metal-on-metal is the serum metal ion level. This may be an issue, particularly with patients who are more active, including those who regularly participate in exercise.[39] In February 2011, the US Food and Drug Administration (FDA) issued an informational bulletin regarding the effectiveness of metal-on-metal hip implant systems.[40] They also made suggestions for patients and surgeons regarding the use of and follow-up after metal-on-metal hip implantation surgery. This included particular follow-up for patients with the "development of local signs or symptoms." In May 2011, the FDA ordered safety studies for metal-on-metal hip replacements to be required of manufacturers because of concerns about "potential problems with the device, including loosening, adverse local tissue reactions, and increased metal ion concentrations in the blood."[41] However, De Haan et al[42] found no increase in serum cobalt chrome levels in a triathlete around the time of training for a triathalon. Serum concentrations in this triathlete were similar to those in patients who were less active. Urine concentrations were elevated for a prolonged period of time, however. It is unclear what the long-term implications may be for increased serum metal ion levels and their excretion.

Despite the encouraging data on implant longevity and wear rates with newer bearing surfaces, activity following THA is not without risk. McGrory[43] reported on two cases of active patients who sustained periprosthetic femur fractures around uncemented stems following THA after a return to recreational winter activities. Arthroplasty patients are certainly not protected from sustaining the same injuries that afflict other sports participants. Moreover, treating these injuries, such as fractures or ligament injuries around a prosthesis, may present difficult challenges for the orthopaedist.

Hip Resurfacing

Surface replacement arthroplasty of the hip has many key theoretical benefits: increased head size and range of motion, decreased dislocation rate, decreased wear rate of a metal-on-metal articulation, and less femoral bone resection. However, hip resurfacing has been limited by several factors: increased acetabular bone resection, femoral neck fractures, nerve injuries, metal hypersensitivity, pseudotumors, a high failure rate in women, and high early failure rates of several devices. Additionally, there have been unpublished reports of femoral neck stress fractures after hip resurfacing. Some surgeons suggest waiting 6 months before returning to high-level or high-impact activity following hip resurfacing to allow for neck remodeling. Hip resurfacing is also a technically demanding procedure that requires greater exposure than THA.

The marketing literature for hip resurfacing suggests that this procedure allows patients greater activity; however, no good evidence exists that gives an advantage to hip resurfacing over THA with regard to postoperative sports activity. In a level IV study, Naal et al[44] surveyed 112 patients to determine their sports activities after surface replacement at a mean of 23.5 months after surgery. They reported that 105 patients engaged in an average of 4.8 sports disciplines preoperatively, whereas 110 patients participated in an average of 4.6 sports disciplines after surgery. They established that patients were able to return to a high level of sports after hip resurfacing arthroplasty. The authors acknowledge that the effect of this activity, including high-impact activity, on joint loosening and revision rates is unknown. Narvani et al[45] reported an increase in participation in athletic activity after resurfacing, from 65% preoperatively to 92% postoperatively. Khan et al[46] found that with athletic activity, cobalt ion levels increased in patients after surface replacement. No data are available to suggest that the interface between a surface replacement and the remaining femoral head and neck can better withstand the forces of a patient performing high-impact or contact sports than can a THA. The available data suggest that surgeons should be cautious in allowing their patients to resume high-impact or contact sports.

Total Knee Arthoplasty

Concerns exist regarding activity levels following TKA, as with THA. Retrospective studies and surveys exist to guide the surgeon in educating patients regarding appropriate postoperative expectations and limitations. Bradbury et al[47] retrospectively reviewed 160 patients after TKA. They noted that 65% of patients who participated in sports preoperatively returned to sports postoperatively. In patients without comorbidities, that number increased to 75%.

Dahm et al[48] surveyed more than 1,200 TKA patients to determine their level of postoperative activity. Despite more than 50% of the respondents being limited by pain in other joints, they reported activities consistent with an average University of California Los Angeles (UCLA) score of 7.1, which correlates with regular participation in activities such as cycling. Age younger than 70 years, male sex, body mass index less than or equal to 30 kg/m^2, and unilateral knee arthroplasty without other joint limitations were factors that correlated with a higher activity level. Sixteen percent of respondents participated in heavy manual labor or sports considered "not recommended" by Knee Society members.[49]

Mont et al[50] evaluated 46 USTA tennis players after TKA. Only 21% reported that their surgeons permitted high-impact activity such as singles tennis; 45% said their surgeons allowed doubles tennis. Although there is significant selection bias in this study, they showed that players were able to return to their presymptomatic level of play with an improvement in all mobility parameters. This included hitting, running, ground strokes, moving forward after serves to volley, stopping abruptly, and changing direction. They noted a 4% revision rate with a mean follow-up of 7 years.

Mont et al[51] also compared groups of matched low- and high-activity patients after TKA. No differences in overall satisfaction scores, radiographic parameters, or longevity were seen. The high-activity group reported better functionality and independence in their personal and social activities. This was an older group (mean age, 70 years), and none participated in high-impact activities such as jogging, skiing, or team sports. The authors suggested that sustained levels of athletic activity such as biking, hiking, swimming, tennis, and dancing do not have a detrimental effect on the outcome of TKA in the midterm. They further evaluated patients who participated in high-impact activities four times per week.[52] Four percent of all patients with TKAs performed over an 8-year period participated in these activities. The most common activities were singles tennis, jogging, high-impact aerobics, and racquetball. These patients had excellent clinical outcomes; 32 of 33 had good to excellent results. There was one revision in a patient who ran three times per week and played racquetball three times per week. The authors noted that patients who participate in high-impact activities might enjoy excellent clinical outcomes at 4-year follow-up. Although the authors reported favorable midterm results in this active group, they did not advocate these activities for their patients.

Mallon et al[26] studied golf after TKA. They noted a rise in handicap and a decrease in drive length. Although most patients (87%) used a golf cart, approximately 16% reported a mild ache while playing and 36% had an ache after playing. Of note, the lead leg was most often involved, which may be explained by the findings that increased torque is placed on the lead leg during the golf swing.[53] Additionally, D'Lima et al[54] instrumented the tibial stem in three patients to measure knee forces and moments in vivo. The authors noted an increase in tibial forces of greater than 4 times body weight (BW) in the lead leg during a golf swing. This corroborates the findings of the study by Mallon et al. D'Lima et al[54] evaluated other activities besides golf. Walking was associated with forces of 1.8 to 2.5 times BW; this increased to 2 times BW on a treadmill. Increasing the speed to 4 mph increased forces to 2.8 times BW. Jogging was associated with 40% higher forces than walking. Stationary bicycling was associated with a peak force of 1.3 times BW. Increased speed did

not seem to change this, and there was low anterior shear stress. Tennis was associated with forces of nearly 4 times BW. Serving and forehand strokes were associated with higher force generation than the backhand stroke. Actual play was associated with forces 12% higher than those generated during simulated strokes in the laboratory. Other notable activities were rowing (0.85 × BW), elliptical trainer (2.24 × BW with low anterior tibial shear stress), and stair-climber (2.5 × BW at low levels, but >3 × BW at higher levels).

Although epidemiologic data are not available regarding injuries following TKA, it can be assumed that there is a risk of periprosthetic fracture and ligamentous injury. Treating such injuries following TKA in an active population may present some unique difficulties and certainly warrants discussion during preoperative patient counseling.

Unicompartmental Knee Arthroplasty

Unicompartmental knee arthroplasty (UKA) has potential advantages over TKA. UKA shares with TKA an excellent 10-year survivorship of greater than 90% in the appropriately selected patient,[55-58] but it can be performed through a limited incision with a quicker recovery of quadriceps function and stair-climbing ability,[59] and it may show improved range of motion.[60] The cruciate ligaments are spared, allowing for more normal kinematics.[61] The Oxford mobile-bearing design (Biomet, Warsaw, IN) has demonstrated low polyethylene wear rates over time when impingement is avoided at the time of surgery.[62,63] Fisher et al[64] evaluated 71 consecutive Oxford medial UKAs (66 patients) for return to sports. The mean age was 64 years, and follow-up was very short, at 18 months. UCLA scores improved from a mean of 4.2 to 6.5, and the mean postoperative Oxford score was 18.1. The authors noted that patients who participated in postoperative sports had a statistically significant higher postoperative knee score compared with those who did not. Of the 66 patients, 42 (64%) participated in some form of sport or physical activity before becoming symptomatic preoperatively. Only 15 patients were actually participating in sports 3 months before surgery. Of the 42 who participated preoperatively, 39 (93%) returned to their regular activity postoperatively. The authors noted that this was higher than the percentage of patients reported to return to their preoperative sport after TKA. Although in this study more than 90% of patients who underwent a UKA returned to their preoperative activities, the study has a very short follow-up and cannot be used to evaluate for implant survival.

Naal et al[65] evaluated a fixed-bearing UKA with an all-polyethylene tibial component in 83 patients. Patients were stratified by age and were followed for a short period (mean follow-up, 18 months). Patients were generally healthier and had higher Short Form-36 scores compared with a matched referenced population. A very high percentage of patients returned to activities (73 of the 77 who participated preoperatively [95%]). The authors noted that, interestingly, the older group of patients had a higher frequency of activity than the younger group. The most common activities that patients returned to were hiking, cycling, and swimming. Several high-impact activities (downhill and cross-country skiing) had a decrease in participation. No implant failures were reported with these very early results. The authors allow their patients to participate in any sport or activity that they wish to as long as they stay asymptomatic. They recommend low- and mid-impact activities such as cycling, swimming, hiking, weight training, golf, and cross-country and downhill skiing (except short turns and moguls) and recommend avoiding high-impact activities such as running and jumping. They also recommend that patients rehabilitate appropriately before restarting sports, including sufficient restoration of quadriceps and hamstring strength. The authors also believe that close clinical and radiographic surveillance is important.

These studies indicate that a high percentage of patients can return to sporting activities after UKA. However, with only 18-month follow-up in both studies, mid- and long-term implant survival remains unknown. The authors of both studies recommend low- to mid-impact activities following UKA.

Total Shoulder Arthroplasty

Total shoulder arthroplasty (TSA) is widely used in the United States to treat symptomatic shoulder arthritis. Its reported 10-year survival rate is greater than 90%.[66-69] It is estimated that 10,000 TSAs are performed in the United States each year. Similar to THA and TKA, TSA and shoulder hemiarthroplasty have been shown to improve pain and function and to be cost effective for improving quality of life.[70] Data are limited regarding athletic activity after TSA.

Jensen and Rockwood[71] retrospectively reviewed 24 golfers who underwent TSA with an average follow-up of 53.4 months. Twenty-three returned to golf. The mean time to return to golf following arthroplasty was 4.5 months. The golfers improved 4.9 strokes and increased their drives 12.2 yards. They played 1.6 to 2 rounds per week. Three had a mild ache while playing and six had an ache after playing. Playing golf did not seem to increase radiographic evidence of loosening. No increase in lucent lines was noted over time when compared with a control group. In the same study, the authors used a mailed questionnaire to poll American Shoulder and Elbow Surgeons members for expert opinion. Recommendations were as follows: 91% allowed patients to return to golf; return to play was recommended at a mean of 4.3 months (similar to what was found in the retrospective portion of the study); and 60% placed no limit on golf rounds played weekly. The overall recommendations were to begin putting and short chipping before progressing to longer iron shots, to avoid taking divots by teeing the ball up high, and to delay hitting a driver until the patient was comfortable with hitting long irons. Some recommended modifying the golf swing. Two out of three believed that it was not detrimental to carry a golf bag.

McCarty et al[72] performed a retrospective review of sports after TSA with an average follow-up of 3.7 years. Two-thirds of the patients underwent a TSA to be able to return to sports. Fishing showed the highest percentage of return, at 92%. Swimming, golf, and tennis had high rates of return to sports (>75%), but only 40% returned to bowling and 20% to softball. Nineteen percent did not return to athletics after TSA. The mean time to participate at least partially in sports was 3.6 months, and the mean time required to full return to sports was 5.8 months. The mean number of days per week that sports were played increased from 0.7 to 1.7. No differences were noted between TSA and hemiarthroplasty. The authors also noted a decrease in the need for medication to participate in sports, from 71% preoperatively to 39% postoperatively. There were 4 secondary surgeries in this group of 75 patients: 3 arthroscopic débridements and 1 glenoid removal for

Table 1: Results of The Hip Society Survey Regarding Activities Allowed After Total Hip Arthroplasty[a]

	Allowed			Allowed With Experience		
	1999	2005		1999	2005	
Stationary cycling	x	x	Bowling	x		
Ballroom dancing	x	x	Canoeing	x		
Golf	x	x	Road cycling	x		
Shuffleboard	x	x	Hiking	x		
Swimming	x	x	Horseback riding	x	x	
Doubles tennis	x		Cross-country skiing	x	x	
Normal walking	x	x	Rowing		x	
Bowling		x	Ice skating		x	
Canoeing		x	Roller skating		x	
Road cycling		x	Downhill skiing		x	
Square dancing		x	Stationary skiing		x	
Hiking		x	Doubles tennis		x	
Speed walking		x	Weight lifting		x	
			Weight machine		x	

[a]This table is constructed to accurately compare the 1999 and 2005 Hip Society surveys. The 1999 survey asked about croquet (allowed), horseshoes (allowed), shooting (allowed), and lacrosse (not recommended), which were not included in the 2005 survey. The 1999 survey asked about high-impact aerobics (not recommended) and low-impact aerobics (allowed with experience). The 2005 survey combined these activities and asked about aerobics (allowed with experience). The 2005 survey asked about yoga (allowed with experience), which was not included in the 1999 survey.
Adapted with permission from Healy WL, Sharma S, Schwartz B, Iorio R: Athletic activity after total joint arthroplasty. *J Bone Joint Surg Am* 2008;90(10):2245-2252.

loosening. There were no other cases of aseptic loosening. Patients in this study regularly returned to fishing, tennis, golf, and swimming, which indicates that even repetitive activities such as swimming can be accomplished after TSA. More strenuous shoulder activities such as bowling and weight lifting were harder to return to. Despite the low rate of secondary surgery in this study, it must be noted that this is a retrospective study that did not include clinical or radiographic follow-up and had a follow-up period of less than 4 years.

Expert Opinion

Given the lack of high-level evidence to support recommendations regarding athletic activity after joint arthroplasty, expert opinion can be helpful. McGrory et

Table 1: (*continued*)

No Consensus			Not Recommended		
	1999	2005		1999	2005
Square dancing	x		Baseball	x	
Fencing	x	x	Basketball	x	x
Rowing	x		Football	x	x
Ice skating	x		Gymnastics	x	
Downhill skiing	x		Handball	x	
Stationary skiing	x		Hockey	x	
Speed walking	x		Jogging	x	x
Weight lifting	x		Rock climbing	x	
Weight machine	x		Soccer	x	x
Baseball		x	Squash/raquetball	x	
Gymnastics		x	Singles tennis	x	
Handball		x	Volleyball	x	
Hockey		x			
Rock climbing		x			
Squash/raquetball		x			
Singles tennis		x			
Volleyball		x			

al[73] surveyed orthopaedic surgeons at the Mayo Clinic, including staff surgeons, residents, and fellows. Their recommendations for THA and TKA allowed for, and encouraged, low-impact sports including bowling, cycling, golfing, sailing, scuba diving, and swimming. Participation in high-impact sports—specifically, baseball, basketball, football, handball, hockey, karate, racquetball, running, soccer, and water skiing—was discouraged. Staff surgeons allowed cross-country skiing more often than did fellows or residents.

Healy et al surveyed Hip Society and Knee Society members regarding 43 athletic activities in 1999[49] and repeated the study, with a few modifications, in 2005[74] (**Tables 1** and **2**). The authors stratified responses into "allowed," "allowed with experience," and "not recommended." To be classified into a specific recommendation, the activity needed a 73% response. The authors

noted a change in recommendations, as the respondents allowed more activities in 2005 than in 1999.[75] When polled, however, 80% of those who participated did not believe that they changed their recommendations. Activities that were consistently allowed include stationary cycling, ballroom dancing, golfing, shuffleboard, swimming, and normal walking. Basketball, football, jogging, and soccer were not recommended in either study. Interestingly, baseball, gymnastics, handball, hockey, rock climbing, squash, racquetball, and singles tennis, which were not recommended in 1999, had no consensus in the 2005 study.

Klein et al[76] performed a study similar to those of Healy et al. Questionnaires were sent to members of The Hip Society and the American Association of Hip and Knee Surgeons. The survey listed 30 groups of activities with 37 specific sports. Surgeons who did not

Table 2: Results of The Knee Society Survey Regarding Activities Allowed After Total Knee Arthroplasty[a]

Allowed	1999	2005	Allowed With Experience	1999	2005
Bowling	x	x	Canoeing	x	
Stationary cycling	x	x	Road cycling	x	
Ballroom dancing	x	x	Hiking	x	
Golf	x	x	Rowing	x	x
Horseback riding	x		Ice skating	x	x
Shuffleboard	x	x	Cross-country skiing	x	x
Swimming	x	x	Stationary skiing	x	x
Normal walking	x	x	Doubles tennis	x	x
Canoeing		x	Speed walking	x	
Road cycling		x	Downhill skiing	x	
Square dancing		x	Weight machine	x	
Hiking		x	Horseback riding		x
Speed walking		x	Downhill skiing		x

[a]This table is constructed to accurately compare the 1999 and 2005 Knee Society surveys. The 1999 survey asked about croquet (allowed), horseshoes (allowed), shooting (allowed), and lacrosse (not recommended), which were not included in the 2005 survey. The 1999 survey asked about high-impact aerobics (not recommended) and low-impact aerobics (allowed with experience). The 2005 survey combined these activities and asked about aerobics (allowed with experience). The 2005 survey asked about yoga (allowed with experience), which was not included in the 1999 survey.

Adapted with permission from Healy WL, Sharma S, Schwartz B, Iorio R: Athletic activity after total joint arthroplasty. *J Bone Joint Surg Am* 2008;90(10):2245-2252.

perform THA were asked not to respond. More than 500 surgeon responses were available for analysis. For each activity, the survey asked for an "allowed," "allowed with experience," "not allowed," or "undecided" response. A power analysis was performed to determine the response rate needed to reach a consensus. The authors found no significant differences between the two societies, with only minor differences in their recommendations. Recommendations differed for stair climbing, doubles tennis, using weight machines, snowboarding, and rowing, but both societies either allowed these activities or allowed them with experience. Racquetball, squash, baseball, softball, and snowboarding were not allowed (**Table 3**).

These studies demonstrate that over the last 10 to 15 years, surgeons are allowing more activities following total joint arthroplasty. This trend may be influenced by several factors, including patient goals[4,77] and surgeon confidence based on improved implant survivorship and durability. As more data are reported regarding activity after joint arthroplasty, with positive results, we may see more activities allowed by surgeons.

Summary

Many patients choose to have total joint arthroplasty to maintain an active and athletic lifestyle. As with most athletes, the postarthroplasty athlete may benefit from

Table 2: (*continued*)

	No Consensus			Not Recommended	
	1999	2005		1999	2005
Square dancing	x		Baseball	x	
Fencing	x	x	Basketball	x	x
Roller skating	x	x	Football	x	x
Downhill skiing	x		Gymnastics	x	
Weight lifting	x	x	Handball	x	
Baseball		x	Hockey	x	
Gymnastics		x	Jogging	x	x
Handball		x	Rock climbing	x	
Hockey		x	Soccer	x	x
Rock climbing		x	Squash/raquetball	x	
Squash/raquetball		x	Singles tennis	x	
Singles tennis		x	Volleyball	x	x
Weight machine		x			

activity-specific training, general conditioning, and core strengthening. It is not clear whether remaining active after total joint arthroplasty will be detrimental to implant longevity in the short- and midterm. Patients should be warned, however, that the risks of high-impact activities are not well defined and so these activities cannot be comfortably recommended. They should also be made aware of the risks of periprosthetic fracture and ligament injury and the difficulties in treating these injuries. The data on the safety of metal ions released from metal-on-metal implants and its effect on health are still being accumulated. Patients who choose and receive these implants need to be aware of this concern. More latitude may be given to highly trained athletes returning to their particular sport, as they seem less at risk than people inexperienced in that particular sport. The cardiovascular and mental health benefits and the enjoyment of athletic activity must be balanced with the potential risk of reduced survival of the joint arthroplasty.

References

1. Mendenhall S: 2009 hip and knee implant review. *Orthopedic Network News*. July 2009, p 1.

2. Kurtz SM, Ong KL, Schmier J, Zhao K, Mowat F, Lau E: Primary and revision arthroplasty surgery caseloads in the United States from 1990 to 2004. *J Arthroplasty* 2009;24(2):195-203.

3. Mont MA, LaPorte DM, Mullick T, Silberstein CE, Hungerford DS: Tennis after total hip arthroplasty. *Am J Sports Med* 1999;27(1):60-64.

4. Mancuso CA, Graziano S, Briskie LM, et al: Randomized trials to modify patients' preoperative expectations of hip and knee arthroplasties. *Clin Orthop Relat Res* 2008;466(2):424-431.

5. Barry HC, Eathorne SW: Exercise and aging: Issues for the practitioner. *Med Clin North Am* 1994;78(2): 357-376.

6. Paffenbarger RS Jr, Hyde RT, Wing AL, Hsieh CC: Physical activity, all-cause mortality, and longevity of college alumni. *N Engl J Med* 1986;314(10):605-613.

Table 3: Consensus Guidelines for Return to Activities After Total Hip Arthroplasty[a]

Allowed	Allowed With Experience	Not Allowed	Undecided
Golf	*Downhill skiing*[b]	Raquetball/squash	Martial arts
Swimming	Cross-country skiing	Jogging	*Singles tennis*[c]
Doubles tennis	*Weight lifting*[b]	Contact sports (football, basketball, soccer)	
Stair climber	*Ice skating/rollerblading*[b]	High-impact aerobics	
Walking	Pilates	Baseball/softball	
Speed walking[b]		Snowboarding	
Hiking[d]			
Stationary skiing[b]			
Bowling[d]			
Treadmill			
Road cycling[d]			
Stationary bicycling			
Elliptical			
Low-impact aerobics[d]			
Rowing[b]			
Dancing (ballroom, jazz, square)[b]			

[a]Based on a survey by the members of The Hip Society and the American Association of Hip and Knee Surgeons. Italic type denotes classification change from a previous study by Healy[74]: *b* = change from undecided; *c* = change from not allowed; *d* = change from allowed with experience. Underlining denotes activity not previously described. Adapted with permission from Klein GR, Levine BR, Hozack WJ, et al: Return to athletic activity after total hip arthroplasty: Consensus guidelines based on a survey of the Hip Society and American Association of Hip and Knee Surgeons. *J Arthroplasty* 2007;22(2):171-175.

7. Pollock M, Wilmore J: *Exercise in Health and Disease: Evaluation and Prescription for Prevention and Rehabilitation*, ed 2. Philadelphia, PA, WB Saunders, 1990, pp 1-2.

8. Ries MD, Philbin EF, Groff GD, Sheesley KA, Richman JA, Lynch F Jr: Improvement in cardiovascular fitness after total knee arthroplasty. *J Bone Joint Surg Am* 1996;78(11):1696-1701.

9. Röder C, Staub LP, Eggli S, Dietrich D, Busato A, Müller U: Influence of preoperative functional status on outcome after total hip arthroplasty. *J Bone Joint Surg Am* 2007;89(1):11-17.

10. Zeni JA Jr, Snyder-Mackler L: Most patients gain weight in the 2 years after total knee arthroplasty: Comparison to a healthy control group. *Osteoarthritis Cartilage* 2010;18(4):510-514.

11. Chandler HP, Reineck FT, Wixson RL, McCarthy JC: Total hip replacement in patients younger than thirty years old: A five-year follow-up study. *J Bone Joint Surg Am* 1981;63(9):1426-1434.

12. Dorr LD, Takei GK, Conaty JP: Total hip arthroplasties in patients less than forty-five years old. *J Bone Joint Surg Am* 1983;65(4):474-479.

13. Kilgus DJ, Dorey FJ, Finerman GA, Amstutz HC: Patient activity, sports participation, and impact loading on the durability of cemented total hip replacements. *Clin Orthop Relat Res* 1991;(269):25-31.

14. Mintz L, Tsao AK, McCrae CR, Stulberg SD, Wright T: The arthroscopic evaluation and characteristics of severe polyethylene wear in total knee arthroplasty. *Clin Orthop Relat Res* 1991;(273):215-222.

15. Charnley J, Halley DK: Rate of wear in total hip replacement. *Clin Orthop Relat Res* 1975;(112): 170-179.

16. Schmalzried TP, Szuszczewicz ES, Northfield MR, et al: Quantitative assessment of walking activity after total hip or knee replacement. *J Bone Joint Surg Am* 1998;80(1):54-59.

17. Schmalzried TP, Shepherd EF, Dorey FJ, et al: The John Charnley Award. Wear is a function of use, not time. *Clin Orthop Relat Res* 2000;(381):36-46.

18. Maloney WJ, Paprosky W, Engh CA, Rubash H: Surgical treatment of pelvic osteolysis. *Clin Orthop Relat Res* 2001;(393):78-84.

19. Lavernia CJ, Sierra RJ, Hungerford DS, Krackow K: Activity level and wear in total knee arthroplasty: A study of autopsy retrieved specimens. *J Arthroplasty* 2001;16(4):446-453.

20. Diduch DR, Insall JN, Scott WN, Scuderi GR, Font-Rodriguez D: Total knee replacement in young, active patients: Long-term follow-up and functional outcome. *J Bone Joint Surg Am* 1997;79(4):575-582.

21. Gschwend N, Frei T, Morscher E, Nigg B, Loehr J: Alpine and cross-country skiing after total hip replacement: 2 cohorts of 50 patients each, one active, the other inactive in skiing, followed for 5-10 years. *Acta Orthop Scand* 2000;71(3):243-249.

22. Mont MA, Lee CW, Sheldon M, Lennon WC, Hungerford DS: Total knee arthroplasty in patients </=50 years old. *J Arthroplasty* 2002;17(5):538-543.

23. Kim YH, Kook HK, Kim JS: Total hip replacement with a cementless acetabular component and a cemented femoral component in patients younger than fifty years of age. *J Bone Joint Surg Am* 2002;84-A(5): 770-774.

24. Jones DL, Cauley JA, Kriska AM, et al: Physical activity and risk of revision total knee arthroplasty in individuals with knee osteoarthritis: A matched case-control study. *J Rheumatol* 2004;31(7):1384-1390.

25. Chatterji U, Ashworth MJ, Lewis PL, Dobson PJ: Effect of total hip arthroplasty on recreational and sporting activity. *ANZ J Surg* 2004;74(6):446-449.

26. Mallon WJ, Liebelt RA, Mason JB: Total joint replacement and golf. *Clin Sports Med* 1996;15(1): 179-190.

27. Peters P: Mountain sports and total hip arthroplasty: A case report and review of mountaineering with total hip arthroplasty. *Wilderness Environ Med* 2003;14(2): 106-111.

28. Sechriest VF II, Kyle RF, Marek DJ, Spates JD, Saleh KJ, Kuskowski M: Activity level in young patients with primary total hip arthroplasty: A 5-year minimum follow-up. *J Arthroplasty* 2007;22(1):39-47.

29. Eskelinen A, Paavolainen P, Helenius I, Pulkkinen P, Remes V: Total hip arthroplasty for rheumatoid arthritis in younger patients: 2,557 replacements in the Finnish Arthroplasty Register followed for 0-24 years. *Acta Orthop* 2006;77(6):853-865.

30. Eskelinen A, Remes V, Helenius I, Pulkkinen P, Nevalainen J, Paavolainen P: Total hip arthroplasty for primary osteoarthrosis in younger patients in the Finnish arthroplasty register. 4,661 primary replacements followed for 0-22 years. *Acta Orthop* 2005;76(1):28-41.

31. Lombardi AV Jr, Berend KR, Mallory TH, Skeels MD, Adams JB: Survivorship of 2000 tapered titanium porous plasma-sprayed femoral components. *Clin Orthop Relat Res* 2009;467(1):146-154.

32. Davies AJ, Ollivere B, Motha J, Porteous M, August A: Successful performance of the bi-metric uncemented femoral stem at a minimum follow-up of 13 years in young patients. *J Arthroplasty* 2010;25(2):186-190.

33. Healy WL, Tilzey JF, Iorio R, Specht LM, Sharma S: Prospective, randomized comparison of cobalt-chrome and titanium trilock femoral stems. *J Arthroplasty* 2009;24(6):831-836.

34. Glyn-Jones S, Isaac S, Hauptfleisch J, McLardy-Smith P, Murray DW, Gill HS: Does highly cross-linked polyethylene wear less than conventional polyethylene in total hip arthroplasty? A double-blind, randomized, and controlled trial using roentgen stereophoto-grammetric analysis. *J Arthroplasty* 2008;23(3): 337-343.

35. D'Antonio JA, Manley MT, Capello WN, et al: Five-year experience with Crossfire highly cross-linked polyethylene. *Clin Orthop Relat Res* 2005;441:143-150.

36. McCalden RW, MacDonald SJ, Rorabeck CH, Bourne RB, Chess DG, Charron KD: Wear rate of highly cross-linked polyethylene in total hip arthroplasty: A randomized controlled trial. *J Bone Joint Surg Am* 2009;91(4):773-782.

37. Bradford L, Baker D, Ries MD, Pruitt LA: Fatigue crack propagation resistance of highly crosslinked polyethylene. *Clin Orthop Relat Res* 2004;(429):68-72.

38. D'Antonio JA, Sutton K: Ceramic materials as bearing surfaces for total hip arthroplasty. *J Am Acad Orthop Surg* 2009;17(2):63-68.

39. Khan M, Takahashi T, Kuiper JH, Sieniawska CE, Takagi K, Richardson JB: Current in vivo wear of metal-on-metal bearings assessed by exercise-related rise in plasma cobalt level. *J Orthop Res* 2006;24(11):2029-2035.

40. US Food and Drug Adminstration (FDA): Medical Devices: Information for Orthopaedic Surgeons about Metal-on-Metal Hip Implant Surgery. February 10, 2011. http://www.fda.gov/MedicalDevices/ ProductsandMedicalProcedures/Implantsand Prosthetics/MetalonMetalHipImplants/ucm241667. htm. Accessed October 18, 2011.

41. Nelson R: FDA Orders Safety Studies for Metal-on-Metal Hip Replacements? *Medscape Medical News*. May 13, 2011. http://www.medscape.com/viewarticle/ 742710. Accessed October 18, 2011.

42. De Haan R, Campbell P, Reid S, Skipor AK, De Smet K: Metal ion levels in a triathlete with a metal-on-metal resurfacing arthroplasty of the hip. *J Bone Joint Surg Br* 2007;89(4):538-541.

43. McGrory BJ: Periprosthetic fracture of the femur after total hip arthroplasty occurring in winter activities: Report of two cases. *J Surg Orthop Adv* 2004;13(2):119-123.

44. Naal FD, Maffiuletti NA, Munzinger U, Hersche O: Sports after hip resurfacing arthroplasty. *Am J Sports Med* 2007;35(5):705-711.

45. Narvani AA, Tsiridis E, Nwaboku HC, Bajekal RA: Sporting activity following Birmingham hip resurfacing. *Int J Sports Med* 2006;27(6):505-507.

46. Khan M, Kuiper JH, Richardson JB: The exercise-related rise in plasma cobalt levels after metal-on-metal hip resurfacing arthroplasty. *J Bone Joint Surg Br* 2008;90(9):1152-1157.

47. Bradbury N, Borton D, Spoo G, Cross MJ: Participation in sports after total knee replacement. *Am J Sports Med* 1998;26(4):530-535.

48. Dahm DL, Barnes SA, Harrington JR, Sayeed SA, Berry DJ: Patient-reported activity level after total knee arthroplasty. *J Arthroplasty* 2008;23(3):401-407.

49. Healy WL, Iorio R, Lemos MJ: Athletic activity after total knee arthroplasty. *Clin Orthop Relat Res* 2000;(380):65-71.

50. Mont MA, Rajadhyaksha AD, Marxen JL, Silberstein CE, Hungerford DS: Tennis after total knee arthroplasty. *Am J Sports Med* 2002;30(2):163-166.

51. Mont MA, Marker DR, Seyler TM, Gordon N, Hungerford DS, Jones LC: Knee arthroplasties have similar results in high- and low-activity patients. *Clin Orthop Relat Res* 2007;460:165-173.

52. Mont MA, Marker DR, Seyler TM, Jones LC, Kolisek FR, Hungerford DS: High-impact sports after total knee arthroplasty. *J Arthroplasty* 2008;23(6, Suppl 1):80-84.

53. Stover CN, Wiren G, Topaz SR: The modern golf swing and stress syndromes. *Phys Sportsmed* 1976;4(9):42-47.

54. D'Lima DD, Steklov N, Patil S, Colwell CW Jr: The Mark Coventry Award: In vivo knee forces during recreation and exercise after knee arthroplasty. *Clin Orthop Relat Res* 2008;466(11):2605-2611.

55. Berger RA, Meneghini RM, Jacobs JJ, et al: Results of unicompartmental knee arthroplasty at a minimum of ten years of follow-up. *J Bone Joint Surg Am* 2005;87(5):999-1006.

56. Emerson RH Jr, Higgins LL: Unicompartmental knee arthroplasty with the oxford prosthesis in patients with medial compartment arthritis. *J Bone Joint Surg Am* 2008;90(1):118-122.

57. Murray DW, Goodfellow JW, O'Connor JJ: The Oxford medial unicompartmental arthroplasty: A ten-year survival study. *J Bone Joint Surg Br* 1998;80(6):983-989.

58. Svärd UC, Price AJ: Oxford medial unicompartmental knee arthroplasty: A survival analysis of an independent series. *J Bone Joint Surg Br* 2001;83(2):191-194.

59. Price AJ, Webb J, Topf H, et al: Rapid recovery after oxford unicompartmental arthroplasty through a short incision. *J Arthroplasty* 2001;16(8):970-976.

60. Yang KY, Wang MC, Yeo SJ, Lo NN: Minimally invasive unicondylar versus total condylar knee

arthroplasty—Early results of a matched-pair comparison. *Singapore Med J* 2003;44(11):559-562.

61. Patil S, Colwell CW Jr, Ezzet KA, D'Lima DD: Can normal knee kinematics be restored with unicompartmental knee replacement? *J Bone Joint Surg Am* 2005;87(2):332-338.

62. Psychoyios V, Crawford RW, O'Connor JJ, Murray DW: Wear of congruent meniscal bearings in unicompartmental knee arthroplasty: A retrieval study of 16 specimens. *J Bone Joint Surg Br* 1998;80(6): 976-982.

63. Argenson JN, O'Connor JJ: Polyethylene wear in meniscal knee replacement: A one to nine-year retrieval analysis of the Oxford knee. *J Bone Joint Surg Br* 1992; 74(2):228-232.

64. Fisher N, Agarwal M, Reuben SF, Johnson DS, Turner PG: Sporting and physical activity following Oxford medial unicompartmental knee arthroplasty. *Knee* 2006;13(4):296-300.

65. Naal FD, Fischer M, Preuss A, et al: Return to sports and recreational activity after unicompartmental knee arthroplasty. *Am J Sports Med* 2007;35(10):1688-1695.

66. Torchia ME, Cofield RH, Settergren CR: Total shoulder arthroplasty with the Neer prosthesis: Long-term results. *J Shoulder Elbow Surg* 1997;6(6):495-505.

67. Sperling JW, Cofield RH, Rowland CM: Neer hemiarthroplasty and Neer total shoulder arthroplasty in patients fifty years old or less: Long-term results. *J Bone Joint Surg Am* 1998;80(4):464-473.

68. Sperling JW, Cofield RH, Rowland CM: Minimum fifteen-year follow-up of Neer hemiarthroplasty and total shoulder arthroplasty in patients aged fifty years or younger. *J Shoulder Elbow Surg* 2004;13(6):604-613.

69. Adams JE, Sperling JW, Schleck CD, Harmsen WS, Cofield RH: Outcomes of shoulder arthroplasty in Olmsted County, Minnesota: A population-based study. *Clin Orthop Relat Res* 2007;455:176-182.

70. Boorman RS, Kopjar B, Fehringer E, Churchill RS, Smith K, Matsen FA III: The effect of total shoulder arthroplasty on self-assessed health status is comparable to that of total hip arthroplasty and coronary artery bypass grafting. *J Shoulder Elbow Surg* 2003;12(2): 158-163.

71. Jensen KL, Rockwood CA Jr: Shoulder arthroplasty in recreational golfers. *J Shoulder Elbow Surg* 1998;7(4): 362-367.

72. McCarty EC, Marx RG, Maerz D, Altchek D, Warren RF: Sports participation after shoulder replacement surgery. *Am J Sports Med* 2008;36(8):1577-1581.

73. McGrory BJ, Stuart MJ, Sim FH: Participation in sports after hip and knee arthroplasty: Review of literature and survey of surgeon preferences. *Mayo Clin Proc* 1995;70(4):342-348.

74. Healy WL, Iorio R, Lemos MJ: Athletic activity after joint replacement. *Am J Sports Med* 2001;29(3): 377-388.

75. Healy WL, Sharma S, Schwartz B, Iorio R: Athletic activity after total joint arthroplasty. *J Bone Joint Surg Am* 2008;90(10):2245-2252.

76. Klein GR, Levine BR, Hozack WJ, et al: Return to athletic activity after total hip arthroplasty: Consensus guidelines based on a survey of the Hip Society and American Association of Hip and Knee Surgeons. *J Arthroplasty* 2007;22(2):171-175.

77. Weiss JM, Noble PC, Conditt MA, et al: What functional activities are important to patients with knee replacements? *Clin Orthop Relat Res* 2002;(404): 172-188.

Chapter 28

Rehabilitation Considerations for Knee Osteoarthritis

Todd R. Hooks, PT, SCS,
  ATC, MOMT, MTC,
  CSCS
Kevin Wilk, PT, DPT

Key Points
- Knee osteoarthritis is one of the most common musculoskeletal conditions, and its prevalence is increasing sharply.
- Risk factors for knee osteoarthritis include increasing age and female sex.
- Varus or valgus malalignment increases by tenfold the risk of further progression of knee osteoarthritis.
- An appropriate rehabilitation program for knee osteoarthritis includes open and closed kinetic chain exercises based on biomechanical considerations and tissue status and allows for a return to sports activity.

Introduction

Osteoarthritis is one of the most common musculoskeletal diseases in all countries and is estimated to affect 13.9% to 15% of all adults and 33.6% of individuals older than 65 years.[1-3] The overall prevalence of osteoarthritis has increased in recent years; in 2008, Lawrence et al[3] estimated that 26.9 million US adults aged 25 and older had clinical osteoarthritis, a considerable increase over the estimated 21 million reported in 1998.[2] The prevalence of this condition is projected to continue to increase. Nearly 67 million people are expected to have some form of physician-diagnosed arthritis by 2030, with more than 50% of the cases occurring in adults older than 65 years.[4]

The knee is one of the joints most commonly affected by osteoarthritis.

The prevalence of knee osteoarthritis increased from approximately 6 million Americans in 1995 to an estimated 9 million in 2005.[2,3,5-7]

Numerous studies have reported on the prevalence of radiographic knee osteoarthritis. Dillon et al[8] reported the prevalence to be 0.9 per 100, with a three times higher prevalence in females. Felson et al[6] reported the prevalence to be 19.2% in adults 45 years or older. Jordan et al[9] recorded a rate of 27.8% in individuals 45 years and older, and a prevalence of 37.4% in individuals 60 years or older. The prevalence of radiographic knee osteoarthritis varies among ethnic groups, affecting African-American women more often than Caucasian women, for example.[9-11] According to the National Health and Nutrition Examination Survey III, 52.4% of African-

Americans, 37.6% of Mexican-Americans, and 36.2% of Caucasians age 60 or older had evidence of radiographic knee osteoarthritis.[8]

Symptomatic knee osteoarthritis has been reported in 16.7% of US adults 45 years or older and 12.1% of those 60 years or older, affecting 4.3 million adults.[8-10] In general, the prevalence of knee osteoarthritis is higher in women than in men, especially after age 50, with men having a 45% lower prevalence compared with women.[12,13] A recent study by the Centers for Disease Control and Prevention (CDC) reported that the lifetime risk of symptomatic knee osteoarthritis is 46%.[5]

With 11% of adults requiring help with personal care and 14% needing assistance with routine activities because of knee osteoarthritis, the condition ranks high in disability-adjusted life years and years lived with disability.[14,15] The CDC reported that total knee arthroplasty (TKA) procedure rates increased eightfold from 1979 to 2002 in individuals 65 years of age or older. The financial costs associated with knee osteoarthritis also have increased, with $14.3 billion spent in 2004 on hospital costs associated with TKA.[5] Currently, approximately 450,000 primary TKAs are performed annually in the United States, and the number is projected to increase to 3.48 million by 2030.[16] Because of the increased prevalence of osteoarthritis in aging patients, the increasing percentage of the older population, and the associated disability and cost incurred with management of this condition, there is a heightened awareness of and attention to the prevention and treatment of osteoarthritis.

Risk Factors

Knee osteoarthritis is initially treated nonsurgically. The healthcare professional should have an understanding of the risk factors associated with this condition so that appropriate treatment can be delivered to address the specific causative factor or factors.

Some risk factors for knee osteoarthritis are nonmodifiable, such as sex and race (the prevalence is lower in some Asian populations), advancing age, family history, and a previous hysterectomy.[2,3,6-13,17,18] Some occupations place an individual at increased risk of developing knee osteoarthritis. Occupations that require hard labor, heavy lifting, and knee bending, such as agriculture, construction, retail, and cleaning, can increase the risk of knee osteoarthritis.[19-21] Although many of these risk factors cannot be altered, it is important to have an appreciation of them so that proper education and counseling can be provided as part of the patient's care.

Numerous modifiable risk factors for knee osteoarthritis have been reported. Healthcare professionals should address these causative factors as part of the nonsurgical management process when applicable. For example, obesity is strongly associated with knee osteoarthritis; it can predispose an individual to knee osteoarthritis, increase by up to eightfold the likelihood of developing knee osteoarthritis, have a negative effect on existing osteoarthritis, and accelerate the progression of joint space narrowing.[22-26] It has been shown that weight reduction can significantly reduce the pain and associated disability of symptomatic knee osteoarthritis.[27,28] Felson et al[28] reported that a loss of 5.1 kg over 10 years reduced symptoms by more than 50%.

Other factors, such as previous knee trauma or ligamentous injury, previous meniscectomy, abnormal joint alignment, current and previous physical activity level, lower extremity strength, ligament laxity, and proprioception, can contribute to the development and progression of knee osteoarthritis. It is therefore important for the healthcare professional to be aware of these intrinsic factors to allow for a comprehensive assessment and treatment of the mature athlete.[29-31]

Individuals who participated in either recreational or competitive sports throughout their youth and young adult years frequently continue these activities as they age. It is therefore important to understand the influence that prior activities and any applicable injuries may have on the development of knee osteoarthritis. Individuals who participated in group sports, especially those considered to be high-risk activities that include collisions or require high loading or torsional movements, are more likely to develop knee osteoarthritis.[32-36] The prevalence of knee osteoarthritis in retired British soccer players has been reported to range from 32% to 49%, which is significantly higher than the 20% prevalance in the general male British population aged 45 to 64 years.[33,37] The incidence of knee osteoarthritis has been reported to be as high as 38% in retired National Football League players, with 16% reporting degenerative joint disease affecting their activities of daily living (ADLs).[32]

Studies have shown that individuals who participate in long-distance running have a lower incidence of knee osteoarthritis than athletes in collision sports or sports that require torsional stresses. Kujala et al[38] reported the prevalence in former athletes and noted a 31% rate in weight lifters, 29% in soccer players, and 14% in runners. The authors also noted that runners with knee osteoarthritis were more likely to have had a previous injury than were runners without knee osteoarthritis. Soccer players were more likely to have tibiofemoral osteoarthritis, whereas weight lifters had a higher prevalence of patellofemoral osteoarthritis. Subjects with prior knee injury, heavy training, activities involving kneeling or squatting, or a high body mass index at age 20 had an increased risk of developing knee osteoarthritis. Other studies comparing the incidence rates of knee osteoarthritis in runners with age-matched nonrunners have shown no difference between these groups.[39,40]

The similar knee osteoarthritis rates in nonrunners and runners would appear to indicate that experienced runners may undergo adaptations that allow them to endure joint loading more effectively than inexperienced runners. In a group of runners with experience ranging from beginner to experienced who were evaluated after a marathon for the presence of joint effusion using MRI, six of seven beginning runners had joint effusion, whereas no joint effusion was detected in eight experienced runners.[41] Researchers also have used MRI to measure the cartilage volume of the patella and tibia as well as the medial and lateral meniscus in experienced runners. They found a significant reduction in volume in all of these structures following a 5-km run; however, following a 10-km run and a 20-km run, only the medial meniscus demonstrated a significant reduction in volume.[42] In addition, following a 1-hour rest, no significant reduction in cartilage volume persisted.[43] Therefore, it appears that experienced runners are able to adapt to the cyclic repetitive loads incurred during running and are able to quickly recover following cessation of exercise to allow for a quicker return to exercise.

History

Upon the initial presentation of the mature athlete for treatment, the physician or allied healthcare provider should obtain a complete history. This is extremely important in the mature athlete because this condition may be long-standing or from a previous trauma that may have occurred many years earlier for which the athlete may or may not have sought treatment. The examiner should ask about all sports the athlete has participated in, the highest level achieved, and the current and previous training levels. Any traumatic or nontraumatic injuries of either or both lower extremities and any treatment received, as well as any prior diagnostic studies and surgical treatment of the affected knee, should be documented. In addition, the patient's family history should be elicited to determine if there is a genetic predisposition to knee osteoarthritis and because medical conditions such as diabetes mellitus or peripheral vascular disease can adversely affect the athlete's healing potential. In addition, the examiner should determine the patient's ADLs and work activities because jobs that require heavy lifting, repeated squatting, or kneeling can cause, aggravate, or affect the healing potential of knee osteoarthritis.

Physical Examination

The examiner should begin the physical examination with a visual observation of the knee. The patient should be instructed to stand with the feet slightly apart while the examiner makes note of any varus or valgus alignment of the lower extremities, the weight-bearing tolerance, any limb-length discrepancy, and any other abnormalities of the lower extremities. If the patient is able to tolerate a gait analysis, this should be performed. The examiner should assess for initial contact through peak knee flexion angle, amount of knee extension present at heel strike, and the presence of any varus or valgus knee thrust. Altered gait kinematics and kinetics are commonly observed in patients with knee osteoarthritis. These patients frequently ambulate with greater knee flexion at heel strike and during early stance, with a greater toe-out angle, and a reduced peak external knee extension moment in late stance. The greater toe out angle significantly affects knee biomechanics, reducing the frontal plane lever by 6.7%, the adduction moment by 11.7%, the peak adduction lever arm by

22.9%, and the peak adduction moment by 34.4%. The increased lateral muscle activation may assist in stabilizing the knee adduction moment.[44,45] A varus or valgus knee thrust can be present in an arthritic knee as a result of an angular deformity at the knee due to either cartilage and bone deterioration followed by secondary stretching of the collateral ligament and joint capsule of the opposite side, or chronic ligamentous instability. This can cause a shift in the load axis of the knee, potentially causing a yaw in the affected side joint compartment and thereby creating instability and buckling of the knee.[46] Chang et al[47] reported a four-fold increase in the progression of medial osteoarthritis with the presence of a varus thrust during ambulation. A medial thrust is indicative of medial collateral and posteromedial capsular laxity; a lateral thrust could be present with lateral collateral ligament and postero-lateral capsular laxity; and a posterior thrust is present with posterior capsule laxity.

The knee joint should be examined for the presence of any joint effusion either by a circumferential measurement at the knee joint line or by compressing the suprapatellar pouch to allow palpatory grading of effusion. The examiner can grade the effusion according to the following criteria: grade 1 (fluid present), grade 2 (slight lift-off of patella), grade 3 (ballotable patella), or grade 4 (tense effusion permitting compression of the patella against the femoral sulcus).[48] The examiner should also palpate the contracted quadriceps musculature and compare it to the contralateral side for differentiation. The circumference of the thigh should also be measured at a determined distance above the joint line and compared with the contralateral thigh. Calf circumference can also be assessed at this time to determine if atrophy is present.

The patellofemoral joint should also be assessed for crepitus during flexion and extension of the knee during both seated knee extension (with and without resistance) and weight-bearing squatting or similar activity. This will allow the examiner to determine during which arc(s) of motion crepitus is present and evaluate the influence weight bearing or increased compression via quadriceps contraction has on crepitus. This can assist the rehabilitation specialist in determining more appropriate and safe exercises, and also exercises and/or activities to avoid as part of the nonsurgical treatment of knee osteoarthritis for the mature athlete. Patellar tracking should be assessed from full extension into flexion. With the knee in full extension, the patella is offset laterally, with the lateral facet making contact with the lateral side of the femoral sulcus; as the knee is brought into flexion, the patella becomes more centrally positioned. The medial and lateral aspects of the patella also should be evaluated for areas of pain/tenderness as the examiner attempts to palpate various proximal and distal aspects of the patella with appreciation of the facet joints. This systematic evaluation of the patellofemoral joint provides information from the passive range of motion (ROM), active ROM, resisted motion, weight-bearing activity, and palpation. We believe that the examiner can extrapolate from this data to determine the movements and ranges/arcs of motion that the patient can tolerate and therefore the ranges of motion to avoid or limit during a rehabilitation program.

The examiner should also determine if any meniscal pathology is present, as well as note any instability of the knee due to ligamentous injury or associated capsular laxity. Therefore, the anterior and posterior cruciate ligaments, as well as the medial and lateral collateral ligaments and the posteromedial and posterolateral capsule, should be assessed. Injury to the meniscus can create increased contact pressures, and damage to any aspect of the ligamentous or joint capsule can affect both the stability and biomechanics of the knee joint, thereby creating excessive wear of the articular cartilage and predisposing the athlete to early knee osteoarthritis.[49-64]

The clinician should also examine the hip joint for mobility and strength. Limitations in ROM and diminished strength of the hip musculature are present with knee osteoarthritis and can directly affect the knee joint via altered kinematics, leading to patient reports of pain and dysfunction.[65-67] Moreover, with hip osteoarthritis or other hip pathology, anteromedial knee pain may actually be referred from the hip by irritation of the obturator nerve. In addition to performing a hip assessment, the examiner should assess the ankle for ROM, joint mobility, and strength, as well as any other possible dysfunction that could place further strain or stress upon the knee joint during ADLs. A typical example would be dorsiflexion of less than 10° from either restricted joint mobility or an adaptively shortened

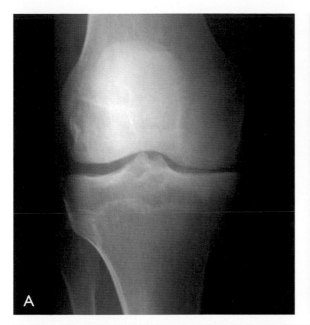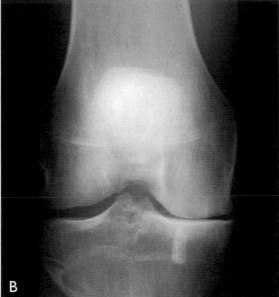

Figure 1 Radiographs of a knee with osteoarthritis. **A,** Weight-bearing AP view reveals some medial joint space narrowing. **B,** Weight-bearing PA view with the knee at 45° of flexion (Rosenberg view) shows significant loss of medial joint space that was not apparent on the view without the knee flexed.

gastrocnemius muscle causing an early heel-off or prolonged subtalar joint pronation during gait to compensate for the lack of adequate talocrural ROM; proximally, this would also cause increased internal rotation of the tibia and a resultant stress at the knee joint.[68-71] This could manifest itself during activities such as squatting or descending stairs. Hindfoot varus or valgus may additionally place undue stress on the medial or lateral compartments of the knee, respectively.

Radiographic examination is commonly included in the assessment of the knee joint for osteoarthritis. A weight-bearing PA view with the knees flexed to 45° (Rosenberg view) is preferred because it provides visualization of the more posterior aspect (30° to 60° flexion zone) of the tibiofemoral joint, which usually demonstrates the earliest and most predominant area of cartilage loss (**Figure 1**).[72-74] Rosenberg et al[74] demonstrated that this view has higher accuracy, sensitivity, and specificity than conventional weight-bearing radiographs in extension when comparing intraoperative cartilage loss with joint space narrowing observed radiographically. In addition to the tibiofemoral joint, the examiner should assess the patellofemoral joint, which can be best viewed using a Merchant view.[75-77] In addition to the Rosenberg view, routine radiographic evaluation should include weight-bearing AP, lateral, and sunrise views. If a determination of the mechanical weight-bearing axis of the limb is desired, a single-leg stance (ie, weight bearing on one limb) hip-knee-ankle radiograph should be obtained.

Nonsurgical Treatment

The overall goals of nonsurgical treatment of knee osteoarthritis in the mature athlete are to reduce pain and disability while improving the patient's overall quality of life. Treatment of these patients can be difficult because of the patient's goals, expectations, and compliance. Patients who have long been active in sports and recreation often have difficulty "slowing it down" or finding other forms of exercise or sports to participate in. Successful nonsurgical treatment of knee osteoarthritis looks similar to successful treatment of any other condition—the patient returns to the desired

Table 1: Tibiofemoral Compressive Loads

Activity	Load[a](× body weight)
Cycling	1.2
Level walking	3.4
Up ramp	4.5
Down ramp	4.5
Down stairs	4.5
Up stairs	4.8
Squat (ascent, 140°)	5.0
Squat (descent, 140°)	5.6
Running	33

[a]Data from Ericson MO, Nisell R: Tibiofemoral joint forces during ergometer cycling. *Am J Sports Med* 1986;14(4):285-290; Morrison JB: The mechanics of the knee joint in relation to normal walking. *J Biomech* 1970;3(1):51-61; Dahlkvist NJ, Mayo P, Seedhom BB: Forces during squatting and rising from a deep squat. *Eng Med* 1982;11(2):69-76.

activity and functional level. The ability to accomplish this is often related to compliance, the severity of the lesion, and any concomitant injuries that may be present.

The treatment plan may include the following interventions: improving overall lower extremity flexibility and strength, changing applied loads, education in modifying the activity levels and lifestyle, medications/injections and supplementation, weight loss, and coping skills. We have designed a four-phase program for the nonsurgical treatment of a patient with knee osteoarthritis, which is described in detail later. This program is designed to address the deficits associated with this condition and prepare the patient for return to activities.

Patient Education

During the initial visit, the patient should be properly educated regarding his or her diagnosis and prognosis.[78] Proper education is valuable in the management of osteoarthritis to address common patient concerns of pain, disability, medications, diet, exercise, and surgery. Patients should be made aware of their condition and its impact on their activities, as this can help the patient self-manage his or her symptoms. The patient should be instructed to minimize activities that cause unnecessary excessive loading of the knee.[79] The patient can be educated on joint protection activities such as incorporating rest breaks into daily activities, the use of a stool when standing for prolonged periods, and avoiding a prolonged flexed-knee position if patellofemoral wear is present. The patient is encouraged to rest for 20 to 30 minutes prior to heavy bouts of loading activity or strenuous exercise, as this may help reduce pain and allow improved activity tolerance. Proper education can assist in the management of arthritis by minimizing causative factors and allowing the patient to understand the associated pain and disability of this condition.[80,81] Patient education interventions can produce a significant reduction in pain.[82] Patients who are able to incorporate cognitive and behavioral coping skills through such actions as less-catastrophic thinking, prayer, ignoring pain, less reinterpretation of pain, or developing a stronger perception of pain control are able to more effectively manage their pain and resultant disability.[83-87]

It is important to educate patients about the compressive loads present during various activities and exercises to allow for modification of activities and activity avoidance. This can allow the patient to make educated decisions about performing ADLs, exercises, and training. **Table 1** lists some common activities and the resultant compressive loads incurred. We believe that informing patients and allowing them to make educated decisions can greatly assist in the rehabilitation process and allows them to feel in control of decision making regarding their individual exercise routines.

Weight Loss

Weight loss should be encouraged in individuals who are obese (body mass index >30 kg/m^2). Weight loss has been shown to reduce the symptomatic reports of knee osteoarthritis and slow the progression of arthrosis.[24,28] An increased body mass may lead to osteoarthritis as a result of increased joint reactive forces, accumulated microtrauma, and interference with normal chondrocyte metabolism. Messier et al[89] demonstrated a direct association between body mass and knee compressive forces, resultant force, abduction moment, and medial rotation moment. They noted that a weight reduction of 9.8 N (1 kg) results in a reduction in compressive forces of 40.6 N, resultant forces of 38.7 N, and a 1.4% reduction in knee abduction moment.[89] Thus, weight loss can have profound effects on minimizing the compressive loads that occur at the knee joint during more strenuous activities such as running, during which loads of up to 33 times body weight at the tibiofemoral joint and 5.6 times body weight at the patellofemoral joint are reported to occur.[88,90] It is clear that weight loss can reduce the magnitude of joint compressive forces that occur as an individual ambulates throughout the day.

Pharmacology and Supplemental Treatment

Over-the-counter supplements and medications, prescription medications, and injections are commonly used in the treatment of arthritic conditions. Physicians often recommend a nonsteroidal anti-inflammatory medication, a corticosteroid or similar intra-articular injection, viscosupplementation, or acetaminophen for control of pain and joint swelling. Ibuprofen and fenoprofen have been shown in vitro to reduce glycosaminoglycan synthesis in canine cartilage, and indomethacin has been shown to speed the progression of osteoarthritis in humans.[91,92] Glucosamine sulfate and chondroitin sulfate are commonly used nutritional supplements that may help in the reduction of pain and retard further articular cartilage degeneration. It appears that these supplements stimulate cartilaginous matrix production, decrease the production of proteolytic enzymes, and improve synovial fluid and anti-inflammatory properties.[93-98] Although good results have been reported with taking glucosamine sulfate alone, results are more favorable when glucosamine sulfate and chondroitin sulfate are taken concomitantly.[99-105] Reginster et al[100] reported in a randomized double-blinded placebo-controlled study that patients with knee osteoarthritis who received glucosamine sulfate and chondroitin sulfate had less joint narrowing and pain and had a 20% improvement in Western Ontario and McMaster Universities Osteoarthritis Index (WOMAC) scores. Patients should be educated that benefits may not become evident until after 4 weeks of continuous use, and to discontinue use if symptoms do not improve within a few months of use.[106,107] Avocado soy bean unsaponifiables (ASUs) are botanicals that appear to be chondroprotective as a result of their anti-inflammatory and proanabolic effect on articular chondrocytes.[108-110] It is important for all healthcare providers to be aware of these products (including side effects, results, contraindications, dosage, etc), as patients commonly ask about the use of these treatments.

Knee Alignment

Biomechanical Implications

As part of the nonsurgical care of the arthritic knee, the rehabilitation specialist should assess both the involved and noninvolved lower extremity for alignment of the foot, knee, and hip. The alignment of the hip, knee, and ankle influences the load and stress distribution that occurs at the knee; an overall varus knee malalignment increases the medial load, and a valgus malalignment increases the lateral load.[111] Having either a varus or valgus malalignment greater than 5° in both knees can lead to a significant functional deterioration as compared with a malalignment of less than than 5°.[111] In the presence of moderate osteoarthritis, the risk of further progression is increased tenfold when varus or valgus malalignment is present.[112] In addition to affecting the tibiofemoral joint, varus or valgus malalignment can also affect patellofemoral osteoarthritis, with varus or valgus malalignment increasing the odds of progression of patellofemoral osteoarthritis isolated in the medial or lateral compartment, respectively.[113] The lower extremity evaluation should assess for any leg-length asymmetry. Golightly et al[114] reported an increased incidence of knee osteoarthritis in association with leg-length inequality of 2 cm or greater. Foot and ankle alignment should be assessed, as patients with increased foot pronation have been shown to have an increased likelihood of developing medial knee osteoarthritis.[115,116] The alignment of the hip and pelvis has also been shown to correlate with the presence of knee osteoarthritis, with patients with lateral compartment osteoarthritis having a wider pelvis and shorter femoral neck and patients with medial compartment osteoarthritis displaying a higher femoral offset.[117]

Diminished Hip and Knee Mobility

ROM defects in the knee can either preceede or be the result of knee osteoarthritis. Knee joint stiffness is one of the most common postoperative complications of surgery of the knee.[118-120] Shelbourne and Gray[121] noted that loss of knee extension greater than 3° (including hyperextension) was the most significant factor associated with lower subjective and objective results in 502 patients at a mean of 14.1 years following anterior cruciate ligament reconstruction; a loss in normal knee flexion was also noted to be significant. These results were adverse, especially when coupled with meniscectomy and articular cartilage damage. A loss in knee extension can also cause increased patellofemoral pain, quadriceps weakness, and an overall poor knee function.[122] Losses in knee flexion, hip internal and external rotation, and hip flexion and extension have been shown to increase the incidence of locomotor disability in knee osteoarthritis.[123,124] Loss of joint motion can cause an altered gait pattern and create increased stress at both the patellofemoral and tibiofemoral joints; therefore, motion should be assessed in both the hip and knee joint to ensure full mobility in all planes.

Strength Assessment

Diminished quadriceps strength is commonly present in patients with knee osteoarthritis. Although some authors report that good quadriceps strength does not diminish the incidence of radiographic knee osteoarthritis, it can help protect against the development of symptomatic knee osteoarthritis by decreasing knee pain and providing overall better physical function.[125-128] A decrease in hip external rotation and abduction strength has been noted in individuals with patellofemoral symptoms.[129] Therefore, the quadriceps, hamstrings, and hip musculature should be assessed to determine any causative factors for knee osteoarthritis and to diminish the symptoms.

Proprioceptive Assessment

Whether diminished proprioception contributes to or is a result of knee osteoarthritis is unclear. Diminished proprioception has been reported as a result of age and injury, suggesting a decreased acuity of movement sense that can lead to joint degeneration.[130-132] Although most authors have reported diminished proprioception

in the presence of knee osteoarthritis,[133-137] other authors have reported no proprioceptive loss.[138] A loss in proprioception can cause the patient to have a diminished gait velocity and stride length, loss in neuromuscular control, and increased potential for further injury.[139] In the presence of pain and inflammation, an inhibitory effect on the neuromuscular system occurs as a result of a decrease in the mechanoreceptor input, the so-called "reflex inhibition."[140] Degenerative arthritis has been shown to lead to muscle inhibition, which could lead to excessive joint overload due to a loss in both force attenuation and dynamic control.[130,131] Proprioceptive defects, altered muscle patterns, and reflex latency delays have been described following rupture of the anterior cruciate ligament.[139-144] Altered muscle activity with increased hamstring activity and decreased quadriceps activity has been shown during gait, stair climbing, and jogging, causing an increase in joint load with a resultant decrease in both ADLs and functional abilities.[145,146] This is thought to contribute to the anterior knee pain commonly experienced after anterior cruciate ligament rupture.

Although studies assessing proprioceptive loss usually are performed with computerized testing, the evaluator can assess clinically for any difference with either a single-limb balance assessment or with a joint replication test, for which the patient is seated. Proprioceptive awareness has been demonstrated to be symmetric between extremities, whether pathologic conditions (either bilateral or unilateral) are present or not.[147] Proprioceptive losses have also been reported in the uninvolved knee in the presence of unilateral knee osteoarthritis;[135,136] this knowledge can assist the evaluator during the evaluation or nonsurgical treatment of the mature athlete with unilateral knee osteoarthritis who cannot assume unilateral stance secondary to pain. The patient can perform this activity on the opposite lower extremity for either assessment or training activities.

Interventions for Malalignment
Patellar Taping

Patellar taping has been used to alter the biomechanics of the knee joint and to provide proprioceptive feedback. Patellar taping has been reported to reduce pain scores and symptoms in patients with patellofemoral arthritis.[148] Hinman et al[149] reported a 73% improvement (as measured by pain scales and patient-perceived rating of change) in individuals with knee osteoarthritis with patellar taping, as compared with 49% with control taping, and 10% improvement with no taping. Patellar taping is thought to reduce pain by providing subtle changes in patellar position, which may alter the stresses or pressures at the patellofemoral joint, diminish the stress at the fat pad, increase proprioception and neuromuscular control of the knee, and improve quadriceps strength.[150-157] Although the exact mechanism is unclear, improving or altering any of these variables could provide symptomatic relief in the arthritic knee by allowing the athlete to perform therapeutic exercises or training with diminished symptoms. Pfeiffer et al[158] have demonstrated that McConnell taping does not maintain median glide after 20 minutes of moderate activity.

Orthoses and Heel Wedges

Orthoses are commonly prescribed in the treatment of unicompartmental knee osteoarthritis to alter the applied forces that occur at the knee with weight bearing by addressing any foot malalignment that may be contributing to the patient's condition. Kerrigan et al[159] reported a significant reduction in knee varus torque with walking in patients with medial knee osteoarthritis with use of both a 5° and 10° lateral heel wedge (6% and 8% reduction, respectively). In individuals with medial compartment osteoarthritis, a lateral heel wedge or custom orthosis can be used to reduce the knee adduction moment, thereby diminishing the medial compartment pressure and load, thus causing a reduction in medial joint line pain.[160,161] Heel wedges have also been shown to diminish the lateral/medial thrust at the knee present in unicompartmental osteoarthritis, with the use of a medial wedge to decrease a medial thrust and a lateral wedge for a lateral thrust.[162] Although the relief is greater in individuals with mild osteoarthritis, patients displaying complete loss of joint space can have some reduction in symptoms.[163-165] This decrease in pain may allow a reduction in the use of NSAIDs.[166,167] It should be noted that some patients experience medial (ie, first or second metatarsophalangeal joint) metatarsalgia due to increased plantar pressure on the forefoot. It also should be noted that the American Academy of

Orthopaedic Surgeons' clinical practice guideline on knee osteoarthritis recommends against prescribing lateral heel wedges for patients with symptomatic medial compartment knee osteoarthritis because of a lack of evidence supporting their use.[168]

Shoe Modification

The patient's daily and training shoewear should be assessed to determine if they are appropriate for that patient. Patients who tend to wear high heels should be informed of the increased varus knee torque, increased forces at the patellofemoral joint, and greater compressive force at the medial knee compartment that occur during ambulation.[169,170] Shoes with variable stiffness may help reduce the knee adduction moment in individuals with medial compartment knee osteoarthritis.[171,172]

Knee Bracing

Functional knee braces that produce a valgus stress at the knee may be effective for the treatment of medial compartment osteoarthritis. These braces attempt to unload the medial compartment of the knee by reducing the knee adduction moment and thereby redistributing the joint load. Asymptomatic walking tolerance, overall function, and mean knee adduction moment during walking and running have been shown to improve with the use of an unloader brace.[173-177] An unloader brace has also been shown to be more effective than a neoprene sleeve in reduction of symptoms following walking and stair climbing.[177]

Rehabilitation for Knee Osteoarthritis

Physical therapy has been shown to be very effective in the treatment of knee osteoarthritis. A physical therapist may incorporate physical modalities (electrical stimulation, heat or cold, ultrasound), ROM, strengthening exercises, flexibility, proprioception, aerobic conditioning, and aquatic therapy activities in the nonsurgical treatment of knee osteoarthritis based on the patient's presentation and current condition. Prior to implementation of an exercise program, the rehabilitation specialist should determine the athlete's impairments, general conditioning, status of the knee ligamentous tissues, and the grade and location (tibia,

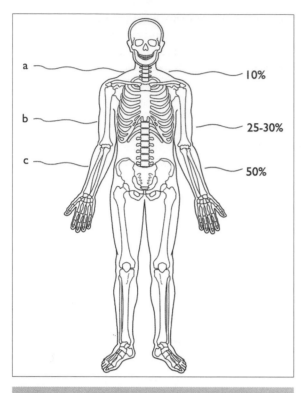

Figure 2   Illustration shows percentage of body weight supported by the lower limbs at various water depths: a, the neck (C7); b, the chest (xiphoid process); and c, the pelvis (anterior superior iliac spine). (Adapted with permission from Bates A, Hanson N, eds: *Aquatic Exercise Therapy*. Philadelphia, PA, Saunders, 1996, p 25.)

femur, patella, or combination) of osteoarthritis in the knee.

Aquatic Therapy

Aquatic therapy is commonly used in the rehabilitation process and can be helpful in the treatment of the mature athlete with knee osteoarthritis. The buoyancy of water allows most individuals to float and therefore can be beneficial in the reduction of weight-bearing forces and stresses at the knee that occur with ambulation and jogging. Individuals who are very lean and need to further decrease the weight-bearing forces on the lower extremity in the pool can use buoyancy assist devices such as a life vest or floats. The depth of water affects the weight-bearing forces: at waist level, a 50%

reduction is produced; at the xiphoid process, a 70% reduction; and at the seventh cervical vertebrae, a 90% decrease in weight-bearing forces is achieved (**Figure 2**).[178]

Other physical properties of water, such as the hydrostatic pressure exerted on the lower extremity, make aquatic therapy advantageous. A pressure of 22.4 mm Hg is exerted per each foot of depth of immersion; as a result, at a depth of 4 feet, the pressure is 89.6 mm Hg, which is greater than the diastolic pressure.[179] This can be beneficial in the rehabilitation process to assist in controlling joint swelling and effusion while the athlete exercises. Performing aquatic therapy in warm water has many physiologic effects on the body, including increased peripheral circulation, muscle relaxation, elevated body temperature, increased sweating, and increased cardiovascular demands.

Hinman et al[180] reported that 75% of subjects with knee osteoarthritis who performed aquatic therapy for 6 weeks had improvements in pain and function, with continued benefits noted at 6 weeks following completion of exercises. Wyatt et al[181] evaluated a land-based program versus an aquatic program and found no significant difference in the improvement in knee ROM, thigh girth, and time for a 1-mile walk; however, the subjects who underwent an aquatic program had significantly lower subjective pain levels compared with the land-based group. Silva et al[182] reported similar findings with a reduction in pain at rest and following a 50-foot walk test, and improvements in WOMAC and Lequesne index scores in both aquatic and land-based rehabiliation groups, although individuals in the aquatic program had a significantly greater decrease in pain before and after the walk test at 18-week follow-up. Conversely, Lund et al[183] reported that compared with control subjects, only subjects undergoing a land-based exercise program showed improvement in pain and muscle strength; no difference was noted with an aquatic program. However, the authors noted that 11 of the 25 patients reported discomfort with a land-based program, compared with 3 of 27 patients in the aquatic program.[183] We commonly use aquatic rehabilitation as an adjunct to land-based therapy in the rehabilitation program to allow the athlete to perform higher level activities than are currently tolerated with land-based therapy and as a form of therapy activity modification.

Biomechanical Considerations for Rehabilitation

In planning a rehabilitation program for the arthritic knee, a multitude of factors should be considered, including the status of the ligamentous tissue and meniscal tissue, and articular cartilage wear. Using these factors to determine the most appropriate exercises for each patient will minimize any deleterious effects that an exercise may have on the arthritic knee. Strength-training exercises are performed in either an open kinetic chain (OKC) or closed kinetic chain (CKC) manner, and it is important for the treating physician to understand the stresses and forces that occur with each of these forms of exercise. CKC exercises are generally prescribed because they replicate functional activities such as stair climbing, whereas OKC exercises are used to isolate specific muscle groups for strength training.[184] To avoid excessive weight bearing or shear forces across the tibiofemoral joint, the rehabilitation specialist may choose a more OKC-focused program; however, consideration should be given to the compressive forces incurred at the patellofemoral joint and excessive anterior or posterior shear forces that are created that could cause unnecessary tibial translation in the presence of joint laxity.

Open Kinetic Chain

Increased anterior shear forces occur between 40° and 0° of OKC knee extension, with stress increasing exponentially along with increased resistance.[185,186] Posterior shear forces can also occur during OKC knee extension, depending on the angle of the knee. High shear forces are noted at 90° to 100° of knee flexion and have been reported to continue until 40° of knee flexion during OKC knee extension.[185-188] These high posterior shear forces are also produced during OKC knee flexion. Lutz et al[188] reported a maximum shear force of 1,780 N at 90° of knee flexion, 1,526 N at 60°, and 939 N at 30° during isometric knee flexion.

The exercise prescriber should also take into consideration the stresses that occur at the patellofemoral joint during OKC knee extension. The greatest amount of patellofemoral contact area (6.0 cm^2) occurs at 90°; at 30° of knee flexion, the contact area decreases to 2.0 cm^2.[189,190] Increased quadriceps force is produced during OKC knee extension as the knee approaches full

knee extension, and this force production is further increased with the addition of external loads.[191] Therefore, greater forces are produced at the patellofemoral joint as the knee nears full extension, which increases as the knee angle becomes less than 57°.[192] In general, the patella begins to articulate with the femur at approximately 10° and 20° of knee flexion, depending on the size of the patella and the length of the patellar tendon.[190] With knee flexion, the contact area migrates proximally upon the inferior aspect of the patella: at 30° of knee flexion, the contact is upon the inferior facets; at 60° of knee flexion, the middle facets of the patella articulate with the trochlea; at 90° of knee flexion, the contact area is at the superior facets; and at 135° of knee flexion, the contact area is at the proximal aspect of the patella at the lateral and odd facet.[190,193] Therefore, in addition to contact forces, the rehabilitation specialist should consider the contact zone of the patella throughout the arc of motion, especially if articular cartilage wear is noted at the patella by making such adjustments as avoiding a particular arc of motion that coincides with the patient's articular cartilage damage. For example, a patient with an isolated lesion on the anterior aspect of the femoral condyle may tolerate exercises at greater flexion angles, whereas a lesion on the posterior condyle may necessitate avoidance of exercises at greater flexion angles because of the rolling-and-sliding component of the articulation that occurs at deeper knee flexion angles.[194]

Closed Kinetic Chain

Wilk et al[185] reported that a posterior tibiofemoral shear force was observed throughout the entire motion for both the squat and leg press (peak 1,500 N). In addition, unlike OKC, the application of external loads does not result in a significant amount of increased anterior shear stress; therefore, it appears that the effect of the compressive body weight load serves as a protective mechanism against anterior stress.[195] When considering the electromyographic activity of the quadriceps and hamstrings, the greatest cocontractions are produced during exercises such as squats and lateral lunges to 30° of knee flexion, whereas exercises such as the leg press and wall squats produce a more isolated quadriceps contraction. Therefore, depending upon such variables as trunk position relative to the knee,

knee flexion angle, and direction of movement (ascending or descending), quadriceps and hamstrings muscle activity during a CKC exercise can vary.[186] Numerous authors have reported relatively low tibiofemoral and patellofemoral joint forces at low angles (0° to 30°); therefore, we initiate exercises such as the leg press and vertical and wall squats within these angles.[189,190,196]

Rehabilitation Program

We have established a four-phase program for the non-surgical treatment of the arthritic knee. The implementation of this program is based on the physical examination, including a biomechanical and musculoskeletal assessment, as well as patient goals. The treatment program has multiple phases and focuses on reducing pain and difficulty with ADLs and recreational activity by incorporating any and all treatment strategies deemed appropriate. The initial goal of treatment is symptom relief. This is accomplished through medications, activity modification, and biomechanical modifications.

Phase I (Acute Phase)

Phase I is focused on restoring/normalizing ROM and flexibility of the lower extremity, beginning muscle-strengthening exercise, modifying the patient's activity level, evaluating for the use of biomechanical unloading devices (orthoses or knee brace), nutritional supplementation, and determining the need for weight reduction. If swelling is noted, the patient's treatment should include swelling reduction techniques such as cryotherapy and a knee compression sleeve. The goal of this initial phase is to return the knee to homeostasis.

To normalize gait/stride length and to decrease the stresses that occur at the knee, it is important that ROM and flexibility are restored in the lower extremity. The athlete is instructed to begin a stretching program for the entire lower extremity to address the entire kinetic chain, including the hip flexors/abductors/adductors, quadriceps, hamstrings, and gastrocnemius-soleus complex. This will allow the musculature to provide more shock absorption at the knee and help to eliminate any compensatory movement patterns as a result of decreased flexibility. Because ROM deficits can also result from joint stiffness, it is important to assess for proper joint mobility of the hip, knee, and ankle. Diminished joint mobility can be the result of injury, or

postoperative or decreased capsular mobility as a result of the arthritic condition. Hip capsular mobility should be assessed for proper joint play in all planes; if diminished mobility is noted, joint mobilization techniques are warranted. The rehabilitation specialist should then evaluate the knee joint for both patellar mobility and tibiofemoral mobility. Decreased patellar mobility can be the result of postoperative complications, such as those after anterior cruciate ligament reconstruction or TKA, or as a result of joint tightness due to knee osteoarthritis. The patella should translate approximately 8 to 10 mm in all directions; if tightness is noted, patellar mobilizations are incorporated into the treatment program and the patient is instructed so that he or she can perform them as part of the home exercise program. If knee ROM is limited in either extension or flexion, the rehabilitation specialist should attempt to regain the lost motion through the use of flexibility exercises, joint mobilization, and low-load long-duration (LLLD) stretches if needed. If limited joint mobility is noted in either flexion or extension, appropriate mobilization techniques should be performed. For a knee extension loss, the tibia can be translated anteriorly on the femur (or the femur posteriorly on the tibia), and tibial external rotation can be performed to improve terminal knee extension. To improve knee flexion, the tibia can be translated posteriorly on the femur (or the femur anteriorly on the tibia), and tibial internal rotation can also be performed to improve the arthokinematic component of knee flexion.

The rehabilitation specialist can also include LLLD knee stretches in the treatment program. The goal of this treatment is to create plastic deformation of the tissue and cause remodeling to occur as a result of creep stress causing tissue change.[197,198] We prefer to have the patient perform LLLD knee extension while supine as opposed to prone because the supine position allows greater relaxation of the hip extensors and hamstring muscle groups and improved patient comfort. This overpressure program can be performed with an ankle weight (2.7 to 5.4 kg [6 to 12 lb]) placed on the knee; treatment sessions last 15 minutes. Ideally, the patient should perform this activity four times per day to allow for a total longer duration at end ROM for greater tissue plastic deformation. This activity can also be performed with the use of commercially available equipment such

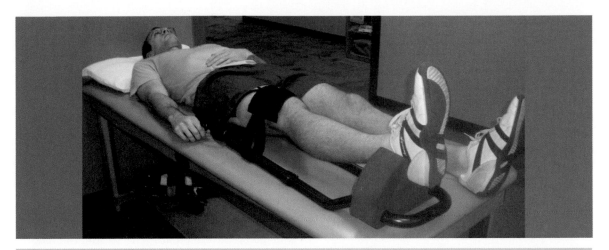

Figure 3   Photograph shows a patient using the ERMI Knee Extensionater (ERMI, Atlanta, GA), used to improve knee extension range of motion.

as the ERMI Knee Extensionater (ERMI, Atlanta, GA; **Figure 3**).

A lower extremity strengthening program should be initiated immediately, with special emphasis on the quadriceps. The patient often will have a decreased ability to voluntarily activate the quadriceps because of pain, inflammation, disuse, decreased patellar mobility, and loss of knee extension.[199] An increase in intra-articular joint temperature has been shown to stimulate proteolytic enzyme activity, causing a deleterious effect on the articular cartilage.[200,201] Petterson et al[202] reported that individuals with unilateral knee osteoarthritis had quadriceps weakness due to decreased volitional muscle activation and smaller lean muscle cross-sectional area compared with the contralateral limb. The authors attributed 40% of the variance in maximal voluntary isometric contraction to volitional muscle activation and 27% to muscle cross-sectional area. Therefore, in this initial phase, we emphasize swelling reduction measures such as cryotherapy, electrical stimulation, and a knee sleeve. It is also important to control volitional quadriceps muscle activation. Neuromuscular electrical stimulation and biofeedback have been shown to augment return of muscle recruitment.[203,204] We have found it beneficial to perform neuromuscular electrical stimulation concomitant with voluntary quadriceps contractions (**Figure 4**). This prevents further muscle atrophy, assists in restoring patellar

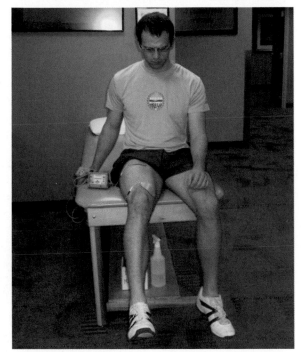

Figure 4   Photograph shows a patient undergoing electrical muscle stimulation using an EMPI PV 300 (EMPI, St. Paul, MN) concomitant with voluntary quadriceps contraction to enhance muscle contraction.

mobility (especially superior), and reduces reports of pain. Once the patient has regained independent muscle activation, biofeedback can be used to facilitate further neuromuscular activation of the quadriceps.[194] The patient will perform strengthening exercises for the entire lower kinetic chain, using OKC and CKC exercises as tolerated. Cardiovascular and muscular endurance exercises should be included in the treatment program. The patient should perform bicycling or pool activities as tolerated without symptoms.

During the initial phases of the rehabilitation program, neuromuscular control drills should be incorporated. Diminished proprioception can occur as a result of injury and advanced age; it is therefore important to incorporate dynamic stability training into the rehabilitation of patients with knee osteoarthritis. The initial goals of this program are to improve proprioception and balance, equalize weight distribution with stance, and normalize the gait pattern. The patient can perform squatting activities on an unstable surface, weight-shifting drills, and forward and lateral cone walking. If the patient is unable to tolerate weight-bearing activities secondary to pain, non–weight-bearing proprioceptive activities can be performed such as joint reproduction drills with the eyes closed and single-leg proprioceptive exercises on the noninvolved lower extremity.

Phase II (Subacute Phase)

The goals of this phase are to continue to enhance lower extremity ROM/flexibility, progress with lower extremity strengthening exercises, and progressively increase weight-bearing activities through CKC and functional activities. Before the patient progresses to phase II, the rehabilitation specialist should ensure that pain/inflammation have diminished, strengthening exercises and neuromuscular control drills have been initiated, and knee ROM has improved to full motion or only a minimum loss in knee mobility. The patient continues with knee ROM techniques such as flexibility exercises, joint mobilization techniques, and the use of LLLD stretches as needed.

The patient continues with a lower extremity strengthening program, advancing the weight-bearing forces and incorporating functional activities as tolerated. The patient performs CKC strengthening exercises consisting of leg presses, squats, and forward and

lateral lunges; an aquatic rehabilitation program can be initiated as well. To offer feedback to the patient, we often perform these CKC exercises on devices that monitor weight disruption (force platforms). We find this form of feedback particularly useful in the patient who has developed a decreased weight-load tolerance with gait secondary to knee pain. The exercises are monitored for patient tolerance with the knee ROM and joint loading adjusted to minimize stress on articular lesions. Patients can also perform these weight-bearing exercises while wearing a brace and/or orthoses to further diminish weight-bearing loads, which can allow the patient to begin CKC exercises/drills sooner with decreased symptoms. The patient continue to perform hip-strengthening exercises (with emphasis on hip abductors/rotators) to ensure proximal stabilization with functional activities such as stair climbing. Balance and proprioceptive drills are progressed with the incorporation of drills such as squats on the Biodex Balance System (Biodex Medical Systems, Shirley, NY) (**Figure 5**) and tilt board, and lunges onto an unstable surface (foam). In addition, the patient should perform exercises for the trunk and core to improve stabilization.

Phase III (Advanced Phase)

Phase III continues with more advanced training and exercise progression. Before beginning phase III, the patient should be pain free, exhibit full knee ROM, and tolerate CKC activities without an increase in symptoms. During this phase, strengthening exercises are progressed, functional activities are implemented, and unilateral weight-bearing activities are initiated to increase the kinetic forces occurring at the knee joint (**Figure 6**). The exercise dosage is gradually increased, with continued joint monitoring by the rehabilitation specialist for joint irritation. This phase includes functional strengthening activities such as cone-stepping drills and forward, backward, and lateral lunges. In addition, proprioceptive and plyometric drills such as the plyometric leg press or lateral lunges/hops can be performed. To minimize joint-reaction forces, the patient can begin pool running, running on a de-weighted treadmill (**Figure 7**), or performing cardiovascular training on an elliptical machine.

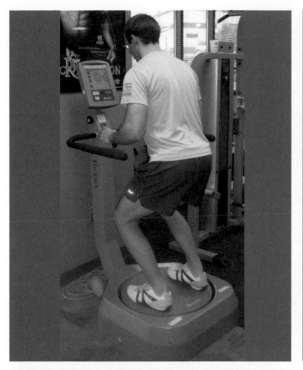

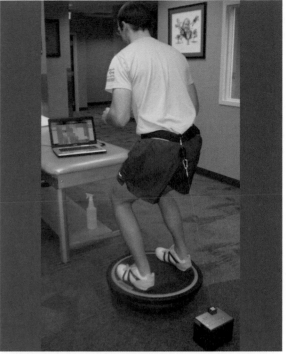

Figure 5 Photograph shows a patient performing squats on a Biodex Balance System (Biodex Medical Systems, Shirley, NY).

Figure 6 Photograph shows a patient performing squats on a stability ball while using a MR Cube (Monitored Rehab Systems, Haarlem, Netherlands) to enhance functional training.

Phase IV (Sport-Specific Activities)

The following criteria must be met before the patient is progressed into the fourth phase of the rehabilitation process: full pain-free knee ROM, minimum to no joint effusion, satisfactory lower extremity strength, and a good tolerance of the current rehabilitation program. The goal of this phase is to return the athlete to a desirable level of athletic competition with an asymptomatic knee. Sport-specific drills and activities are initiated during this phase as well as a running program. We use a gradual and methodical approach to implementing sport-specific activities. The running program is gradually progressed in intensity, duration, and difficulty of running performed. For example, the patient can begin with lateral movement drills, then progress to backward running, and finally progress to forward running. We commonly implement backward running before forward running because increased electromyographic activity of the hamstring and quadriceps and

decreased joint forces occur in backward running compared with forward running.[205] Patients can begin to perform cutting drills (initially 45°, followed by 90°) as needed for their sport, then progress to jumping drills and sport-specific activity. This allows the patient to return to practice and ultimately to competition.

Although the athlete is progressing with functional drills and activities, the flexibility, ROM, and strengthening program should be continued. The ROM and flexibility program is of particular importance because commonly a patient will lose some knee ROM, especially knee extension, once beginning functional activities. This can cause a cascade of problems, potentially returning the patient to the prior level of disability. In addition, because of the high level of training and joint loading that occurs during this phase, we commonly have the athlete perform strengthening exercises and running/functional drills on alternate days. This allows

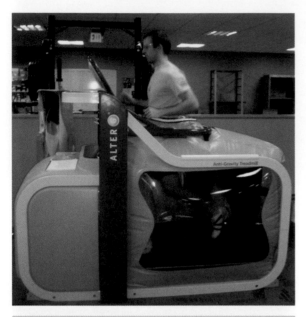

Figure 7   Photograph shows a patient jogging on an AlterG Anti-Gravity Treadmill (Alter-G, Fremont, CA). The treadmill allows specific unweighting of the lower extremities.

greater tissue recovery and minimizes any overuse syndromes.

Return to Sports

Patients can be returned to their sport once they have met the following criteria: full, nonpainful knee ROM; no effusion/inflammation; satisfactory (80% or greater) quadriceps bilateral comparison muscle strength; and completion of an appropriate rehabilitation and sport-specific program. The ultimate goal is an asymptomatic knee joint. The patient should be educated about monitoring the joint line for pain/tenderness following activities once he or she has returned to sporting activities to facilitate constant monitoring of the knee's reaction to intensity of activities.

Summary

Osteoarthritis of the knee is a common disorder, and athletes who participate in contact sports or activities that require excessive joint loading are at a greater risk of developing osteoarthritis. Nonsurgical treatments consisting of weight loss, nutritional supplementation,

medications, and physical therapy are commonly prescribed in the management of this condition. Physical therapy is considered an important aspect of nonsurgical management and should consist of improving lower extremity flexibility, regaining knee ROM, establishing good muscular control, improving proprioceptive control, altering lower extremity joint forces, and modifying the activity level of the patient. Rehabilitation programs appear to be of benefit in the nonsurgical management of knee osteoarthritis and can allow patients to return to their desired level of activity. Moderate-intensity exercise may have a protective effect on articular cartilage and can significantly reduce pain and symptoms associated with osteoarthritis.[206-209] Jan et al[210] compared non–weight-bearing versus weight-bearing exercises and noted equal improvements in WOMAC function score, walking speed, and strength; however, proprioceptive joint reposition sense was greater in the weight-bearing group. Lin et al[211] compared the outcomes of proprioceptive training and strength training in subjects with knee osteoarthritis. Although they reported that both groups had an improved WOMAC function score, the improvement in the strength training group was noted to be a result of a greater increase in knee extensor strength, whereas improvement in the proprioceptive training was reported to be a result of the greater proprioceptive function as demonstrated with improved walking time on a spongy surface and a reduced knee reposition error.[211] We attempt to improve knee mobility, flexibility, strength, and muscular control, as this will allow the athlete to control and dissipate weight-bearing forces at the tibiofemoral joint. We therefore believe an effective nonsurgical rehabilitation program consists of non–weight-bearing, weight-bearing, proprioceptive, and aquatic exercise based on patient presentation and tolerance of activities. We also consider biomechanical modifications, nutritional supplementation, and patient education to allow the mature athlete the greatest opportunity for improvement and return to the desired level of activity.

References

1. van Saase JL, van Romunde LK, Cats A, Vandenbroucke JP, Valkenburg HA: Epidemiology of osteoarthritis: Zoetermeer survey. Comparison of

radiological osteoarthritis in a Dutch population with that in 10 other populations. *Ann Rheum Dis* 1989; 48(4):271-280.

2. Lawrence RC, Helmick CG, Arnett FC, et al: Estimates of the prevalence of arthritis and selected musculoskeletal disorders in the United States. *Arthritis Rheum* 1998;41(5):778-799.

3. Lawrence RC, Felson DT, Helmick CG, et al: Estimates of the prevalence of arthritis and other rheumatic conditions in the United States: Part II. *Arthritis Rheum* 2008;58(1):26-35.

4. Hootman JM, Helmick CG: Projections of US prevalence of arthritis and associated activity limitations. *Arthritis Rheum* 2006;54(1):226-229.

5. Murphy L, Schwartz TA, Helmick CG, et al: Lifetime risk of symptomatic knee osteoarthritis. *Arthritis Rheum* 2008;59(9):1207-1213.

6. Felson DT, Naimark A, Anderson JJ, Kazis L, Castelli W, Meenan RF: The prevalence of knee osteoarthritis in the elderly: The Framingham Osteoarthritis Study. *Arthritis Rheum* 1987;30(8):914-918.

7. Felson DT, Zhang Y, Hannan MT, et al: The incidence and natural history of knee osteoarthritis in the elderly: The Framingham Osteoarthritis Study. *Arthritis Rheum* 1995;38(10):1500-1505.

8. Dillon CF, Hirsch R, Rasch EK, Gu Q: Symptomatic hand osteoarthritis in the United States: Prevalence and functional impairment estimates from the third U.S. National Health and Nutrition Examination Survey, 1991-1994. *Am J Phys Med Rehabil* 2007;86(1):12-21.

9. Jordan JM, Helmick CG, Renner JB, et al: Prevalence of knee symptoms and radiographic and symptomatic knee osteoarthritis in African Americans and Caucasians: The Johnston County Osteoarthritis Project. *J Rheumatol* 2007;34(1):172-180.

10. Dillon CF, Rasch EK, Gu Q, Hirsch R: Prevalence of knee osteoarthritis in the United States: Arthritis data from the third National Health and Nutritional Examination Survey 1991-1994. *J Rheumatol* 2006;33(11):2271-2279.

11. Sowers M, Lachance L, Hochberg M, Jamadar D: Radiographically defined osteoarthritis of the hand and knee in young and middle-aged African American and Caucasian women. *Osteoarthritis Cartilage* 2000;8(2): 69-77.

12. Buckwalter JA, Saltzman C, Brown T: The impact of osteoarthritis: Implications for research. *Clin Orthop Relat Res* 2004;(427 Suppl):S6-S15.

13. Srikanth VK, Fryer JL, Zhai G, Winzenberg TM, Hosmer D, Jones G: A meta-analysis of sex differences prevalence, incidence and severity of osteoarthritis. *Osteoarthritis Cartilage* 2005;13(9):769-781.

14. Guccione AA, Felson DT, Anderson JJ, et al: The effects of specific medical conditions on the functional limitations of elders in the Framingham Study. *Am J Public Health* 1994;84(3):351-358.

15. Michaud CM, McKenna MT, Begg S, et al: The burden of disease and injury in the United States 1996. *Popul Health Metr* 2006;4:11.

16. Kurtz S, Ong K, Lau E, Mowat F, Halpern M: Projections of primary and revision hip and knee arthroplasty in the United States from 2005 to 2030. *J Bone Joint Surg Am* 2007;89(4):780-785.

17. Felson DT, Zhang Y: An update on the epidemiology of knee and hip osteoarthritis with a view to prevention. *Arthritis Rheum* 1998;41(8):1343-1355.

18. Felson DT: Risk factors for osteoarthritis: Understanding joint vulnerability. *Clin Orthop Relat Res* 2004;(427 Suppl):S16-S21.

19. Rossignol M, Leclerc A, Allaert FA, et al: Primary osteoarthritis of hip, knee, and hand in relation to occupational exposure. *Occup Environ Med* 2005; 62(11):772-777.

20. Kellgren JH, Lawrence JS: Rheumatism in miners: II. X-ray study. *Br J Ind Med* 1952;9(3):197-207.

21. Partridge RE, Duthie JJ: Rheumatism in dockers and civil servants: A comparison of heavy manual and sedentary workers. *Ann Rheum Dis* 1968;27(6): 559-568.

22. Davis MA, Neuhaus JM, Ettinger WH, Mueller WH: Body fat distribution and osteoarthritis. *Am J Epidemiol* 1990;132(4):701-707.

23. Dougados M, Gueguen A, Nguyen M, et al: Longitudinal radiologic evaluation of osteoarthritis of the knee. *J Rheumatol* 1992;19(3):378-384.

24. Felson DT, Anderson JJ, Naimark A, Walker AM, Meenan RF: Obesity and knee osteoarthritis: The Framingham Study. *Ann Intern Med* 1988;109(1): 18-24.

25. van Saase JL, Vandenbroucke JP, van Romunde LK, Valkenburg HA: Osteoarthritis and obesity in the general population: A relationship calling for an explanation. *J Rheumatol* 1988;15(7):1152-1158.

26. Leach RE, Baumgard S, Broom J: Obesity: Its relationship to osteoarthritis of the knee. *Clin Orthop Relat Res* 1973;(93):271-273.

27. Sharma L: Nonpharmacologic management of osteoarthritis. *Curr Opin Rheumatol* 2002;14(5): 603-607.

28. Felson DT, Zhang Y, Anthony JM, Naimark A, Anderson JJ: Weight loss reduces the risk for symptomatic knee osteoarthritis in women: The Framingham Study. *Ann Intern Med* 1992;116(7): 535-539.

29. Cooper C, Inskip H, Croft P, et al: Individual risk factors for hip osteoarthritis: Obesity, hip injury, and physical activity. *Am J Epidemiol* 1998;147(6):516-522.

30. Rangger C, Kathrein A, Klestil T, Glötzer W: Partial meniscectomy and osteoarthritis: Implications for treatment of athletes. *Sports Med* 1997;23(1):61-68.

31. Neyret P, Donell ST, Dejour H: Results of partial meniscectomy related to the state of the anterior cruciate ligament: Review at 20 to 35 years. *J Bone Joint Surg Br* 1993;75(1):36-40.

32. Callahan LF, Currey SS, Jones BL, et al: Osteoarthritis in retired National Football League players: The role of injuries and playing position. *Arthritis Rheum* 2002; 46:S415.

33. Drawer S, Fuller CW: Propensity for osteoarthritis and lower limb joint pain in retired professional soccer players. *Br J Sports Med* 2001;35(6):402-408.

34. Kettunen JA, Kujala UM, Kaprio J, Koskenvuo M, Sarna S: Lower-limb function among former elite male athletes. *Am J Sports Med* 2001;29(1):2-8.

35. Deacon A, Bennell K, Kiss ZS, Crossley K, Brukner P: Osteoarthritis of the knee in retired, elite Australian Rules footballers. *Med J Aust* 1997;166(4):187-190.

36. Sandmark H, Vingård E: Sports and risk for severe osteoarthrosis of the knee. *Scand J Med Sci Sports* 1999;9(5):279-284.

37. Kujala UM, Kaprio J, Sarna S: Osteoarthritis of weight bearing joints of lower limbs in former élite male athletes. *BMJ* 1994;308(6923):231-234.

38. Kujala UM, Kettunen J, Paananen H, et al: Knee osteoarthritis in former runners, soccer players, weight lifters, and shooters. *Arthritis Rheum* 1995;38(4): 539-546.

39. Lane NE, Oehlert JW, Bloch DA, Fries JF: The relationship of running to osteoarthritis of the knee and hip and bone mineral density of the lumbar spine: A 9 year longitudinal study. *J Rheumatol* 1998;25(2): 334-341.

40. Chakravarty EF, Hubert HB, Lingala VB, Zatarain E, Fries JF: Long distance running and knee osteoarthritis: A prospective study. *Am J Prev Med* 2008;35(2): 133-138.

41. Hohmann E, Wörtler K, Imhoff A: Osteoarthritis from long-distance running? *Sportverletz Sportschaden* 2005;19(2):89-93.

42. Kessler MA, Glaser C, Tittel S, Reiser M, Imhoff AB: Volume changes in the menisci and articular cartilage of runners: An in vivo investigation based on 3-D magnetic resonance imaging. *Am J Sports Med* 2006; 34(5):832-836.

43. Kessler MA, Glaser C, Tittel S, Reiser M, Imhoff AB: Recovery of the menisci and articular cartilage of runners after cessation of exercise: Additional aspects of in vivo investigation based on 3-dimensional magnetic resonance imaging. *Am J Sports Med* 2008;36(5): 966-970.

44. Jenkyn TR, Hunt MA, Jones IC, Giffin JR, Birmingham TB: Toe-out gait in patients with knee osteoarthritis partially transforms external knee adduction moment into flexion moment during early stance phase of gait: A tri-planar kinetic mechanism. *J Biomech* 2008;41(2):276-283.

45. Heiden TL, Lloyd DG, Ackland TR: Knee joint kinematics, kinetics and muscle co-contraction in knee osteoarthritis patient gait. *Clin Biomech (Bristol, Avon)* 2009;24(10):833-841.

46. Noyes FR, Schipplein OD, Andriacchi TP, Saddemi SR, Weise M: The anterior cruciate ligament-deficient knee with varus alignment: An analysis of gait adaptations and dynamic joint loadings. *Am J Sports Med* 1992;20(6):707-716.

47. Chang A, Hayes K, Dunlop D, et al: Thrust during ambulation and the progression of knee osteoarthritis. *Arthritis Rheum* 2004;50(12):3897-3903.

48. Tria AJ Jr, Klein KS: *An Illustrated Guide to the Knee.* New York, NY, Churchill Livingston, 1992.

49. Bach BR, Warren RF: Radiographic indicators of anterior cruciate ligament injury, in Feagin JA Jr, ed: *The Crucial Ligaments.* New York, NY, Churchill Livingston, 1988, pp 317-327.

50. Feagin JA Jr, Cabaud HE, Curl WW: The anterior cruciate ligament: Radiographic and clinical signs of successful and unsuccessful repairs. *Clin Orthop Relat Res* 1982;(164):54-58.

51. Pavlov H: The radiographic diagnosis of the anterior cruciate ligament deficient knee. *Clin Orthop Relat Res* 1983;(172):57-64.

52. Sherman MF, Warren RF, Marshall JL, Savatsky GJ: A clinical and radiographical analysis of 127 anterior cruciate insufficient knees. *Clin Orthop Relat Res* 1988;227:229-237.

53. Louboutin H, Debarge R, Richou J, et al: Osteoarthritis in patients with anterior cruciate ligament rupture: A review of risk factors. *Knee* 2009;16(4):239-244.

54. Øiestad BE, Engebretsen L, Storheim K, Risberg MA: Knee osteoarthritis after anterior cruciate ligament injury: A systematic review. *Am J Sports Med* 2009;37(7):1434-1443.

55. Roos H, Adalberth T, Dahlberg L, Lohmander LS: Osteoarthritis of the knee after injury to the anterior cruciate ligament or meniscus: The influence of time and age. *Osteoarthritis Cartilage* 1995;3(4):261-267.

56. Keller PM, Shelbourne KD, McCarroll JR, Rettig AC: Nonoperatively treated isolated posterior cruciate ligament injuries. *Am J Sports Med* 1993;21(1):132-136.

57. Allen PR, Denham RA, Swan AV: Late degenerative changes after meniscectomy: Factors affecting the knee after operation. *J Bone Joint Surg Br* 1984;66(5):666-671.

58. Casscells SW: The torn or degenerated meniscus and its relationship to degeneration of the weight-bearing areas of the femur and tibia. *Clin Orthop Relat Res* 1978;(132):196-200.

59. Fairbank TJ: Knee joint changes after meniscectomy. *J Bone Joint Surg Am* 1948;30B(4):664-6708.

60. Fukubayashi T, Kurosawa H: The contact area and pressure distribution pattern of the knee. A study of normal and osteoarthrotic knee joints. *Acta Orthop Scand* 1980;51(6):871-879.

61. McGinity JB, Geuss LF, Marvin RA: Partial or total meniscectomy: a comparative analysis. *J Bone Joint Surg Am* 1977;59(6):763-766.

62. Walker PS, Erkman MJ: The role of the menisci in force transmission across the knee. *Clin Orthop Relat Res* 1975;(109):184-192.

63. Clancy WG Jr: Repair and reconstruction of the posterior cruciate ligament, in Chapman MW, ed: *Operative Orthopedics*. Philadelphia, PA, JB Lippincott, 1988, pp 2093-2107.

64. Clancy WG Jr, Shelbourne KD, Zoellner GB, Keene JS, Reider B, Rosenberg TD: Treatment of knee joint instability secondary to rupture of the posterior cruciate ligament: Report of a new procedure. *J Bone Joint Surg Am* 1983;65(3):310-322.

65. Weidow J, Tranberg R, Saari T, Kärrholm J: Hip and knee joint rotations differ between patients with medial and lateral knee osteoarthritis: Gait analysis of 30 patients and 15 controls. *J Orthop Res* 2006;24(9):1890-1899.

66. Reiman MP, Bolgla LA, Lorenz D: Hip functions influence on knee dysfunction: A proximal link to a distal problem. *J Sport Rehabil* 2009;18(1):33-46.

67. Issa SN, Dunlop D, Chang A, et al: Full-limb and knee radiography assessments of varus-valgus alignment and their relationship to osteoarthritis disease features by magnetic resonance imaging. *Arthritis Rheum* 2007;57(3):398-406.

68. Murray MP: Gait as a total pattern of movement. *Am J Phys Med* 1967;46(1):290-333.

69. Root M, Orien W, Weed J: *Clinical Biomechanics: Normal and Abnormal Function of the Foot.* Los Angeles, CA, Clinical Biomechanics Corp, 1977.

70. Perry J: The mechanics of walking: A clinical interpretation, in Perry J, Hislop HJ, eds: *Principles of Lower Extremity Bracing.* New York, NY, American Physical Therapy Association, 1967, pp 9-32.

71. Seibel MO: *Foot Function.* Baltimore, MD, Williams & Wilkins, 1988.

72. Buckland-Wright JC, Macfarlane DG, Jasani MK, Lynch JA: Quantitative microfocal radiographic assessment of osteoarthritis of the knee from weight bearing tunnel and semiflexed standing views. *J Rheumatol* 1994;21(9):1734-1741.

73. Newhouse KE, Rosenberg TD: Basic radiographic examination of the knee, in Fu FH, Harner CD, Vince KG, eds: *Knee Surgery.* Baltimore, MD, Williams & Wilkins, 1994, pp 313-323.

74. Rosenberg TD, Paulos LE, Parker RD, Coward DB, Scott SM: The forty-five-degree posteroanterior flexion weight-bearing radiograph of the knee. *J Bone Joint Surg Am* 1988;70(10):1479-1483.

75. Fulkerson JP: Imaging the patellofemoral joint, in Fulkerson JP: *Disorders of the Patellofemoral Joint.* Baltimore, MD, Williams & Wilkins, 1997, pp 73-104.

76. Math KR, Ghelman B, Potter HG: Imaging of the patellofemoral joint, in Scuderi BR, ed: *The Patella.* New York, NY, Springer-Verlag, 1995, pp 83-125.

77. Merchant AC, Mercer RL, Jacobsen RH, Cool CR: Roentgenographic analysis of patellofemoral congruence. *J Bone Joint Surg Am* 1974;56(7):1391-1396.

78. Lorig K, Konkol L, Gonzalez V: Arthritis patient education: A review of the literature. *Patient Educ Couns* 1987;10(3):207-252.

79. Lindberg H, Montgomery F: Heavy labor and the occurrence of gonarthrosis. *Clin Orthop Relat Res* 1987;(214):235-236.

80. Stross JK, Mikkelsen WM: Educating patients with osteoarthritis. *J Rheumatol* 1977;4(3):313-316.

81. Muller PD, Laville EA, Biddle AK, Lorig K: Efficacy of psychoeducational interventions on pain, depression, and disability in people with arthritis: A meta-analysis. *J Rheumatol Suppl* 1987;14 Suppl 15:33-39.

82. Superio-Cabuslay E, Ward MM, Lorig KR: Patient education interventions in osteoarthritis and rheumatoid arthritis: A meta-analytic comparison with nonsteroidal antiinflammatory drug treatment. *Arthritis Care Res* 1996;9(4):292-301.

83. Kratz AL, Davis MC, Zautra AJ: Pain acceptance moderates the relation between pain and negative affect in female osteoarthritis and fibromyalgia patients. *Ann Behav Med* 2007;33(3):291-301.

84. Keefe FJ, Brown GK, Wallston KA, Caldwell DS: Coping with rheumatoid arthritis pain: Catastrophizing as a maladaptive strategy. *Pain* 1989;37(1):51-56.

85. Manne SL, Zautra AJ: Coping with arthritis: Current status and critique. *Arthritis Rheum* 1992;35(11):1273-1280.

86. Keefe FJ, Caldwell DS, Queen KT, et al: Pain coping strategies in osteoarthritis patients. *J Consult Clin Psychol* 1987;55(2):208-212.

87. Rapp SR, Rejeski WJ, Miller ME: Physical function among older adults with knee pain: The role of pain coping skills. *Arthritis Care Res* 2000;13(5):270-279.

88. Harrison RN, Lees A, McCullagh PJ, Rowe WB: A bioengineering analysis of human muscle and joint forces in the lower limbs during running. *J Sports Sci* 1986;4(3):201-218.

89. Messier SP, Gutekunst DJ, Davis C, DeVita P: Weight loss reduces knee-joint loads in overweight and obese older adults with knee osteoarthritis. *Arthritis Rheum* 2005;52(7):2026-2032.

90. Flynn TW, Soutas-Little RW: Patellofemoral joint compressive forces in forward and backward running. *J Orthop Sports Phys Ther* 1995;21(5):277-282.

91. Petrella RJ: Hyaluronic acid for the treatment of knee osteoarthritis: Long-term outcomes from a naturalistic primary care experience. *Am J Phys Med Rehabil* 2005;84(4):278-293.

92. Rashad S, Revell P, Hemingway A, Low F, Rainsford K, Walker F: Effect of non-steroidal anti-inflammatory drugs on the course of osteoarthritis. *Lancet* 1989;2(8662):519-522.

93. Bassleer C, Henrotin Y, Franchimont P: In-vitro evaluation of drugs proposed as chondroprotective agents. *Int J Tissue React* 1992;14(5):231-241.

94. Bassleer CT, Combal JP, Bougaret S, Malaise M: Effects of chondroitin sulfate and interleukin-1 beta on human articular chondrocytes cultivated in clusters. *Osteoarthritis Cartilage* 1998;6(3):196-204.

95. Dodge GR, Jimenez SA: Glucosamine sulfate modulates the levels of aggrecan and matrix metalloproteinase-3 synthesized by cultured human osteoarthritis articular chondrocytes. *Osteoarthritis Cartilage* 2003;11(6):424-432.

96. Piperno M, Reboul P, Hellio Le Graverand MP, et al: Glucosamine sulfate modulates dysregulated activities of human osteoarthritic chondrocytes in vitro. *Osteoarthritis Cartilage* 2000;8(3):207-212.

97. Morreale P, Manopulo R, Galati M, Boccanera L, Saponati G, Bocchi L: Comparison of the antiinflammatory efficacy of chondroitin sulfate and diclofenac sodium in patients with knee osteoarthritis. *J Rheumatol* 1996;23(8):1385-1391.

98. Ronca F, Palmieri L, Panicucci P, Ronca G: Anti-inflammatory activity of chondroitin sulfate. *Osteoarthritis Cartilage* 1998;6(Suppl A):14-21.

99. Drovanti A, Bignamini AA, Rovati AL: Therapeutic activity of oral glucosamine sulfate in osteoarthrosis: A placebo-controlled double-blind investigation. *Clin Ther* 1980;3(4):260-272.

100. Reginster JY, Deroisy R, Rovati LC, et al: Long-term effects of glucosamine sulphate on osteoarthritis progression: A randomised, placebo-controlled clinical trial. *Lancet* 2001;357(9252):251-256.

101. Vetter G: Topical therapy of arthroses with glucosamines (Dona 200). *Munch Med Wochenschr* 1969;111(28):1499-1502.

102. Bruyere O, Honore A, Ethgen O, et al: Correlation between radiographic severity of knee osteoarthritis and future disease progression: Results from a 3-year prospective, placebo-controlled study evaluating the effect of glucosamine sulfate. *Osteoarthritis Cartilage* 2003;11(1):1-5.

103. Das A Jr, Hammad TA: Efficacy of a combination of FCHG49 glucosamine hydrochloride, TRH122 low molecular weight sodium chondroitin sulfate and manganese ascorbate in the management of knee osteoarthritis. *Osteoarthritis Cartilage* 2000;8(5): 343-350.

104. Leffler CT, Philippi AF, Leffler SG, Mosure JC, Kim PD: Glucosamine, chondroitin, and manganese ascorbate for degenerative joint disease of the knee or low back: A randomized, double-blind, placebo-controlled pilot study. *Mil Med* 1999;164(2):85-91.

105. Lippiello L, Woodward J, Karpman R, Hammad TA: Beneficial effect of cartilage structure modifying agents tested in chondrocyte cultures and a rabbit instability model of osteoarthrosis. *Arthritis Rheum* 1999;42(suppl):S256.

106. McAlindon TE, LaValley MP, Felson DT: Efficacy of glucosamine and chondroitin for treatment of osteoarthritis. *JAMA* 2000;284(10):1241.

107. Owens S, Wagner P, Vangsness CT Jr: Recent advances in glucosamine and chondroitin supplementation. *J Knee Surg* 2004;17(4):185-193.

108. Maheu E, Mazières B, Valat JP, et al: Symptomatic efficacy of avocado/soybean unsaponifiables in the treatment of osteoarthritis of the knee and hip: A prospective, randomized, double-blind, placebo-controlled, multicenter trial with a six-month treatment period and a two-month followup demonstrating a persistent effect. *Arthritis Rheum* 1988;41(1):81-91.

109. Cake MA, Read RA, Guillou B, Ghosh P: Modification of articular cartilage and subchondral bone pathology in an ovine meniscectomy model of osteoarthritis by avocado and soya unsaponifiables (ASU). *Osteoarthritis Cartilage* 2000;8(6):404-411.

110. Appelboom T, Schuermans J, Verbruggen G, Henrotin Y, Reginster JY: Symptoms modifying effect of avocado/soybean unsaponifiables (ASU) in knee osteoarthritis: A double blind, prospective, placebo-controlled study. *Scand J Rheumatol* 2001;30(4): 242-247.

111. Sharma L, Song J, Felson DT, Cahue S, Shamiyeh E, Dunlop DD: The role of knee alignment in disease progression and functional decline in knee osteoarthritis. *JAMA* 2001;286(2):188-195.

112. Cerejo R, Dunlop DD, Cahue S, Channin D, Song J, Sharma L: The influence of alignment on risk of knee osteoarthritis progression according to baseline stage of disease. *Arthritis Rheum* 2002;46(10):2632-2636.

113. Cahue S, Dunlop D, Hayes K, Song J, Torres L, Sharma L: Varus-valgus alignment in the progression of patellofemoral osteoarthritis. *Arthritis Rheum* 2004;50(7):2184-2190.

114. Golightly YM, Allen KD, Renner JB, Helmick CG, Salazar A, Jordan JM: Relationship of limb length inequality with radiographic knee and hip osteoarthritis. *Osteoarthritis Cartilage* 2007;15(7): 824-829.

115. Anne Reilly K, Louise Barker K, Shamley D, Sandall S: Influence of foot characteristics on the site of lower limb osteoarthritis. *Foot Ankle Int* 2006;27(3): 206-211.

116. Reilly K, Barker K, Shamley D, Newman M, Oskrochi GR, Sandall S: The role of foot and ankle assessment of patients with lower limb osteoarthritis. *Physiotherapy* 2009;95(3):164-169.

117. Weidow J, Mars I, Kärrholm J: Medial and lateral osteoarthritis of the knee is related to variations of hip and pelvic anatomy. *Osteoarthritis Cartilage* 2005; 13(6):471-477.

118. Shelbourne KD, Patel DV, Martini DJ: Classification and management of arthrofibrosis of the knee after anterior cruciate ligament reconstruction. *Am J Sports Med* 1996;24(6):857-862.

119. Noyes FR, Berrios-Torres S, Barber-Westin SD, Heckmann TP: Prevention of permanent arthrofibrosis after anterior cruciate ligament reconstruction alone or combined with associated procedures: A prospective study in 443 knees. *Knee Surg Sports Traumatol Arthrosc* 2000;8(4):196-206.

120. Harner CD, Irrgang JJ, Paul J, Dearwater S, Fu FH: Loss of motion after anterior cruciate ligament reconstruction. *Am J Sports Med* 1992;20(5):499-506.

121. Shelbourne KD, Gray T: Minimum 10-year results after anterior cruciate ligament reconstruction: How the loss of normal knee motion compounds other factors related to the development of osteoarthritis after surgery. *Am J Sports Med* 2009;37(3):471-480.

122. Sachs RA, Daniel DM, Stone ML, Garfein RF: Patellofemoral problems after anterior cruciate ligament reconstruction. *Am J Sports Med* 1989; 17(6):760-765.

123. Steultjens MP, Dekker J, van Baar ME, Oostendorp RA, Bijlsma JW: Range of joint motion and disability in patients with osteoarthritis of the knee or hip. *Rheumatology (Oxford)* 2000;39(9):955-961.

124. Odding E, Valkenburg HA, Algra D, Vandenouweland FA, Grobbee DE, Hofman A: The association of abnormalities on physical examination of the hip and knee with locomotor disability in the Rotterdam Study. *Br J Rheumatol* 1996;35(9): 884-890.

125. Diraçoglu D, Baskent A, Yagci I, Ozçakar L, Aydin R: Isokinetic strength measurements in early knee osteoarthritis. *Acta Reumatol Port* 2009;34(1):72-77.

126. Amin S, Baker K, Niu J, et al: Quadriceps strength and the risk of cartilage loss and symptom progression in knee osteoarthritis. *Arthritis Rheum* 2009;60(1): 189-198.

127. Segal NA, Torner JC, Felson D, et al: Effect of thigh strength on incident radiographic and symptomatic knee osteoarthritis in a longitudinal cohort. *Arthritis Rheum* 2009;61(9):1210-1217.

128. Brandt KD, Heilman DK, Slemenda C, et al: Quadriceps strength in women with radiographically progressive osteoarthritis of the knee and those with stable radiographic changes. *J Rheumatol* 1999; 26(11):2431-2437.

129. Ireland ML, Willson JD, Ballantyne BT, Davis IM: Hip strength in females with and without patellofemoral pain. *J Orthop Sports Phys Ther* 2003;33(11):671-676.

130. Sharma L, Pai YC: Impaired proprioception and osteoarthritis. *Curr Opin Rheumatol* 1997;9(3): 253-258.

131. Skinner HB, Barrack RL, Cook SD: Age-related decline in proprioception. *Clin Orthop Relat Res* 1984;(184):208-211.

132. Kaplan FS, Nixon JE, Reitz M, Rindfleish L, Tucker J: Age-related changes in proprioception and sensation of joint position. *Acta Orthop Scand* 1985;56(1): 72-74.

133. Lund H, Juul-Kristensen B, Hansen K, et al: Movement detection impaired in patients with knee osteoarthritis compared to healthy controls: A cross-sectional case-control study. *J Musculoskelet Neuronal Interact* 2008;8(4):391-400.

134. Sharma L: Proprioceptive impairment in knee osteoarthritis. *Rheum Dis Clin North Am* 1999; 25(2):299-314, vi.

135. Garsden LR, Bullock-Saxton JE: Joint reposition sense in subjects with unilateral osteoarthritis of the knee. *Clin Rehabil* 1999;13(2):148-155.

136. Sharma L, Pai YC, Holtkamp K, Rymer WZ: Is knee joint proprioception worse in the arthritic knee versus the unaffected knee in unilateral knee osteoarthritis? *Arthritis Rheum* 1997;40(8):1518-1525.

137. Koralewicz LM, Engh GA: Comparison of proprioception in arthritic and age-matched normal knees. *J Bone Joint Surg Am* 2000;82-A(11):1582-1588.

138. Bayramoglu M, Toprak R, Sozay S: Effects of osteoarthritis and fatigue on proprioception of the knee joint. *Arch Phys Med Rehabil* 2007;88(3): 346-350.

139. Lephart SM, Fu FH: *Proprioception and Neuromuscular Control in Joint Stability*. Champaign, IL, Human Kinetics, 2000.

140. Beard DJ, Kyberd PJ, Fergusson CM, Dodd CA: Proprioception after rupture of the anterior cruciate ligament: An objective indication of the need for surgery? *J Bone Joint Surg Br* 1993;75(2):311-315.

141. Hurley MV, Newham DJ: The influence of arthrogenous muscle inhibition on quadriceps rehabilitation of patients with early, unilateral osteoarthritic knees. *Br J Rheumatol* 1993;32(2): 127-131.

142. Beynnon BD, Good L, Risberg MA: The effect of bracing on proprioception of knees with anterior cruciate ligament injury. *J Orthop Sports Phys Ther* 2002;32(1):11-15.

143. Beard DJ, Dodd CA, Trundle HR, Simpson AH: Proprioception enhancement for anterior cruciate ligament deficiency: A prospective randomised trial of two physiotherapy regimes. *J Bone Joint Surg Br* 1994;76(4):654-659.

144. Williams GN, Chmielewski T, Rudolph KS, Buchanan TS, Snyder-Mackler L: Dynamic knee stability: Current theory and implications for clinicians and scientists. *J Orthop Sports Phys Ther* 2001;31(10):546-566.

145. Limbird TJ, Shiavi R, Frazer M, Borra H: EMG profiles of knee joint musculature during walking: Changes induced by anterior cruciate ligament deficiency. *J Orthop Res* 1988;6(5):630-638.

146. Andriacchi TP, Birac D: Functional testing in the anterior cruciate ligament-deficient knee. *Clin Orthop Relat Res* 1993;(288):40-47.

147. Barrack RL, Skinner HB, Cook SD, Haddad RJ Jr: Effect of articular disease and total knee arthroplasty on knee joint-position sense. *J Neurophysiol* 1983; 50(3):684-687.

148. Cushnaghan J, McCarthy C, Dieppe P: Taping the patella medially: A new treatment for osteoarthritis of the knee joint? *BMJ* 1994;308(6931):753-755.

149. Hinman RS, Crossley KM, McConnell J, Bennell KL: Efficacy of knee tape in the management of osteoarthritis of the knee: Blinded randomised controlled trial. *BMJ* 2003;327(7407):135.

150. McConnell J: Management of patellofemoral problems. *Man Ther* 1996;1(2):60-66.

151. Duri ZA, Aichroth PM, Dowd G: The fat pad: Clinical observations. *Am J Knee Surg* 1996;9(2): 55-66.

152. Callaghan MJ, Selfe J, Bagley PJ, Oldham JA: The effects of patellar taping on knee joint proprioception. *J Athl Train* 2002;37(1):19-24.

153. Handfield T, Kramer J: Effect of McConnell taping on perceived pain and knee extensor torques during isokinetic exercise performed by patients with patellofemoral pain syndrome. *Physiother Canada* 2000;52:39-44.

154. Herrington L: The effect of patellar taping on quadriceps peak torque and perceived pain: A preliminary study. *Phys Ther Sport* 2001;2(1):23-28.

155. Gilleard W, McConnell J, Parsons D: The effect of patellar taping on the onset of vastus medialis obliquus and vastus lateralis muscle activity in persons with patellofemoral pain. *Phys Ther* 1998;78(1):25-32.

156. Cowan SM, Bennell KL, Hodges PW: Therapeutic patellar taping changes the timing of vasti muscle activation in people with patellofemoral pain syndrome. *Clin J Sport Med* 2002;12(6):339-347.

157. Christou EA: Patellar taping increases vastus medialis oblique activity in the presence of patellofemoral pain. *J Electromyogr Kinesiol* 2004;14(4):495-504.

158. Pfeiffer RP, DeBeliso M, Shea KG, Kelley L, Irmischer B, Harris C: Kinematic MRI assessment of McConnell taping before and after exercise. *Am J Sports Med* 2004;32(3):621-628.

159. Kerrigan DC, Lelas JL, Goggins J, Merriman GJ, Kaplan RJ, Felson DT: Effectiveness of a lateral-wedge insole on knee varus torque in patients with knee osteoarthritis. *Arch Phys Med Rehabil* 2002;83(7): 889-893.

160. Butler RJ, Marchesi S, Royer T, Davis IS: The effect of a subject-specific amount of lateral wedge on knee mechanics in patients with medial knee osteoarthritis. *J Orthop Res* 2007;25(9):1121-1127.

161. Crenshaw SJ, Pollo FE, Calton EF: Effects of lateral-wedged insoles on kinetics at the knee. *Clin Orthop Relat Res* 2000;(375):185-192.

162. Ogata K, Yasunaga M, Nomiyama H: The effect of wedged insoles on the thrust of osteoarthritic knees. *Int Orthop* 1997;21(5):308-312.

163. Keating EM, Faris PM, Ritter MA, Kane J: Use of lateral heel and sole wedges in the treatment of medial osteoarthritis of the knee. *Orthop Rev* 1993;22(8): 921-924.

164. Sasaki T, Yasuda K: Clinical evaluation of the treatment of osteoarthritic knees using a newly designed wedged insole. *Clin Orthop Relat Res* 1987;(221):181-187.

165. Tohyama H, Yasuda K, Kaneda K: Treatment of osteoarthritis of the knee with heel wedges. *Int Orthop* 1991;15(1):31-33.

166. Gélis A, Coudeyre E, Aboukrat P, Cros P, Hérisson C, Pélissier J: Feet insoles and knee osteoarthritis: evaluation of biomechanical and clinical effects from a literature review. *Ann Readapt Med Phys* 2005;48(9): 682-689.

167. Maillefert JF, Hudry C, Baron G, et al: Laterally elevated wedged insoles in the treatment of medial knee osteoarthritis: A prospective randomized controlled study. *Osteoarthritis Cartilage* 2001; 9(8):738-745.

168. American Academy of Orthopaedic Surgeons: *Clinical Practice Guideline on the Treatment of Osteoarthritis (OA) of the Knee.* Rosemont, IL, American Academy of Orthopaedic Surgeons, December 2008. http://www.aaos.org/research/guidelines/OAKguideline.pdf. Accessed October 3, 2011.

169. Kerrigan DC, Johansson JL, Bryant MG, Boxer JA, Della Croce U, Riley PO: Moderate-heeled shoes and knee joint torques relevant to the development and

progression of knee osteoarthritis. *Arch Phys Med Rehabil* 2005;86(5):871-875.

170. Kerrigan DC, Todd MK, Riley PO: Knee osteoarthritis and high-heeled shoes. *Lancet* 1998;351(9113):1399-1401.

171. Erhart JC, Mündermann A, Elspas B, Giori NJ, Andriacchi TP: A variable-stiffness shoe lowers the knee adduction moment in subjects with symptoms of medial compartment knee osteoarthritis. *J Biomech* 2008;41(12):2720-2725.

172. Fisher DS, Dyrby CO, Mündermann A, Morag E, Andriacchi TP: In healthy subjects without knee osteoarthritis, the peak knee adduction moment influences the acute effect of shoe interventions designed to reduce medial compartment knee load. *J Orthop Res* 2007;25(4):540-546.

173. Fantini Pagani CH, Potthast W, Brüggemann GP: The effect of valgus bracing on the knee adduction moment during gait and running in male subjects with varus alignment. *Clin Biomech (Bristol, Avon)* 2010;25(1):70-76.

174. Pollo FE, Otis JC, Backus SI, Warren RF, Wickiewicz TL: Reduction of medial compartment loads with valgus bracing of the osteoarthritic knee. *Am J Sports Med* 2002;30(3):414-421.

175. Hewett TE, Noyes FR, Barber-Westin SD, Heckmann TP: Decrease in knee joint pain and increase in function in patients with medial compartment arthrosis: A prospective analysis of valgus bracing. *Orthopedics* 1998;21(2):131-138.

176. Lindenfeld TN, Hewett TE, Andriacchi TP: Joint loading with valgus bracing in patients with varus gonarthrosis. *Clin Orthop Relat Res* 1997;(344):290-297.

177. Kirkley A, Webster-Bogaert S, Litchfield R, et al: The effect of bracing on varus gonarthrosis. *J Bone Joint Surg Am* 1999;81(4):539-548.

178. Harrison RA, Hillman M, Bulstrode S: Loading of the lower limb when walking partially immersed: Implications for clinical practice. *Physiotherapy* 1992;78:164-166.

179. Becker BE: Aquatic physics, in Ruoti RG, Morris DM, Cole AJ, eds: *Aquatic Rehabilitation*, ed 1. Philadelphia, PA, Lippincott Williams & Wilkins, 1997, p 15.

180. Hinman RS, Heywood SE, Day AR: Aquatic physical therapy for hip and knee osteoarthritis: Results of a single-blind randomized controlled trial. *Phys Ther* 2007;87(1):32-43.

181. Wyatt FB, Milam S, Manske RC, Deere R: The effects of aquatic and traditional exercise programs on persons with knee osteoarthritis. *J Strength Cond Res* 2001;15(3):337-340.

182. Silva LE, Valim V, Pessanha AP, et al: Hydrotherapy versus conventional land-based exercise for the management of patients with osteoarthritis of the knee: A randomized clinical trial. *Phys Ther* 2008;88(1):12-21.

183. Lund H, Weile U, Christensen R, et al: A randomized controlled trial of aquatic and land-based exercise in patients with knee osteoarthritis. *J Rehabil Med* 2008;40(2):137-144.

184. Wilk KE, Reinold MM: Closed kinetic chain exercises and plyometrics activities, in Bandy WD, Sanders B, eds: *Therapeutic Exercise: Techniques for Intervention*. Baltimore, MD, Lippincott Williams & Wilkins, 2001, pp 179-211.

185. Wilk KE, Escamilla RF, Fleisig GS, Barrentine SW, Andrews JR, Boyd ML: A comparison of tibiofemoral joint forces and electromyographic activity during open and closed kinetic chain exercises. *Am J Sports Med* 1996;24(4):518-527.

186. Beynnon BD, Johnson RJ, Fleming BC, Stankewich CJ, Renström PA, Nichols CE: The strain behavior of the anterior cruciate ligament during squatting and active flexion-extension: A comparison of an open and a closed kinetic chain exercise. *Am J Sports Med* 1997;25(6):823-829.

187. Kaufman KR, An KN, Litchy WJ, Morrey BF, Chao EY: Dynamic joint forces during knee isokinetic exercise. *Am J Sports Med* 1991;19(3):305-316.

188. Lutz GE, Palmitier RA, An KN, Chao EY: Comparison of tibiofemoral joint forces during open-kinetic-chain and closed-kinetic-chain exercises. *J Bone Joint Surg Am* 1993;75(5):732-739.

189. Huberti HH, Hayes WC: Patellofemoral contact pressures: The influence of q-angle and tendofemoral contact. *J Bone Joint Surg Am* 1984;66(5):715-724.

190. Hungerford DS, Barry M: Biomechanics of the patellofemoral joint. *Clin Orthop Relat Res* 1979;(144):9-15.

191. Grood ES, Suntay WJ, Noyes FR, Butler DL: Biomechanics of the knee-extension exercise: Effect of

cutting the anterior cruciate ligament. *J Bone Joint Surg Am* 1984;66(5):725-734.

192. Escamilla RF, Fleisig GS, Zheng N, Barrentine SW, Wilk KE, Andrews JR: Biomechanics of the knee during closed kinetic chain and open kinetic chain exercises. *Med Sci Sports Exerc* 1998;30(4):556-569.

193. Fulkerson JP, Hungerford DS: Biomechanics of the patellofemoral joint, in *Disorders of the Patellofemoral Joint*, ed 2. Baltimore, MD, Williams & Wilkins, 1990, pp 25-39.

194. Reinold MM, Wilk KE, Macrina LC, Dugas JR, Cain EL: Current concepts in the rehabilitation following articular cartilage repair procedures in the knee. *J Orthop Sports Phys Ther* 2006;36(10):774-794.

195. Fleming BC, Beynnon BD, Renstrom PA, et al: The strain behavior of the anterior cruciate ligament during stair climbing: An in vivo study. *Arthroscopy* 1999;15(2):185-191.

196. Steinkamp LA, Dillingham MF, Markel MD, Hill JA, Kaufman KR: Biomechanical considerations in patellofemoral joint rehabilitation. *Am J Sports Med* 1993;21(3):438-444.

197. Fung YC: *Biomechanics: Material Properties of Living Tissue*. New York, NY, Springer-Verlag, 1981.

198. McClure PW, Blackburn LG, Dusold C: The use of splints in the treatment of joint stiffness: Biologic rationale and an algorithm for making clinical decisions. *Phys Ther* 1994;74(12):1101-1107.

199. Spencer JD, Hayes KC, Alexander IJ: Knee joint effusion and quadriceps reflex inhibition in man. *Arch Phys Med Rehabil* 1984;65(4):171-177.

200. Horvath SM, Hollander JL: Intra-articular temperature as a measure of joint reaction. *J Clin Invest* 1949;28(3):469-473.

201. Osbahr DC, Cawley PW, Speer KP: The effect of continuous cryotherapy on glenohumeral joint and subacromial space temperatures in the postoperative shoulder. *Arthroscopy* 2002;18(7):748-754.

202. Petterson SC, Barrance P, Buchanan T, Binder-Macleod S, Snyder-Mackler L: Mechanisms underlying quadriceps weakness in knee osteoarthritis. *Med Sci Sports Exerc* 2008;40(3):422-427.

203. Snyder-Mackler L, Delitto A, Bailey SL, Stralka SW: Strength of the quadriceps femoris muscle and functional recovery after reconstruction of the anterior cruciate ligament: A prospective, randomized clinical trial of electrical stimulation. *J Bone Joint Surg Am* 1995;77(8):1166-1173.

204. Delitto A, Rose SJ, McKowen JM, Lehman RC, Thomas JA, Shively RA: Electrical stimulation versus voluntary exercise in strengthening thigh musculature after anterior cruciate ligament surgery. *Phys Ther* 1988;68(5):660-663.

205. Flynn TW, Soutas-Little RW: Mechanical power and muscle action during forward and backward running. *J Orthop Sports Phys Ther* 1993;17(2):108-112.

206. Otterness IG, Eskra JD, Bliven ML, Shay AK, Pelletier JP, Milici AJ: Exercise protects against articular cartilage degeneration in the hamster. *Arthritis Rheum* 1998;41(11):2068-2076.

207. Kiviranta I, Tammi M, Jurvelin J, Säämänen AM, Helminen HJ: Moderate running exercise augments glycosaminoglycans and thickness of articular cartilage in the knee joint of young beagle dogs. *J Orthop Res* 1988;6(2):188-195.

208. Newton PM, Mow VC, Gardner TR, Buckwalter JA, Albright JP: Winner of the 1996 Cabaud Award: The effect of lifelong exercise on canine articular cartilage. *Am J Sports Med* 1997;25(3):282-287.

209. Minor MA: Exercise in the treatment of osteoarthritis. *Rheum Dis Clin North Am* 1999;25(2):397-415.

210. Jan MH, Lin CH, Lin YF, Lin JJ, Lin DH: Effects of weight-bearing versus nonweight-bearing exercise on function, walking speed, and position sense in participants with knee osteoarthritis: A randomized controlled trial. *Arch Phys Med Rehabil* 2009;90(6):897-904.

211. Lin DH, Lin CH, Lin YF, Jan MH: Efficacy of 2 non-weight-bearing interventions, proprioception training versus strength training, for patients with knee osteoarthritis: A randomized clinical trial. *J Orthop Sports Phys Ther* 2009;39(6):450-457.

Chapter 29
Microfracture

J. Richard Steadman, MD
William G. Rodkey, DVM
Karen K. Briggs, MPH

Key Points

- In patients older than 45 years, traumatic or chronic cartilage lesions of the knee may be present, and many of these lesions can be treated with the microfracture technique.
- Previous partial or total meniscectomy is commonly found in the "baby boomer" population and should be considered when recommending the microfracture procedure.
- Neutral or near-neutral alignment is necessary for the microfracture procedure to succeed.
- The key to the microfracture procedure is to establish the marrow clot to provide the optimal environment for the body's own pluripotential marrow cells (mesenchymal stem cells or progenitor cells) to differentiate into stable tissue within the lesion.
- Performing an adequate microfracture is more difficult in chronic degenerative chondral lesions because of the eburnated bone and bony sclerosis with thickening of the subchondral plate.
- Appropriate rehabilitation is crucial to the success of the microfracture technique.

Introduction

Trauma to the articular cartilage of the knee is a common component of injuries in active patients older than 45 years. Articular cartilage has poor capacity to heal itself, which creates a challenge in the treatment of these lesions.[1,2] In older patients, cartilage injuries may be caused by acute trauma. This acute event may result in an isolated full thickness defect or start a degenerative cascade that can lead to chronic full-thickness loss.[3] The degenerative cascade typically includes early softening and fibrillation (grade I); fissures and cracks in the surface of the cartilage (grade II); severe fissures and cracks with a "crabmeat" appearance (grade III); and, finally, exposure of the subchondral bone (grade IV).[3] Many patients older than 45 years who had knee injuries in their twenties underwent a partial or total meniscectomy. Studies have shown that knees with loss of meniscus tissue may have increased risk of degenerative changes in the articular cartilage.[4]

The microfracture technique has been demonstrated to be an effective arthroscopic treatment for full-thickness chondral lesions and knees with degenerative lesions.[5-13] This technique is cost-effective, techni-

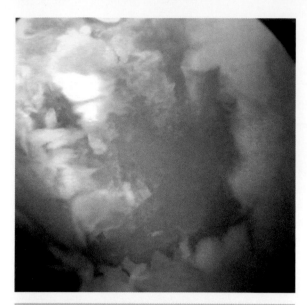

Figure 1   Arthroscopic view shows damaged cartilage of the lateral femoral condyle in a 57-year-old woman with neutral alignment. The lesion has thin edges, but they are adequate to hold the clot.

cally not complicated, has an extremely low rate of associated patient morbidity, and does not burn any bridges for further treatment. Microfracture is not tissue replacement; rather, it should be considered tissue repair. Microfracture relies on a "marrow-based" strategy for the tissue repair. For tissue to regenerate, cells must be present. In this procedure, the creation of controlled "microfractures" through the subchondral bone allows access to marrow-based mesenchymal stem cells and growth factors. A fibrin clot is formed at the base of a prepared chondral lesion.[13] These cells proliferate and differentiate into cells with morphologic features of chondrocytes and produce a cartilaginous repair tissue that fills the chondral defect.[14]

Indications and Contraindications

General indications for microfracture include a full-thickness defect, unstable cartilage that overlies the subchondral bone, and a partial-thickness lesion in which, when probed, the cartilage simply scrapes off down to bone.

Malalignment is a primary contraindication to the microfracture procedure. A history of partial or com-

plete medial meniscectomy may be associated with malalignment. The lack of meniscal tissue also results in lack of protection of the repair tissue that is formed with microfracture. The joint with previous surgery and malalignment may create a hostile environment that may be amenable to an arthroscopic treatment protocol that treats the pain generators to provide symptomatic relief (see chapter 35 on arthroscopic treatment of the degenerative knee). Patient age is not a specific contraindication. One study reported that with acute lesions, patients younger than 35 years showed greater improvement; however, older patients also improved.[10] In a study of patients with degenerative changes treated with microfracture, age was not a predictor of success.[8]

The size of the lesion is not a contraindication to microfracture.[10] In previous studies, we have shown that large acute lesions respond well to microfracture; however, it has been shown that lesions smaller than 400 mm^2 tend to respond better to microfracture than do lesions larger than 400 mm^2, although we have not observed this difference to be statistically significant.[8,10] More important than size of the lesion is the height of the rim of the lesion. When the microfracture is complete, a clot is formed. It is crucial to have adequate depth of cartilage on the rim of the lesion to hold the clot in place (**Figure 1**). Often, the cartilage surrounding a degenerative lesion is thin and not able to stabilize the clot. This is a contraindication to the microfracture technique.

Other specific contraindications to microfracture include a patient who is unwilling or unable to follow the required strict and rigorous rehabilitation protocol or a patient who is unable to use the opposite leg for weight bearing during the minimal or non–weight-bearing period. Patients' expectations also should be considered in the patient selection process. These expectations include recovery time, symptom relief, and return to activity.

In the treatment of chronic degenerative lesions, other specific contraindications include any systemic immune-mediated disease, disease-induced arthritis, or cartilage disease. A relative contraindication is a patient older than 65 years, because we have observed that some patients older than 65 experience difficulty with crutch-walking and the required rigorous rehabilitation. Another contraindication to microfracture is global degenerative osteoarthrosis.

Preoperative Considerations

Initial evaluation of patients who present with knee joint pain includes a thorough physical and musculoskeletal examination, as well as an evaluation of their symptoms. These symptoms may include pain, swelling, stiffness, and mechanical symptoms. It is important on the initial evaluation to determine the patient's activity level and expectations. Identification of point tenderness over a femoral condyle or tibial plateau is a useful finding, but in itself it is not diagnostic. If compression of the patella elicits pain, this finding might be indicative of a patellar or trochlear lesion. At times, the physical diagnosis can be difficult and elusive, especially if only an isolated chondral defect is present.

Patients with chronic or degenerative chondral lesions often are treated nonsurgically for at least 12 weeks after initial diagnosis. This treatment regimen includes activity modification, physical therapy, nonsteroidal anti-inflammatory drugs, joint injections, and perhaps dietary supplements that may have cartilage-stimulating properties. If nonsurgical treatment is not successful, then surgical treatment is considered. A crucial factor in the older patient is acceptable biomechanical alignment of the knee. We use weight-bearing hip-knee-ankle radiographs to determine angular deformity and joint space narrowing that is indicative of loss of articular cartilage and to determine the weight-bearing characteristics at the knee. A line is drawn on the radiograph from the center of the hip to the center of the ankle. This weight-bearing line across the tibial plateau determines axial alignment. If the line falls within 25% of the neutral line, then the patient's alignment is acceptable for the microfracture technique.[13] If mechanical alignment is deemed unacceptable, consideration should be given to concomitant realignment (eg, femoral or tibial osteotomy).

Surgical Technique

Acute Injury

A thorough diagnostic arthroscopic examination of the knee is performed through three portals (inflow cannula, arthroscope, and working instruments). We inspect the suprapatellar pouch, the medial and lateral gutters, the patellofemoral joint, the intercondylar notch and its contents, and the medial and lateral compartments, including the posterior horns of both menisci. Particular attention should be paid to anterior interval scarring, plicae, and the lateral retinaculum, which have the potential to increase compression between cartilage surfaces. Microfracture is the final intra-articular procedure performed. This sequence is followed to help prevent loss of visualization with blood and fat droplets entering the knee from the microfracture.

After identification of the full-thickness articular cartilage lesion, all remaining unstable cartilage is removed. A handheld curved curet and a full-radius resector can be used to remove the loose or marginally attached cartilage back to a stable rim of cartilage (**Figure 2**). The calcified cartilage layer that remains as a cap to many lesions must be removed, preferably by using a curet. Thorough and complete removal of the calcified cartilage layer is extremely important based on animal studies we have completed.[15,16] The integrity of the subchondral plate should be maintained. It is important that the defect be débrided deep enough to remove the calcified cartilage layer but not so deep as to damage the subchondral plate. This prepared lesion, with a stable perpendicular edge of healthy well-attached viable cartilage surrounding the defect (**Figure 2, A**), provides a pool that helps hold the marrow clot, or "super clot" as we have termed it, as it forms.

Arthroscopic awls are used to make multiple holes, or "microfractures" (**Figure 2, B**). An angled awl, typically 30° or 45°, permits the tip to be perpendicular to the bone as it is advanced. A 90° awl is used for the patella or other soft bone; however, it should be advanced only manually, not with a mallet. Starting at the periphery, microfracture holes are made, finishing with holes toward the center of the defect. The holes are made far enough apart that they do not break into each other, as this could damage the subchondral plate between them. Fat droplets from the marrow cavity are seen when the appropriate depth (approximately 2 to 4 mm) has been reached. When creation of the microfracture holes has been completed, the irrigation fluid pump pressure is reduced to observe the release of marrow fat droplets and blood from the holes. Micro-

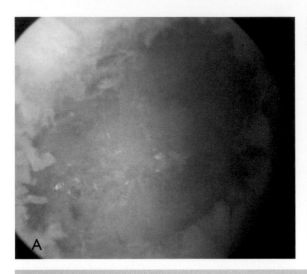
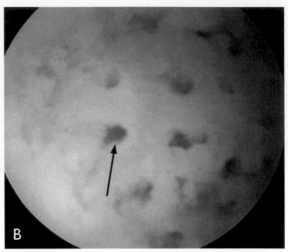

Figure 2   Arthroscopic views of the same chondral defect seen in Figure 1. **A,** The lesion has been débrided and is ready to be microfractured. The microfracture holes are started at the periphery of the defect adjacent to the stable cartilage. **B,** The microfracture procedure has been completed. Note the proximity of the microfracture holes, usually no more than 3 to 4 mm apart. Marrow elements, including blood and fat droplets, accessed by the subchondral bone microfracture can be seen egressing from the microfracture holes (arrow).

fracture creates a rough surface in the defect. This surface should not be débrided or shaved further to make it smooth. This rough surface allows the marrow clot to adhere more easily, yet the integrity of the subchondral plate is maintained for joint surface shape. Intra-articular drains should not be used because the goal is for the surgically induced marrow clot, rich in marrow elements, to form and stabilize while covering the lesion. The key to the microfracture procedure is to establish the marrow clot, which provides the optimal environment for the body's mesenchymal stem cells or progenitor cells to differentiate into stable tissue within the lesion[15,16] (**Figure 3**).

Chronic Lesions

The surgical technique for chronic lesions follows the same steps as the protocol for traumatic lesions. However, performing an adequate microfracture is more difficult in chronic degenerative chondral lesions because of the eburnated bone and bony sclerosis with thickening of the subchondral plate[8,17] (**Figure 4,** *A*). After the lesion has been débrided to stable edges, a few microfracture holes are made to assess the thickness of the subchondral plate. A motorized burr can be used to

remove the sclerotic bone until punctate bleeding is seen (**Figure 4,** *B*). After the bleeding appears uniformly over the surface of the lesion, a microfracture procedure can be performed as described above. Cartilage surrounding the defect must be thick enough to hold the marrow clot. In patients with thin cartilage, such as that seen in advanced degenerative lesions, we would likely not do a microfracture.

Postoperative Management

The postoperative program is designed to promote the ideal physical environment in which the newly recruited mesenchymal stem cells from the marrow can differentiate into the appropriate articular cartilage–like cell lines.[18-20] These differentiation and maturation processes must occur slowly but consistently. Our animal studies have confirmed that both cellular and molecular changes are an essential part of the development of a durable repair tissue.[15,16]

Patients are counseled carefully so they understand that they likely will not start to experience improvement in their knees for at least 6 months after microfracture. It has been our experience, confirmed by our clinical

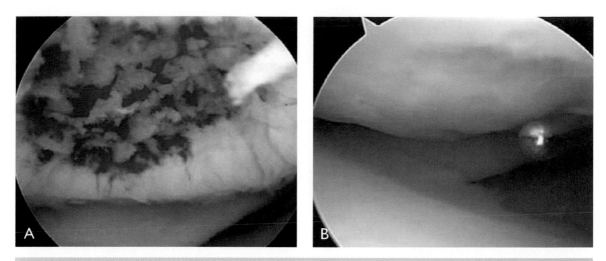

Figure 3   Arthroscopic views of a lateral femoral condyle lesion in a 27-year-old patient. **A,** The lesion at the time of microfracture. Note the rough surface, which allows the clot to attach to the lesion. **B,** At 4 months following microfracture, the lesion shows fill tissue with immature repair cartilage.

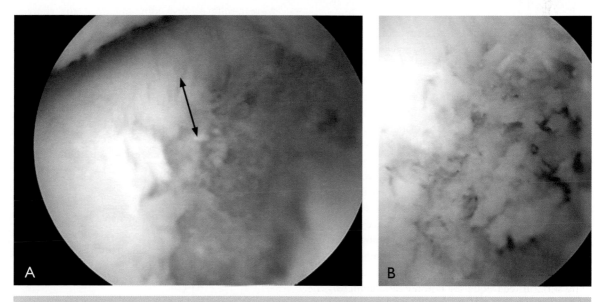

Figure 4   Arthroscopic views of a trochlear groove lesion in a 47-year-old patient. **A,** Note the rim height (double arrow). Yellow degenerative changes are seen at the base of the defect. **B,** At completion of the microfracture, blood is seen egressing from microfracture holes and burring of the defect. A rough surface is left following microfracture, which helps the clot attach to the lesion.

research data, that improvement can be expected to occur slowly and steadily for at least 2 years.[8,10,11] During this protracted period, the repair tissue matures, pain and swelling resolve, and the patient regains confidence and comfort in the knee during increased levels of activity.

The postoperative rehabilitation program after microfracture necessitates consideration of several factors.[13,21-23] The specific protocol recommended depends on both the anatomic location and the size of the defect.[13] These factors are critical to determine the ideal postoperative plan. For example, if other intra-articular procedures are done concurrently with microfracture, such as anterior cruciate ligament reconstruction, rehabilitation programs are customized as necessary.

Lesions on the Femoral Condyles or Tibial Plateau

After microfracture of lesions on the weight-bearing surfaces of the femoral condyles or tibial plateau, use of a continuous passive motion (CPM) machine is started in the recovery room. The initial range of motion (ROM) typically is 30° to 70°; it is increased as tolerated by 10° to 20° until full passive ROM is achieved. The rate of the machine is usually 1 cycle/min, but the rate can be varied based on patient preference and comfort. Many patients tolerate use of the CPM machine at night. The goal is to have the patient in the CPM machine for 6 to 8 hours every 24 hours. Cold therapy is used for 1 to 7 days postoperatively.

We prescribe crutch-assisted, touch-down weight-bearing ambulation for 6 to 8 weeks, depending on the size of the lesion. Patients with lesions on the femoral condyles or tibial plateaus rarely use a brace during the initial postoperative period. However, we now prescribe an unloading-type brace when the patient becomes more active and the postoperative swelling has resolved.

We begin mobilization immediately after surgery with an emphasis on ROM and patellar and patellar tendon motion and mobility. Patients typically begin stationary biking without resistance and a deep-water exercise program at 1 to 2 weeks after the microfracture procedure. Patients usually progress to full weight bearing after about 8 weeks and start more vigorous biking with increasing resistance. They also begin knee flexion exercises at approximately 8 weeks after microfracture.

A detailed description of the progression of the rehabilitation program has been published previously.[21] Depending on the clinical examination, size of the patient, the sport, and the size of the lesion, we usually recommend that patients do not return to sports that involve pivoting, cutting, or jumping until at least 4 to 9 months after microfracture.

Patellofemoral Lesions

All patients treated by microfracture for patellofemoral lesions must use a brace locked at 0° for 6 to 8 weeks. This brace limits compression of the regenerating surfaces of the trochlea or patella, or both. We allow passive motion with the brace removed, but otherwise the brace must be worn at all times. Patients with patellofemoral lesions are placed into a CPM machine immediately postoperatively. We also use cold therapy for 1 to 7 days postoperatively. With this regimen, patients typically obtain a pain-free, full passive ROM shortly after surgery.

We carefully observe joint angles at the time of arthroscopy to determine where the defect comes into contact with the patellar facet or the trochlear groove. We make certain to avoid these areas during strength training for approximately 4 months. This avoidance allows for training in the 0° to 20° range immediately postoperatively because there is minimal compression of these chondral surfaces with such limited motion.

Weight bearing is allowed as tolerated in the brace 2 weeks after surgery. It is essential for patients to use a brace that prevents placing excessive shear force on the maturing marrow clot in the early postoperative period. We routinely lock the brace between 0° and 20° ROM to prevent flexion past the point where the median ridge of the patella engages the trochlear groove. After 8 weeks, we open the knee brace gradually before it is discontinued. When the brace is discontinued, patients are allowed to advance their training progressively.

Outcomes Measures
Lysholm Score

In our database, the Lysholm knee score is used to measure knee function. The scale of Lysholm and Gillquist[24] consists of eight domains related to function of the knee: walking with a limp, support, locking, instability, pain, swelling, stair climbing, and squatting.

Pain and instability receive the highest point allocation, followed by locking, swelling, and stair climbing. A total score of 95 to 100 is associated with normal function, 84 to 94 indicates symptoms related to vigorous activity, and a score less than 84 suggests symptoms related to activities of daily living.

Kocher et al[25] determined the reliability, validity, and responsiveness of the Lysholm score for the treatment of chondral defects. These psychometric properties were analyzed in a group of 1,657 patients with chondral disorders of the knee. Test-retest, which entailed the same patient completing the questionnaire twice within 4 weeks, determined the reproducibility of the score between patients, or the reliability. Validity of the score, which included content validity, criterion validity, and construct validity, also was measured. To determine if the score can assess change, the responsiveness was determined. Acceptable test-retest reliability was found for the overall Lysholm scale and six of the eight domains. Internal consistency was acceptable. Floor (0%) and ceiling (0.7%) effects for the overall Lysholm scale were acceptable, but there were high floor effects for the domain of squatting and high ceiling effects for the domains of limp, instability, support, and locking. Criterion validity was acceptable, with significant ($P < 0.05$) correlations between the overall Lysholm scale and the physical functioning domain of the Short Form–12 scale; the pain, stiffness, and function domains of the Western Ontario and McMaster Universities Osteoarthritis Index (WOMAC); and the Tegner activity scale. Construct validity was acceptable. Responsiveness to change for the overall Lysholm scale was acceptable (effect size = 1.16; standardized response mean = 1.10). This study showed that the overall Lysholm score performed acceptably for the assessment of outcome following treatment of chondral disorders but some individual domains of the score did not perform as well.[25]

Tegner Activity Scale

In our database, activity level is measured with the Tegner activity scale.[26] With the Tegner scale, a numerical value of 0 to 10 is assigned to specific activities. An activity level of 10 corresponds to competitive sports, including soccer, American football, and rugby at the elite level; an activity level of 6 corresponds to recre-ational sports; and a level of 0 corresponds to a person on sick leave or disability because of knee problems. Activity levels of 5 to 10 can be achieved only if the patient participates in recreational or competitive sports. The Tegner activity scale is easy to use; however, not all sports are represented in the categories.[26]

WOMAC

In studies documenting the outcomes of patients with osteoarthritis of the knee, we use the WOMAC score in addition to the previously mentioned scores. The WOMAC is a general musculoskeletal instrument for patients who have osteoarthritis of the hip or knee.[27] It has been validated in randomized clinical trials and has been shown to be a responsive tool in measuring outcomes following treatment of osteoarthritis of the knee.[27] The WOMAC has 3 domains: pain (5 items), stiffness (2 items), and physical functioning (17 items). The questions are ranked on a 5-point Likert scale (0 = none, 1 = slight, 2 = moderate, 3 = severe, and 4 = extreme). The score is reported as the sum of the scores for each domain.[27]

Patient Satisfaction

Recognizing that health care is becoming more patient-driven is a major objective of our data collection assessing patient satisfaction. Our objectives are to evaluate patient satisfaction with outcomes of treatment and to identify parameters that are related to such satisfaction. With determinants of patient satisfaction from these studies, we can identify the elements that are most important to the patients following surgery. We measure satisfaction with outcomes of treatment on a scale of 1 to 10, with 10 being very satisfied and 1 being dissatisfied.

Results of Microfracture

Outcomes following microfracture in the degenerative knee have been reported in a recent study. We documented the outcomes at 2 years in patients with degenerative chondral lesions treated with microfracture.[8] Patients showed improvement in their function and had decreased symptoms with proper surgical technique, and patients were compliant with a well defined rehabilitation program. Average Lysholm scores improved from 54 to 83, and the mean Tegner activity score at follow-up was 4.5. Factors that were associated with less Lysholm improvement included bipolar lesions, lesions larger than 400 mm^2, and knees with absent menisci. Repeat arthroscopy was reported in 15.5% of these patients. Failure, as defined by revision microfracture or total knee arthroplasty, was documented in 6% of the patients.

Another study on microfracture looked at the long-term outcomes of microfracture. Using longitudinal analysis, patients were tracked over 10 years.[28] The analysis showed that age was not a factor in the outcomes of microfracture. Although degenerative lesions did not show the same improvement, improvement was seen and maintained over the long term.

Summary

In conclusion, the microfracture procedure is a safe and effective method to treat cartilage defects of the knee. Knee alignment, the depth of the cartilage rim surrounding the lesion, and patient compliance with rehabilitation are a few of the factors that can affect the outcomes following microfracture.

References

1. Mankin HJ: The response of articular cartilage to mechanical injury. *J Bone Joint Surg Am* 1982;64(3):460-466.

2. Buckwalter JA: Articular cartilage: Injuries and potential for healing. *J Orthop Sports Phys Ther* 1998;28(4):192-202.

3. Mankin HJ: The reaction of articular cartilage to injury and osteoarthritis (second of two parts). *N Engl J Med* 1974;291(25):1335-1340.

4. McDermott ID, Amis AA: The consequences of meniscectomy. *J Bone Joint Surg Br* 2006;88(12):1549-1556.

5. Blevins FT, Steadman JR, Rodrigo JJ, Silliman J: Treatment of articular cartilage defects in athletes: An analysis of functional outcome and lesion appearance. *Orthopedics* 1998;21(7):761-768.

6. Knutsen G, Drogset JO, Engebretsen L, et al: A randomized trial comparing autologous chondrocyte implantation with microfracture: Findings at five years. *J Bone Joint Surg Am* 2007;89(10):2105-2112.

7. Knutsen G, Engebretsen L, Ludvigsen TC, et al: Autologous chondrocyte implantation compared with microfracture in the knee: A randomized trial. *J Bone Joint Surg Am* 2004;86(3):455-464.

8. Miller BS, Steadman JR, Briggs KK, Rodrigo JJ, Rodkey WG: Patient satisfaction and outcome after microfracture of the degenerative knee. *J Knee Surg* 2004;17(1):13-17.

9. Rodrigo JJ, Steadman JR, Silliman JF, Fulstone HA: Improvement of full-thickness chondral defect healing in the human knee after debridement and microfracture using continuous passive motion. *Am J Knee Surg* 1994;7:109-116.

10. Steadman JR, Briggs KK, Rodrigo JJ, Kocher MS, Gill TJ, Rodkey WG: Outcomes of microfracture for traumatic chondral defects of the knee: Average 11-year follow-up. *Arthroscopy* 2003;19(5):477-484.

11. Steadman JR, Miller BS, Karas SG, Schlegel TF, Briggs KK, Hawkins RJ: The microfracture technique in the treatment of full-thickness chondral lesions of the knee in National Football League players. *J Knee Surg* 2003;16(2):83-86.

12. Steadman JR, Rodkey WG: Microfracture in chondral defects of the knee, in Micheli LJ, Kocher M, eds: *The Pediatric and Adolescent Knee*. Philadelphia, PA, Saunders Elsevier, 2006, pp 308-311.

13. Steadman JR: The microfracture technique, in Steadman JR, Feagin JA, eds: *The Crucial Principles in Care of the Knee*. Philadelphia, PA, Lippincott Williams & Wilkins, 2007, pp 129-151.

14. Frisbie DD, Trotter GW, Powers BE, et al: Arthroscopic subchondral bone plate microfracture technique augments healing of large chondral defects in the radial carpal bone and medial femoral condyle of horses. *Vet Surg* 1999;28(4):242-255.

15. Frisbie DD, Morisset S, Ho CP, Rodkey WG, Steadman JR, McIlwraith CW: Effects of calcified cartilage on healing of chondral defects treated with microfracture in horses. *Am J Sports Med* 2006;34(11):1824-1831.

16. Frisbie DD, Oxford JT, Southwood L, et al: Early events in cartilage repair after subchondral bone microfracture. *Clin Orthop Relat Res* 2003;(407):215-227.

17. Johnson LL: The sclerotic lesion: Pathology and the clinical response to arthroscopic abrasion arthroplasty, in Ewing JW, ed: *Articular Cartilage and Knee Joint Function: Basic Science and Arthroscopy*. New York, NY, Raven Press, 1990, pp 319-333.

18. Helminen HJ, Kiviranta I, Saamanen AM, et al: Effect of motion and load on articular cartilage in animal models, in Kuettner K, ed: *Articular Cartilage and Osteoarthritis*. New York, NY, Raven Press, 1992, pp 503-510.

19. Li KW, Williamson AK, Wang AS, Sah RL: Growth responses of cartilage to static and dynamic compression. *Clin Orthop Relat Res* 2001;(391 Suppl): S34-S48.

20. Radin EL, Martin RB, Burr DB, Caterson B, Boyd RD, Goodwin C: Effects of mechanical loading on the tissues of the rabbit knee. *J Orthop Res* 1984;2(3): 221-234.

21. Hagerman GR, Atkins JA, Dillman C: Rehabilitation of chondral injuries and chronic degenerative arthritis of the knee in the athlete. *Oper Tech Sports Med* 1995;3:127-135.

22. Irrgang JJ, Pezzullo D: Rehabilitation following surgical procedures to address articular cartilage lesions in the knee. *J Orthop Sports Phys Ther* 1998;28(4):232-240.

23. Ohkoshi Y, Ohkoshi M, Nagasaki S, Ono A, Hashimoto T, Yamane S: The effect of cryotherapy on intraarticular temperature and postoperative care after anterior cruciate ligament reconstruction. *Am J Sports Med* 1999;27(3):357-362.

24. Lysholm J, Gillquist J: Evaluation of knee ligament surgery results with special emphasis on use of a scoring scale. *Am J Sports Med* 1982;10(3):150-154.

25. Kocher MS, Steadman JR, Briggs KK, Sterett WI, Hawkins RJ: Reliability, validity, and responsiveness of the Lysholm knee scale for various chondral disorders of the knee. *J Bone Joint Surg Am* 2004;86(6):1139-1145.

26. Tegner Y, Lysholm J: Rating systems in the evaluation of knee ligament injuries. *Clin Orthop Relat Res* 1985;(198):43-49.

27. Bellamy N, Buchanan WW, Goldsmith CH, Campbell J, Stitt LW: Validation study of WOMAC: A health status instrument for measuring clinically important patient relevant outcomes to antirheumatic drug therapy in patients with osteoarthritis of the hip or knee. *J Rheumatol* 1988;15(12):1833-1840.

28. Miller B, Briggs K, Steadman JR: Clinical outcomes following the microfracture procedure for chondral defects of the knee: A longitudinal data analysis. *Cartilage* 2010;1:108-112.

Chapter 30

Autologous Chondrocyte Implantation in the Mature Athlete

Andreas H. Gomoll, MD
Nicholas A. DiNubile, MD

Key Points

- Physiologic age, rather than chronologic age, is a key factor in deciding whether a patient is a candidate for cartilage repair. Physiologic age includes general state of health, activity level, and weight.
- There is no set age limit for autologous chondrocyte implantation (ACI). However, because of the complex and long recovery, some of the benefits of ACI in very young patients (eg, delaying arthroplasty until a more appropriate age) obviously decrease with advancing age. Therefore, time should be spent discussing arthroplasty alternatives with older patients, and expectations should be adjusted.
- Aggressive correction of malalignment and maltracking is crucial with ACI; failure to do so will result in a lower success rate.
- All degenerative tissue should be débrided, even if doing so enlarges the defect substantially. Inadequate débridement is associated with a higher failure rate of ACI.
- Defect size is not related to failure rate of ACI.
- The high reoperation rate after ACI can be lowered significantly by the use of a collagen membrane in place of a periosteal patch; however, this currently is an off-label use and therefore must be emphasized in the informed consent process.
- Setbacks are frequent in the postoperative recovery period, but they generally are only temporary and do not negatively impact the ultimate outcome.

Dr. Gomoll or an immediate family member is a member of a speakers' bureau or has made paid presentations on behalf of Genzyme; serves as a paid consultant to or is an employee of Tigenix, Arthrex, and Mentice; and has received research or institutional support from Genzyme and Conformis.
Dr. DiNubile or an immediate family member is a member of a speakers' bureau or has made paid presentations on behalf of Genzyme and serves as a paid consultant to or is an employee of Genzyme and H-Wave.

Introduction

Osteoarthritis is a prevalent[1-4] disease that is expected to become symptomatic in almost half the US population within their lifetimes.[5-7] It may cause considerable pain, symptoms of depression, functional limitations, and deterioration of health-related quality of life.[8-14] This is especially worrisome for physiologically young patients with early degenerative changes because of their high functional demands and long, active lifespan. These patients in their 40s and 50s, sometimes referred to as "tweeners," often find themselves in a "treatment hiatus": the knee is symptomatic with daily pain and functional limitations, but nonsurgical management options such as injections and physical therapy have been exhausted and prosthetic replacement is either not yet indicated, because of young age and/or well-preserved joint spaces, or is rejected by the patients as a treatment option. The originally held belief that arthroscopic débridement could offer relief for these patients was shaken by several studies that demonstrated little or no benefit of arthroscopic intervention in these patients, although the methodology and conclusions of these studies remain a subject of debate.[15-20] (See the AAOS clinical practice guideline regarding osteoarthritis of the knee.[21]) Traditionally, these patients were recommended to restrict their activities to keep their pain at the lowest, and hopefully tolerable, level. Increasingly, however, the active aging population is less willing to accept activity restrictions, which are also medically undesirable because of the substantial health benefits of cardiovascular exercise, especially in the setting of a virtual epidemic of obesity in the United States. Clearly, new treatment options are needed for physiologically young and active patients in their 40s and early 50s with cartilage defects and early degenerative changes. Partial and total joint arthroplasty have seen substantial improvements over the last decade with the introduction of more wear-resistant bearing surfaces, minimally invasive and extensor mechanism–sparing approaches, and custom-design implants that are more bone-preserving. Fairly significant activity restrictions still apply after joint arthroplasty, however, and revision surgery is virtually guaranteed in this younger age group. Although the outcomes of primary total knee arthroplasty are among the best of any orthopaedic procedure, revision arthroplasty is associated with substantially worse outcomes.[22] Orthopaedic surgeons therefore routinely attempt to delay arthroplasty as long as possible, oftentimes at great cost to the patient in terms of persistent pain, limited function, and pain medication use. Cartilage repair has recently gained increased attention as a bridging treatment to preserve the natural knee for as long as possible, with the goal of delaying joint arthroplasty to a time that decreases, or even obviates, the need for revision surgery in the patient's lifetime.

ACI (Carticel; Genzyme Biosurgery, Cambridge, MA) is a cell-based treatment modality for the treatment of medium to large full-thickness, focal chondral defects. The technique produces hyaline cartilage–like repair tissue.[23,24] Multiple studies with up to 10 years of follow-up have reported promising clinical results and substantial functional improvement;[13,25-32] however, some have demonstrated a trend toward worse outcomes in patients older than the relatively young age of 30 years.[33] In older patients, metabolic cell activity is assumed to be lower and defects are often large and chronic in nature, adding to concerns over the efficacy of cartilage repair procedures in these patients. Furthermore, the classic indications for ACI have excluded multifocal and bipolar defects, which represent an early stage in the wide spectrum of disease included in the term osteoarthritis, and are commonly seen in the patient population discussed here. Treatment of older patients with cartilage defects has therefore traditionally consisted of palliation, osteotomy, or joint arthroplasty. Arthroplasty in particular is perceived as being associated with faster recovery and more predictable outcomes. An increasing number of older patients wish to remain active and are less willing to accept the limitations associated with multimodal nonsurgical treatment or joint arthroplasty, or dislike the comparatively large angular corrections of isolated osteotomy. Occasionally, these older patients who wish to avoid prosthetic replacement are deemed to be candidates for cartilage repair because of their activity level, young physiologic age, and good health. Increasingly, data have become available on the use of ACI in chondral defects that suggest this intervention can reduce symptoms and increase function even in this difficult patient group.[34-37]

This chapter discusses the indications and contraindications for ACI, outlines the diagnostic workup for potential cartilage defects, and describes the technique of ACI in this challenging patient population. It also reviews the results of two recent studies focusing on the outcomes of ACI in older patients and in patients with early degenerative changes. Many of the described indications and techniques—including the use of ACI in bipolar, patellar, and tibial defects, as well as its use for the treatment of degenerative joint disease—deviate from the US Food and Drug Administration (FDA)–approved indications for ACI.

Indications and Contraindications

Because of the invasiveness of the procedure, ACI is mainly indicated for the treatment of larger lesions, generally those larger than 4 cm^2. ACI is FDA approved for unipolar chondral lesions located on the femoral condyles and the trochlea; treatment of bipolar, patellar, and tibial plateau lesions with ACI is off-label. Ideally, the lesion is contained, thus providing a stable rim of intact cartilage to support the periosteal sutures. Defects that extend deep into the subchondral bone occasionally require staged or concomitant bone grafting. Articular comorbidities, such as malalignment, ligamentous instability, and meniscal insufficiency, are contraindications to ACI, unless corrected in a staged or concomitant fashion. Advanced degenerative changes, including joint space narrowing of more than 50%, are relative contraindications. Complete loss of joint space is an absolute contraindication, except possibly in salvage situations in the youngest of patients without other treatment options.

Examination and Diagnostic Workup

Patients with cartilage defects frequently present with knee pain and swelling, especially with weight-bearing and impact activities. A history of knee injury or prior surgical procedures such as meniscectomy or anterior cruciate ligament reconstruction is common. No examination findings are pathognomonic for cartilage defects; however, the examiner often encounters activity-related soft-tissue swelling and joint effusion, quadriceps atrophy, tenderness with palpation of the joint line and femoral condyle, and, occasionally, mild laxity due to loss of cartilage and/or meniscal substance. Motion is generally preserved except in more advanced cases of osteoarthritis or adhesions from prior surgery. Patellar tracking should be carefully evaluated, including specific questioning for a history of patellar subluxation or dislocation. Physical examination findings that are concerning for tracking abnormalities include an increased quadriceps (Q) angle at 30° of knee flexion, a J-sign in terminal extension, and increased patellar mobility and apprehension with lateral displacement of the patella. The patient's gait should be evaluated for varus or valgus thrust, which could be indicative of ligamentous instability that would require concomitant or staged reconstruction.

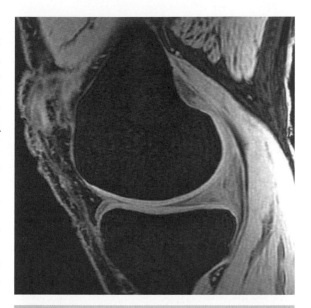

Figure 1 High-resolution sagittal dual-echo steady-state (DESS) MRI of a normal knee captured on a 3-T magnet. The articular cartilage is clearly visible and intact.

The diagnostic workup includes standard weight-bearing AP radiographs in extension, PA views in 45° of flexion, flexion lateral, and axial sunrise views. Double-stance weight-bearing long-leg (ie, hip-knee-ankle) radiographs are obtained to assess lower extremity alignment to determine if corrective osteotomy is necessary. MRI is useful for the evaluation of associated pathology of the meniscal and ligamentous structures; however, high-resolution (≥1.5-T) MRI (**Figure 1**), ideally with advanced cartilage-specific sequences such as T2 mapping, T1-rho, or intravenous/intra-articular gadolinium contrast enhancement (delayed gadolinium-enhanced MRI of cartilage [dGEMRIC]), is required to accurately assess articular cartilage.

Informed Consent Process

ACI is associated with substantial morbidity and a high incidence of subsequent surgical procedures in any age group. Therefore, a careful and detailed discussion with the patient and family is critical to establish reasonable expectations and provide an overview of the projected postoperative course. This discussion should include the extended weight-bearing restrictions; use of a continuous passive motion (CPM) device; the length and extent of rehabilitative exercises; estimated time to return to activities of daily living and sports; complications; and use of the collagen membrane in off-label fashion, if this portion of the procedure is to be performed. In particular, patients approaching the appropriate age for knee arthroplasty require careful counseling with regard to these issues, and we routinely discuss prosthetic replacement as an alternative treatment. When deciding whether to recommend ACI or arthroplasty, we consider several patient- and joint-specific factors; these include positive factors such as a physiologically young patient with a high activity level, and negative factors such as morbid obesity, smoking, and unwillingness or inability to participate in the complex rehabilitation. Positive joint factors include preserved joint space (>50%) on weight-bearing radiographs and focal lesions, whereas near-complete or complete loss of joint space constitutes an indication for either osteotomy or joint arthroplasty.

Articular Comorbidities

Most chondral defects not caused by acute trauma, such as anterior cruciate ligament tear or patellar dislocation, are associated with other intra-articular comorbidities that increase or induce abnormal forces on the articular cartilage and thus lead to accelerated degeneration. These comorbidities include coronal plane malalignment, patellar maltracking, and ligamentous or meniscal insufficiency. Coronal plane malalignment and patellar maltracking shift the load-bearing axis, thus resulting in local overload and accelerated degeneration of the articular surface. Ligamentous insufficiency, most commonly of the anterior cruciate ligament, increases shear forces in the knee joint and thus contributes to chondral wear. Meniscal insufficiency as a result of total meniscectomy increases contact stresses by up to 300% in the respective compartment[38] and is predictably associated with the development of osteoarthritis. Unless these comorbidities are corrected in staged or concomitant procedures, cartilage repair is likely to fail in short- to midterm follow-up. Older patients tend to present with more chronic (rather than acute traumatic) defects, and critical evaluation and aggressive treatment of any and all articular comorbidities is vitally important to the success of any type of cartilage repair. Coro-

nal plane mechanical malalignment of more than 2° may be corrected with high tibial osteotomy (most commonly opening wedge) for varus alignment and distal femoral osteotomy for valgus alignment. Patellofemoral cartilage defects, particularly bipolar defects, may undergo concomitant distal realignment with anteromedialization tibial tubercle osteotomy. Lateral meniscal deficiency results in comparatively larger increases in contact stresses and therefore may require lateral meniscal allograft transplantation to protect the cartilage repair; otherwise, the implant will fail rapidly.[39] Medial meniscal deficiency, because of the better congruency of the medial compartment, is better tolerated,[39] and in our experience, a meniscal transplant is not obligatory, as long as the alignment is corrected through osteotomy. In this case, we recommend slight overcorrection to the lateral tibial spine.

Technique

Diagnostic Arthroscopy and Cartilage Biopsy

A diagnostic arthroscopy is performed to evaluate the defect and assess the joint for any potential comorbidities. If the defects are found to be amenable to ACI, a full-thickness cartilage biopsy is removed with a sharp gouge from the superior aspect of the intercondylar notch or the peripheral aspect of the trochlea. The biopsy specimen should measure approximately 5 mm wide by 10 mm long and weigh 200 to 300 mg. After removal from the joint, the biopsy specimen is placed in sterile medium supplied by Genzyme Biosurgery and shipped. At the Genzyme facility, the cartilage matrix is enzymatically digested and the approximately 200,000 to 300,000 cells contained within are grown to 4 vials of approximately 12 million cells each in a 4- to 6-week process. This process can be interrupted after 2 weeks and the cells placed in cryopreservation for up to 2 years.

Concomitant Procedures

Articular comorbidities such as malalignment and meniscal or ligamentous deficiencies require concomitant or staged correction. In the author's experience, concomitant correction is preferable to avoid multiple operations with prolonged weight-bearing restrictions, leading to more profound deconditioning. When staging procedures, the biomechanical environment should

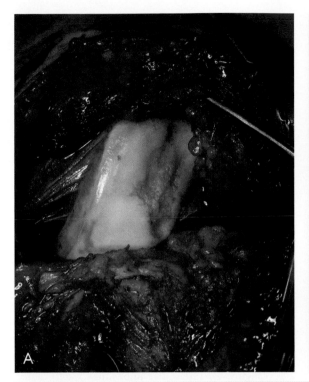 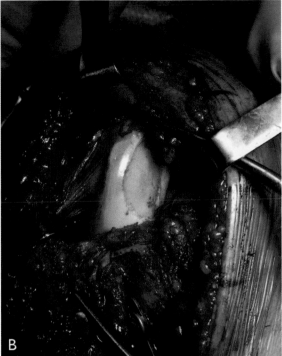

Figure 2   Intraoperative photographs show a large chondral defect of the medial femoral condyle. **A,** The defect is exposed through a medial subvastus approach. **B,** The defect after careful débridement.

be corrected first, with cartilage repair as the last step. For example, an osteotomy or meniscal transplantation can be performed at the time of cartilage biopsy, followed by cartilage repair at a later stage.

Implantation

Surgical steps for cell implantation include arthrotomy, defect preparation, periosteal patch harvest, patch fixation, and chondrocyte implantation.

Arthrotomy

For single lesions of the femoral condyles, a limited medial or lateral parapatellar arthrotomy is used. Adequate exposure is critical, and it may become necessary to mobilize the meniscus by incising the coronary ligament and taking down the intermeniscal ligament and anterior meniscal root with subsequent repair at the end of the procedure, particularly when tibial plateau lesions are treated. For multiple defects, a standard medial parapatellar arthrotomy or subvastus approach is per-

formed with lateral subluxation or dislocation of the patella.

Defect Preparation

Careful defect preparation, in particular for degenerative lesions without clearly defined borders (**Figure 2,** *A*), is one of the most crucial technical aspects to ensure a successful long-term outcome. The defect bed is débrided of all degenerative tissue to achieve a stable rim with vertical shoulders. This is performed by first outlining the defect with a scalpel, aggressively including all unstable, softened, fissured, or undermined areas of surrounding cartilage. This necessarily increases the size of the lesion, often by a considerable margin, but any degenerated cartilage left behind will fail in a matter of years, increasing the short-term failure rate of ACI because of progression of disease beyond the area of the original ACI graft. Occasionally, it may be advisable to leave a small rim of degenerated tissue to sew into, rather than using bone tunnels or suture anchors. The

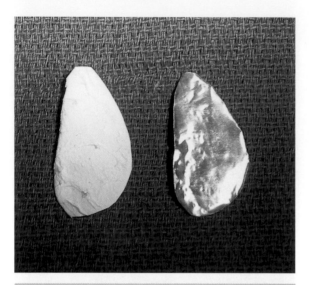

Figure 3   Aluminum foil template (right) and corresponding collagen membrane (left). These were prepared for a different defect than the one depicted in Figure 2.

degenerative cartilage is then débrided with small-ring or conventional curets. During débridement, it is essential to maintain an intact subchondral plate, as bleeding would result in migration of a mixed stem cell population from the marrow cavity into the chondral defect in addition to the end-differentiated chondrocytes grown in vitro. Minor bleeding from the subchondral bone can usually be controlled with thrombin or epinephrine soaked sponges, or electrocautery. Once a healthy defect bed is prepared (**Figure 2, *B***), it is measured and templated with glove paper or aluminum foil suture packaging (**Figure 3**). If periosteum is used, the template should be oversized by 2 mm in both length and width to allow for shrinkage.

Periosteal Patch Harvest

The most accessible site for periosteal harvest is the proximal medial tibia, which can be accessed through enlargement of the arthrotomy incision or by adding a second, more distal incision. A wet sponge can be used to gently sweep away loose adipose tissue. The periosteal patch is outlined with the scalpel according to the template and then mobilized with a small, sharp periosteal elevator. After harvesting, the periosteum should

be spread out on a moist sponge to avoid desiccation and reduce shrinkage. If a tourniquet has been used, it can be deflated at this point for the remainder of the procedure.

Patch Fixation

Minor punctate bleeding from the defect bed is common and can be controlled with epinephrine- or thrombin-soaked sponges, or fibrin glue. Once the defect is completely dry, the periosteal patch is retrieved from the back table and placed over the defect, with the cambium layer facing in. Suturing is performed with 6-0 braided absorbable suture that has been immersed in mineral oil or glycerin for better handling. The sutures are placed first through the periosteum and then the articular cartilage, exiting approximately 3 mm from the defect edge, everting the periosteal edge slightly to provide a better seal against the defect wall. The knots are tied on the defect side, thus remaining below the level of the adjacent cartilage. An opening wide enough to accept an angiographic catheter is left in the highest aspect of the defect to inject the chondrocytes (**Figure 4**). The suture line is now waterproofed with fibrin glue. If there are any concerns about the tightness of the suture line, a water tightness test should be performed by slowly injecting saline into the covered defect with a tuberculin syringe and plastic 18-gauge angiographic catheter. Any leakage should be addressed with additional sutures or fibrin glue as needed. Lastly, the saline is reaspirated and the chondrocytes are slowly injected into the defect. One or two additional sutures and fibrin glue are then used to close the injection site.

Treatment of Osteochondral Defects

Osteochondral defects deeper than approximately 8 to 10 mm, as measured from the cartilage surface, should be treated by either staged or concomitant bone grafting. Bone graft can be obtained from the distal femur or proximal tibia through a cortical window, obviating the need for iliac crest bone graft. The defect bed is prepared by perforating the often sclerotic bone with a small drill, Kirschner wire, or microfracture pick to stimulate bleeding. The cancellous bone is morcellized, compacted into the defect with a bone tamp to be flush with the surrounding subchondral plate, and covered with a membrane, either periosteum or collagen. If performed concomitant with cartilage repair, standard ACI is now performed as outlined above. If performed in a staged fashion, which is rarely done, an interval of 6 to 9 months should be allowed before second-stage chondral repair to permit the cancellous bone graft to harden and form a new "subchondral bone plate"; otherwise, significant bleeding can be encountered during preparation of the defect bed.

Evolving Techniques

Periosteal Substitutes

Membranes composed of porcine type I/III collagen were developed in an attempt to decrease the high reoperation rate due to periosteal hypertrophy. These membranes obviate the need for periosteal harvesting, are more robust than the delicate periosteum, and completely resorb within a matter of months. Short-term outcomes have been reported in European studies, with results similar to conventional ACI and virtual elimination of hypertrophy-related reoperation.[27,40] Currently, no collagen membranes are approved by the FDA for use with ACI; however, several similar xenograft membranes that are commercially available and approved for procedures such as rotator cuff repair and dental reconstruction are being used in an off-label fashion, with results comparable to the European experience.[41]

Matrix-Assisted ACI

Matrix-assisted ACI (MACI) was developed to address several limitations of ACI, such as the risk of cell leakage from the defect and the potentially uneven cell distribution within the defect. In addition, the use of a collagen matrix virtually eliminates the risk of hypertrophy. Similar to ACI, MACI involves culturing of biopsied chondrocytes for several weeks. Several days before delivery, the chondrocytes are seeded onto a type I/type III porcine-derived collagen carrier matrix. This carrier matrix is sized to match the defect and then implanted either through a minimally invasive open procedure or arthroscopically with fibrin-glue fixation, decreasing surgical time and morbidity associated with a wide exposure. European studies of MACI have shown clinical results that were comparable to current ACI techniques, with lower reoperation rates for graft hypertrophy.[42,43] MACI has been used in Europe for several years, but it is not currently available in the United

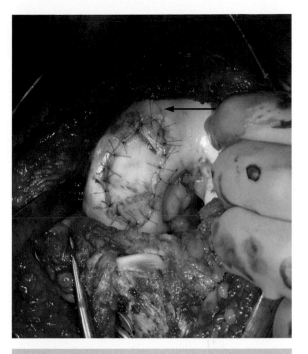

Figure 4 Intraoperative photograph of the same defect shown in Figure 2 after the collagen membrane has been sutured in place. (The patella is now subluxated laterally, improving exposure.) A suture has been passed at the highest point but left untied (arrow) to allow injection of the chondrocytes.

States. A prospective randomized trial of MACI versus microfracture completed enrollment in Europe in 2010. The data will be used to support a submission to the FDA in 2012 or 2013.

Postoperative Regimen

Adherence to the specific, staged rehabilitation protocol is just as important as the surgical procedure in terms of achieving optimal clinical and functional results. The biology of the repair process dictates the rehabilitation sequence. Tissue maturation, and therefore rehabilitation, after ACI is divided into three phases: proliferation, transition, and remodeling. During the first phase, the implant is vulnerable to shear and compression forces, so the focus of rehabilitation in this period is to protect the graft. Patients are maintained in touch down weight bearing on two crutches and use CPM for 6 to 8 hours per day for 6 weeks after surgery. A small, inexpensive child's skateboard can be substituted as an alternative for those who need to get back to work or are unable to be near their CPM machine the necessary amount of time. Patients are asked to perform the "skateboard slide," in which the operated-side foot is placed on the skateboard and a gentle rocking motion is started, simulating CPM movement. Patients can keep the skateboard under a desk or in places in the home where they sit often. Alternately, patients can sit on a table with the knee flexed 90° and use the normal leg to passively extend and flex the operated leg.

The exercise protocol is determined by the defect location: condylar defects are allowed full range of motion, whereas patellofemoral defects are limited to passive extension only, to protect the graft. Likewise, CPM is advanced as tolerated to 90° for condylar lesions but is held at 40° for patellofemoral defects to minimize repetitive shear and compressive forces on the patellofemoral graft caused by the CPM, with one cycle per minute. To avoid arthrofibrosis, patients are asked to dangle the leg over the side of the bed at least three to five times per day to achieve 90° of flexion by 3 weeks. In addition, the patella is passively mobilized side to side and up and down three times per day. During the second phase (7 to 12 weeks postoperatively), patients gradually transition to full weight bearing at 2 to 3 months and begin closed-chain strengthening exercises, depending on the size and location of lesion(s). The third and last phase marks a slow return to activities of daily living, and additional strengthening and proprioceptive exercises are added to the regimen. Patients are restricted from impact activities such as basketball or running for 12 to 18 months and from cutting sports for at least 18 months.

Because of the lengthy rehabilitation and long time until the patient can return to full activities, creativity is often needed to keep these individuals not only motivated but also active and fit, while still protecting the operated knee—specifically the repair tissue—through its maturation phases to a durable hyaline cartilage–like material. To potentially help with this repair process, patients are also placed on a high-quality joint supplement containing glucosamine and chondroitin sulfate, although it should be noted that there is a lack of clinical data to support this procedure.

Results

Multiple studies have demonstrated good and excellent results after ACI in more than 70% to 80% of patients; however, these studies focused on younger patients with focal defects. The findings discussed here in more detail are from two studies that investigated the outcome of ACI specifically in the "baby boomer" age group[44] and in those with early degenerative changes.[36]

The first study described the failure rate and outcomes of ACI specifically in patients 45 years or older at the time of implantation; 56 patients (36 men and 20 women) were treated with ACI.[44] The mean patient age was 48.6 years (range, 45 to 60 years), and outcomes were reported at a minimum of 2 years and mean of 4.7 years (range, 2 to 11 years). The mean transplant size was 4.7 cm^2 per defect (range, 1 to 15.0 cm^2) and 9.8 cm^2 per knee (range, 2.5 to 31.6 cm^2). Twenty-eight patients underwent concomitant osteotomies to address malalignment. There were 8 failures: 6 of 15 in patients receiving workers' compensation and 2 of 41 in non–workers' compensation patients. Surprisingly, only 1 failure occurred in the 16 patients treated for kissing lesions, resulting in a failure rate (6%) lower than the average failure rate across all patients; however, the low numbers in this subcategory make a meaningful statistical interpretation impossible. Among the eight knees in which the procedure failed, four improved before failure and four never improved. Three failed knees underwent revision with repeat ACI, three underwent patellofemoral prosthetic replacement, and there was one case each of total knee arthroplasty and osteochondral allograft transplantation. Additional arthroscopic surgical procedures were required in 24 patients for periosteal-related problems and adhesions; 88% of these patients experienced lasting improvement. At their latest available follow-up, activity levels as reflected by the modified Cincinnati score improved, from an average of 3.6 ("no sports possible") to 5.9 ("some limitations with sports but I can participate"); 78% of patients felt improved by the surgery; and 81% would choose to undergo ACI again. Eight percent felt their knee was worse than before the surgery, and these 8% also would not choose to have ACI again if they were in a similar situation. These findings are comparable to patient satisfaction with total knee arthroplasty, which for patient satisfaction has been reported as 73%

to 85%.[45-47] Functional scores showed significant improvements at the time of latest follow-up, and, importantly, no significant relationship was found between complexity of defect and clinical outcome.

Overall, this study demonstrated a failure rate and satisfaction that was comparable with previous reports of ACI in younger patient cohorts. Even in patients who traditionally have been considered too old, ACI can provide results that are comparable to those in younger patients if associated malalignment, instability, and degenerative changes are treated with concomitant procedures.

The second study[36] focused on the results of ACI in patients traditionally excluded from cartilage repair—those with early degenerative changes such as osteophytes, bipolar lesions, and joint space narrowing. Minas et al[36] prospectively followed 153 patients (155 knees) for up to 11 years after treatment with ACI for early-stage osteoarthritis, defined radiographically by the presence of peripheral intra-articular osteophyte formation and/or 0% to 50% joint-space narrowing (Ahlbäck stage 0 or 1 classification), and clinically by the presence of bipolar (kissing) lesions or generalized chondromalacia noted at the time of surgery. The mean patient age at the time of ACI was 38.3 years. On average, 2.1 defects were treated per knee with a mean defect size of 4.9 cm^2 and total area per knee of 10.4 cm^2. Twelve knees (8%) were revised to joint arthroplasties and were therefore considered treatment failures; the remaining 92% of patients experienced 50% to 75% improvement in Western Ontario and McMaster Universities Osteoarthritis Index (WOMAC) subscales. Furthermore, 91.6% of patients were satisfied with their outcome after treatment with ACI, 90.2% rated their knees better than before the surgery, and 91.3% would undergo the same procedure again. These findings suggest that ACI results in clinically relevant reductions in pain and improvement in function even in patients with early osteoarthritis who were previously not considered candidates for cartilage repair. At an average of 5 years postoperatively, 92% of patients were functioning well and were able to delay the need for joint arthroplasty. An additional study that specifically investigated the outcomes of ACI after prior treatment with marrow stimulation techniques (MST) such as microfracture, drilling, or abrasion arthroplasty

has challenged the conventional wisdom that regards these techniques as being non–bridge-burning treatment options.[48] Two groups were compared: one underwent ACI after MST, and one had been treated previously with débridement only. The failure rate was tripled in the previously marrow-stimulated patients. Marrow stimulation techniques are acceptable treatment options for smaller defects (< 3 to 4 cm^2) because good outcomes have been demonstrated in the literature, but larger defects should be approached with caution. Not only have outcomes in these larger lesions been less predictable with microfracture,[49,50] it also appears that the failure rate of subsequent cartilage repair with ACI is increased.

Mithoefer et al[51] looked at return to sports participation following ACI. Based on Tegner scores (an ordinal scale from 0 to 10 points based on athletic activity), many athletes can return to their endeavors following ACI. The time until return to sports after ACI is long (18 months), but ACI is more durable than other techniques; more than 90% of those returning to sport remain so at an average of 50 months.

Summary

Patients older than 45 years, in particular those with early degenerative changes such as multiple or bipolar large cartilage defects, present a challenge to conventional treatment algorithms. Many wish to maintain a physically active lifestyle and therefore prefer to avoid or at least delay joint arthroplasty surgery, but they find little pain relief with nonsurgical interventions. Traditionally, orthopaedic surgeons had little to offer this demanding patient population besides osteotomy or arthroscopic débridement, and the efficacy of the latter has been called into question. Cartilage repair with ACI is an invasive procedure with a long recovery, but recent studies have demonstrated that this technique can be applied successfully even in relatively older patients, as well as in those with early degenerative changes. Careful and thorough discussion of the invasive nature of the surgical procedure, its complex rehabilitation, and its long recovery, as well as the high likelihood of repeat surgery, is paramount to ensure a reasonable level of patient expectations and satisfaction with the outcome. Given the limited treatment options for this subset of patients, ACI may be a viable treatment even for older patients with early osteoarthritic changes to delay the need for joint arthroplasty surgery in hopes of obviating subsequent revision surgery, which is associated with much less satisfactory outcomes than primary procedures.

References

1. Arøen A, Løken S, Heir S, et al: Articular cartilage lesions in 993 consecutive knee arthroscopies. *Am J Sports Med* 2004;32(1):211-215.

2. Centers for Disease Control and Prevention (CDC): Prevalence of disabilities and associated health conditions among adults—United States, 1999. *MMWR Morb Mortal Wkly Rep* 2001;50(7):120-125.

3. Centers for Disease Control and Prevention (CDC): Prevalence of self-reported arthritis or chronic joint symptoms among adults—United States, 2001. *MMWR Morb Mortal Wkly Rep* 2002;51(42):948-950.

4. Centers for Disease Control and Prevention (CDC): Prevalence of doctor-diagnosed arthritis and possible arthritis—30 states, 2002. *MMWR Morb Mortal Wkly Rep* 2004;53(18):383-386.

5. Felson DT: An update on the pathogenesis and epidemiology of osteoarthritis. *Radiol Clin North Am* 2004;42(1):1-9.

6. Mankin HJ, Mow VC, Buckwalter JA: Articular cartilage repair and osteoarthritis, in Buckwalter JA, Einhorn TA, Simon SR, eds: *Orthopaedic Basic Science: Biology and Biomechanics of the Musculoskeletal System*, ed 2. Rosemont, IL, American Academy of Orthopaedic Surgeons, 2000, pp 471-488.

7. Murphy L, Schwartz TA, Helmick CG, et al: Lifetime risk of symptomatic knee osteoarthritis. *Arthritis Rheum* 2008;59(9):1207-1213.

8. Buckwalter JA: Articular cartilage: Composition, structure, response to injury, and methods of facilitating repair, in Ewing J, ed: *Articular Cartilage and Knee Joint Function: Basic Science and Arthroscopy*. New York, NY, Raven Press, 1990, pp 19-56.

9. de Bock GH, Kaptein AA, Touw-Otten F, Mulder JD: Health-related quality of life in patients with osteoarthritis in a family practice setting. *Arthritis Care Res* 1995;8(2):88-93.

10. Dexter P, Brandt K: Distribution and predictors of depressive symptoms in osteoarthritis. *J Rheumatol* 1994;21(2):279-286.

11. Ethgen O, Vanparijs P, Delhalle S, Rosant S, Bruyère O, Reginster JY: Social support and health-related quality of life in hip and knee osteoarthritis. *Qual Life Res* 2004;13(2):321-330.

12. Mankin HJ: The response of articular cartilage to mechanical injury. *J Bone Joint Surg Am* 1982; 64(3):460-466.

13. Minas T: Autologous chondrocyte implantation for focal chondral defects of the knee. *Clin Orthop Relat Res* 2001;(391 Suppl):S349-S361.

14. Yelin E, Lubeck D, Holman H, Epstein W: The impact of rheumatoid arthritis and osteoarthritis: The activities of patients with rheumatoid arthritis and osteoarthritis compared to controls. *J Rheumatol* 1987;14(4): 710-717.

15. Moseley JB, O'Malley K, Petersen NJ, et al: A controlled trial of arthroscopic surgery for osteoarthritis of the knee. *N Engl J Med* 2002;347(2):81-88.

16. Kalunian KC, Moreland LW, Klashman DJ, et al: Visually-guided irrigation in patients with early knee osteoarthritis: A multicenter randomized, controlled trial. *Osteoarthritis Cartilage* 2000;8(6):412-418.

17. Ravaud P, Mouliner L, Giraudeau B, et al: Effects of joint lavage and steroid injection in patients with osteoarthritis of the knee: Results of a multicenter randomized, controlled trial. *Arthritis Rheum* 1999; 42(3):475-482.

18. Laupattarakasem W, Laopaiboon M, Lapattarakasem P, Sumananont C: Arthroscopic debridement for knee osteoarthritis. *Cochrane Database Syst Rev* 2008; (1): CD005118.

19. Hubbard MJ: Articular debridement versus washout for degeneration of the medial femoral condyle: A five-year study. *J Bone Joint Surg Br* 1996;78(2):217-219.

20. Kirkley A, Birmingham TB, Litchfield RB, et al: A randomized trial of arthroscopic surgery for osteoarthritis of the knee. *N Engl J Med* 2008;359 (11):1097-1107.

21. American Academy of Orthopaedic Surgeons: *Guideline on the Treatment of Osteoarthritis (OA) of the Knee*. Rosemont, IL, American Academy of Orthopaedic Surgeons, December 2008. http://www.aaos.org/ research/guidelines/OAKguideline.pdf. Accessed March 2, 2011.

22. Robertsson O, Dunbar M, Pehrsson T, Knutson K, Lidgren L: Patient satisfaction after knee arthroplasty: A report on 27,372 knees operated on between 1981 and

1995 in Sweden. *Acta Orthop Scand* 2000;71(3): 262-267.

23. Brittberg M, Lindahl A, Nilsson A, Ohlsson C, Isaksson O, Peterson L: Treatment of deep cartilage defects in the knee with autologous chondrocyte transplantation. *N Engl J Med* 1994;331(14):889-895.

24. Minas T, Peterson L: Advanced techniques in autologous chondrocyte transplantation. *Clin Sports Med* 1999;18(1):13-44.

25. Bentley G, Biant LC, Carrington RW, et al: A prospective, randomised comparison of autologous chondrocyte implantation versus mosaicplasty for osteochondral defects in the knee. *J Bone Joint Surg Br* 2003;85(2):223-230.

26. Brittberg M, Tallheden T, Sjögren-Jansson B, Lindahl A, Peterson L: Autologous chondrocytes used for articular cartilage repair: An update. *Clin Orthop Relat Res* 2001;(391 Suppl)S337-S348.

27. Gooding CR, Bartlett W, Bentley G, Skinner JA, Carrington R, Flanagan A: A prospective, randomised study comparing two techniques of autologous chondrocyte implantation for osteochondral defects in the knee: Periosteum covered versus type I/III collagen covered. *Knee* 2006;13(3):203-210.

28. Micheli LJ, Browne JE, Erggelet C, et al: Autologous chondrocyte implantation of the knee: Multicenter experience and minimum 3-year follow-up. *Clin J Sport Med* 2001;11(4):223-228.

29. Mithöfer K, Peterson L, Mandelbaum BR, Minas T: Articular cartilage repair in soccer players with autologous chondrocyte transplantation: Functional outcome and return to competition. *Am J Sports Med* 2005;33(11):1639-1646.

30. Peterson L, Brittberg M, Kiviranta I, Akerlund EL, Lindahl A: Autologous chondrocyte transplantation: Biomechanics and long-term durability. *Am J Sports Med* 2002;30(1):2 12.

31. Peterson L, Minas T, Brittberg M, Lindahl A: Treatment of osteochondritis dissecans of the knee with autologous chondrocyte transplantation: Results at two to ten years. *J Bone Joint Surg Am* 2003;85-A(2, Suppl 2)17-24.

32. Peterson L, Minas T, Brittberg M, Nilsson A, Sjögren-Jansson E, Lindahl A: Two- to 9-year outcome after autologous chondrocyte transplantation of the knee. *Clin Orthop Relat Res* 2000;(374):212-234.

33. Knutsen G, Engebretsen L, Ludvigsen TC, et al: Autologous chondrocyte implantation compared with microfracture in the knee: A randomized trial. *J Bone Joint Surg Am* 2004;86-A(3):455-464.

34. Minas T: Autologous chondrocyte implantation in the arthritic knee. *Orthopedics* 2003;26(9):945-947.

35. Minas T: Autologous chondrocyte implantation in the osteoarthritic knee, in Cole BJ, Malek MM, eds: *Articular Cartilage Lesions: A Practical Guide to Assessment and Treatment.* New York, NY, Springer, 2004, pp 105-118.

36. Minas T, Gomoll AH, Solhpour S, Rosenberger R, Probst C, Bryant T: Autologous chondrocyte implantation for joint preservation in patients with early osteoarthritis. *Clin Orthop Relat Res* 2010; 468(1):147-157.

37. Saleh KJ, Arendt EA, Eldridge J, Fulkerson JP, Minas T, Mulhall KJ: Symposium: Operative treatment of patellofemoral arthritis. *J Bone Joint Surg Am* 2005; 87(3):659-671.

38. Baratz ME, Fu FH, Mengato R: Meniscal tears: The effect of meniscectomy and of repair on intraarticular contact areas and stress in the human knee: A preliminary report. *Am J Sports Med* 1986;14(4): 270-275.

39. Peña E, Calvo B, Martinez MA, Palanca D, Doblaré M: Why lateral meniscectomy is more dangerous than medical meniscectomy: A finite element study. *J Orthop Res* 2006;24(5):1001-1010.

40. Haddo O, Mahroof S, Higgs D, et al: The use of chondrogide membrane in autologous chondrocyte implantation. *Knee* 2004;11(1):51-55.

41. Gomoll AH, Probst C, Farr J, Cole BJ, Minas T: The use of a type I/III bilayer collagen membrane to decrease reoperation rates for symptomatic hypertrophy after autologous chondrocyte implantation. *Am J Sports Med* 2009;37 Suppl 1:20S-23S.

42. Bartlett W, Skinner JA, Gooding CR, et al: Autologous chondrocyte implantation versus matrix-induced autologous chondrocyte implantation for osteochondral defects of the knee: A prospective, randomised study. *J Bone Joint Surg Br* 2005;87(5):640-645.

43. Behrens P, Bitter T, Kurz B, Russlies M: Matrix-associated autologous chondrocyte transplantation/implantation (MACT/MACI)—5-year follow-up. *Knee* 2006;13(3):194-202.

44. Rosenberger RE, Gomoll AH, Bryant T, Minas T: Repair of large chondral defects of the knee with autologous chondrocyte implantation in patients 45 years or older. *Am J Sports Med* 2008;36(12): 2336-2344.

45. Baker PN, van der Meulen JH, Lewsey J, Gregg PJ, National Joint Registry for England and Wales, Data from the National Joint Registry for England and Wales: The role of pain and function in determining patient satisfaction after total knee replacement. *J Bone Joint Surg Br* 2007;89(7):893-900.

46. Bullens PH, van Loon CJ, de Waal Malefijt MC, Laan RF, Veth RP: Patient satisfaction after total knee arthroplasty: A comparison between subjective and objective outcome assessments. *J Arthroplasty* 2001; 16(6):740-747.

47. Hawker G, Wright J, Coyte P, et al: Health-related quality of life after knee replacement. *J Bone Joint Surg Am* 1998;80(2):163-173.

48. Minas T, Gomoll AH, Rosenberger R, Royce RO, Bryant T: Increased failure rate of autologous chondrocyte implantation after previous treatment with marrow stimulation techniques. *Am J Sports Med* 2009;37(5):902-908.

49. Mithoefer K, Williams RJ III, Warren RF, Wickiewicz TL, Marx RG: High-impact athletics after knee articular cartilage repair: A prospective evaluation of the microfracture technique. *Am J Sports Med* 2006; 34(9):1413-1418.

50. Asik M, Ciftci F, Sen C, Erdill M, Atalar A: The microfracture technique for the treatment of full-thickness articular cartilage lesions of the knee: Midterm results. *Arthroscopy* 2008;24(11):1214-1220.

51. Mithoefer K, Hambly K, Della Villa S, Silvers H, Mandelbaum BR: Return to sports participation after articular cartilage repair in the knee: Scientific evidence. *Am J Sports Med* 2009;37 Suppl 1:167S-176S.

Chapter 31

The Future of Cartilage Repair: Tissue Engineering

Victor M. Goldberg, MD

Key Points

- Articular cartilage has a limited capacity to heal.
- Strategies to repair articular cartilage include stimulation of the marrow and transplantation of cells/tissues.
- Tissue engineering using cells, scaffolds, and signaling molecules is a new approach to articular cartilage restoration.
- Cell sources include differentiated chondrocytes and mesenchymal stem cells.
- Scaffolds or delivery vehicles can be natural, such as hyaluronic acid (HA), or synthetic, such as polymers of lactic and glycolic acid.
- Signaling molecules (bioactive factors) used include transforming growth factor-β (TGF-β), bone morphogenetic protein-2 (BMP-2), and BMP-7.
- The biochemical and biomechanical properties of articular cartilage are complex, so the application of tissue engineering to clinical problems is difficult.

Introduction

The articular cartilage of the mature athlete has a limited capability to heal after significant injury, and osteoarthritis may result. Full-thickness injuries that have access to the bone marrow do have some capacity to heal, but typically this tissue is comprised mostly of fibrocartilage and fibrous tissue and is functional for only a limited period of time. Untreated injuries confined to the cartilage alone with destruction of both the cells and matrix have no potential to heal in the adult athlete. Although the relationship between the original articular trauma and subsequent osteoarthritis is difficult to define, studies suggest that an individual who sustains trauma to the articular surface of the knee as an adult has almost twice the chance of exhibiting osteoarthritis by age 65.[1] Early, accurate MRI assessment of the type, location, and severity of the articular surface damage is central to treating these lesions in order to reduce the risk of subsequent osteoarthritis. Treatment approaches in the mature athlete are directed toward restoring joint alignment, stability, and congruency. Contemporary treatment has been successful in short-term follow-up; however, longer follow-up is required. A newer treatment concept in the mature athlete that attempts to restore the articular cartilage to its pre-injury state uses tissue engineering principles and may provide the best approach to preventing osteoarthritis.

Articular Cartilage

Structure

Articular cartilage is a complex tissue that is not uniform in structure or function and has a limited capacity to heal.[2,3] The surface layer of the articular surface has cells with a flattened appearance, whereas the cells in the deeper layer are rounded. The extracellular matrix also has nonuniform composition and properties. For example, the deeper layers have collagen that is vertically oriented and acts as scaffolding material, whereas the superficial layers are randomly distributed but usually parallel to the surface and may have load-bearing function.

These structural differences of hyaline cartilage give rise to four zones. The superficial zone, known as the lamina splendens, is cell free. The transitional zone contains chondrocytes that are parallel to the surface and collagen fibers that are tangential to the superficial zone. The radial zone contains chondrocytes that are larger and arranged in columns and collagen fibers that are vertically oriented. The basal (fourth) layer is the calcified zone. It is separated from the third zone by a border known as the tidemark. This calcified zone is an important transition to the subchondral bone and is central in maintaining the mechanical and biologic integrity of the articular hyaline cartilage.

Cartilage Injuries

Lesions of the articular cartilage are a significant problem in medical practice, with approximately 1 million patients treated annually and almost 250,000 surgical procedures performed.[4,5] These injuries can be characterized in several ways.[2,6] Lesions may be superficial and confined to the articular hyaline cartilage, or they may be full thickness and include the adjacent subchondral bone. The first type has little capacity to heal, but the full-thickness defects may heal with a mixture of fibrocartilage and hyaline cartilage.

Cartilage injuries also can be characterized by their potential for healing.[4,6,7] In one type, the mechanical

damage is confined to loss of the matrix components, without damage to the chondrocytes or collagen scaffold. In this situation, the chondrocytes are able to synthesize new proteoglycans, and the hyaline cartilage can be completely restored. In the second type of cartilage injury, there is mechanical destruction of the cells and matrix, including the collagen. In this circumstance, the chondrocytes may have the potential to repair, depending on the extent of the injury as well as the location of the injury. When trauma extends into the subchondral vascular bone marrow, healing is directed by the resident progenitor cells that do have the capacity to repair.

Cartilage Response to Injury

The classic response to injury is divided into four stages—necrosis, inflammation, repair, and scar remodeling—and requires active participation of the vascular system.[3,7,8] The inability of articular cartilage to heal centers on its lack of blood supply. An important concept for restoration of a functional tissue is the distinction between repair and regeneration.[3,8] Repair replaces the damaged or lost cells or matrix with new cells or matrix but does not necessarily restore this tissue to its original structure and function. In contrast, regeneration is a complete replacement of the damaged tissue with new cells and matrix identical to the original tissue, with structure and function that is identical to the normal hyaline cartilage. Hyaline cartilage that undergoes repair but not regeneration with a mixture of fibrocartilage and hyaline cartilage can be clinically functional, but it will degenerate in the long term because of its lack of biologic and mechanical integrity.

Strategies to Restore Articular Cartilage

Although the focus of this chapter is on tissue engineering as a means of biologically restoring articular cartilage, it is helpful to understand other approaches to restoring articular cartilage.[5,6,9] Each strategy can be characterized as one of two major types: stimulation of the underlying marrow or transplantation of cells or tissues.

Stimulation of the marrow uses the intrinsic capabilities of the diarthrodial joint to repair itself. This method is directed toward accessing the subchondral vascularity and marrow, using varied techniques such as drilling of the subchondral bone, or microfracture.[5,6,10] In conjunction with obtaining access to the subchondral bone marrow, removal of loose cartilage particles and joint lavage is performed. The repair tissue is usually fibrocartilaginous-like, with both type I and type II collagen, and does not have the biochemical or biomechanical properties of normal hyaline cartilage. The short-term outcomes are usually satisfactory, with reduction in pain and improvement in function; however, the long-term outcomes are unpredictable.[10] Another approach that uses stimulation of the intrinsic repair capabilities of cartilage is the application of growth factors such as fibroblastic growth factor, insulin-like growth factor, transforming growth factor (TGF), and bone morphogenetic proteins (BMPs).[11] Several studies suggest that the local treatment of partial- and full-thickness articular cartilage defects with growth factors such as BMP can stimulate regeneration of the articular surface.[12] However, it is unlikely that these factors alone can restore the complexity and mechanical function of the hyaline cartilage.

The second strategy for biologically restoring articular cartilage is transplantation of cells or tissues. One technique of cell transplantation using autologous chondrocytes (autologous chondrocyte implantation [ACI]) was first performed by Peterson.[13,14] Cartilage is obtained at an initial procedure, culture expanded ex vivo, and then injected into the articular cartilage defect under a patch of periosteum or tissue membrane (see chapter 30). The clinical results to date have been encouraging.[13,15,16] Good or excellent clinical outcomes were reported in more than 80% of the defects repaired with this technique. Biopsies from the treated lesions demonstrated a mixture of hyaline and fibrocartilage. One randomized study compared the outcome of ACI with microfracture in 80 patients without generalized osteoarthritis with a stable single symptomatic cartilage defect on the femoral condyle.[17] At 5 years after surgery, satisfactory results were observed in 77% of the patients with no significant differences in clinical or radiographic outcomes. Early radiographic signs of osteoarthritis were seen in one third of the patients. Long-term follow-up is still required to determine the role of these treatment modalities in prevention or modifying osteoarthritis of the knee.[18] Another approach using cell-based technology was reported recently using culture-expanded autologous bone marrow stem cells to repair cartilage defects after tibial osteotomy.[19] No difference in clinical outcome was reported when compared with controls treated with osteotomy alone. Tissue transplantation using either periosteum or perichondrium has been used for many years with variable results.[6,20,21] An alternative approach has been the transplantation of autologous osteochondral plugs harvested from presumably normal, but minimally loaded, regions of the knee joint.[22,23] This technique, also known as mosaicplasty, usually is recommended for defects from 1 to 4 cm^2. The early clinical results have been satisfactory, with more than 80% of patients who underwent mosaicplasty of the femoral condyle, tibial plateau, or patellofemoral joint demonstrating improved function and reduced pain. The biologic survival of these osteochondral grafts has not been reported, however, and the long-term clinical issues are yet to be delineated. In summary, although many of these procedures have reported clinically satisfactory outcomes, the ultimate biologic restoration and long-term functioning have not been demonstrated.

Tissue Engineering

Tissue engineering is an interdisciplinary field that applies the principles of engineering and life sciences to the development of biologic substitutes that restore, maintain, or improve tissue function.[8,24,25] The basic concept of this strategy is the use, either in combination or separately, of cells, biomatrices/scaffolds/delivery vehicles, and signaling molecules that provide the biologic cues for the progression of cell differentiation to phenotypically functional cells.

Central to this strategy is the need for a cell source.[3,8,26,27] Differentiated chondrocytes have been used, but these are less responsive to the necessary biologic and mechanical cues. By contrast, osteoprogenitor cells or mesenchymal stem cells have the appropriate developmental potential and appear to be responsive to local stimuli as well as capable of ultimately differentiating into the desired phenotype. Other important issues that relate to cells include the source of the cells and their number, density, age, phenotypic character, and developmental potency. Many questions remain to be answered before the correct cell strategy is defined.

Biomatrices or scaffolds may be made of either synthetic or natural material and can be used as delivery vehicles for signaling molecules, cytokines, or cells.[25,28-30] The optimal properties of these biomatrices should include consideration of their biodegradability, porosity, bonding capabilities, remodeling capacity, surface characteristics, and overall architecture. These vehicles have multifactoral properties that allow for early inductive capabilities and modulation, and they should contribute to the control of integration of the newly formed tissue into the host. The natural materials that are available for articular cartilage tissue engineering are extracellular matrix–like materials, such as collagen and hyaluronic acid (HA).[3,9] HA is a glycosaminoglycan composed of repeated disaccharide units to form a linear polymer and is an important component of the extracellular matrix of articular cartilage. HA has several functions that may enhance mesenchymal stem cell differentiation into adult hyaline cartilage. These include a supportive network for cell-matrix interaction, chondroinductivity, antiangiogenicity, and chondroprotection. Further, hyaluronic acid (HA) is an important feature of the embryonic environment when active tissue formation occurs. Collagen, either type II or type I in a gel form, has been used for several tissue-engineering applications, including cartilage regeneration.[4,9,31] Collagen is degraded in vivo, is capable of integrating into the host, and is highly supportive of cellular differentiation.

Synthetic biomaterials that have been used in tissue-engineering applications include polymers of lactic and glycolic acid, hydrogels, and carbon-based materials.[9,25,30] Polymers have been widely used because they are easily integratable, biocompatible, and biodegradable. Further, these synthetic materials can be formulated to deliver growth factors such as TGF-β. Polylactic acid has been found to be less toxic to human chondrocytes then polyglycolic acid.[9] Both natural and synthetic materials provide many characteristics necessary for tissue-engineered cartilage.

Bioactive factors are another important aspect of tissue engineering, as successful regenerative tissue depends on a sequence of events directed by biologic agents that are able to enhance cellular differentiation into hyaline cartilage.[11] The molecules most studied both in vitro and in vivo are TFG-β, fibroblastic bone factor, and BMPs.[4] These molecules have been successful in directing the repair of articular cartilage; however, several significant questions need to be answered to understand the function of these bioactive factors. These issues include the choice of specific molecules, dosing, timing, and sequence of administration.

The complexity of the biochemical and biomechanical properties of articular cartilage makes the application of tissue-engineering principles for its regeneration difficult. One important question that remains is whether the composite of cells, scaffolds, and bioactive molecules should be introduced to the repair site, allowing the environment to provide the necessary mechanical and biologic cues, or whether these events should be controlled in vitro using bioreactors.[8,24]

Several experimental and clinical studies have used tissue-engineering principles to regenerate articular cartilage. Wakitani et al[31] reported on the use of osteochondral progenitor cells isolated from periosteum and bone marrow in type I collagen gel and transplanted into large full-thickness defects of articular cartilage in rabbits. Within the first month, these chondroprogenitor cells had differentiated into chondrocytes and the articular surface appeared to be hyaline cartilage. A satisfactory integration of the neotissue with the host occurred. No evidence of osteoarthrosis was seen, and the subchondral bone was completely regenerated. The authors expanded their experimental studies using bone-marrow–derived mesenchymal cells transplanted in a collagen gel to repair articular cartilage defects in osteoarthritis.[19] Although histology was consistent with hyaline cartilage at 1 year, there was no significant clinical benefit when compared to controls. Marcacci et al[32] reported their experience with 141 patients who were treated using a combination of autologous chondrocytes that were grown on a scaffold of an HA derivative (HYAFF 11; Fidia Advanced Biopolymers, Abano Terme, Italy) and then transplanted into articular surface defects. The clinical results were encouraging, with subjective improvement in patient function and reduction of pain at an average 38-month follow-up. Second-look arthroscopy in 55 patients graded the cartilage as normal in 96% of the treated knees. Biopsy of the repaired site in 22 patients demonstrated hyaline-like cartilage. These results are encouraging, but long-term studies are required to establish this approach as a viable treatment alternative.

In summary, the goal of tissue engineering is the regeneration of articular cartilage defects with cells and matrix identical to the native tissue. The complete integration of the regenerated tissue is critical to the load-bearing function of articular cartilage. This neo-cartilage must respond to the same regulation of its growth and remodeling as the host tissue. Specific pre-cepts must be followed to develop a successful cell-based tissue-engineering strategy. These include the re-placement of the excised tissue with biologically matched tissue, requiring that precise and discrete boundaries be established to fit the volume required by the excised or damaged tissue, and the seamless integra-tion of the neotissue with the host tissue. It is critical to understand the scale of tissue that is being replaced by the engineered tissue because this may require special design features to promote the survivability of the cells following implantation. One approach to tissue regen-eration involves understanding key features of embry-onic tissue development that may be used in designing tissue-engineering strategies. Embryonic development has been shown to be a sequence of genetically pro-grammed changes that produce specific tissues. Under-standing the important biologic cues in accomplishing this tissue formation in the embryo may be important in designing a tissue-engineered replacement in the adult. Because cartilage is avascular, the accessibility of nutrients to the new tissue is difficult. This requires the appropriate design of delivery vehicles that can be made to enhance accessibility to appropriate molecular nutri-ents. Other remaining concerns for the success of tissue-engineering strategies include the place of bioreactors, the relevant experimental defects in animal models to be studied, the source of cells, the cell carrier system, signaling molecules, and the mechanical competence and quality of the regenerated tissue. Finally, the trans-fer of this treatment modality to clinical problems is a large step that will require significant financial investment.

References

1. Davis MA, Ettinger WH, Neuhaus JM, Cho SA, Hauck WW: The association of knee injury and obesity with unilateral and bilateral osteoarthritis of the knee. *Am J Epidemiol* 1989;130(2):278-288.

2. Buckwalter J: Articular cartilage: Overview, in Goldberg V, Caplan A, eds: *Orthopaedic Tissue Engineering*. New York, NY, Marcel Dekker, Inc, 2004, pp 179-200.

3. Caplan AI, Elyaderani M, Mochizuki Y, Wakitani S, Goldberg VM: Principles of cartilage repair and regeneration. *Clin Orthop Relat Res* 1997(342): 254-269.

4. Hunziker EB: Articular cartilage repair: Basic science and clinical progress. A review of the current status and prospects. *Osteoarthritis Cartilage* 2002;10(6):432-463.

5. Smith GD, Knutsen G, Richardson JB: A clinical review of cartilage repair techniques. *J Bone Joint Surg Br* 2005;87(4):445-449.

6. Goldberg VM, Caplan AI: Biologic restoration of articular surfaces. *Instr Course Lect* 1999;48:623-627.

7. Hunziker EB: Articular cartilage repair: Are the intrinsic biological constraints undermining this process insuperable? *Osteoarthritis Cartilage* 1999;7(1):15-28.

8. Goldberg VM, Caplan AI: Principles of tissue engineering and regeneration of skeletal tissues, in Goldberg V, Caplan A, eds: *Orthopaedic Tissue Engineering*. New York, NY, Marcel Dekker, Inc, 2004, pp 1-10.

9. Kinner B, Spector M: Cartilage: Current applications, in Goldberg V, Caplan A, eds: *Orthopaedic Tissue Engineering*. New York, NY, Marcel Dekker, Inc, 2004, pp 201-236.

10. Steadman JR, Briggs KK, Rodrigo JJ, Kocher MS, Gill TJ, Rodkey WG: Outcomes of microfracture for traumatic chondral defects of the knee: Average 11-year follow-up. *Arthroscopy* 2003;19(5):447-484.

11. Reddi AH: Tissue engineering and morphogenesis: Role of morphogenetic proteins, in Goldberg V, Caplan A, eds: *Orthopaedic Tissue Engineering*. New York, NY, Marcel Dekker, Inc, 2004, pp 11-20.

12. Rosen V: BMP2 signaling in bone development and repair. *Cytokine Growth Factor Rev* 2009;20(5-6): 475-480.

13. Minas T: Autologous chondrocyte implantation for focal chondral defects of the knee. *Clin Orthop Relat Res* 2001;391 Suppl:S349-S361.

14. Peterson L, Minas T, Brittberg M, Nilsson A, Sjögren-Jansson E, Lindahl A: Two- to 9-year outcome after autologous chondrocyte transplantation of the knee. *Clin Orthop Relat Res* 2000;374:212-234.

15. Minas T, Gomoll AH, Solhpour S, Rosenberger R, Probst C, Bryant T: Autologous chondrocyte implantation for joint preservation in patients with early osteoarthritis. *Clin Orthop Relat Res* 2010;468(1):147-157.

16. Peterson L, Brittberg M, Kirvanta I, Akerlund EL, Lindahl A: Autologous chondrocyte transplantation: Biomechanics and long-term durability. *Am J Sports Med* 2002;30(1):2-12.

17. Knutsen G, Engebretsen L, Ludvigsen TC, et al: Autologous chondrocyte implantation compared with microfracture in the knee: A randomized trial. *J Bone Joint Surg Am* 2004;86-A(3):455-464.

18. Gelber AC, Hochberg MC, Media LA, Wang NY, Wigley FM, Klag MJ: Joint injury in young adults and risk for subsequent hip osteoarthritis. *Ann Intern Med* 2000;133(5):321-328.

19. Wakitani S, Imoto K, Yamamoto T, Saito M, Murata N, Yoneda M: Human autologous culture expanded bone marrow mesenchymal cell transplantation for repair of cartilage defects in osteoarthritic knees. *Osteoarthritis Cartilage* 2002;10(3):199-206.

20. Homminga GN, Bulstra SK, Bouwmeester PS, van der Linden AJ: Perichondral grafting for cartilage lesions of the knee. *J Bone Joint Surg Br* 1990;72(6):1003-1007.

21. Bouwmeester P, Kuijer R, Terwindt-Rouwenhorst E, van der Linden T, Bulstra S: Histological and biochemical evaluation of perichondrial transplants in human articular cartilage defects. *J Orthop Res* 1999;17(6):843-849.

22. Hangody L, Kish G, Kárpáti Z, Szerb I, Udvarhelyi I: Arthroscopic autogenous osteochondral mosaicplasty for the treatment of femoral condylar articular defects: A preliminary report. *Knee Surg Sports Traumatol Arthrosc* 1997;5(4):262-267.

23. Hangody L, Füles P: Autologous osteochondral mosaicplasty for the treatment of full-thickness defects of weight-bearing joints: Ten years of experimental and clinical experience. *J Bone Joint Surg Am* 2003;85-A Suppl 2:25-32.

24. Lumelsky NL: Commentary: Engineering of tissue healing and regeneration. *Tissue Eng* 2007;13(7):1393-1398.

25. Johnson PC, Mikos AG, Fisher JP, Jansen JA: Strategic directions in tissue engineering. *Tissue Eng* 2007;13(12):2827-2837.

26. Huang JI, Yoo J, Goldberg VM: Orthopedic applications of stem cells, in Lanza R, ed: *Essentials of Stem Cell Biology*. Amsterdam, The Netherlands, Elsevier Academic Press, 2006, pp 449-456.

27. Caterson EJ, Taun RS, Bruder S: Cell-based approaches to orthopaedic tissue engineering, in Goldberg V, Caplan A, eds: *Orthopaedic Tissue Engineering*. New York, NY, Marcel Dekker, Inc, 2004, pp 21-50.

28. Meister K, Cobb A, Bentley G: Treatment of painful articular cartilage defects of the patella by carbon-fibre implants. *J Bone Joint Surg Br* 1998;80(6):965-970.

29. Ochi M, Uchio Y, Kawasaki K, Wakitani S, Iwasa J: Transplantation of cartilage-like tissue made by tissue engineering in the treatment of cartilage defects of the knee. *J Bone Joint Surg Br* 2002;84(4):571-578.

30. Frenkel SR, Di Cesare PE: Scaffolds for articular cartilage repair. *Ann Biomed Eng* 2004;32(1):26-34.

31. Wakitani S, Goto T, Pineda SJ, et al : Mesenchymal cell-based repair of large, full-thickness defects of articular cartilage. *J Bone Joint Surg Am* 1994;76(4):579-592.

32. Marcacci M, Berruto M, Brochetta D, et al: Articular cartilage engineering with Hyalograft C: 3-year clinical results. *Clin Orthop Relat Res* 2005;435:96-105.

Chapter 32

Meniscal Tears: Débridement, Repair, and Transplantation

Atul F. Kamath, MD
Brian J. Sennett, MD

Key Points

- The ability of meniscal tissue to heal after a tear relates to the location, size, and complexity of the tear, as well as host factors such as age.
- In the presence of pain and mechanical symptoms, and in the appropriate clinical setting, the treatment of meniscal pathology with débridement versus repair shows promising results.
- Traditionally, results after meniscal interventions have been less successful in older patients, which may be related to a more advanced degree of underlying arthritis and/or degenerative tissue.
- Meniscal repair presents an opportunity for primary healing of meniscal tissue.
- Meniscal transplantation, in the appropriate patient, is an option for addressing the clinical problem of a meniscus-deficient knee.
- The role of meniscal repair or transplantation in the aging (>45 years) athlete is relatively understudied.
- The treatment of meniscal pathology should be based on the individual patient and his or her functional demands and expectations, along with the particular characteristics of the meniscal tear.
- Future directions will address biocompatible and tissue-engineered options for meniscal repair and replacement. The risks and benefits of these advances in surgical technique and implants must be carefully weighed in the aging athlete.

Introduction

Tears of the knee menisci represent common musculoskeletal injuries, and meniscectomy continues to be one of the most frequently performed orthopaedic procedures in the United States.[1] Once thought to be vestigial structures, the crescent- and wedge-shaped menisci[2] are now well known to provide support and transmit load within the tibiofemoral joint.[3,4] Importantly, the menisci play an integral role in maintaining proper joint dynamics, lubrication, and nutritive support.

Compromise of joint alignment and stability may predispose the knee to secondary arthritis and regional soft-tissue problems. Osteoarthritis is common after total meniscectomy and, to a lesser extent, after partial meniscectomy.[5-7] Postmeniscectomy knees may be more prone to accelerated malalignment or ligament insufficiency problems. Meniscectomy has been implicated in accelerated osteoarthritis,[8] and this has been demonstrated in animal models of disease progression.[9,10] The goal of arthroscopy is to conserve as much meniscal tissue as possible to prevent functional and pain-related adverse outcomes.

Recent advances in surgical technique and technology attempt to improve the long-term functional outcomes after meniscal tears. More recently, several treatment options—including meniscal transplantation—have been explored for the management of meniscal pathology. With a better understanding of the biology of meniscal damage and subsequent reparative processes, meniscal repair and transplantation have played a more important, and clinically successful, role.

Although meniscal repair and transplantation show promise in selected younger patients, the role of these modalities in the management of middle-aged and elderly patients is unclear. Specifically, as the demands of the older athlete are increasing, the treatment algorithm for these patients is continually challenged. The roughly 80 million American baby boomers account for a large proportion of sports-related injuries.[11] Sports-related injuries in the aging population rose 33% from 1990 to 1996, accounting for more than $18 billion in medical costs.[12] For these middle-aged patients affected by "boomeritis,"[13] the orthopaedic surgeon must carefully weigh the risks and benefits for the individual patient when considering broadening the indications for newer treatment options.

Meniscal Tears in the Aging Population

Meniscal tears are classified according to location and type. The integrity and vascular supply of the tissue must be assessed carefully. Tears located at peripheral attachment sites are referred to as outer-third, or "red-red," tears because the vascular supply is generally preserved. Middle-third tears can be grouped into "red-white" (more peripheral, approximately 4 mm from the meniscal attachment) or "white-white" (minimally vas-

cular) tears. The inner third of the meniscus is avascular, so tears in this region are solely white-white. Experimental studies demonstrate poor spontaneous healing responses in these avascular regions.[14,15]

The treatment ladder for the aging athlete is similar to that for the younger patient. Initial management should consist of oral nonsteroidal anti-inflammatory medications. Physical therapy may prove beneficial in certain patients, especially those without significant underlying degenerative joint disease. Cortisone injections may be most effective for acute episodes or flares, rather than chronic symptoms. The role of nutraceuticals, viscosupplementation, and bracing (including unloader braces) has not been established in the setting of meniscal pathology without concomitant arthritis. Surgical arthroscopy—including meniscal débridement versus repair—and open surgical procedures are reserved for those patients in whom nonsurgical treatment modalities fail.

Meniscal Débridement

Arthroscopic partial meniscectomy is one of the most common orthopaedic procedures. When performed for the proper indications, namely joint line pain and/or mechanical symptoms in the absence of extensive degenerative disease, this procedure can be highly successful. Krüger-Franke et al[16] reported excellent clinical results in 96% of patients.

Meniscal tears in baby boomers present unique challenges. The aging body undergoes general physiologic changes, along with specific musculoskeletal alterations.[17] Meniscal tissue degenerates, and the healing milieu for tears is generally less robust. Advancing arthritis presents not only a mechanically unfavorable environment for tissue healing but also a source of chronic pain, even if meniscal pathology is addressed. Musculoskeletal manifestations of aging include effects on bone, cartilage, and connective tissue (**Table 1**).[18]

Factors that commonly place a patient at risk for the development of complications following partial meniscectomy include advancing age, increasing body mass index, and workers' compensation status.[19] This is in line with the increasing risk of complications and/or poor outcomes with increasing age in patients undergoing arthroscopic procedures.[20,21] Conversely, it has been shown that patients with higher preoperative

Table 1: Musculoskeletal Manifestations of Aging	
Area	**Effects of Aging**
Bone	Progressive loss of mineral density "Tubularization" of diaphyseal bone
Ligaments and tendons	Decreased fiber compliance Stiffness of ligaments and tendons Increased susceptibility to catastrophic failure Decreased glycosaminoglycan concentration Decreased collagen fiber bundle thickness Decreased vascularity
Meniscus	Intrasubstance degeneration Loss of ability to dissipate stress Increased propensity to degenerative tears
Articular cartilage	Decreased concentration of chondroitin sulfate, relative increase in keratan sulfate (nonosteoarthritic) Relative increase in chondroitin sulfate (osteoarthritic) Chondromalacia (cumulative damage)
Skeletal muscle	Sarcopenia (decreased type I and II muscle fiber) Volumetric loss of individual fiber size Progressive muscle denervation Decreased mitochondrial volume Increased collagen content Degenerative ultrastructural changes Decreased muscle flexibility

Adapted from Chen AL, Mears SC, Hawkins RJ: Orthopaedic care of the aging athlete. *J Am Acad Orthop Surg* 2005;13(6):407-416.

activity levels, including participation in sports, had better outcomes after arthroscopic partial medial meniscectomy.[10]

In broadening surgical indications to include patients of advancing age, the treating surgeon may see less favorable outcomes. Persistent symptoms after meniscectomy include recurrence, alteration of joint mechanics, and progression of osteoarthritis. Following meniscectomy, the tibiofemoral contact area decreases by approximately 50% and the contact forces increase two- to threefold.[22] Removal of as little as 15% to 34% of a meniscus increases contact pressures by more than 350%.[23] In 1948, Fairbank[5] described radiographic changes that occur after meniscectomy, including flattening of the femoral condyle, joint space narrowing,

and "ridge formation" (osteophytes); these are now termed "Fairbank changes" (**Figure 1**). The radiographic appearance of degenerative joint disease at 4 years after arthroscopic partial medial and lateral meniscectomy has been reported as 38% and 24%, respectively.[24]

Meniscal Repair

Indications

Traditional indications for meniscal repair include patient age up to about 40 years; activity level is an equally important factor. Minimum vascularity needed for healing is generally seen in red-white tears in the middle and outer thirds of the meniscus. Regardless of suitabil-

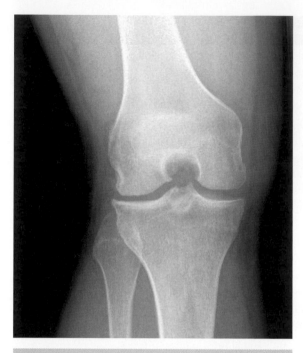

Figure 1 Fairbank changes (flattening of the femoral condyle, joint space narrowing, and ridge formation) of the lateral hemijoint seen on a flexion PA weight-bearing radiograph.

ity of the meniscal tear for repair, the individual patient must be made aware of and should be willing to comply with postoperative restrictions, such as brace wear and avoidance of deep knee flexion postoperatively.

As patient age increases and/or physiologic activity level or activity demands decrease, the patient may be considered less suitable for repair. In these cases, partial meniscectomy may be a better option. Avascular tears, poorly vascularized peripheral meniscal tears, and chronic degenerative tears are not suitable for repair. Likewise, secondary, complex, or multifragmented tears (in patients of any age) or those that are not easily apposed are generally not amenable to repair. As with younger patients, older patients unwilling to comply with postoperative rehabilitation regimens should not be considered for meniscal repair (**Table 2**).

In comparing partial meniscectomy versus repair of bucket-handle medial meniscus tears at the time of anterior cruciate ligament (ACL) reconstruction, one study found that clinical outcomes of repair were not superior to partial meniscectomy.[25] Furthermore, degenerative medial meniscal tears, when repaired, fared worse than repaired nondegenerative tears. In a long-term radiographic follow-up study comparing meniscal repair versus meniscectomy, more joint space was seen to be preserved in the repaired meniscus at 7-year follow-up;[26] however, at 13-year follow-up, no significant difference in joint space narrowing was seen, even when only the successful repairs were compared with meniscectomy.

Surgical Techniques

Several surgical options, techniques, and approaches exist for meniscal repair. No substantial prospective level 1 evidence exists to definitively support a particular fixation device or technique.[27] Suture fixation approaches include open, outside-in, all-inside, and inside-out repair. When compared with open vertical mattress suturing, certain all-inside fixation devices have shown worse clinical outcomes and complications,[28] along with inferior biomechanical properties and failure mechanisms.[29]

Healing rates of meniscal repair peformed with concomitant ACL reconstruction have been shown to be superior to those seen with isolated meniscal repair. This is presumably due to the presence of blood and growth factors released with the ACL reconstruction. Thus, to improve the theoretical healing response in the setting of meniscal repair, several adjuvant techniques have been tried. These include meniscal rasping to stimulate bleeding,[30] trephination,[31] and methods to form a perimeniscal fibrin clot.[32] Other options include application of growth factors,[33] tissue-engineered cells incorporated into scaffolds,[34] mesenchymal stem cells,[35] and platelet-rich plasma.[36]

Meniscal Transplantation

Allograft meniscal transplantation provides an opportunity for restoration of meniscal biomechanics while aiming to alleviate the pain of the meniscus-deficient or postmeniscectomy knee. Although the technique was developed more than 30 years ago, the long-term clinical outcomes after transplantation have not been excellent. Furthermore, the role of meniscal transplantation in the aging athlete is poorly understood. In the baby boomer, it may provide only short-term relief of

Table 2: Indications and Pearls for Arthroscopic Meniscal Repair

Patient age	Tears in younger patients more likely to heal, but repair considered in any active patient <60 years of age • Age <30 years: 12% failure rate • Age >30 years: 33% failure rate
Tear location	Red-red and red-white tears within 3 to 4 mm of periphery • White-white zone tear or incomplete radial tear that does not extend into outer-third region is contraindication to repair • Repair of medial tear within 4 to 5 mm of rim considered if concomitant anterior cruciate ligament repair
Tear anatomy	Tears <1 cm usually stable Repairable tear types: • Peripheral single longitudinal tear (red-red) in one plane; repairable in all cases, with high success rates • Red-white tear in middle-third region with vascular supply present • Tear in outer- and middle-third regions (red-white) in one plane (longitudinal, radial, or horizontal); often repairable • Complex tear in multiple planes (double or triple longitudinal or flap tear) in outer-third and middle-third regions (red-white); repair rather than excision Peripheral 2 to 3 mm ideal • 50% success rate in tears outside 4-mm periphery • Popliteal region can make repair difficult; contraindication to repair
Meniscal healing	Vascular supply/access: within 3 mm of periphery Lateral meniscus has greater healing potential Acute injury favorable • Chronic degenerative tear with tissue of poor quality not amenable to suture repair
Timing	Acute: ideal <3 to 4 weeks (usually <8 weeks) for repair
Concomitant injuries	Combined injuries more likely acute/traumatic • Success rate of repair higher in setting of concurrent alignment/instability correction Isolated tears often chronic/degenerative in white-white, red-white zones
Patient activity level	Repair contraindicated in sedentary patient (unless repair necessary to save meniscus) or patient who will not be compliant with postoperative rehabilitation protocol

Adapted from Noyes FR, Barber-Westin SD, Chen RC: Repair of complex and avascular meniscal tears and meniscal transplantation. *Instr Course Lect* 2011;60:415-437; and Griffin JR: Meniscal preservation/transplantation, in *Boomeritis: Musculoskeletal Care of the Mature Athlete.* Course syllabus. Rosemont, IL, American Academy of Orthopaedic Surgeons, 2010, pp 109-116.

Table 3: Indications and Contraindications for Meniscal Transplantation

Indications

Pain in meniscus-deficient or postmeniscectomy tibiofemoral compartment

Patient age <50 years

No radiographic evidence of advanced joint deterioration, ≥2 mm of tibiofemoral joint space on 45° weight-bearing PA radiographs

No or only minimal bone exposed on tibiofemoral surfaces

Normal axial alignment

Ligamentous stable knee

Appropriate range of motion, muscular strength

Graft factors: sizing, processing (fresh, cryopreserved, fresh-frozen), bone plugs

Contraindications

Advanced knee joint arthrosis with flattening of femoral condyle, concavity of tibial plateau, osteophytes that prevent anatomic seating of meniscal transplant

Symptomatic noteworthy deterioration of patellofemoral articular cartilage

Articular cartilage Outerbridge changes greater than grade 2

Uncorrected varus or valgus axial malalignment

Uncorrected knee joint instability, anterior cruciate ligament deficiency

Knee arthrofibrosis or substantial muscular atrophy

Prior joint infection with subsequent arthritis

Obesity (body mass index >30 kg/m^2)

Prophylactic procedure (asymptomatic patient with no articular cartilage damage)

Host-graft mismatch, poor graft viability

Unwillingness to comply with postoperative restrictions or rehabilitation

Adapted from Noyes FR, Barber-Westin SD, Chen RC: Repair of complex and avascular meniscal tears and meniscal transplantation. *Instr Course Lect* 2011;60:415-437; and Griffin JR: Meniscal preservation/transplantation, in *Boomeritis: Musculoskeletal Care of the Mature Athlete.* Course syllabus. Rosemont, IL, American Academy of Orthopaedic Surgeons, 2010, pp 109-116.

symptoms or may serve as a bridge to more definitive treatment of underlying pathology or concomitant arthritis.

Indications

Clinical indications for meniscal transplantation mirror those of meniscal repair (**Table 3**). Asymptomatic patients may be followed clinically or with yearly MRI to detect early chondral changes. Transplantation in asymptomatic individuals is not currently recom-

mended. Symptomatic younger patients (generally <50 years of age) with meniscus-deficient knees (**Figure 2**) are potential surgical candidates. Ideal joint space is greater than 2 mm on weight-bearing views. Diagnostic arthroscopy provides perhaps the best evaluation of articular quality.

Meniscus transplantation should be reserved for patients with early hyaline cartilage degeneration (Outerbridge[37] grade 1 or 2; **Table 4**), given poor clinical outcomes in the setting of advanced arthrosis.[38] Ex-

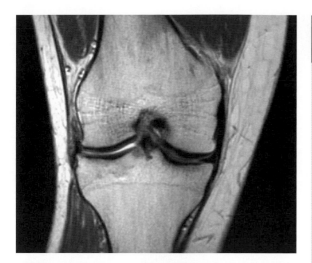

Figure 2   Coronal MRI of a lateral meniscus–deficient knee.

Table 4: Outerbridge Grading System for Chondral Lesions[a]	
Grade	Characteristics of Articular Cartilage Damage
0	Normal cartilage
1	Chondromalacia: softening/swelling of articular surface
2	Surface fissuring and partial-thickness defect Lesion <15 mm in diameter Lesion does not extend to subchondral bone
3	Defect extends to subchondral bone Lesion diameter greater than 15 mm
4	Exposed subchondral bone

[a]Modified Outerbridge classification, adapted with permission from Crook TB, Ardolino A, Williams LAP, Barlow IW: Meniscal allograft transplantation: A review of the current literature. *Ann R Coll Surg Engl* 2009;91:361-365.

posed subchondral bone (Outerbridge grade 4) on imaging studies or diagnostic arthroscopy should be a contraindication to transplantation. Arthrofibrosis, muscle atrophy, and history of joint sepsis are other contraindications.[39]

Timing of Transplantation

Advances in MRI of cartilage have shed light on articular collagen structure (T2-weighted sequences) and proteoglycan content (T1-weighted rho sequence). Bone scans also may aid in diagnosing subtle articular changes[39] in the hope of identifying meniscal transplant candidates earlier.

Lateral meniscal deficiency causes more rapid arthrosis than medial meniscal deficiency,[40] as the lateral compartment transmits more weight during locomotion.[41] Therefore, meniscus replacement may be considered earlier in the lateral meniscus–deficient knee.

Another consideration is the timing/sequence of combined procedures to address concomitant knee instability or axial malalignment. No clear consensus exists on this issue. The decision to stage procedures versus using a single-stage approach is based on surgeon experience and preference, along with the complexities associated with the particular procedures needed. Osteotomy may be performed before or in conjunction with meniscal transplant and/or cartilage resurfacing.

Allograft Choices: Cellularity and Viability

It is difficult to draw definitive conclusions regarding the role of graft processing on the clinical outcome based on the current literature. Small patient numbers and the numerous confounding variables are a likely explanation for the lack of significant differences between different graft types. The most commonly used allografts for transplantation are cryopreserved and fresh-frozen.

Fresh and cryopreserved allografts contain viable cells, whereas fresh-frozen and lyophilized allografts are acellular. In a goat model, donor cells in fresh allograft were completely replaced by host cells within 4 weeks.[42] Although fresh grafts contain viable cells, concerns include transportation issues and surgical timing, along with increased disease transmission risk. Cryopreservation maintains cell viability and affords longer storage time by use of controlled freezing. The freezing process for fresh-frozen graft production destroys all donor

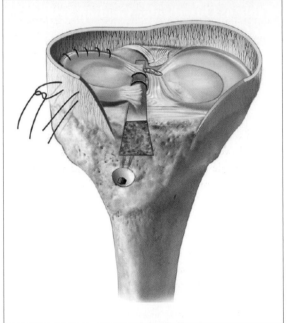

Figure 3   Lateral meniscus allograft implantation. (Reproduced with permission from Noyes FR, Barber-Westin SD: Meniscus transplantation: Diagnosis, operative techniques, and clinical outcomes, in Noyes FR, Barber-Westin SD, eds: *Noyes' Knee Disorders: Surgery, Rehabilitation, Clinical Outcomes*. Philadelphia, PA, Saunders, 2009, pp 772-805.)

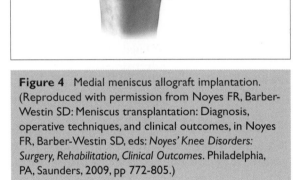

Figure 4   Medial meniscus allograft implantation. (Reproduced with permission from Noyes FR, Barber-Westin SD: Meniscus transplantation: Diagnosis, operative techniques, and clinical outcomes, in Noyes FR, Barber-Westin SD, eds: *Noyes' Knee Disorders: Surgery, Rehabilitation, Clinical Outcomes*. Philadelphia, PA, Saunders, 2009, pp 772-805.)

cells. Fresh-frozen grafts are less expensive than cryopreserved grafts, and lack of donor cell viability in fresh-frozen grafts has not been a problem: Fabbriciani et al[43] found no advantages between cryopreserved and deep-frozen grafts in goats.

Ethylene oxide sterilization should not be performed on fresh or cryopreserved allografts because the process destroys viable cells, and ethylene oxide may increase the risk of graft-associated synovitis.[44] Gamma irradiation may alter the graft material properties. Lyophilization may increase the susceptibility to altered material properties like shrinkage.[45]

Concomitant Procedures

Lateral (**Figure 3**) or medial (**Figure 4**) meniscal transplantation may be performed in isolation, or it may be combined with several procedures to address specific cartilage, ligamentous, or osteochondral pathology. The need to address articular cartilage damage, limb malalignment, or an ACL tear in the setting of meniscal deficiency must be evaluated with respect to the individual patient.

Articular Cartilage Lesion Resurfacing

Cartilage lesion size must be carefully evaluated. Healthy articular cartilage around a lesion may dissipate stress depending on the size of the lesion and its location. Attention must be paid to the weight-bearing contact areas, as the zone of highest contact stresses in the lateral hemijoint moves posteriorly with increasing knee flexion and femoral rollback.[46] Osteochondral tissue transfer may be needed for lesions greater than 1 cm in diameter, but microfracture techniques may be suitable for lesions less than 1 cm in diameter.

The meniscal transplant and the cartilage environment play symbiotic roles. The meniscal transplant protects healing cartilage lesions by decreasing contact stresses; likewise, a healing articular surface will aid in the future protection of the meniscal graft.

Axial Malalignment Correction

Meniscal transplantation must be performed in a stable knee with normal axial alignment. The normal mechanical axis passes through or just medial to the midpoint between the tibial spines.

Varus deformity and medial hemijoint arthrosis may be treated with a valgus-producing osteotomy and medial meniscal transplantation. Likewise, for a valgus knee with lateral compartment arthrosis, a varus-producing osteotomy is performed in conjunction with lateral meniscal transplantation.

Ligament Reconstruction for Instability

In knees with ACL tears, the medial meniscus is a secondary restraint to translational moments.[47] The medial meniscus serves to decrease forces across the ACL in both cadaveric[48] and clinical[49] studies. Therefore, early arthritis is commonly seen in the setting of chronic ACL insufficiency, and concomitant ACL reconstruction with medial meniscal transplantation may restore this chondral protection and knee stability.

Postoperative Care

The principles used for rehabilitation after meniscal repair can provide some guidance for determining the ideal postoperative management after meniscal transplantation. A hinged knee brace is used for the first 6 weeks, with gradual progression of weight bearing allowed after 4 weeks and up to 6 weeks. Some clinicians advocate the use of an unloader brace for an additional 4 to 6 weeks after the start of full weight-bearing activities.

Early range-of-motion exercise is started immediately. Flexion is limited to 90° during the first 4 to 6 weeks, because deep knee flexion may cause posterior horn impingement/shearing[50] and strain on the meniscocapsular junction.[51] Closed kinetic chain strengthening exercises and avoidance of open chain flexion exercises, as described by Fritz et al,[52] are used. Sport-related activities and running are generally not recommended

until after 4 or 5 months postoperatively, and patients are not allowed to perform deep knee bends/squats for at least 6 months. If concomitant procedures are performed (eg, ACL reconstruction), the rehabilitation program is modified accordingly.

Clinical Results

Meniscal transplantation has been shown to provide statistically significant improvements in pain and function. However, the outcomes literature is limited by small sample sizes, lack of controls, and variability in clinical outcome tools used. Subject heterogeneity, degree of underlying arthritis, surgical technique, and concomitant procedures also affect the ability to make definitive conclusions on the efficacy of transplantation. Furthermore, not all studies provide direct, validated evaluations of implanted meniscal tissue, and end points and definitions of failure differ across studies.

Fresh Meniscal Transplants

Verdonk et al[53] reported on 100 fresh meniscal transplants at a mean of 7.2 years (range, 0.5 to 14.5 years) postoperatively. The mean age of the patients was 35 years (range, 16 to 50 years). The failure rate was 28% for medial meniscal transplants (mean time to failure, 6.0 ± 8.8 years) and 16% for lateral meniscal transplants (mean time to failure, 4.8 ± 2.8 years). Medial meniscal transplantation performed with high tibial osteotomy increased the 10-year cumulative survival rate from 74.2% to 83.3%.

Verdonk et al[54] presented another 38 patients (39 fresh meniscal allografts) 10 to 14.8 years postoperatively. The average age of the patients was 35.2 years (range, 22 to 50 years), and most patients (67%) had grade 3 or higher chondrosis. At time of follow-up, radiographs revealed no further decrease in the tibiofemoral joint space in 41% of knees. Eighteen percent of transplants failed, with failure defined as conversion to total knee arthroplasty. Radiographic and MRI parameters did not correlate with clinical outcome.

Cryopreserved Meniscal Transplants

A prospective study of 38 patients (40 cryopreserved medial/lateral transplants) was presented at a mean of 3.3 years (range, 24 to 69 months) postoperatively.[55] The mean age at surgery was 30 years (range, 14 to

49 years), and cartilage resurfacing and ACL reconstruction were performed in several patients. At the time of follow-up, 76% of patients were participating in light, low-impact sports. Transplant failure occurred in 44% of patients with moderate arthritis and in 14% of patients with mild arthritis. One patient had total knee arthroplasty 35 months after transplantation.

A 45% survival rate was reported in a cohort of 22 cryopreserved meniscal transplants at a mean follow-up of 11.8 years (range, 9.6 to 13.9 years).[56] The mean age of the patients was 32 years (range, 17 to 46 years). Lysholm and pain scores improved in 90% of patients. Interval joint space narrowing was seen in 10 of 15 patients. Another study presented 23 patients followed 13 to 69 months after implantation of cryopreserved menisci.[57] The average age of the patients was 31 years (range, 20 to 42 years). At 5 to 28 months postoperatively, 35% of patients needed a second operation for meniscal symptoms. Rath et al[58] reported the results of 22 cryopreserved meniscal transplants at 2 to 8 years after the procedure. The average age of the patients was 30 years (range, 19 to 41 years). ACL reconstruction was performed in 11 of the 18 patients at time of transplant. There was a 36% failure rate of the transplants, although all patients except one experienced significant improvements in outcome scores.

van Arkel et al[59] reported the results of 19 cryopreserved meniscal transplants followed 14 to 55 months after surgery. The average age of the patients was 40 years (range, 30 to 54 years). Three transplants were deemed clinical failures, and eight transplants were considered failures by shrinkage on MRI. A separate survival analysis of 57 patients followed 63 cryopreserved transplants at an average of 5 years (range, 0.3 to 10.5 years).[60] The mean age of the patients was 39 years (range, 26 to 55 years). The 10-year survival rates of lateral, medial, and combined transplants were 76%, 50%, and 67%, respectively.

Fresh-Frozen Meniscal Transplants

A prospective study looked at the results of 96 fresh-frozen irradiated transplants in 82 patients at 2- to 5-year follow-up.[61] Failure was significantly related to the degree of underlying arthritis on MRI: 6% for normal or mild arthritis, 45% for moderate arthritis,

and 80% for severe arthritis. No differences in scores were seen between transplants that failed or survived.

Another study examined 33 fresh-frozen, nonirradiated transplants at greater than 2 years of follow-up.[62] Twenty-four patients had grade 3 or higher chondrosis preoperatively, with no significant change in joint space at time of follow-up. Seven of 33 transplants failed, with a higher percentage failing in patients with grade 4 chondrosis.

Medial Versus Lateral Meniscal Transplantation

Most studies comparing medial and lateral meniscal transplantation have failed to find any significant differences, although several studies have found that lateral transplants survive longer and have better clinical results.[55,60]

Sekiya et al[63] studied 25 lateral cryopreserved transplants, with an average patient age of 30 years (range, 19 to 45 years). Radiographic joint space narrowing of the lateral compartment was associated with outcome scoring. Another study presented 14 lateral transplantations after resection of lateral discoid menisci. The average age of the patients was 27.9 years (range, 17 to 41 years), and mean follow-up was 4.8 years (range, 1.75 to 8.75 years).[64] Modified Lysholm scores improved significantly, and no joint space changes were seen in 11 patients.

Data from 21 lateral transplants were extracted from a prospective study of 44 meniscal transplants (39 patients) in a study by Cole et al.[65] The mean age of the patients was 31 years (range, 16 to 48 years); 16% of grafts failed at a mean follow-up of only 2.8 years. Significant improvements were seen in outcomes across groups, and isolated lateral transplants demonstrated a trend toward greatest improvement.

Concomitant Procedures

Several studies have evaluated the clinical outcomes involving procedures in conjunction with meniscal transplantation. Rueff et al[66] reported on outcomes of ACL reconstruction with meniscal transplants or partial meniscectomy/meniscal repair. The groups had similar improvements in outcome scores, but the transplant group saw greater improvement in pain. Graf et al[67] examined eight medial meniscal cryopreserved (seven irradiated) transplants combined with ACL reconstruction. At a mean of 9.7 years, there was improvement in pain, stability, and function. Another study analyzed KT-1000 arthrometer (MEDmetric, San Diego, CA) measurements in patients who underwent ACL reconstruction with and without concomitant transplantation; patients with combined procedures had significantly improved arthrometer results,[68] findings similar to those of other studies looking at anterior stability following transplantation.[38]

Few studies on combined meniscal transplantation and chondral resurfacing are available in the literature. A prospective study of 29 meniscal transplants combined with resurfacing was reported at a mean follow-up of 3.1 years (range, 1.9 to 5.6 years).[69] Of the 15 autologous chondrocyte implantation (ACI) and 14 osteochondral allograft procedures, the absolute outcome scores were better for ACI versus osteochondral allograft (percentage improvement from the preoperative scores did not differ significantly). No difference was reported in outcomes between the medial and lateral groups, and the combined procedure groups did not have an increase in complications. Another study looked at 33 cases of combined meniscal transplant and ACI at minimum follow-up of 2 years.[70] Mean outcomes scores improved, although four grafts failed before the 2-year follow-up and were excluded. Bhosale et al[71] studied eight cryopreserved transplants combined with ACI. Six of the eight patients reported improved pain relief and function at 1 year; at a mean of 3.2 years (range, 2 to 6 years), functional improvement was seen in five of eight patients. Stone et al[72] evaluated 47 transplants (29 cryopreserved, 18 fresh-frozen) at an average 5.8-year follow-up (range, 2 to 7.25 years). The mean age was 48 years (range, 14 to 69 years); all patients had at least grade 3 arthritis, and 81% had grade 4. Outcome measures improved, but no difference was seen between concomitant procedure groups. Failures were all limited to grade 4 patients.

It is unclear whether combining meniscal transplantation with osteotomy delays joint degeneration. A report of 23 cryopreserved transplants, at a minimum 2-year follow-up, showed that all transplant failures were related to malalignment.[38] Accordingly, knee outcome scores were higher for patients with neutral alignment. Verdonk et al[54] reported results after 27 medial meniscal transplants. Concomitant high tibial os-

teotomy afforded significantly greater pain and functional score improvements versus isolated transplantation. In another study, the same group reported 10-year survival rates of 83.3% for combined medial meniscal transplant and osteotomy versus 74.2% for isolated medial meniscal transplant.[53] Whether clinical improvement was due to the transplantation or the osteotomy could not be definitely determined from the study. Another study of 34 knees after combined transplantation and osteotomy demonstrated good or excellent results in 85% of patients.[73]

Magnetic Resonance Imaging

Systems for the classification of meniscal transplant characteristics involve findings on MRI, clinical examination and symptoms, and follow-up arthroscopy (when performed). MRI has been used to measure transplant parameters, including displacement, during full or partial weight bearing,[74] as well as capsular attachments and surrounding chondral surface integrity.[75] Postoperative alterations in the signal intensity of meniscal transplants on MRI have been frequently reported.[57] Potter et al[76] evaluated 29 meniscal transplants with MRI and clinical examination 3 to 41 months postoperatively. All of the patients had moderate or severe chondral degeneration, and graft displacement was seen in 11 patients. In other studies, MRI has also been shown to correlate with arthroscopic transplant evaluation.[64,75] In a sheep model, Kelly et al[77] also demonstrated correlations between T2-weighted MRI cartilage evaluation and other evaluation measures. However, other authors have failed to find a correlation between MRI/arthroscopy evaluation and clinical outcome.[78]

Future Directions

A recent development, the Menaflex scaffold implant (ReGen Biologics, Hackensack, NJ), is used for partial meniscal deficiencies. In a prospective randomized study, Menaflex improved activity when compared with repeat partial meniscectomy for chronic meniscal injury.[79] The Menaflex implant is not currently approved by the US Food and Drug Administration (FDA) for use in the United States, but results from Europe have been encouraging. Long-term effects continue to be studied.

Other scaffolding materials under study include bioresorbable porous polyurethane[80] and synthetic hydrogel meniscal implants,[81] such as the hydrogel meniscal replacement (Salumedica, Atlanta, GA), in animal models.[82] Long-term durability and clinical efficacy in humans are still unknown.

Future efforts will continue with tissue engineering, scaffolding, and synthetic biomaterials. Options for meniscal replacement or regeneration may arise from advancements in protein biology or stem cell biology. The role of basic science studies and histologic analysis, along with animal models and biomechanical cadaveric models, will certainly increase. Translational research issues of transplant remodeling, resistance to in vivo shear and compressive forces, and collagen/matrix structural properties and cellularity will be ongoing challenges.

Summary

The short-term results after meniscal repair and transplantation have shown that most patients have improved knee function and relief of pain. The long-term chondroprotective effects of meniscal transplantation remain unknown, but outcomes at present demonstrate eventual degeneration of the implant and clinical loss of function. Although meniscal repair and transplantation show promise in selected younger patients, the role of these modalities in the management of middle-aged and elderly patients is unclear.

As the demands of the older athlete increase, the treatment algorithm for meniscal tears in these patients is continually challenged. The orthopaedic surgeon must carefully weigh the risks and benefits for each individual when considering broadening the indications for newer techniques. Patients should be advised that meniscal transplantation may have only short-term benefits and, in the long term, additional surgery is likely to be required. More studies are needed in older populations, along with longitudinal studies in younger patients to evaluate the survivorship and long-term clinical outcomes after meniscal repair and transplantation. Broadening indications, refined surgical techniques, and advances in biomedical/tissue-engineering science will likely play important roles in the treatment of both the young patient and the aging athlete.

References

1. McCarty EC, Marx RG, DeHaven KE: Meniscus repair: Considerations in treatment and update of clinical results. *Clin Orthop Relat Res* 2002;(402): 122-134.

2. McMurray TP: The semilunar cartilages. *Br J Surg* 1942;29:407-414.

3. Messner K, Gao J: The menisci of the knee joint: Anatomical and functional characteristics, and a rationale for clinical treatment. *J Anat* 1998; 193(pt 2):161-178.

4. Ahmed AM: The load-bearing role of the knee menisci, in Mow VC, Arnoczky SP, Jackson DW, eds: *Knee Meniscus: Basic and Clinical Foundation.* New York, NY, Raven Press, 1992, pp 59-73.

5. Fairbank TJ: Knee joint changes after meniscectomy. *J Bone Joint Surg Br* 1948;30(4):664-670.

6. Hede A, Larsen E, Sandberg H: Partial versus total meniscectomy: A prospective, randomised study with long-term follow-up. *J Bone Joint Surg Br* 1992;74(1): 118-121.

7. McGinity JB, Geuss LF, Marvin RA: Partial or total meniscectomy: A comparative analysis. *J Bone Joint Surg Am* 1977;59(6):763-766.

8. Baratz ME, Fu FH, Mengato R: Meniscal tears: The effect of meniscectomy and of repair on intraarticular contact areas and stress in the human knee. A preliminary report. *Am J Sports Med* 1986;14(4): 270-275.

9. Messner K, Fahlgren A, Persliden J, Andersson BM: Radiographic joint space narrowing and histologic changes in a rabbit meniscectomy model of early knee osteoarthrosis. *Am J Sports Med* 2001;29(2):151-160.

10. Shapiro F, Glimcher MJ: Induction of osteoarthrosis in the rabbit knee joint. *Clin Orthop Relat Res* 1980;(147): 287-295.

11. Pennington B: Baby boomers stay active, and so do their doctors. *New York Times.* April 16, 2006. http://www.nytimes.com/2006/04/16/sports/16boomers.html?_r=1. Accessed April 25, 2010.

12. Rutherford GW Jr, Schroeder TJ: *Sports-Related Injuries to Persons 65 Years of Age and Older.* Washington, DC, United States Consumer Product Safety Commission, April 1998. http://www.cpsc.gov/cpscpub/pubs/grand/aging/injury65.PDF. Accessed April 25, 2010.

13. DiNubile N: Boomeritis: What is it??? *Dr. Nick.com.* http://www.drnick.com/boomeritis. Accessed September 17, 2010.

14. Arnoczky SP, Warren RF: The microvasculature of the meniscus and its response to injury: An experimental study in the dog. *Am J Sports Med* 1983;11(3):131-141.

15. Zhang ZN, Tu KY, Xu YK, Zhang WM, Liu ZT, Ou SH: Treatment of longitudinal injuries in avascular area of meniscus in dogs by trephination. *Arthroscopy* 1988;4(3):151-159.

16. Krüger-Franke M, Siebert CH, Kugler A, Trouillier HH, Rosemeyer B: Late results after arthroscopic partial medial meniscectomy. *Knee Surg Sports Traumatol Arthrosc* 1999;7(2):81-84.

17. Menard D, Stanish WD: The aging athlete. *Am J Sports Med* 1989;17(2):187-196.

18. Chen AL, Mears SC, Hawkins RJ: Orthopaedic care of the aging athlete. *J Am Acad Orthop Surg* 2005;13(6):407-416.

19. Meredith DS, Losina E, Mahomed NN, Wright J, Katz JN: Factors predicting functional and radiographic outcomes after arthroscopic partial meniscectomy: A review of the literature. *Arthroscopy* 2005;21(2):211-223.

20. Chatain F, Robinson AH, Adeleine P, Chambat P, Neyret P: The natural history of the knee following arthroscopic medial meniscectomy. *Knee Surg Sports Traumatol Arthrosc* 2001;9(1):15-18.

21. Chatain F, Adeleine P, Chambat P, Neyret P, Société Française d'Arthroscopie: A comparative study of medial versus lateral arthroscopic partial meniscectomy on stable knees: 10-year minimum follow-up. *Arthroscopy* 2003;19(8):842-849.

22. Kurosawa H, Fukubayashi T, Nakajima H: Load-bearing mode of the knee joint: Physical behavior of the knee joint with or without menisci. *Clin Orthop Relat Res* 1980;(149):283-290.

23. Seedhom BB, Hargreaves DJ: Transmission of the load in the knee joint with special reference to the role of the menisci: Part II. Experimental results, discussion, and conclusions. *Eng Med* 1979;8:220-228.

24. Rangger C, Klestil T, Gloetzer W, Kemmler G, Benedetto KP: Osteoarthritis after arthroscopic partial meniscectomy. *Am J Sports Med* 1995;23:240-244.

25. Shelbourne KD, Carr DR: Meniscal repair compared with meniscectomy for bucket-handle medial meniscal tears in anterior cruciate ligament-reconstructed knees. *Am J Sports Med* 2003;31(5):718-723.

26. Rockborn P, Messner K: Long-term results of meniscus repair and meniscectomy: A 13-year functional and radiographic follow-up study. *Knee Surg Sports Traumatol Arthrosc* 2000;8(1):2-10.

27. Lozano J, Ma CB, Cannon WD: All-inside meniscus repair: A systematic review. *Clin Orthop Relat Res* 2007;455:134-141.

28. Lee GP, Diduch DR: Deteriorating outcomes after meniscal repair using the Meniscus Arrow in knees undergoing concurrent anterior cruciate ligament reconstruction: Increased failure rate with long-term follow-up. *Am J Sports Med* 2005;33(8):1138-1141.

29. Rankin CC, Lintner DM, Noble PC, Paravic V, Greer E: A biomechanical analysis of meniscal repair techniques. *Am J Sports Med* 2002;30(4):492-497.

30. Okuda K, Ochi M, Shu N, Uchio Y: Meniscal rasping for repair of meniscal tear in the avascular zone. *Arthroscopy* 1999;15(3):281-286.

31. Ritchie JR, Miller MD, Bents RT, Smith DK: Meniscal repair in the goat model: The use of healing adjuncts on central tears and the role of magnetic resonance arthrography in repair evaluation. *Am J Sports Med* 1998;26(2):278-284.

32. Port J, Jackson DW, Lee TQ, Simon TM: Meniscal repair supplemented with exogenous fibrin clot and autogenous cultured marrow cells in the goat model. *Am J Sports Med* 1996;24(4):547-555.

33. Pangborn CA, Athanasiou KA: Growth factors and fibrochondrocytes in scaffolds. *J Orthop Res* 2005;23(5):1184-1190.

34. Weinand C, Peretti GM, Adams SB Jr, Bonassar LJ, Randolph MA, Gill TJ: An allogenic cell-based implant for meniscal lesions. *Am J Sports Med* 2006;34(11):1779-1789.

35. Izuta Y, Ochi M, Adachi N, Deie M, Yamasaki T, Shinomiya R: Meniscal repair using bone marrow-derived mesenchymal stem cells: Experimental study using green fluorescent protein transgenic rats. *Knee* 2005;12(3):217-223.

36. Ishida K, Kuroda R, Miwa M, et al: The regenerative effects of platelet-rich plasma on meniscal cells in vitro and its in vivo application with biodegradable gelatin hydrogel. *Tissue Eng* 2007;13(5):1103-1112.

37. Outerbridge RE: The etiology of chondromalacia patellae. *J Bone Joint Surg Br* 1961;43(4):752-757.

38. van Arkel ER, de Boer HH: Human meniscal transplantation: Preliminary results at 2 to 5-year follow-up. *J Bone Joint Surg Br* 1995;77(4):589-595.

39. Packer JD, Rodeo SA: Meniscal allograft transplantation. *Clin Sports Med* 2009;28(2):259-283.

40. McNicholas MJ, Rowley DI, McGurty D, et al: Total meniscectomy in adolescence: A thirty-year follow-up. *J Bone Joint Surg Br* 2000;82(2):217-221.

41. Walker PS, Erkman MJ: The role of the menisci in force transmission across the knee. *Clin Orthop Relat Res* 1975;(109):184-192.

42. Jackson DW, Whelan J, Simon TM: Cell survival after transplantation of fresh meniscal allografts: DNA probe analysis in a goat model. *Am J Sports Med* 1993;21(4):540-550.

43. Fabbriciani C, Lucania L, Milano G, Schiavone Panni A, Evangelisti M: Meniscal allografts: Cryopreservation vs deep-frozen technique. An experimental study in goats. *Knee Surg Sports Traumatol Arthrosc* 1997;5(2):124-134.

44. Jackson DW, Windler GE, Simon TM: Intraarticular reaction associated with the use of freeze-dried, ethylene oxide-sterilized bone-patella tendon-bone allografts in the reconstruction of the anterior cruciate ligament. *Am J Sports Med* 1990;18(1):1-11.

45. Wirth CJ, Peters G, Milachowski KA, Weismeier KG, Kohn D: Long-term results of meniscal allograft transplantation. *Am J Sports Med* 2002;30(2):174-181.

46. Li G, DeFrate LE, Park SE, Gill TJ, Rubash HE: In vivo articular cartilage contact kinematics of the knee: An investigation using dual-orthogonal fluoroscopy and magnetic resonance image-based computer models. *Am J Sports Med* 2005;33(1):102-107.

47. Allen CR, Wong EK, Livesay GA, Sakane M, Fu FH, Woo SL: Importance of the medial meniscus in the anterior cruciate ligament-deficient knee. *J Orthop Res* 2000;18(1):109-115.

48. Papageorgiou CD, Gil JE, Kanamori A, Fenwick JA, Woo SL, Fu FH: The biomechanical interdependence between the anterior cruciate ligament replacement graft and the medial meniscus. *Am J Sports Med* 2001;29(2):226-231.

49. Shelbourne KD, Gray T: Results of anterior cruciate ligament reconstruction based on meniscus and articular cartilage status at the time of surgery: Five- to fifteen-year evaluations. *Am J Sports Med* 2000;28(4):446-452.

50. Thompson WO, Thaete FL, Fu FH, Dye SF: Tibial meniscal dynamics using three-dimensional reconstruction of magnetic resonance images. *Am J Sports Med* 1991;19(3):210-216.

51. Morgan CD, Wojtys EM, Casscells CD, Casscells SW: Arthroscopic meniscal repair evaluated by second-look arthroscopy. *Am J Sports Med* 1991;19(6):632-638.

52. Fritz JM, Irrgang JJ, Harner CD: Rehabilitation following allograft meniscal transplantation: A review of the literature and case study. *J Orthop Sports Phys Ther* 1996;24(2):98-106.

53. Verdonk PC, Demurie A, Almqvist KF, Veys EM, Verbruggen G, Verdonk R: Transplantation of viable meniscal allograft: Survivorship analysis and clinical outcome of one hundred cases. *J Bone Joint Surg Am* 2005;87(4):715-724.

54. Verdonk PC, Verstraete KL, Almqvist KF, et al: Meniscal allograft transplantation: Long-term clinical results with radiological and magnetic resonance imaging correlations. *Knee Surg Sports Traumatol Arthrosc* 2006;14(8):694-706.

55. Noyes FR, Barber-Westin SD, Rankin M: Meniscal transplantation in symptomatic patients less than fifty years old. *J Bone Joint Surg Am* 2004;86(7):1392-1404.

56. Hommen JP, Applegate GR, Del Pizzo W: Meniscus allograft transplantation: Ten-year results of cryo-preserved allografts. *Arthroscopy* 2007;23(4):388-393.

57. Stollsteimer GT, Shelton WR, Dukes A, Bomboy AL: Meniscal allograft transplantation: A 1- to 5-year follow-up of 22 patients. *Arthroscopy* 2000;16(4):343-347.

58. Rath E, Richmond JC, Yassir W, Albright JD, Gundogan F: Meniscal allograft transplantation: Two- to eight-year results. *Am J Sports Med* 2001;29(4):410-414.

59. van Arkel ER, Goei R, de Ploeg I, de Boer HH: Meniscal allografts: Evaluation with magnetic resonance imaging and correlation with arthroscopy. *Arthroscopy* 2000;16(5):517-521.

60. van Arkel ER, de Boer HH: Survival analysis of human meniscal transplantations. *J Bone Joint Surg Br* 2002;84(2):227-231.

61. Noyes FR, Barber-Westin SD, Butler DL, Wilkins RM: The role of allografts in repair and reconstruction of knee joint ligaments and menisci. *Instr Course Lect* 1998;47:379-396.

62. Rodeo SA: Meniscal allografts—where do we stand? *Am J Sports Med* 2001;29(2):246-261.

63. Sekiya JK, West RV, Groff YJ, Irrgang JJ, Fu FH, Harner CD: Clinical outcomes following isolated lateral meniscal allograft transplantation. *Arthroscopy* 2006;22(7):771-780.

64. Kim JM, Bin SI: Meniscal allograft transplantation after total meniscectomy of torn discoid lateral meniscus. *Arthroscopy* 2006;22(12):1344-1350, e1.

65. Cole BJ, Dennis MG, Lee SJ, et al: Prospective evaluation of allograft meniscus transplantation: A minimum 2-year follow-up. *Am J Sports Med* 2006; 34(6):919-927.

66. Rueff D, Nyland J, Kocabey Y, Chang HC, Caborn DN: Self-reported patient outcomes at a minimum of 5 years after allograft anterior cruciate ligament reconstruction with or without medial meniscus transplantation: An age-, sex-, and activity level-matched comparison in patients aged approximately 50 years. *Arthroscopy* 2006;22(10):1053-1062.

67. Graf KW Jr, Sekiya JK, Wojtys EM: Long-term results after combined medial meniscal allograft transplantation and anterior cruciate ligament reconstruction: Minimum 8.5-year follow-up study. *Arthroscopy* 2004;20(2):129-140.

68. Garrett J: Meniscal transplantation, in Aichroth P, Cannon W, eds: *Knee Surgery: Current Practice.* London, United Kingdom, Martin Dunitz, Ltd, 1992, pp 95-103.

69. Rue JP, Yanke AB, Busam ML, McNickle AG, Cole BJ: Prospective evaluation of concurrent meniscus transplantation and articular cartilage repair: Minimum 2-year follow-up. *Am J Sports Med* 2008;36(9): 1770-1778.

70. Farr J, Rawal A, Marberry KM: Concomitant meniscal allograft transplantation and autologous chondrocyte implantation: Minimum 2-year follow-up. *Am J Sports Med* 2007;35(9):1459-1466.

71. Bhosale AM, Myint P, Roberts S, et al: Combined autologous chondrocyte implantation and allogenic meniscus transplantation: A biological knee replacement. *Knee* 2007;14(5):361-368.

72. Stone KR, Walgenbach AW, Turek TJ, Freyer A, Hill MD: Meniscus allograft survival in patients with moderate to severe unicompartmental arthritis: A 2- to 7-year follow-up. *Arthroscopy* 2006;22(5):469-478.

73. Cameron JC, Saha S: Meniscal allograft transplantation for unicompartmental arthritis of the knee. *Clin Orthop Relat Res* 1997;(337):164-171.

74. Rankin M, Noyes FR, Barber-Westin SD, Hushek SG, Seow A: Human meniscus allografts' in vivo size and motion characteristics: Magnetic resonance imaging assessment under weightbearing conditions. *Am J Sports Med* 2006;34(1):98-107.

75. Potter HG, Linklater JM, Allen AA, Hannafin JA, Haas SB: Magnetic resonance imaging of articular cartilage in the knee: An evaluation with use of fast-spin-echo imaging. *J Bone Joint Surg Am* 1998;80(9):1276-1284.

76. Potter HG, Rodeo SA, Wickiewicz TL, Warren RF: MR imaging of meniscal allografts: Correlation with clinical and arthroscopic outcomes. *Radiology* 1996; 198(2):509-514.

77. Kelly BT, Potter HG, Deng XH, et al: Meniscal allograft transplantation in the sheep knee: Evaluation of chondroprotective effects. *Am J Sports Med* 2006; 34(9):1464-1477.

78. Noyes FR, Barber-Westin SD: Irradiated meniscus allografts in the human knee: A two to five year follow-up study. *Orthop Trans* 1995;19:417.

79. Rodkey WG, DeHaven KE, Montgomery WH III, et al: Comparison of the collagen meniscus implant with partial meniscectomy: A prospective randomized trial. *J Bone Joint Surg Am* 2008;90(7):1413-1426.

80. Ramrattan NN, Heijkants RG, van Tienen TG, Schouten AJ, Veth RP, Buma P: Assessment of tissue ingrowth rates in polyurethane scaffolds for tissue engineering. *Tissue Eng* 2005;11(7-8):1212-1223.

81. Kobayashi M, Toguchida J, Oka M: Development of an artificial meniscus using polyvinyl alcohol-hydrogel for early return to, and continuance of, athletic life in sportspersons with severe meniscus injury: II. Animal experiments. *Knee* 2003;10(1):53.

82. Kelly BT, Robertson W, Potter HG, et al: Hydrogel meniscal replacement in the sheep knee: Preliminary evaluation of chondroprotective effects. *Am J Sports Med* 2007;35(1):43-52.

Chapter 33

Anterior Cruciate Ligament Tears in the Mature Athlete

J. Richard Steadman, MD
Ryan Miyamoto, MD
Karen K. Briggs, MPH

Dr. Steadman or an immediate family member serves as a board member, owner, officer, or committee member of the Vail Valley Surgical Center; has received royalties from Linvatec and Össur; serves as a paid consultant to or is an employee of Össur and Regen Biologics; has received research or institutional support from Arthrex, Össur, Smith & Nephew, and Siemens; and owns stock or stock options in Regeneration Technologies and Regen Biologics. Dr. Briggs or an immediate family member has received research or institutional support from Smith & Nephew, Össur, Genzyme, Arthex, and Siemens. Neither Dr. Miyamoto nor any immediate family member has received anything of value from or owns stock in a commercial company or institution related directly or indirectly to the subject of this chapter.

Key Points

- Increased activity levels and exercise patterns in older patients highlight the importance of knee stability.
- Nonsurgical treatment may be a good option for less active patients.
- Special knee considerations need to be addressed before surgically reconstructing anterior cruciate ligament (ACL)–deficient knees in older patients.
- ACL repair using the healing response technique has significant advantages in patients with a proximal ACL tear.
- Clinical results for ACL reconstruction in patients older than 40 years are excellent in the appropriate patient.
- ACL reconstruction can result in functional stability of the knee, regardless of the patient's age.

Introduction

Many older people today lead very active lifestyles that may include skiing, mountain biking, hunting, fitness programs, running, and golf. ACL ruptures occur in an active older population, as they do in younger patients.

The standard course of treatment for an ACL-deficient knee in younger active patients is reconstruction to restore knee stability, with the ultimate goals of preventing further damage to the knee, reducing the risk of future arthritis, and helping the patient return to the desired activity level. Some studies have suggested that older patients do not return to their preinjury level of activity.[1-3] The current dilemma is whether sur-gical ACL reconstruction is the best course of treatment for mature patients.

The treatment of ACL injuries in the mature athlete remains a controversial topic. Issues such as activity level, arthrofibrosis, chondral defects, arthritic changes, alignment, patient expectations, and overall health status all must be taken into consideration.[4,5] An increasing number of people continue to stay active into their later years, and this change in exercise patterns has highlighted the importance of maintaining knee stability in these athletes.

In 2003, Marx et al[6] published the results of a survey of a random sampling of members of the American Academy of Orthopaedic

Surgeons (AAOS) to determine attitudes regarding the ACL-deficient knee. The authors found that approximately 83% of the respondents thought that ACL disruption was associated with an increased arthrosis, and 81% thought that ACL-deficient individuals were more symptomatic than non–ACL-deficient individuals. Eighty-eight percent of the surveyed surgeons reported that bracing was useful for nonsurgical treatment. Disagreement was evident among surgeons who routinely did ACL surgery, citing that patient age older than 40 years was a factor that influenced their decision as to whether to perform ACL reconstruction.

More recently, Seng et al[7] used an expected-value decision analysis with sensitivity analysis to evaluate surgical versus nonsurgical treatment of ACL tears in patients 40 years and older. They evaluated 69 subjects and showed that these individuals are averse to accepting possible knee instability, preferring ACL reconstruction despite the potential risk of surgical complications. This finding lends further credence to the idea that surgical reconstruction for patients with ACL tears in this age group should at the very least be an option that is seriously considered for the appropriate patient.

Many surgeons have concerns that surgical reconstruction of the ACL in older patients may result in higher rates of postoperative arthrofibrosis, with a decrease in range of motion (ROM). However, multiple studies of older patients have demonstrated rates of arthrofibrosis to be comparable to or lower than the rates in younger patients.[8-10] Sterett et al[11] also reported no difference in the prevalence of arthrofibrosis based on the timing of surgery following injury. In this study, patients who had surgery within 3 weeks of injury and patients who had surgery after 3 weeks of injury showed no significant difference in the development of arthrofibrosis, provided specific criteria are used to determine the knee's readiness for surgery.

As our active population ages, they have a growing expectation that their medical treatment will return them pain-free to their previous activity level. We recommend the following clinical options based on the individual patient factors; however, age is not a limiting factor.

Clinical Options for Treatment of ACL Tears

Nonsurgical Treatment

Although surgical results are encouraging, it is imprudent to presume that every middle-aged patient with an ACL rupture is a surgical candidate.[1,2] Nonsurgical management should be strongly considered in patients who participate primarily in cycling, swimming, and walking or whose lifestyle does not require significant knee stability. In acute cases, nonsurgical treatment should concentrate on certain objectives, namely: (1) decreasing swelling and inflammation; (2) regaining full ROM (minimum active ROM of 0° to 120°); and (3) strengthening, with special emphasis on the hamstrings and quadriceps.

Bracing also can be helpful, particularly during higher risk activities involving significant pivoting or cutting, as opposed to full-time wear. In chronic cases, similar principles apply; however, further attention should be paid to other potential pathology about the knee including meniscus damage, degenerative joint disease, limb malalignment, and patellofemoral compartment changes. Recent studies have also shown that patients who return to their preinjury level of activity on a knee with continued instability may be at significant risk for reinjury.[1-3,5] Additionally, the use of a knee brace might not be successful in preventing reinjury. Reinjury rates can lead to dissatisfaction among both patients and surgeons.

Once the appropriate workup is completed, including an MRI scan to determine the morphology of the tear and identify other intra-articular pathology, a thorough discussion with the patient should occur. This conversation should include topics such as the patient's goals and expectations and the potential risks of surgery. All options other than surgical intervention should be discussed before going into the specifics of the surgical procedure. Additionally, if significant meniscus or cartilage damage is noted on physical examination or MRI, early surgery may be indicated to address this pathology, as an ACL reconstruction may decrease shear stresses on the defects.

Surgical Intervention

If acute surgery (within the first 3 weeks after injury) is warranted, the environment of the knee joint must be appropriate for ligament reconstruction. This includes full or near-full ROM with excellent patella mobility as compared to the uninjured knee, as well as quadriceps muscle tone. Additionally, a significant palpable temperature difference between knees is a contraindication to surgery, as this is an indication of inflammation and could increase the risk of arthrofibrosis.

Once the surgical option is chosen, the graft choice for the aging athlete is a crucial consideration. A variety of autografts and allografts is available, and many of the early series showed success in this age group using bone–patellar tendon–bone (BPTB) autografts for the ACL reconstruction.[12,13] Other options include autologous hamstring and quadriceps tendons, as well as BPTB, hamstring, and Achilles allografts.

Although there is no "wrong" graft choice, we strongly suggest considering allograft for patients who have concomitant degenerative joint disease (DJD) of the knee, particularly in the patellofemoral compartment. In the presence of DJD, special considerations include malalignment, contracture, cartilage loss, inflammation, and pain. A knee contracture of 5° compared to the uninjured knee is usually a contraindication to ligament reconstruction. Additionally, if there is significant arthritis in the medial or lateral compartment along with limb malalignment, our preferred treatment is to perform a staged procedure. The first procedure consists of an osteotomy and treatment of the DJD including possible chondroplasty, microfracture, or other cartilage-sparing or restoring procedures. The primary stage is meant to create the best possible environment for reconstruction. The second stage consists of ligament reconstruction, once appropriate knee ROM has been regained and bony consolidation of the osteotomy has occurred. A similar two-stage procedure may also be indicated if microfracture of the trochlea or patella is required. Occasionally, these two procedures can be performed at the same time.

Our two-incision technique has been previously published.[14] There are several keys to success when performing an ACL reconstruction. The tunnels must be properly positioned to ensure ideal graft length (**Figure 1**, *A*), the graft must have adequate strength, and

impingement must be avoided. The fixation of the graft in the tunnels must allow for early ROM (**Figure 1**, *B*). The reconstruction must restore normal biomechanics of soft tissue. When a patellar tendon autograft is used, steps should be taken to avoid a deficit in the donor site. To minimize the risk of scarring after the graft, the patient should avoid excessive strain early, for up to 6 to 12 weeks. To avoid scarring and joint stiffness, all patients undergo patellar mobilization exercises in addition to early ROM.[15] Full extension and flexion is important. Strengthening exercises are avoided until ROM and patellar mobility are achieved. Other solutions used to avoid anterior knee pain include grafting defects with bone from the tunnel drilling (**Figure 1**, *C*), and loose partial-thickness closure of the patellar tendon defect (**Figure 1**, *D*). Lateral patellofemoral retinacular release is also routinely performed. This consists of incising the lateral retinaculum from the lower patella to the superior patella. Using this regimen, the senior author (J.R.S.) has reported graft-site morbidity of less than 3%.[14]

The Arthritic Knee

If arthritis is present in the joint, it is important to address the joint environment to ensure good clinical results. If there is patellofemoral joint arthritis, the healing response technique (see section below) is a viable surgical alternative. Medial or lateral compartment arthritis with malalignment may require an osteotomy first. If ACL reconstruction requires an osteotomy because of malalignment, or if DJD is present, a two-stage approach is frequently used. After first-stage procedures, rehabilitation is critical to achieve maximal ROM before the ACL is reconstructed. If there is no malalignment, the best graft choice in the presence of DJD is usually an allograft (BPTB, Achilles, or other tendon). Joint contracture is frequently a contraindication to ACL reconstruction. Special considerations in the arthritic knee include malalignment, contracture, cartilage loss, inflammation, and pain.

Healing Response

As an alternative to reconstruction in the setting of an unstable knee in which MRI shows a proximal tear of the ACL, we commonly use the healing response tech-

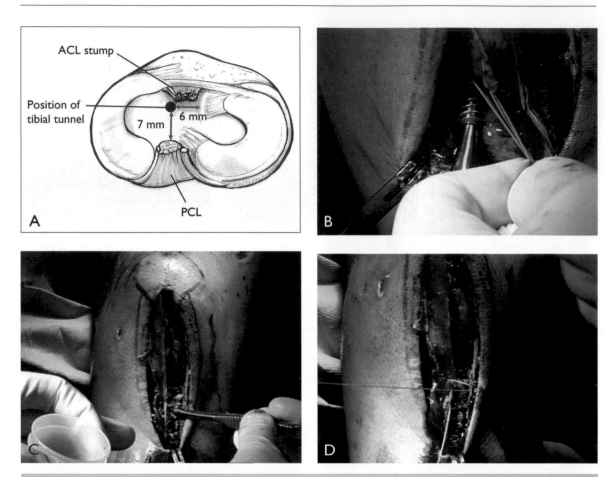

Figure 1 Anterior cruciate ligament (ACL) reconstruction. **A,** Drawing shows the position of the tibial tunnel 6 mm lateral to the medial wall and 7 to 9 mm anterior to the posterior cruciate ligament (PCL). **B,** Intraoperative photograph shows placement of the femoral 9-mm interference screw alongside guidewires inserted parallel and posterior to the bone blocks. Intraoperative photographs show grafting the site of the patellar tendon graft harvest with bone from the tibial tunnel (**C**) and loose partial-thickness closure of the patellar tendon defect (**D**). (Panel A reproduced with permission from Steadman JR: Anterior cruciate ligament reconstruction, in Feagin JA, Steadman JR, eds: *The Crucial Principles in Care of the Knee.* Philadelphia, PA, Lippincott Williams & Wilkins, 2008, pp 117-128.)

nique.[16,17] This technique is a primary treatment that is the equivalent of a microfracture procedure at the anatomic site of the ACL in the notch, along with perforations made in the body of the ligament.[16-18]

The healing response technique was originally conceived by the senior author (J.R.S.) for proximal one-third ACL lesions, the type frequently seen in skiers.[16-18] It has proven its usefulness in many other ACL injuries, regardless of the injury mechanism. The healing response technique has significant advantages

that offset its possible shortcomings. It is a technically easy arthroscopic procedure with minimal downside; in particular, it does not preclude and minimally affects future ligament reconstruction, if necessary. An experimental study of dogs investigated the morphologic, cellular, and molecular events that occur within the surgically induced clot and ligament during the healing process.[18] This knowledge of the basic science of the healing response technique led to a better understanding of clinical observations in patients.[16,17]

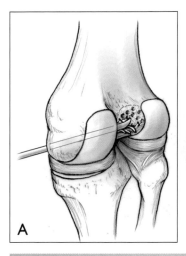
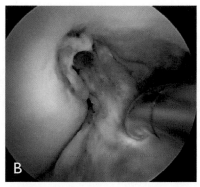
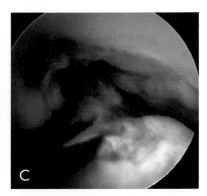

Figure 2 Healing response technique. **A,** Illustration shows creation of six to ten holes in the cortical bone at the origin of the disrupted ligament. **B,** The awl is used to perforate the distal stump of the ligament multiple times over its entire length to aid blood-clot invasion. **C,** Arthroscopic view shows a completed healing response, with blood at the femoral attachment and in holes in the ligament. (Reproduced with permission from Steadman JR, Rodkey WG: The healing response technique: A minimally invasive procedure to stimulate healing of anterior cruciate ligament injuries using the microfracture technique, in Feagin JA, Steadman JR, eds: *The Crucial Principles in Care of the Knee*. Philadelphia, PA, Lippincott Williams & Wilkins, 2008, pp 153-162.)

The healing response technique is an all-arthroscopic surgical procedure.[16] The technique uses an arthroscopic microfracture awl with an angle that allows the tip of the awl to be perpendicular to the femoral attachment site of the ACL. With the awl, six to ten holes (2 to 3 mm in diameter and 3 to 4 mm deep) are made into the cortical bone at the origin of the disrupted ligament (**Figure 2,** *A*). The ligament distal stump is also perforated with the awl multiple times over its entire length to aid blood-clot invasion (**Figure 2,** *B*). Care is taken to ensure that the disrupted end of the ligament is manipulated into the correct anatomic location with a probe before wound closure. No further manipulation of the ligament or the marrow clot is needed, and no fixation devices are used. The marrow clot surrounds the end of the ligament and holds it in place[16] (**Figure 2,** *C*). A great deal of caution should be taken to ensure that in younger patients an open growth plate is not penetrated with the microfracture awl. If the physis is open, the awl is advanced without the use of a mallet to avoid impaction injury to the growth plate.

Postoperative Care

Patients are braced immediately postoperatively. The brace is locked in full extension to help stabilize the ligament ends with the marrow clot. Patients wear the brace for 6 weeks and are transitioned into an ACL brace. Initial weight bearing is toe-touch with crutches; gradually increased weight bearing continues over 6 weeks. Physical therapy is initiated within 24 hours of surgery. Week 1 is focused on gentle 0° to 90° passive ROM, quadriceps control, gait training, and swelling control. During weeks 2 through 6, patients begin full passive ROM and active-assisted ROM, isometrics, and low-resistance closed kinetic chain activities. After 6 weeks, crutches should be discontinued. Weeks 6 through 12 are focused on progressive strengthening, eccentric loading, and initiation of open-chain exercises, with special attention directed to avoiding patellofemoral pain. Stationary biking starts at 6 weeks. Weeks 12 through 24 focus on continued strengthening, sport-specific conditioning, agility, and proprioceptive training. Patients are allowed to return to full activity after 24 weeks. Use of an ACL brace during athletic activities is recommended for the first year, and on an ongoing basis for high-risk activity.

Early postoperative rehabilitation should focus on regaining ROM and decreasing swelling before beginning strengthening exercises. Patellar mobilization is also emphasized to prevent scarring in the anterior interval.[19] By week 6, we begin to add resistance to stationary bike exercise, and at week 8, uphill treadmill use is allowed at a slow speed at a grade no higher than 7%. The elliptical machine is allowed at 10 weeks, with jogging permitted at week 16. At 6 months, change of direction with elastic resistance bands begins, with a goal of return to sport by 6 months for autograft ACL reconstructions, and 6 to 8 months for allograft reconstructions.

Outcomes

Plancher et al[12] reviewed the outcomes of 72 patients older than 40 years who underwent BPTB ACL reconstructions; mean follow-up was 55 months. Only three patients had reported pain or swelling, and none had symptoms of giving way or patellofemoral pain. Marked improvements were noted in postoperative Lysholm scores, Hospital for Special Surgery scores, and International Knee Documentation Committee (IKDC) scores, and all patients were satisfied with the results of the procedure. In this study, bicycling was resumed at an average of 4 months, jogging at 9 months, skiing at 10 months, and tennis at 12 months. The authors noted that the outcomes in their cohort were at least as good as those in younger patients and were superior to those in middle-aged patients managed nonsurgically.

Similar results in patients older than 40 years have been documented by others.[13,20-26] Adams and Moore[20] reviewed outcomes at minimum follow-up of 9 months in 13 patients 40 to 53 years of age who underwent BPTB ACL reconstruction for instability. All patients had significant reduction in pain, an increase in occupational and physical activity, and a high level of satisfaction. None experienced clinically significant (>10°) flexion contracture. Deakon and Zarnett[13] reported on 80 patients who underwent autologous BPTB ACL reconstruction, half of whom were older than 40 years. At an average follow-up of 26 months, no

differences were seen in postoperative course, rates of arthrofibrosis, or complications, outcomes, or return to sport between patients older than 40 and those younger than 40. Barber et al[21] compared 33 patients older than 40 who underwent ACL reconstruction with BPTB autograft or allograft or Achilles allograft with 133 patients younger than 40 who underwent the same procedure. At an average follow-up of 21 months, both groups showed significant improvement in Lysholm and Tegner scores, as well as arthrometric, radiographic, and clinical examinations. In the older group, 89% had excellent/good results versus 91% in the younger group. Because the outcomes between the groups were not statistically significant, the authors concluded that an age of 40 years is not a barrier to successful ACL reconstruction. Heier et al[22] reviewed the results of 45 consecutive patients over the age of 40 who underwent ACL reconstruction with autologous BPTB grafts. At an average follow-up of 37 months, 76% had returned to their preoperative activity levels.

Recently, Javernick et al[26] reported on the results of ACL reconstruction using autologous hamstring graft in 84 patients 40 years and older. Significant improvements in Lysholm scores, Short Form-36 scores, and Tegner activity scale scores were noted, and 87% of patients were satisfied and stated they would have the surgery again under similar circumstances. No patient reported anterior knee pain or symptomatic loss of ROM, and no major surgical complications occurred.

In the series reported by Steadman and Rodkey[16] of 198 patients older than 40 years who underwent a healing response procedure for a proximally torn ACL, only 5 patients (2.5%) subsequently sustained a reinjury that necessitated an ACL reconstruction. The average Lysholm score increased from 63 to 94, and 95% of the cohort reported no symptoms of giving way of the knee. The average patient's satisfaction was 9.1 (with 10 being very satisfied), and on arthrometer testing, the manual maximum difference between the two sides improved from 5.0 mm preoperatively to 1.9 mm postoperatively. Similar success with the healing response for proximal ACL ruptures has also been seen in a younger cohort of patients treated by the senior author (J.R.S.).[17]

Summary

Changes in activity levels and exercise patterns in older patients highlight the importance of knee stability. Results of ACL surgical intervention in mature athletes mirror those in younger patients. Nonsurgical treatment and bracing may be a good option for less active patients who participate in low-impact sports or whose lifestyles do not require significant knee stability, but reliance on a brace to return to preinjury level of activity with continuing knee instability may lead to significant reinjury rates. Surgical intervention in older patients should address the joint environment—malalignment, contracture, cartilage loss, inflammation, and pain—to ensure good clinical results. The healing response technique should be considered in patients with the appropriate surgical indications. ACL reconstruction results in functional stability of the knee and high patient satisfaction, regardless of the patient's age.

References

1. Bonamo JJ, Fay C, Firestone T: The conservative treatment of the anterior cruciate deficient knee. *Am J Sports Med* 1990;18(6):618-623.

2. Ciccotti MG, Lombardo SJ, Nonweiler B, Pink M: Non-operative treatment of ruptures of the anterior cruciate ligament in middle-aged patients: Results after long-term follow-up. *J Bone Joint Surg Am* 1994;76(9): 1315-1321.

3. Finsterbush A, Frankl U, Matan Y, Mann G: Secondary damage to the knee after isolated injury of the anterior cruciate ligament. *Am J Sports Med* 1990;18(5): 475-479.

4. Ichiba A, Kishimoto I: Effects of articular cartilage and meniscus injuries at the time of surgery on osteoarthritic changes after anterior cruciate ligament reconstruction in patients under 40 years old. *Arch Orthop Trauma Surg* 2009;129(3):409-415.

5. Noyes FR, Matthews DS, Mooar PA, Grood ES: The symptomatic anterior cruciate-deficient knee: Part II. The results of rehabilitation, activity modification, and counseling on functional disability. *J Bone Joint Surg Am* 1983;65(2):163-174.

6. Marx RG, Jones EC, Angel M, Wickiewicz TL, Warren RF: Beliefs and attitudes of members of the American Academy of Orthopaedic Surgeons regarding the treatment of anterior cruciate ligament injury. *Arthroscopy* 2003;19(7):762-770.

7. Seng K, Appleby D, Lubowitz JH: Operative versus nonoperative treatment of anterior cruciate ligament rupture in patients aged 40 years or older: An expected-value decision analysis. *Arthroscopy* 2008;24(8): 914-920.

8. Strum GM, Friedman MJ, Fox JM, et al: Acute anterior cruciate ligament reconstruction: Analysis of complications. *Clin Orthop Relat Res* 1990;(253): 184-189.

9. Harner CD, Irrgang JJ, Paul J, Dearwater S, Fu FH: Loss of motion after anterior cruciate ligament reconstruction. *Am J Sports Med* 1992;20(5):499-506.

10. Fisher SE, Shelbourne KD: Arthroscopic treatment of symptomatic extension block complicating anterior cruciate ligament reconstruction. *Am J Sports Med* 1993;21(4):558-564.

11. Sterett WI, Hutton KS, Briggs KK, Steadman JR: Decreased range of motion following acute versus chronic anterior cruciate ligament reconstruction. *Orthopedics* 2003;26(2):151-154.

12. Plancher KD, Steadman JR, Briggs KK, Hutton KS: Reconstruction of the anterior cruciate ligament in patients who are at least forty years old: A long-term follow-up and outcome study. *J Bone Joint Surg Am* 1998;80(2):184-197.

13. Deakon RT, Zarnett ME: ACL reconstruction in patients over 40 years of age using autogenous bone-patellar tendon-bone. *Arthroscopy* 1996;12(3):388.

14. Steadman JR: Anterior cruciate ligament reconstruction, in Feagin JA, Steadman JR, eds: *The Crucial Principles in Care of the Knee*. Philadelphia PA, Lippincott Williams & Wilkins, 2008, pp 117-128.

15. Stalzer S, Atkins J, Hagerman G: Rehabilitation principles, in Feagin JA, Steadman JR, eds: *The Crucial Principles in Care of the Knee*. Philadelphia, PA, Lippincott Williams & Wilkins, 2008, pp 203-219.

16. Steadman JR, Rodkey WG: The healing response technique: A minimally invasive procedure to stimulate healing of anterior cruciate ligament injuries using the microfracture technique, in Feagin JA, Steadman JR, eds: *The Crucial Principles in Care of the Knee*. Philadelphia PA, Lippincott Williams & Wilkins, 2008, pp 153-162.

17. Steadman JR, Cameron-Donaldson ML, Briggs KK, Rodkey WG: A minimally invasive technique ("healing response") to treat proximal ACL injuries in skeletally immature athletes. *J Knee Surg* 2006;19(1):8-13.

18. Rodkey WG, Arnoczky SP, Steadman JR: Healing of a surgically created partial detachment of the posterior cruciate ligament using marrow stimulation: An experimental study in dogs. *J Knee Surg* 2006;19(1):14-18.

19. Steadman JR, Dragoo JL, Hines SL, Briggs KK: Arthroscopic release for symptomatic scarring of the anterior interval of the knee. *Am J Sports Med* 2008;36(9):1763-1769.

20. Adams MA, Moore KD: Abstract: Intra-articular ACL reconstruction in the over 40-year-old patient. *Arthroscopy* 1995;11:374.

21. Barber FA, Elrod BF, McGuire DA, Paulos LE: Is an anterior cruciate ligament reconstruction outcome age dependent? *Arthroscopy* 1996;12(6):720-725.

22. Heier KA, Mack DR, Moseley JB, Paine R, Bocell JR: An analysis of anterior cruciate ligament reconstruction in middle-aged patients. *Am J Sports Med* 1997;25(4):527-532.

23. Viola R, Vianello R: Intra-articular ACL reconstruction in the over-40-year-old patient. *Knee Surg Sports Traumatol Arthrosc* 1999;7(1):25-28.

24. Brandsson S, Kartus J, Larsson J, Eriksson BI, Karlsson J: A comparison of results in middle-aged and young patients after anterior cruciate ligament reconstruction. *Arthroscopy* 2000;16(2):178-182.

25. Kuechle DK, Pearson SE, Beach WR, et al: Allograft anterior cruciate ligament reconstruction in patients over 40 years of age. *Arthroscopy* 2002;18(8):845-853.

26. Javernick MA, Potter BK, Mack A, Dekay KB, Murphy KP: Autologous hamstring anterior cruciate ligament reconstruction in patients older than 40. *Am J Orthop (Belle Mead NJ)* 2006;35(9):430-434.

Chapter 34
The Arthritic Patellofemoral Joint

Daniel Fulham O'Neill, MD, EdD

Key Points

- Arthritic changes of the patellofemoral joint develop in most people, and a substantial percentage of these knees become symptomatic.
- Since the early 1980s, the recommended treatment of patellofemoral pain has emphasized activity modification and specific exercise programs. This recommendation remains in effect today.
- Working with a knowledgeable trainer, physical therapist, or coach in all aspects of sports and exercise can often allow high levels of activity despite arthritic changes in the patellofemoral joint.
- Effective treatment can be as simple as correcting a flexion contracture or as complex as a revision total knee arthroplasty.
- Most patellofemoral pain can at least be lessened with a coordinated program of care.
- Isolated patellofemoral joint arthroplasty should be reserved for patients younger than 60 years with isolated patellofemoral disease.

Dr. O'Neill or an immediate family member is a member of a speakers' bureau or has made paid presentations on behalf of Ferring Pharmaceuticals.

Introduction

The patellofemoral joint has been the bane of active people and their physicians since well before the dawn of sports medicine. Similar to the lumbar spine, the patella, with its intricate array of static and dynamic components, seems to have a questionable design, as humans of all ages struggle with patellofemoral problems. In older athletes, however, osteoarthritis is the leading cause of patellofemoral pain.[1] In fact, studies have found that 50% to 80% of knees in individuals older than 60 years have some degree of osteoarthritis, although it is not always clinically significant.[2-4]

Determining whether the etiology of knee pain is overuse or osteoarthritis is not always easy to quantify. Although exercise is generally assumed to be good for joints and overall health, it is not clear how much exercise is beneficial, especially on already compromised joints. In one long-term Finnish study, signs of hip and knee osteoarthritis were evaluated in individuals who had been elite-level athletes in their youth and were now older than 60 years. Only team athletes (ie, participants in sports with a high percentage of knee injuries—soccer, hockey, basketball) had a greater degree of knee disability than a less athletic control group.[5] The endurance and track-and-field athletes actually had less knee and hip disability than did the control subjects. Given the many confounding factors (eg, general fitness), quantifying what is good for the knee and specifically what is healthy for the patellofemoral joint continues to be a work in progress.

Historical Perspective

The good news is that older athletes are playing sports and staying active in greater numbers.[6] The bad news is that, similar to the Finnish team-sports athletes, these activities are often being performed on already compromised joints. As a result, many of these patients seek medical attention in the hope of increasing activities that have been slowed by their knees. Many years ago, one of my mentors, Stan James, referred to the patellofemoral joint as the "black hole of orthopaedics," and so it remains today.[7] In the 1960s, baby boomers underwent the Elmslie-Trillat, Maquet, Hauser, and other procedures that were done with the best of intentions but not always based on the best science.[8] It is hoped that as this younger generation ages, they will benefit from a growing understanding of the anatomy, physiology, and biomechanics of the patellofemoral joint.

In 1954, DePalma wrote[9]:

Degenerative alterations of the osseous and the cartilaginous components of the knee joint and the synovialis occur naturally with advancing age, [T]hey increase in severity from decade to decade, and the changes are more pronounced in those areas subject to the greatest stresses, such as the articular surface of the patella.

When discussing treatment of chondromalacia of the patella, he wrote, "in the future patellar prostheses such as the one designed by D. C. McKeever will supplant all other operative procedures."[9]

In the 1970s, O'Donoghue[10] described three classes of patellar "malacia": (1) traumatic, (2) disturbance of rhythm of the patellar function, and (3) primary malacia. He went on to note:

Treatment of the knee having these conditions of the patella is surgical. True enough, the symptoms may be ameliorated somewhat by nonsurgical treatment but the future is bleak indeed since the defect in the patella remains and the

symptoms will promptly recur with resumption of activity.

Insall's *Surgery of the Knee*[11] was published in 1984. In those early days of sports medicine, a clear scientific sensibility was beginning to take shape with regard to thinking about the patellofemoral joint. When discussing disorders of the patella, Insall stated:

The patients are middle-aged or older and very seldom give a long history of knee pain beginning in adolescence. Rather, these patients usually have symptoms of relatively brief duration before presenting for examination, which typically indicates well-advanced changes of osteoarthritis.

Although multiple pages were devoted to some of the now-discredited surgical procedures alluded to previously, "conservative treatment" was first discussed. Under the category "usually helpful," Insall listed activity modification, knee braces, anti-inflammatory agents, orthoses, and, importantly, exercise, noting, "It is our experience that symptoms secondary to patellofemoral arthrosis respond best to exercise."

Anatomy and Physiology

With upward of two thirds of all people older than 60 years having some type of cartilage injury in the patellofemoral joint, this damage might be considered more physiologic than pathologic.[4,12] Most athletic movements take place from 20° to 40° of knee flexion, and many of our sports such as skiing, hiking, tennis, and cycling load the patella at even greater angles. As a result, it is no surprise that pain in this area can make it difficult to remain active.[13] Discussions of anatomic variations such as congruence and morphology are interesting and provide a better understanding of how the joint functions, but these are academic discussions and do not help patients get back to their desired activities.[14,15]

Perhaps most analogous to the shoulder, the patellofemoral joint is a sensitive design that depends on bony and soft-tissue balance for optimal function. Unlike the shoulder, however, the patellofemoral joint, being located in the middle of the lower extremity kinetic chain, is sensitive to abnormalities remote from the joint. The patella has a thick but uneven layer of articular cartilage that glides in the trochlear grove, the morphology of which varies from person to person.[16,17] Factors to be considered include alignment (especially varus/valgus); rotational issues stemming from the pelvis, hips, ankles, and the rest of the lower extremity; plus a person's natural bony asymmetry. The picture is complicated even without considering the soft-tissue restraints. The primary ligamentous stabilizers are the lateral patellofemoral ligament, the patellar tendon, and the recently well-described medial patellofemoral ligament.[18] The neuromuscular elements compromise the dynamic element of the patellofemoral joint. Finally, the importance of hip and other "core" musculature on the performance and subsequent pathology of the patellofemoral joint is beginning to be appreciated.

History and Physical Examination

History

The evaluation of the older athlete always begins with a proper history. This is described elsewhere in this book, so the discussion here is limited to the patellofemoral joint. The history and physical examination are more complicated than in the younger athlete because the older knee has had more years of use and possible abuse. Thus, in addition to previous injuries, years of asymmetric general wear and tear may have occurred.

It is imperative to obtain a clear history of injuries, surgeries, and activities and to understand the patient's plans for the future. Specific details about the patient's activities—whether at home, at work, in the gym, in the yard, or in other sports—should be elicited, with attention paid to any red flags that might signal knee abuse that might have simple solutions. For example, a patient who walks his or her dog up and down a hilly road that leads from the house might be advised to drive to a flatter area to walk the dog. Although this solution may be cumbersome, it might be all that is needed to alleviate much of the patient's pain. Reviewing any previous surgical notes or arthroscopic photographs can be especially useful. For example, arthroscopy would be unlikely to produce long-term relief in a knee in which grade III or IV patellofemoral changes were documented 5 years ago, despite present reports of mechanical symptoms.

One common and easily remedied cause of patellofemoral pain is abusive exercise routines, from open-chain knee extension exercises starting at 90° of knee flexion to plyometric jumps on a cement floor. Performing any exercise with the knee flexed beyond 45° should be discouraged, whether squatting, sled work, lunges, or knee extensions. The treating physician is encouraged to ask specifically about such activities during the history. Toward this end, masters athletes should consider an annual evaluation with a qualified personal trainer, coach, or physical therapist to check position and technique for their exercise routines. The athlete should find someone with solid background and experience in working with older athletes in that particular sport. The patient should be educated about periodization that includes cross-training, which avoids exposing joints to the same stresses week after week. If patients are using equipment at home, they should have the trainer come to the home to provide instruction. Many baby boomers are injured while using exercise equipment, and such preventive measures can be a simple and efficient way to keep them participating safely.

A pioneer in the treatment of patellofemoral joint disorders, Fulkerson[19] suggested asking the patient several questions to help lead to the often subtle diagnosis of patellofemoral pain: (1) describe the onset and the type of pain, (2) detail the association of pain with activity, and (3) point with one finger to the location of the pain. Although such questions appear on many knee history and physical examination forms, diagnosing patellofemoral joint disorders is challenging and often requires substantial clinical acumen and diagnostic skill. The more information the physician has at the end of the examination, the greater the chance of coordinating a positive outcome for these sometimes mysterious cases.

Finally, the patient should be asked what physical activity he or she hopes to participate in. Patients who plan to run a 100-km ultramarathon (as one of my 67-year-old patients recently announced) are going to be disappointed with the results of most treatment modalities and need to be counseled about realistic expectations early in the relationship.

Physical Examination

When examining the patellofemoral joint, it is important to examine all elements of the lower extremity kinetic chain, from the foot to the lumbar spine. During the physical examination, the clinician must always think anatomically and systematically to rule out each tissue as a source of pain: bone, cartilage, ligament, tendon, fascia, neurovascular structures, bursa, and skin. Even the brain, in terms of psychology, should be considered. (The psychology of the aging athlete is discussed in chapter 13.) Shoe wear should be evaluated, and the patient should be asked about the use of orthoses or other insoles. Such devices in masters athletes should be evaluated by a trained orthotist at least every 3 years but more often in runners or those who participate in other pounding sports.

The examination should begin with the patient standing. Functional testing should be routine and can be performed relatively quickly and efficiently. In addition to gait, single-leg balance, squatting, and duck-walking should be assessed. Balance and flexibility are two muscle qualities that are lost with aging and thus should be evaluated and discussed specifically with older athletes. Spine evaluation, including evaluation of range of motion (ROM) and scoliosis, is then performed while the patient is still standing. Leg-length assessment is performed with the patient standing, sitting, and supine, to differentiate between real and "virtual" limb-length discrepancies. Regardless of whether the discrepancy is real or virtual, however, it can be worthwhile to begin correction with a 1/4-in lift to see if the patient notes any clinical improvement. In more significant cases of limb-length discrepancy, hip radiographs or scanograms can be ordered. Patellofemoral pain can start anywhere in the kinetic chain and manifest at the knee.

For the next part of the examination, the patient is seated. Motion of the patella is evaluated with inspection and palpation. Maltracking (as evidenced by a positive J sign), crepitus, swelling, asymmetry, tibial alignment, scars, rashes, and other abnormalities are noted. This is also a good time to reevaluate the hips, ankles, and feet for ROM, strength, sensation, flexibility, and any other issues.

With the patient supine, a standard knee examination is performed. As with all knee symptoms, significant time is spent at the patellofemoral joint, as pathology here can masquerade as other problems. Inspection and palpation with active and passive motion will reveal the patellofemoral issue in the vast majority of patients.

Patellar position, tracking, and mobility, as well as apprehension, quadriceps tone, and pathology at the patellar tendon, fat pad, and tibial tubercle are assessed. Hypermobility and apprehension have clearly been shown to be related to knee pain.[20] Quantitative measurements of the quadriceps bulk and quadriceps angles (Q-angles) should be recorded.

Particular attention is given to ROM. Any limitation of hyperextension, especially when compared with the opposite knee (assuming it is without pathology), is a significant problem. Limitation of hyperextension is a red flag and should be treated aggressively to have any hope of a relatively symptom-free knee.[21] The patient should be educated about regaining motion using both passive and active stretches.[21,22] Many flexion contractures will respond to aggressive use of extension boards or other similar devices.

Ankle ROM and hip ROM are checked again with the patient supine. Although this rechecking might seem excessive, it can be accomplished quite quickly once it becomes habitual. Evaluating the entire lower extremity in numerous positions helps limit surprises. Hamstring flexibility was assessed during the functional testing. Quadriceps flexibility can now be evaluated, first with the patient on his or her side and then, if any issue is suspected, in the prone position. Like limited extension, decreased quadriceps flexibility can be related to patellofemoral pain.[23] Finally, rotational deformities of the femur, particularly when combined with weak hip internal rotation, can lead to increased lateral patellar loading and be a potential source of pain.[24,25]

In addition to a complete knee examination—and it should be noted that the preceding text is not meant to be a comprehensive discussion of a knee evaluation—examination for patellofemoral joint problems in an older athlete needs to involve more than just the knee. All aspects of the athlete's life and physiology must be considered. In some cases, simply regaining extension or making a change in activities will cure the problem. In the vast majority of older athletes, the diagnosis will contain some element of osteoarthritis. Therefore, even if malalignment is present, the treatment will probably differ from that for a teenage nonarthritic knee with a similar malalignment.

Radiographic Evaluation

Because most issues with the patellofemoral joint in elderly athletes are related to degeneration, plain radiographs are usually the only imaging studies needed for diagnosis and treatment planning. A standard protocol includes an AP weight-bearing view and a bilateral PA weight-bearing view at 45° of flexion. Significant joint space narrowing that is not appreciated on the AP view can be seen remarkably often on the PA view; this reflects damage to the distal posterior aspects of the femoral condyles. The lateral view is taken in full extension, ideally with the posterior aspects of the femoral condyles superimposed. Trochlear dysplasia can be determined on the lateral view by the crossing sign (the convergence of the trochlea and lateral femoral condyle).[26] Such dysplasia can lead to instability, malalignment, dislocation, and ultimately the breakdown of articular cartilage.[15] A bilateral Merchant view also is obtained.[4]

Other studies, such as bone scans,[27] MRI, and CT, have been used to assess the patellofemoral joint. Measurements such as the sulcus angle[4] and tibial tubercle–trochlear groove[28] offset have been used by many practitioners to guide treatment, but these measurements do not always give a clear picture of the patellofemoral joint in vivo.[29] In addition to evaluating for problems such as arthritic changes, loose bodies, and subluxation, this is also an excellent time to assess for osteopenia and begin a discussion with the patient regarding possible dual-energy x-ray absorptiometry (DEXA) scanning and other modalities to assess and potentially prevent osteoporosis.

Extensor Mechanism Injuries

Extensor mechanism injuries, whether due to quadriceps or patellar tendon ruptures, are more common in older age groups, causing most treatment protocols to be developed for "older athletes" by necessity. In a recent paper that examined motion after patella and quadriceps tendon repair in 50 patients injured during sports, the average age was 55 years.[30] Treatment of these masters athletes is no different from treatment of any other population; however, it is worthwhile to keep in mind the psychologic trauma the patient will endure through the loss of their normal physical activities[31] (see chapter 13). As a result, it is incumbent upon physicians

who treat older athletes to suggest alternative activities to maintain cardiovascular, musculoskeletal, and mental fitness during this time. Early mobilization is possible with the use of transosseous fixation; however, considerable healing and rehabilitation time is still required. It can be helpful to quantify the program as much as possible so that improvement—whether ROM, weight bearing, or strength gains—can be easily appreciated by the athlete.

Treatment of Patellofemoral Disorders

Footwear

As noted previously, the simplest of treatments, such as a change of footwear, can sometimes bring the patellofemoral joint into what has been described by Dye and Vaupel[6] as the "envelope of function." I am invariably told by patients when I point out their ancient footwear that "I just threw these on to come to this appointment." If that's the case, it should be easy to discard the shoes upon returning home! Although fashion-conscious teenagers may not comply when advised to change their footwear, adults should be encouraged to make sensible shoe choices. All athletes, especially those playing sports with cleated shoes that rarely have proper support, should "customize" their new shoes while still at the shoe store. Excellent off-the-shelf insoles are available, and a knowledgeable salesperson can be helpful. A lift can be fitted at the same time if a limb-length discrepancy has been diagnosed. Patients should be advised to not be in a hurry when buying shoes. They should buy later in the day, when the feet are larger, and take the time to carefully evaluate both shoes and insoles. The purchase of shoes over the Internet should be discouraged in patients who have orthopaedic issues.

When a patient has significant asymmetry or pes planus (pronation, navicular drop), calcaneal valgus, bunion, or other deformity, it may be more efficient to have the patient see a trained orthotist, ie, someone trained in shoe fitting and custom insole fabrication.[32] Orthotists have been vital to the development of a comfortable ski boot fit for many years and are useful for shoe fitting in all sports and physical activities, as well as work boots. Although orthoses have been recommended for many years to treat patellofemoral issues, their use has more "face validity" than data from a true prospective study.[33] The use of specific wedges, most commonly lateral heel wedges for varus knees, has a similar lack of research when addressing the knee joint.[34,35] Wedges are, however, relatively benign, inexpensive, and might be worthwhile in some patients, especially when combined with knee bracing.[35] It should be noted, however, that the American Academy of Orthopaedic Surgeons (AAOS) does not advocate the use of heel wedges for the treatment of knee osteoarthritis as there is a paucity of data to support or discourage their use.[36]

Canes, Crutches, and Walking Sticks

Although decidedly "low tech" and perhaps shunned by some patients, canes, crutches, and walking sticks can be used to decrease stress across the knee by the reduction of ground reaction forces and should be considered. The use of a cane in the hand opposite the painful knee has been shown to alleviate tibiofemoral joint pain and improve function in the patellofemoral joint as well, largely by shifting the center of gravity to the opposite limb.[35] The use of crutches, a walking stick, or hiking poles can have a similar effect. As has been noted repeatedly in this chapter, active older patients should be offered strategies to deal with their arthritis that allow them to continue their lifestyle with less pain. The use of a cane or crutches does not have to be an all-or-none proposition. By using a cane for an activity that may require a significant amount of standing and walking, such as traveling by plane, the patient might prevent irritation to the knee so that he or she can enjoy the activities planned for the following day. The use of hiking poles, especially on downhill sections, has become commonplace for active walkers of all ages. Adjustable-length hiking poles confer the additional advantage of allowing the patient to shorten or lengthen the pole height for uphill or downhill efforts, respectively.

Activity Modification and Physical Therapy

The discussion of a patient's activity profile is perhaps the most important aspect of the evaluation and treatment of patellofemoral pain in the older athlete.[37] The "intrinsic" issues in the older knee with osteoarthritis are less likely to be modifiable, but "extrinsic" variables, such as how much stress is placed across the joint in the course of the day, can be changed, as with walking aids. The difficulty is that each patient deals with a unique amount of pathology, and no one has a "pop-up timer" to know when to stop an activity.[21] Patients should attempt to quantify their activities so that they have some idea of the load they are putting on their knees. One simple rule that can be followed easily is that pain and swelling the next day means activity should be decreased. By making adjustments to the load, whether by decreasing the volume or decreasing the intensity, patients can often find a level of participation their knees can tolerate. Top athletes keep training logs to quantify their preparation; recreational masters athletes also can benefit from this tool. By reading a training log, the physician often can see where the athlete overstressed the joint, make adjustments for recovery, and provide notes to avoid such overload in the future. Training logs can be especially important for the patient coming back from injury, dealing with chronic disabilities, or recovering from surgery.[22]

Traditionally, the staple for treating any malady of the knee joint involved a physical therapy consult that emphasized quadriceps strengthening.[38-40] Ensuring a strong, contracted quadriceps with the knee fully extended is vital when performing quadriceps setting or leg-raising exercises. Having the patient manually feel the muscle and compare it with the unaffected leg can provide feedback that the exercise is being done correctly. As noted earlier, limiting knee flexion to 45° with any resistive exercises will usually allow strengthening without irritation. Most patients can get to this angle without encountering crepitus from the patellofemoral joint.

As knowledge has been gained in the field of knee mechanics and rehabilitation, flexibility, hamstring strength, hip strength, attention to other "core" musculature, and aerobic conditioning also have been shown to be potentially useful in both treating and possibly avoiding patellofemoral pain and injury.[21,41-43] Initial strengthening should begin with closed-chain exercises (ie, the foot firmly planted on the ground or a firm surface), as cocontraction from the antagonist muscle group (hamstrings) can be protective and less painful than open-chain exercises. By using more physiologic loading during closed-chain motions, the patella is thought to have more contact in the trochlea, resulting in the distribution of force over a greater area.[44] Hip involvement in patellofemoral pain has received significant research attention. Weakness in abduction and external hip rotators is thought to predispose to lateral patellar tracking.[42,45] Gains in hip external rotation and abduction strength appear to benefit not only the patellofemoral joint but also can globally improve knee pain as the kinetic chain is strengthened proximally.[46,47] Whether hip weakness is a result or a cause of knee pain is not known, but certainly studies point to the hip and other core musculature as being important in any patellofemoral rehabilitation.[48,49]

Spending time discussing "soft" workouts can be exceedingly valuable for the elderly patient population. Some patients will respond only to their doctor's encouragement to stop running or participating in other high-impact activities. Although patients may not stop entirely, most will at least compromise and do some "running" workouts in water or use a bike. For patients to enjoy cycling or any new activity, they must have the right equipment and be adequately coached. The patient should see a knowledgeable person for a proper bike fit. Adjusting the seat approximately 2 cm higher than the ideal cycling position initially will decrease irritation of the knee by decreasing knee flexion and motion arc while the patient is learning proper pedaling and riding techniques. This can also be an opportune time to impress upon the athlete that resistive exercise is vital for maintaining muscle and bone mass. A resistive or weight-training program developed with a professional can also help keep tendons and other connective tissues strong enough to participate in golf, tennis, skiing, and other recreational activities.[50]

Weight loss is perhaps both the simplest and the most difficult way to reduce stress on the knee. Although being told they are overweight is not news to most patients, it can be useful to point out the significant decrease in irritation to the knee that is realized with even limited weight loss. Although walking on level ground causes little stress across the patellofemoral joint because the patella is not engaged firmly in the trochlea, stair climbing can place stress equivalent to three to four times body weight on the joint; getting up from a chair can represent eight times body weight.[14] Because load across the patellofemoral joint is directly related to weight, weight loss can mean an exponential decrease in forces and potential pain over the course of the day. Although the literature on weight loss and diet is confusing at best, encouraging fitness (ie, improved strength, coordination, balance, endurance, flexibility, and quickness) is part of the responsibilities of medical caregivers and will often lead to losing weight.[20,22] Moreover, one study found that osteoarthritis of the knee was associated with falls and resulting hip fractures.[2] Although this study was done in an elderly, nonathletic population, gaining muscle qualities such as balance and flexibility through exercise can have far-reaching positive effects on one's life.

In summary, making changes in the exercise program is key for long-term improvement of patellofemoral problems. Many athletes focus on the technique of their sport, but it is also important that they examine training routines for issues that might aggravate the patellofemoral joint or other parts of their anatomy, such as the lumbar spine. Patients should be encouraged to fine-tune all of their training with the help of a physical therapist, trainer, coach, or other expert who can give feedback and evaluate technique. In other words, the patient should not resume prior routines after the knee symptoms subside. Ultimately, doctors, physical therapists, and athletic trainers only serve as guides. The patient is the one who must make the changes and put in the work to improve and hopefully avoid injury. Although many of these masters athletes have been training and exercising for many years and understand what an exercise program should look like, they are seeking medical advice because they are now in pain, so the clinician's job is to break this cycle of abuse. A visit to a physical therapist is often the first step. In addition, during the office visit, the patient should be provided with exercises and guidance to begin the process of rehabilitation and decreasing inflammation.

Anti-Inflammatory Drugs and Injections

Oral joint health supplements such as glucosamine and chondroitin have been widely available for many years as treatments of osteoarthritis.[51] The literature on this subject is confusing and is discussed in more detail in chapter 5. Because of their ready availability and what is thought to be a minimal "downside," oral joint health supplements should at least be considered and understood, as many patients will have questions regarding their use.

Nonsteroidal anti-inflammatory drugs (NSAIDs) such as ibuprofen and naproxen have been a mainstay of osteoarthritis management for decades but have well-known drawbacks. Gastrointestinal issues are seen in a significant percentage of long-term users of these medications and often lead to bleeding and toxicity.[52] The hope was that the cyclooxygenase-2 (COX-2) selective inhibitors such as celecoxib would obviate many of these problems, but concerns regarding cardiovascular complications have arisen. Although gastrointestinal issues have decreased, questions about the safety of COX-2 selective inhibitors still remain, and, as with any long-term medication, these drugs must be used with caution and be monitored closely.

A certain mystery surrounds the mechanism of corticosteroid injections, particularly with a joint that is not obviously swollen or otherwise inflamed; however, they continue to be used daily in orthopaedic offices. Aside from the effect of corticosteroids on synovial vasodilation and vascular permeability, part of their effectiveness may be due to the aspiration of irritating intra-articular enzymes and the postinjection instructions, which instruct the patient to avoid aggressive movements for 3 to 5 days, apply ice to the knee, take a short course of an NSAID such as ibuprofen, and then slowly return to activity, often with the guidance of a physical therapist. Many patients report immediate improvement in pain, but perhaps it is the entire program that helps these patients feel better over time.

Because of the problems that can arise from long-term use of NSAIDs, injection therapy can be a safer approach for many patients. Hyaluronic acid injections have been found to be safe and effective for many athletes dealing with patellofemoral problems,[52-54] one to five injections are recommended, depending on the formulation (or product). As with all treatments for patellofemoral pain, patient selection is vital.[55] I do not recommend hyaluronic acid injections until the patient has achieved rehabilitation goals of close to normal ROM, especially in extension, and improved quadriceps flexibility and tone.[56] Injection of corticosteroid concomitant with the initial hyaluronate injection may have a synergistic effect, immediately decreasing inflammation and pain. After the injections of hyaluro-

nate, patients are again advised to follow the postinjection instructions, particularly after the first injection, to try to avoid any potential inflammatory reaction.

Taping, Sleeves, and Braces

Patellar taping is another modality commonly used by physical therapists that has shown promising results in some patients, although no study has looked specifically at older patients.[57] As with other alignment adjustments, the concept is to increase the surface area of contact, thereby decreasing loading of painful arthritic points. Although similar improvements in pain have not been seen when patients themselves do the taping, taping can be viewed in the same light as many other temporary modalities. Achieving a temporary reduction in patellofemoral joint symptoms, whether for days, weeks, or months, allows treatment that may result in longer term gains in flexibility, strength, and other muscle qualities.

The use of knee sleeves, with or without metal hinges and with or without patella-stabilizing straps, is a treatment that physicians appear to have tried without a great deal of supporting data.[34] If a patient is having chronic effusions, using a soft compression sleeve can be helpful, along with other anti-inflammatory measures such as ice, NSAIDs, or injections. These sleeves, which are sized to the patient, are pulled on in the morning and are usually well tolerated. For knees that are inflamed enough that there is an element of quadriceps inhibition, these sleeves provide a sense of security and "stability" that can make activities that do not involve high angles of knee flexion more pleasant. Sleeves with metal stays are generally not recommended for patellofemoral pain because these can shift position and potentially exacerbate the problem.

Specific patellar bracing that directs a force, most often medially, on the patella can be of use in some patients, especially those with symptoms of patellar instability.[19] The patient should think of this brace not necessarily as keeping the knee in place but as another item in the "education" of the patellofemoral joint, in addition to exercises and physical therapy.

Most unloading hinged braces are directed at misalignments of the tibiofemoral joint, not the patellofemoral joint, but of course they could have an effect on patellofemoral joint mechanics.[35] These braces are generally tolerated only by knees of certain shapes, despite custom fitting. Ramsey et al[58] suggests that less expensive, neutrally aligned hinged braces can provide some benefit for medial compartment disease.

Arthroscopy and Lateral Release

Arthroscopic surgery with or without articular cartilage stimulation in the treatment of knee osteoarthritis has been highly controversial since the report published by Moseley et al[59] in 2002 that showed no significant differences among knees treated with placebo surgery, arthroscopic lavage, and arthroscopic débridement. Although this study has been criticized for its methodologic flaws and did not specifically address patients with isolated patellofemoral arthrosis, the conclusions drawn should apply. Other studies have shown, perhaps not surprisingly, that patients with at least 3 mm of tibiofemoral joint space (ie, less severe osteoarthritis) have better outcomes after arthroscopy than do patients with more severe disease.[60] Again, as with any surgical procedure treating the wide range of pathology found in the patellofemoral joint, patient selection is paramount.[34] Patients with mechanical symptoms, such as those due to an unstable flap of cartilage or loose body, and no significant grade IV lesions should respond well to arthroscopic débridement.[60]

Lateral retinacular release for patellofemoral disease has a similarly confusing history, as historically this procedure was done without sufficient regard to the anatomy and pathology.[19] It has become clear that this can be an effective procedure for a sagittally aligned but tilted patella with isolated lateral patella facet arthrosis, as decompression of the mechanical loads on an already compromised area may result in symptomatic relief.

Autologous Chondrocyte Implantation and Other Cartilage Procedures

Autologous chondrocyte implantation (ACI) is an exciting technology, but most older athletes do not have isolated lesions that would be amenable to this operation. One recent study that looked at the outcomes of the procedure when it was used for lesions specifically in the patellofemoral joint showed promising results, but the patients were young (mean age, 31.2 years), with the oldest patient only 55 years.[61] Not surprisingly, isolated lesions fared better than multiple lesions and traumatic

lesions did better than degenerative lesions, and results deteriorated over time. In another multicenter study looking specifically at trochlear lesions, the conclusion was that ACI is a good procedure for "young to middle-aged" patients.

Isolated (ie, without concomitant osteotomy) microfracture, ACI, and mosaicplasty procedures all have been used for the patellofemoral joint, but the results have been guarded in all patients and must be considered particularly unpredictable in older athletes.[62-64] At best, these patients should be prepared for a less than excellent outcome, even if they adhere to a long postoperative program of crutches, passive motion, and limited activities.

Realignment Procedures

Most knees that undergo total knee arthroplasty (TKA) need some form of realignment; this is additional evidence that malalignment is a risk factor in the development of arthrosis.[65] A detailed discussion of malalignment etiologies such as trochlear dysplasia is beyond the scope of this chapter. It is clear, however, that there is a connection between dysplasia and patellar instability and, concomitantly, between instability and osteoarthritis. In fact, dysplasia is not always solely related to the knee but can be due to hip and femoral torsion.[25]

Although realignment procedures have a checkered history, in theory, a patient with isolated patellofemoral osteoarthritis and pain due to malalignment should respond to a tibial tubercle transfer or other realignment procedure.[66] The trick is making sure (1) that the osteoarthritis is isolated to the patellofemoral joint and (2) that the tibiofemoral compartments are not also overloaded and thus will soon become arthritic.[14] Again, because the knee is a dynamic system, static measurements of alignment will not always coincide with symptoms, and thus a detailed picture of the anatomy and biomechanics of the patient's knee must be clear before proceeding with these formidable operations.[7]

One of the main issues with misalignment is defining what qualifies as pathologic alignment, as many variations of alignment can be considered "normal." As with scoliosis, pes planus, and many other orthopaedic conditions, knee alignment can vary widely without being deemed pathologic unless a thorough evaluation of the entire kinetic chain reveals problems.[65] A patellofemoral joint that can perform the activities required of it without pain or swelling should be the goal, not meeting specific clinical or radiologic criteria. This is not to say that lateral patellar displacement and other malalignment are not significantly associated with cartilage lesions in some cases.[15] Similarly, femoral anteversion has been related to adult patellofemoral pain.[24] Most studies have been performed with younger patients; consequently, interventions such as osteotomies that might be effective for patients younger than 40 years might not be appropriate for the older athlete with more comorbidity and less plasticity.[34,67] In theory, a tibial tubercle transfer will unload the damaged lateral and distal portions of the patella toward the less diseased cartilage. Unfortunately, in older knees, the risk is that the resulting forces will be placed on already compromised cartilage (ie, proximal and medial).[28] As a result, without concomitant patellar instability, a tibial tubercle transfer, even when combined with a cartilage restoration procedure, is rarely indicated in the older athlete.[19]

Patellofemoral Arthroplasty

As noted previously, isolated patellofemoral joint arthroplasty has been in the knee surgeon's armamentarium for many years.[9] Unfortunately, results have been mixed at best. Longer term follow-up and new outcomes instruments, however, have helped quantify results of patellofemoral arthroplasty. Most of these studies included a relatively small number of patients, resulting in a narrow list of indications for this procedure.

One recent retrospective study from Utukuri et al[68] looked at 17 patients who underwent patellofemoral arthroplasty, 16 of whom were women. All results were good or excellent at a mean follow-up of 52.5 months, with a mean Knee Osteoarthritis Outcome Score (KOOS) of 57.4% (with 100% indicating no knee problems) for function in sports and recreation. Another report by Kooijman et al[69] showed similar long-term results. In this study, 51 patients with a mean age of 50 years were treated with a Richards prosthesis (Smith & Nephew, Memphis, TN). The mean follow-up was 17 years. Although the reoperation rate was greater than 20%, 86% of the patients eventually had a good or excellent result. Loosening was rare, and ROM was excellent. Once again, determining that the patient had isolated patellofemoral disease was the most difficult issue.[69]

A 2005 study from France reported on unilateral patellofemoral arthroplasty performed in 66 patients, 9 of whom died of unrelated causes.[70] In the 57 living patients, revision was required in 14 for tibiofemoral osteoarthritis at a mean of 7.3 years and in 11 for loosening at a mean of 4.5 years. Of the 29 patients with prostheses that survived to follow-up at the 16-year mark, 21 had no knee pain. Along with the risk of arthritic progression in other parts of the knee, the authors warn against this procedure in cases of patellofemoral malalignment and patients with previous patellar fractures. These authors suggest this procedure for patients younger than 60 years who meet their criteria.

Like osteotomies done for malalignment, patellofemoral arthroplasty achieves good results if done in the setting of isolated patellofemoral osteoarthritis, as the main reason for failure is pain in other parts of the knee. In elderly athletes, isolated disease tends to be the exception, so this procedure should probably be reserved for those toward the "middle age" of the masters athlete spectrum (ie, younger than 60 years).[71] Also, no study has been large enough to provide reliable data regarding how active these patients can safely be after this procedure. Because of the significant complication rate, patellofemoral arthroplasty should be considered predominantly a temporizing measure to treat knee osteoarthritis on the road to probable TKA.[72]

Leadbetter et al[73] compiled a list of contraindications to patellofemoral arthroplasty gleaned from an analysis of numerous studies. In addition to the previously discussed issues of tibiofemoral arthrosis, malalignment, and limited nonsurgical care, the authors added multiple other conditions that could adversely affect outcome, such as obesity, male sex, quadriceps atrophy, and unrealistic patient expectations.

Ultimately, patellofemoral arthroplasty is an operation that should be performed as a last resort in a patient ideally between the ages of 40 and 60 years by someone with significant experience in all aspects of patellofemoral joint surgery. For the older athlete, TKA is still the treatment of choice. Regardless of the procedure—whether TKA or patellofemoral arthroplasty—

returning to aggressive athletic activities cannot be recommended with confidence. (For additional discussion of athletic activity after joint arthroplasty, see chapter 27.)

Total Knee Arthroplasty

No large studies have quantified the activity level of older athletes with TKA; thus, most recommendations are based on the personal experience of the surgeon.[37] TKA is the gold standard and the most common surgical choice for advanced patellofemoral athrosis.[73,74] The main goal of knee arthroplasty is to allow activities of daily living to be performed without pain, but baby boomers with TKAs are "pushing the envelope," engaging in aggressive activities despite the lack of complete consensus in the medical community regarding which activities are recommended.[50] Traditionally, aggressive cutting and jumping sports such as basketball, running, soccer, and racket sports were not recommended.[50,75] Interestingly, Jackson et al[76] reported that although golfers had relief of pain after TKA, most still chose to use a cart while playing, thus mitigating some of the potential health benefits of this activity. Deciding which sports and activities should be recommended and which not recommended will no doubt be a major topic as the population ages, prosthetic designs evolve, and more and more primary and revision TKAs are performed.

Conclusions

Baby boomers and those older than 65 years are increasingly heeding the call to become more active. Unfortunately, sometimes this increased activity involves more than just fitness and leads to participation in sports that have an inherently high risk of injuries. In addition, most of the population will develop osteoarthritis of the patellofemoral joint. Knee pain, much of which is patellofemoral in origin, whether in athletes or the general population, has been shown to be a barrier to a healthy life. Knee pain also has been found to be a significant factor in the risk of falling. Thus, not only can such pain be an issue regarding sports participation, but it could be a factor in further injury. Furthermore, severe knee pain is related to loss of mobility, and any such limitation in the elderly is associated with multiple physical and psychologic problems.[77]

As knowledge about the patellofemoral joint increases, the question becomes whether that knowledge can be translated into ways to alleviate pain and avoid future injury. Cartilage has little regenerative potential in any age group, but especially in the older athlete. Although understanding of the etiology of patellofemoral osteoarthritis has improved, effective treatment of the end result—osteoarthritis—is lacking. Therefore, these masters athletes and their treating physicians must be especially respectful of the biology of cartilage degeneration when planning for the future. Should aggressive realignment or other procedures be considered in patients with high activity profiles but no symptoms? Would it be reasonable to limit a young person's activities based on what is expected to happen to the joint 20 or 30 years hence? Certainly, it would be easier if cartilage restoration technology improved to the point where surgeons could wait until lesions developed before undertaking a significant surgery.

The underlying problem continues to be lack of understanding of the etiology of specific pathologies. Perhaps future imaging technology will be able to evaluate patients as they climb stairs, ski, and run, to provide a dynamic picture of what happens in the patellofemoral joint. That would allow the tailoring of rehabilitation or surgical procedures to a specific problem. As is true in the treatment of virtually all conditions, patient selection is the key to success.

Dye and Vaupel[6] opined in 1994 that "The principles of treatment in most patients with patellofemoral pain consist of protection of sensitive tissues from excessive loading, appropriate anti-inflammatory therapy, and nonirritating rehabilitation." Certainly, despite the research and advances since that statement was made, this is still the best initial approach to these patients.

Although prevention of patellofemoral osteoarthritis is rarely possible once the older athlete presents with knee symptoms, the treating physician can counsel the patient on how to live with a deteriorating joint while remaining active and engaged. Perhaps equally important is the discussion with senior patients that issues such as osteoarthritis and osteoporosis can be diseases that start in the teenage years. Educating the dedicated and energetic master athlete on the care of the musculoskeletal system is vital so that this knowledge can be passed on, hopefully so that future generations can avoid such damage.

References

1. Leveille SG, Jones RN, Kiely DK, et al: Chronic musculoskeletal pain and the occurrence of falls in an older population. *JAMA* 2009;302(20):2214-2221.

2. Arden NK, Crozier S, Smith H, et al: Knee pain, knee osteoarthritis, and the risk of fracture. *Arthritis Rheum* 2006;55(4):610-615.

3. Lamb SE, Guralnik JM, Buchner DM, et al: Factors that modify the association between knee pain and mobility limitation in older women: The Women's Health and Aging Study. *Ann Rheum Dis* 2000; 59(5):331-337.

4. Davies AP, Vince AS, Shepstone L, Donell ST, Glasgow MM: The radiologic prevalence of patellofemoral osteoarthritis. *Clin Orthop Relat Res* 2002;(402):206-212.

5. Kettunen JA, Kujala UM, Kaprio JK, Koskenvuo M, Sarna S: Lower-limb function among former elite male athletes. *Am J Sports Med* 2001;29(1):2-8.

6. Dye SF, Vaupel GL: The pathophysiology of patellofemoral pain. *Sports Med Arthrosc Rev* 1994;2(3):203-210.

7. Dye SF: Patellofemoral pain current concepts: An overview. *Sports Med Arthrosc Rev* 2001;9(4):264-272.

8. Rutherford GW Jr, Schroeder TJ: *Sports-Related Injuries to Persons 65 Years of Age and Older*. Washington, DC, US Consumer Product Safety Commission, 1998.

9. DePalma AF: *Diseases of the Knee: Management in Medicine and Surgery*. Philadelphia, PA, JB Lippincott Co, 1954.

10. O'Donoghue DH: *Treatment of Injuries to Athletes*. Philadelphia, PA, WB Saunders Company, 1976.

11. Insall JN: *Surgery of Knee*. New York, NY, Churchill Livingstone Inc, 1984.

12. Saleh KJ, Arendt EA, Eldridge J, Fulkerson JP, Minas T, Mulhall KJ: Symposium: Operative treatment of patellofemoral arthritis. *J Bone Joint Surg Am* 2005; 87(3):659-671.

13. Ruffin MT V, Kiningham RB: Anterior knee pain: The challenge of patellofemoral syndrome. *Am Fam Physician* 1993;47(1):185-194.

14. Grelsamer RP, Dejour D, Gould J: The pathophysiology of patellofemoral arthritis. *Orthop Clin North Am* 2008;39(3):269-274.

15. Yang B, Tan H, Yang L, Dai G, Guo B: Correlating anatomy and congruence of the patellofemoral joint with cartilage lesions. *Orthopedics* 2009;32(1):20.

16. Stäubli HU, Dürrenmatt U, Porcellini B, Rauschning W: Anatomy and surface geometry of the patellofemoral joint in the axial plane. *J Bone Joint Surg Br* 1999;81(3):452-458.

17. Kwak SD, Colman WW, Ateshian GA, Grelsamer RP, Henry JH, Mow VC: Anatomy of the human patellofemoral joint articular cartilage: Surface curvature analysis. *J Orthop Res* 1997;15(3):468-472.

18. Bicos J, Fulkerson JP, Amis A: Current concepts review: The medial patellofemoral ligament. *Am J Sports Med* 2007;35(3):484-492.

19. Fulkerson JP: Diagnosis and treatment of patients with patellofemoral pain. *Am J Sports Med* 2002;30(3): 447-456.

20. Witvrouw E, Lysens R, Bellemans J, Cambier D, Vanderstraeten G: Intrinsic risk factors for the development of anterior knee pain in an athletic population: A two-year prospective study. *Am J Sports Med* 2000;28(4):480-489.

21. Weng MC, Lee CL, Chen CH, et al: Effects of different stretching techniques on the outcomes of isokinetic exercise in patients with knee osteoarthritis. *Kaohsiung J Med Sci* 2009;25(6):306-315.

22. O'Neill DF: *Knee Surgery: The Essential Guide to Total Knee Recovery*. New York, NY, St. Martin's Press, 2008.

23. Witvrouw E, Lysens R, Bellemans J, Peers K, Vanderstraeten G: Open versus closed kinetic chain exercises for patellofemoral pain: A prospective, randomized study. *Am J Sports Med* 2000;28(5): 687-694.

24. Lee TQ, Anzel SH, Bennett KA, Pang D, Kim WC: The influence of fixed rotational deformities of the femur on the patellofemoral contact pressures in human cadaver knees. *Clin Orthop Relat Res* 1994; (302):69-74.

25. Eckhoff DG, Montgomery WK, Kilcoyne RF, Stamm ER: Femoral morphometry and anterior knee pain. *Clin Orthop Relat Res* 1994;(302):64-68.

26. Grelsamer RP, Tedder JL: The lateral trochlear sign: Femoral trochlear dysplasia as seen on a lateral view roentgenograph. *Clin Orthop Relat Res* 1992;(281): 159-162.

27. Dye SF, Chew MH: The use of scintigraphy to detect increased osseous metabolic activity about the knee. *J Bone Joint Surg Am* 1993;75(9):1388-1406.

28. Colvin AC, West RV: Patellar instability. *J Bone Joint Surg Am* 2008;90(12):2751-2762.

29. Smith TO, Davies L, Toms AP, Hing CB, Donell ST: The reliability and validity of radiological assessment for patellar instability: A systematic review and meta-analysis. *Skeletal Radiol* 2011;40(4):399-414.

30. West JL, Keene JS, Kaplan LD: Early motion after quadriceps and patellar tendon repairs: Outcomes with single-suture augmentation. *Am J Sports Med* 2008; 36(2):316-323.

31. Jones EA, McBeth J, Nicholl BA, et al: What characterizes persons who do not report musculoskeletal pain? Results from a 4-year population-based longitudinal study (the Epifund study). *J Rheumatol* 2009;36(5):1071-1077.

32. Tiberio D: The effect of excessive subtalar joint pronation on patellofemoral mechanics: A theoretical model. *J Orthop Sports Phys Ther* 1987;9(4):160-165.

33. Insall J: "Chondromalacia patellae": Patellar malalignment syndrome. *Orthop Clin North Am* 1979;10(1):117-127.

34. Richmond J, Hunter D, Irrgang J, et al: Treatment of osteoarthritis of the knee (nonarthroplasty). *J Am Acad Orthop Surg* 2009;17(9):591-600.

35. Gross KD, Hillstrom HJ: Noninvasive devices targeting the mechanics of osteoarthritis. *Rheum Dis Clin North Am* 2008;34(3):755-776.

36. American Academy of Orthopaedic Surgeons: Clinical Practice Guideline on Treatment of Osteoarthritis of the Knee (non-arthroplasty). Rosemont, IL, American Academy of Orthopaedic Surgeons. http://www.aaos. org/Research/guidelines/OAKguideline.pdf.

37. Best TM, Hart L: A growing concern: the older athlete. *Clin J Sport Med* 2008;18(6):477-478.

38. Fithian DC, Powers CM, Khan N: Rehabilitation of the knee after medial patellofemoral ligament reconstruction. *Clin Sports Med* 2010;29(2):283-290.

39. Syme G, Rowe P, Martin D, Daly G: Disability in patients with chronic patellofemoral pain syndrome: A randomised controlled trial of VMO selective training versus general quadriceps strengthening. *Man Ther* 2009;14(3):252-263.

40. Kannus P, Natri A, Paakkala T, Järvinen M: An outcome study of chronic patellofemoral pain syndrome: Seven-year follow-up of patients in a randomized, controlled trial. *J Bone Joint Surg Am* 1999;81(3):355-363.

41. Boling MC, Padua DA, Marshall SW, Guskiewicz K, Pyne S, Beutler A: A prospective investigation of biomechanical risk factors for patellofemoral pain syndrome: The Joint Undertaking to Monitor and Prevent ACL Injury (JUMP-ACL) cohort. *Am J Sports Med* 2009;37(11):2108-2116.

42. Nakagawa TH, Muniz TB, Baldon Rde M, Dias Maciel C, de Menezes Reiff RB, Serrão FV: The effect of additional strengthening of hip abductor and lateral rotator muscles in patellofemoral pain syndrome: A randomized controlled pilot study. *Clin Rehabil* 2008;22(12):1051-1060.

43. Okada T, Huxel KC, Nesser TW: Relationship between core stability, functional movement, and performance. *J Strength Cond Res* 2011;25(1):252-261.

44. Besier TF, Draper CE, Gold GE, Beaupré GS, Delp SL: Patellofemoral joint contact area increases with knee flexion and weight-bearing. *J Orthop Res* 2005; 23(2):345-350.

45. Baldon Rde M, Nakagawa TH, Muniz TB, Amorim CF, Maciel CD, Serrão FV: Eccentric hip muscle function in females with and without patellofemoral pain syndrome. *J Athl Train* 2009;44(5):490-496.

46. Bennell KL, Hunt MA, Wrigley TV, et al: Hip strengthening reduces symptoms but not knee load in people with medial knee osteoarthritis and varus malalignment: A randomised controlled trial. *Osteoarthritis Cartilage* 2010;18(5):621-628.

47. Sled EA, Khoja L, Deluzio KJ, Olney SJ, Culham EG: Effect of a home program of hip abductor exercises on knee joint loading, strength, function, and pain in people with knee osteoarthritis: A clinical trial. *Phys Ther* 2010;90(6):895-904.

48. Hinman RS, Hunt MA, Creaby MW, Wrigley TV, McManus FJ, Bennell KL: Hip muscle weakness in individuals with medial knee osteoarthritis. *Arthritis Care Res (Hoboken)* 2010;62(8):1190-1193.

49. Willson JD, Binder-Macleod S, Davis IS: Lower extremity jumping mechanics of female athletes with and without patellofemoral pain before and after exertion. *Am J Sports Med* 2008;36(8):1587-1596.

50. American Academy of Family Physicians, American Academy of Orthopaedic Surgeons, American College of Sports Medicine, et al: Selected issues for the master athlete and the team physician: A consensus statement. *Med Sci Sports Exerc* 2010;42(4):820-833.

51. DiNubile NA: A potential role for avocado- and soybean-based nutritional supplements in the management of osteoarthritis: A review. *Phys Sportsmed* 2010;38(2):71-81.

52. Bert JM, Gasser SI: Approach to the osteoarthritic knee in the aging athlete: Debridement to osteotomy. *Arthroscopy* 2002;18(9, Suppl 2)107-110.

53. Kirchner M, Marshall D: A double-blind randomized controlled trial comparing alternate forms of high molecular weight hyaluronan for the treatment of osteoarthritis of the knee. *Osteoarthritis Cartilage* 2006;14(2):154-162.

54. Bellamy N, Campbell J, Robinson V, Gee T, Bourne R, Wells G: Viscosupplementation for the treatment of osteoarthritis of the knee. *Cochrane Database Syst Rev* 2006;2:CD005321.

55. Briem K, Axe MJ, Snyder-Mackler L: Functional and perceived response to intra-articular hyaluronan injection in patients with knee osteoarthritis: Persistence of treatment effects over 5 months. *Knee Surg Sports Traumatol Arthrosc* 2009;17(7):763-769.

56. Migliore A, Granata M: Intra-articular use of hyaluronic acid in the treatment of osteoarthritis. *Clin Interv Aging* 2008;3(2):365-369.

57. Warden SJ, Hinman RS, Watson MA Jr, Avin KG, Bialocerkowski AE, Crossley KM: Patellar taping and bracing for the treatment of chronic knee pain: A systematic review and meta-analysis. *Arthritis Rheum* 2008;59(1):73-83.

58. Ramsey DK, Briem K, Axe MJ, Snyder-Mackler L: A mechanical theory for the effectiveness of bracing for medial compartment osteoarthritis of the knee. *J Bone Joint Surg Am* 2007;89(11):2398-2407.

59. Moseley JB, O'Malley K, Petersen NJ, et al: A controlled trial of arthroscopic surgery for osteoarthritis of the knee. *N Engl J Med* 2002;347(2):81-88.

60. Aaron RK, Skolnick AH, Reinert SE, Ciombor DM: Arthroscopic débridement for osteoarthritis of the knee. *J Bone Joint Surg Am* 2006;88(5):936-943.

61. Gobbi A, Kon E, Berruto M, et al: Patellofemoral full-thickness chondral defects treated with second-generation autologous chondrocyte implantation: Results at 5 years' follow-up. *Am J Sports Med* 2009; 37(6):1083-1092.

62. Saris DB, Vanlauwe J, Victor J, et al: Treatment of symptomatic cartilage defects of the knee: Characterized chondrocyte implantation results in better clinical outcome at 36 months in a randomized trial compared to microfracture. *Am J Sports Med* 2009;37(1, Suppl 1)10S-19S.

63. Pascual-Garrido C, Slabaugh MA, L'Heureux DR, Friel NA, Cole BJ: Recommendations and treatment outcomes for patellofemoral articular cartilage defects with autologous chondrocyte implantation: Prospective evaluation at average 4-year follow-up. *Am J Sports Med* 2009;37(1, Suppl 1)33S-41S.

64. Van Assche D, Van Caspel D, Vanlauwe J, et al: Physical activity levels after characterized chondrocyte implantation versus microfracture in the knee and the relationship to objective functional outcome with 2-year follow-up. *Am J Sports Med* 2009;37(1, Suppl 1): 42S-49S.

65. Arendt E: Anatomy and malalignment of the patellofemoral joint: Its relation to patellofemoral arthrosis. *Clin Orthop Relat Res* 2005;(436):71-75.

66. Rue JP, Colton A, Zare SM, et al: Trochlear contact pressures after straight anteriorization of the tibial tuberosity. *Am J Sports Med* 2008;36(10):1953-1959.

67. O'Neill DF, James SL: Valgus osteotomy with anterior cruciate ligament laxity. *Clin Orthop Relat Res* 1992; (278):153-159.

68. Utukuri MM, Khanduja V, Somayaji HS, Dowd GS: Patient-based outcomes in patellofemoral arthroplasty. *J Knee Surg* 2008;21(4):269-274.

69. Kooijman HJ, Driessen AP, van Horn JR: Long-term results of patellofemoral arthroplasty: A report of 56 arthroplasties with 17 years of follow-up. *J Bone Joint Surg Br* 2003;85(6):836-840.

70. Argenson JN, Flecher X, Parratte S, Aubaniac JM: Patellofemoral arthroplasty: An update. *Clin Orthop Relat Res* 2005;440:50-53.

71. Ackroyd CE, Chir B: Development and early results of a new patellofemoral arthroplasty. *Clin Orthop Relat Res* 2005;(436):7-13.

72. Lonner JH: Patellofemoral arthroplasty. *J Am Acad Orthop Surg* 2007;15(8):495-506.

73. Leadbetter WB, Ragland PS, Mont MA: The appropriate use of patellofemoral arthroplasty: An analysis of reported indications, contraindications, and failures. *Clin Orthop Relat Res* 2005;(436):91-99.

74. Dalury DF: Total knee replacement for patellofemoral disease. *J Knee Surg* 2005;18(4):274-277.

75. Healy WL, Iorio R, Lemos MJ: Athletic activity after joint replacement. *Am J Sports Med* 2001;29(3):377-388.

76. Jackson JD, Smith J, Shah JP, Wisniewski SJ, Dahm DL: Golf after total knee arthroplasty: Do patients return to walking the course? *Am J Sports Med* 2009; 37(11):2201-2204.

77. Chodzko-Zajko WJ, Proctor DN, Fiatarone Singh MA, et al: American College of Sports Medicine position stand: Exercise and physical activity for older adults. *Med Sci Sports Exerc* 2009;41(7):1510-1530.

Chapter 35

The Arthroscopic Package: A Systematic Approach to Treating the Degenerative Knee

J. Richard Steadman, MD
Christopher B. Dewing, MD
William G. Rodkey, DVM

Dr. Steadman or an immediate family member serves as a board member, owner, officer, or committee member of the Vail Valley Surgery Center; has received royalties from ConMed Linvatec and Össur; serves as a paid consultant to or is an employee of Össur and ReGen Biologics; has received research or institutional support from Arthrex, Össur, Smith & Nephew, and Siemens; and owns stock or stock options in Regeneration Technologies and ReGen Biologics. Dr. Rodkey or an immediate family member serves as a paid consultant to or is an employee of ReGen Biologics; has received research or institutional support from Össur, Regen Biologics, Smith & Nephew, Arthrex, Genzyme, Siemens Medical Solutions USA, and OrthoRehab; owns stock or stock options in Johnson & Johnson and ReGen Biologics; and has received non-income support (such as equipment or services), commercially derived honoraria, or other non–research-related funding (such as paid travel) from ReGen Biologics. Neither Dr. Dewing nor any immediate family member has received anything of value from or owns stock in a commercial company or institution related directly or indirectly to the subject of this chapter.

Key Points

- The "arthroscopic package" is not a simple débridement/lavage procedure, but rather a carefully tailored and systematic arthroscopic treatment that addresses the specific degenerative findings.
- Scarring of the anterior interval of the knee is a common cause of pain, disordered patellofemoral tracking, and diminished motion.
- The key to improving function and relieving pain in the degenerative knee is improving and maintaining joint volume.
- Correct rehabilitation is essential to preserve the surgical gains in joint volume and range of motion.

Introduction

Osteoarthritis, or degenerative joint disease, is a chronic problem resulting from the thinning of the articular cartilage within the knee joint. Knee osteoarthritis has a greater prevalence among older adults, with 16% of adults age 45 and older having symptoms of the disease.[1] The symptoms of osteoarthritis include pain, swelling, stiffness, and mechanical symptoms. Pain in osteoarthritis is generated by various combinations of stiffness, synovitis, loose bodies, meniscal tears, closed spaces, and contractures.[2] Chondral defects or flaps can also be a source of pain.

In the past decade, two well-designed randomized, prospective studies have shown no lasting benefit to the patient from knee arthroscopy for the treatment of knee osteoarthritis.[3,4] The first trial compared patients receiving arthroscopic débridement and lavage with placebo treatment (skin incisions only without insertion of arthroscope) and showed no difference between groups over a 2-year period.[3] The second trial compared physical therapy and medical treatment alone with arthroscopic débridement and/or lavage followed by the same physical therapy protocol and showed no difference between the groups by validated outcomes measures over a 2-year period.[4] On the basis of these studies, a recent editorial comment in a leading orthopaedic journal went so far as to claim that "...it is clear that orthopaedic surgeons should no longer use arthroscopy to treat osteoarthritis of the knee, even if the patient has mechanical symptoms."[5] Furthermore, the American Academy of Orthopaedic Surgeons has recently updated its guideline on the treatment of osteoarthritis of the knee, recommending against arthroscopy with débridement or lavage in patients with a primary diagnosis of symptomatic knee osteoarthritis.[6]

Our own experience with a systematic arthroscopic treatment package for patients with symptomatic osteoarthritis of the knee should serve as a counterpoint to such broad condemnation.[7] We understand why arthroscopic débridement and lavage alone failed to provide a lasting benefit. In fact, débridement and lavage represent only one sixth of our arthroscopic package approach. This technique addresses all aspects of pain and stiffness in the degenerative knee: (1) joint space expansion by insufflation; (2) débridement, removal of loose bodies, and limited chondroplasty; (3) partial meniscectomies as indicated by unstable tears; (4) comprehensive lysis of adhesions, including anterior interval release;[8] (5) meticulous synovectomy by thermal ablation; and, finally, (6) excision of anterior osteophytes that block knee extension. This treatment package focuses on increasing joint volume to improve range of motion and is coupled with comprehensive rehabilitation that maintains this improved joint volume and prevents scar reformation. In our study, this tailored approach to treat the degenerative knees of active, mature patients who might otherwise be considered candidates for total knee arthroplasty has yielded good results in more than 70% of patients at 5 years.[7] The success of the procedure is clearly dependent on a methodical rehabilitation program that has evolved contemporaneously with our surgical algorithm.

Patient Evaluation and Education

The systematic package treatment can be successfully applied to patients of all ages who have painful degenerative knees that have failed to respond to an optimized nonsurgical regimen, including physical therapy, intra-articular steroid injections, viscosupplementation, and activity modifications. The package addresses the pain generators that are specific to osteoarthritis, which is more common in adults age 45 and older.

We do not exclude patients with advanced osteoarthritis. In fact, a large percentage of our patients have been previously counseled that, because of their advanced osteoarthritis, their only option is total knee arthroplasty. We do not ask our patients to give up an active lifestyle. To the contrary, we counsel them that when such nonsurgical measures have failed, arthroscopic surgery may be the only means to restore mobility and function to the degenerative knee without prosthetic replacement. Moreover, unlike after prosthetic replacement, the patient may ultimately be able to return to full activity, including higher impact and risky activities that may not be recommended after knee arthroplasty. The package is not just débridement and lavage. It is a series of steps designed to treat arthrofibrosis, capsular contraction, osteophytes (which block extension), symptomatic meniscal tears, painful cartilage fragments and loose bodies, and synovitis. It also frees the patella of contractures.

All patients undergo a comprehensive radiographic examination, including weight-bearing AP, lateral, flexed PA, long weight-bearing, and patellar views. The long weight-bearing view is critical for assessing axial alignment. In our study, patient satisfaction was not affected by a shift in alignment of up to 50%, but postoperative Lysholm scores were diminished in patients with greater malalignment.[7] If significant malalignment exists, corrective osteotomy is discussed with patients who may be good candidates for such procedures. The 45° PA flexion weight-bearing radiographic view demonstrates significant posterior wear and arthritis when present. Patellar views highlight patellofemoral arthritis, patellar tilt, and/or subluxation. Lateral views provide evidence of patella infera, often a subtle finding associated with anterior interval adhesions or scarring.[2,7,8]

After patients complete comprehensive intake questionnaires, we obtain a complete history of their knee symptoms, including their preferred athletic and recreational activities. We carefully evaluate their subjective assessment of their own disability and subsequently determine their willingness to comply with our specific protocol for rehabilitation.

A comprehensive lower extremity examination begins with a careful assessment of the patient's gait. Hip range of motion and strength are documented. The knee is examined initially with the patient seated on the examination table with legs hanging free. We ask the patient to actively extend and flex both knees while we visually and by palpation assess patellar tracking and quadriceps tone. Then, with the patient supine, we perform a comprehensive examination of the ligamentous stability of the knee. Range of motion is carefully measured in both knees, and the presence of any contracture is documented. Particular attention is paid to patellar mobility, both medial and lateral, as well as superior-inferior motion. The patellar tendon is carefully palpated for focal tenderness and mobility. Diminished mobility below the patella suggests adhesions posterior to the tendon, significant infrapatellar and/or suprapatellar plicae, and/or anterior interval scarring. Previous surgical incisions are documented, and a full neurovascular examination of both extremities is completed.

Based on the history and physical and radiographic examinations, we may recommend MRI. MRI helps confirm our presumptive diagnoses and may reveal other pathologic conditions such as loose bodies in the posterior joint capsule, posterior horn meniscal tears that have extruded posteriorly, subclinical ligament tears, and high-grade focal chondral lesions that may necessitate adding microfracture.[9,10] The microfracture procedure may be staged because increased patellar mobility, joint volume, and range of motion likely improve outcomes of cartilage regeneration.

We review all diagnoses with patients to ensure their understanding and informed consent. We carefully explain the package procedure in simple terms, such as: "Your knee space is surrounded by a thickened capsule and is being squeezed on all sides. By doing the surgery, we can increase volume to your joint and take pressure off the areas of cartilage that have been worn down." We also describe the specific pain generators in the patient's knee, including synovitis, chondral damage, meniscal tears, loose bodies, and adhesions. Providing this information to patients helps them prepare for the surgery and subsequent rehabilitation.

Patients are given their choice of anesthesia; most cases are performed under general or spinal anesthesia. Regional anesthesia is not typically performed. Patients are positioned supine with a lateral post. A tourniquet is placed but rarely used. All patients are meticulously examined under anesthesia for range of motion, patellar mobility, and ligamentous stability.

The Treatment Package

Step 1: Knee Insufflation

Initially, we slowly and carefully carefully expand the intra-articular space with sterile normal saline, injected from a superolateral position with an 18-gauge needle on a 60-mL syringe. Care is taken not to pass through the back wall of the joint capsule, which, if infiltrated, might obscure the view of the suprapatellar space. If the needle remains intra-articular, there will be an easy flow from the syringe that may be palpated on the medial aspect of the knee. Insufflation continues until the joint is completely distended and much greater manual pressure is needed to continue insufflation. Adequate pressure can be visually confirmed by removing the syringe and observing a jet of fluid leaving the needle. This point may be reached rapidly in knees with more advanced osteoarthritis at volumes of 60 to 90 mL. We have observed that normal knees typically accept volumes of about 180 mL. Overinsufflating the knee is detrimental if capsular rupture occurs and subsequent bleeding compromises any temporary gains in joint distention. When insufflation is performed carefully, however, the capsule is stretched and knee volume is increased and is maintained by fluid inflow during the arthroscopy and by meticulous postoperative patellar mobilization and rehabilitation.

Steps 2 and 3: Diagnostic Arthroscopy, Débridement, Chondroplasty, and Partial Meniscectomies as Indicated

An inflow portal is made superomedially just medial to the quadriceps tendon. With inflow maintained at 60 mL/min, a lateral peripatellar portal is made at the distended soft spot, slightly more lateral and more superior than is typical. This position facilitates a better view of the anterior interval and any adhesions and/or scar tissue posterior to the patellar tendon (**Figure 1**).

A meticulous arthroscopic examination of the entire knee joint is performed in a systematic fashion. First, the patellofemoral joint is examined and chondral wear patterns are assessed. Grooving or chondral injury from engaging plicae is noted. Then, both medial and lateral gutters are explored, loose bodies are removed, meniscal extrusions are noted, osteophytes are documented, and synovitis is noted. The suprapatellar space is subsequently explored, and particular care is taken to exam-

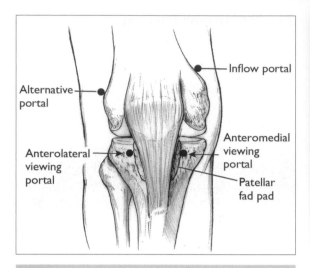

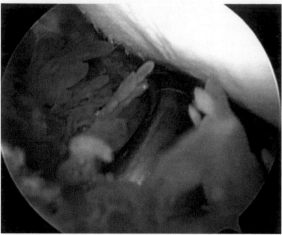

ine the space for compartmentalization or adhesions. The space should easily extend proximally by four fingerbreadths above the patella, and the quadriceps tendon should be easily visualized.

A medial peripatellar portal is made under direct visualization. The intercondylar notch is examined, and the infrapatellar plicae are excised. The anterior cruciate ligament is probed and examined at both origin and insertion. The anterior tibial plateau is examined for the presence of prominent osteophytes, which may block extension. Osteophytes are typically excised as the final intra-articular procedure so as not to obscure visibility by bleeding. The anterior interval is then examined, but scar release is deferred until later in the case (see step 5).

The lateral compartment is then examined, and any unstable cartilage is débrided only to the unstable edges.

A similar "less is more" approach is used for meniscal tears, removing only unstable torn portions.

The same process is repeated in the medial compartment of the knee and then in the patellofemoral joint. Larger loose bodies that are not easily evacuated through the outflow cannula are removed with pituitary rongeurs and/or a high-speed shaver.

Step 4: Synovectomy

Dye[11] suggests that a significant portion of pain in the degenerative knee stems from synovitis. Therefore, a meticulous synovectomy is essential to the success of the package. We use a 70° radiofrequency (RF) wand to carefully brush the surfaces of the inflamed synovium. This instrument is particularly useful in the knee joint because its gentle curvature, accompanied by knee extension, facilitates atraumatic access to the medial and lateral gutters, areas of synovitis often overlooked (**Figure 2**). Care is taken not to penetrate the capsule of the knee or to touch the cartilage surfaces with the RF

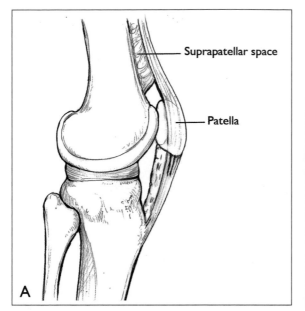
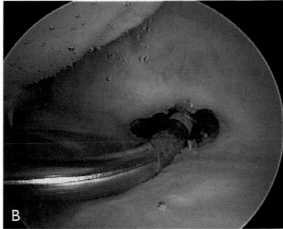

Figure 3   Lysis of adhesions (step 5 of the arthroscopic package). **A,** Illustration shows adhesions in the suprapatellar space. **B,** Arthroscopic view shows the division of adhesion tissue using a radiofrequency ablation device. (Reproduced with permission from Steadman JR: Arthroscopic treatment of the degenerative knee, in Feagin J, Steadman JR, eds: *The Crucial Principles in Care of the Knee.* Philadelphia, PA, Lippincott Williams & Wilkins, 2008, p 182.)

wand. Focal areas of hypertrophic synovium are more completely débrided. Meticulous hemostasis is achieved during the synovectomy. We specifically address inflamed synovium in the medial and lateral gutters and in the suprapatellar pouch. We focus particularly on areas of reactive synovium adjacent to meniscus or chondral pathology.

Step 5: Lysis of Adhesions and Anterior Interval Release

We routinely excise infrapatellar plicae, which have been noted to alter patellofemoral kinematics and may be a cause of retropatellar pain.[12] Medial and/or lateral plicae are also excised, usually by RF to ensure hemostasis. We take care not to violate normal native capsule during the excision, which can lead to localized arthrofibrosis or plicae recurrence.

Adhesions in the suprapatellar space are often not fully recognized and adequately treated. These small, white, thickened bands may significantly tether the patella and alter tracking (**Figure 3,** *A*). We carefully release these adhesions without injuring the capsule beneath and simultaneously observe the effect on the space between the patella and the anterior femur with the knee in extension. One may be able to observe an increase in this "floating space" as the adhesions are lysed.

If we observe an abnormally shortened suprapatellar space (less than four fingerbreadths above the patella), we suspect a compartmentalization of the pouch. The pouch may be partially or completely compartmentalized by this veil of adhesion tissue (**Figure 3,** *B*). We divide this tissue in cruciate fashion and débride the edges to fully open the proximal part of the pouch. Loose bodies may be trapped within this space and should be removed.

After completing the suprapatellar lysis of adhesions, we dynamically assess patellar tracking by bringing the knee from extension to flexion and back with the arthroscope positioned at the base of the trochlea. This maneuver helps to ensure that we have optimized tracking.

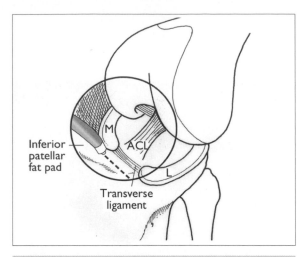

Figure 4   Illustration of anterior interval release (step 5 of the arthroscopic package). The release is completed in a stepwise fashion from medial (M) to lateral (L), just anterior to the peripheral rim of the anterior horn of each meniscus, and from proximal to 1 cm distal along the anterior tibial cortex. Hemostasis should be obtained to prevent postoperative bleeding or recurrent scarring. ACL = anterior cruciate ligament. (Reproduced with permission from Steadman JR: Arthroscopic treatment of the degenerative knee, in Feagin J, Steadman JR, eds: *The Crucial Principles in Care of the Knee.* Philadelphia, PA, Lippincott Williams & Wilkins, 2008, p 181.)

Next, the anterior interval of the knee is examined, specifically the space that normally should be present between the fat pad and the anterior aspect of the tibia, the anterior meniscal horns, and the intermeniscal ligament. Scarring of this space can cause abnormal joint mechanics in the patellofemoral joint and the tibiofemoral joint.[12] In the normal knee, this interval should open approximately 1.5 cm as the knee is ranged from full extension to 120° of flexion. In the degenerative or postoperative knee, however, the interval is often closed by adhesions between a scarred infrapatellar fat pad and the anterior tibia, or even to the tibial insertional fibers of the anterior cruciate ligament.

An arthroscopic probe is used to inspect the extent and density of adhesions in the interval and to better define the anterior horns of the menisci and the anterior attachment of the medial meniscus. When the interval is closed by a hypertrophic fat pad, motion can be assessed by observing the normal motion of the medial meniscus as the knee is flexed and extended.

When interval scarring is present, the RF wand is used to carefully divide the scar tissue in a transverse fashion just anterior to the intermeniscal ligament and at least 1 cm distally, to the level of the anterior tibial periosteum, which should not be violated. The release is completed in a step-wise fashion from medial to lateral, and the motion of the interval is assessed as we continue lysing scar tissue (**Figure 4**).

Step 6: Excision of Anterior Tibial Osteophytes

If a large anterior osteophyte is identified, dynamic examination is performed to evaluate for impingement against the trochlea in terminal extension. Impingement may be evidenced by focal chondral damage or grooving at the trochlea. The offending osteophyte is skeletonized with RF and then resected with a high-speed oval burr. Meticulous hemostasis is maintained, but to ensure adequate evacuation of any marrow elements from the osteophyte bed, a small intra-articular drain is placed and then removed before patient discharge.

Postoperative Care and Rehabilitation

Appropriate rehabilitation is essential to preserve the surgical gains in joint volume and range of motion and to prevent stiffness. This structured postoperative rehabilitation program includes range-of-motion exercises, icing, patellar mobilization, protected weight bearing (if indicated), stretching, and gradual strengthening. If microfracture was also performed, a different rehabilitation regimen is prescribed.

Patients begin rehabilitation with continuous passive motion (CPM) at a slow rate from 30° to 70° immediately in the recovery unit. The CPM may be advanced as tolerated. Recirculating ice cuffs are also used for patient comfort and diminished postoperative bleeding. Patients are discharged to their initial physical therapy consultation either the same day or within 23 hours. They are provided a careful description, both written and verbal, of their tailored therapy and the recommended duration of restricted weight bearing before leaving the therapy unit.

We keep most patients 30% weight bearing for 7 to 14 days or until effusions have resolved and motion has been restored to at least near full extension and 120° of flexion. CPM is recommended for 6 to 8 hours a day for the first 2 weeks. Extensor mechanism stretches of the patella and patellar tendon are also included in the initial rehabilitation program.

The focus during the first postoperative month is placed on maintaining joint volume and mobility through passive and active range of motion and patellar mobility. Stationary bicycling with no resistance is started early and continued throughout the first month. Strengthening is limited to isometric sets for the quadriceps and hamstrings.

Functional strengthening begins at 6 weeks postoperatively and includes uphill treadmill walking, elastic resistance bands, and double-leg 30° knee bends. Pain with any increased activity serves as a clear guide to return to the previous level of rehabilitation that elicits no discomfort. The patient and the physical therapist thus tailor the rehabilitation to fit the recovery progress. Three months postoperatively, single-leg strengthening and more advanced fitness regimens are started. Full weight training is allowed after 4 months, and return to higher level sports such as skiing and tennis is allowed at approximately 5 months if full range of motion has been achieved.

Outcomes and Conclusions

The arthroscopic package provides orthopaedic surgeons and their patients with osteoarthritic knees a viable treatment alternative to total knee arthroplasty. Severity of osteoarthritis is not a contraindication to treatment with the package. In our population of patients with severe osteoarthritis who were candidates for total knee arthroplasty, Lysholm scores following the arthroscopic package improved an average of 25 points. Of the patients with severe degenerative osteoarthritis, only 17% required arthroplasty at 3 years,[7] and 30% required arthroplasty at 5 years. Patients who required subsequent arthroplasty at 3 years were significantly older (64 years) than those who did not (55 years).[7] For older patients with advanced degenerative arthritis of the knee, our systematic approach is an effective alternative intervention to decrease knee pain, aid in continuation of an active lifestyle, and defer knee replacement.

References

1. Jordan JM, Helmick CG, Renner JB, et al: Prevalence of knee symptoms and radiographic and symptomatic knee osteoarthritis in African Americans and Caucasians: The Johnston County Osteoarthritis Project. *J Rheumatol* 2007;34(1):172-180.

2. Steadman JR: Arthroscopic treatment of the degenerative knee, in Feagin JA, Steadman JR, eds: *The Crucial Principles in Care of the Knee*. Philadelphia, PA, Lippincott Williams & Wilkins, 2008, pp 177-184.

3. Moseley JB, O'Malley K, Petersen NJ, et al: A controlled trial of arthroscopic surgery for osteoarthritis of the knee. *N Engl J Med* 2002;347(2):81-88.

4. Kirkley A, Birmingham TB, Litchfield RB, et al: A randomized trial of arthroscopic surgery for osteoarthritis of the knee. *N Engl J Med* 2008;359(11):1097-1107.

5. Moseley B: Arthroscopic surgery did not provide additional benefit to physical and medical therapy for osteoarthritis of the knee. *J Bone Joint Surg Am* 2009;91(5):1281.

6. American Academy of Orthopaedic Surgeons: Clinical Practice Guideline on Treatment of Osteoarthritis of the Knee (non-arthroplasty). Rosemont, IL, American Academy of Orthopaedic Surgeons. http://www.aaos.org/research/guidelines/OAKguideline.pdf.

7. Steadman JR, Ramappa AJ, Maxwell RB, Briggs KK: An arthroscopic treatment regimen for osteoarthritis of the knee. *Arthroscopy* 2007;23(9):948-955.

8. Steadman JR, Dragoo JL, Hines SL, Briggs KK: Arthroscopic release for symptomatic scarring of the anterior interval of the knee. *Am J Sports Med* 2008;36(9):1763-1769.

9. Steadman JR: Microfracture, in Feagin JA, Steadman JR, eds: *The Crucial Principles in Care of the Knee*. Philadelphia, PA, Lippincott Williams & Wilkins, 2008, pp 129-151.

10. Miller BS, Steadman JR, Briggs KK, Rodrigo JJ, Rodkey WG: Patient satisfaction and outcome after microfracture of the degenerative knee. *J Knee Surg* 2004;17(1):13-17.

11. Dye SF: The pathophysiology of patellofemoral pain: A tissue homeostasis perspective. *Clin Orthop Relat Res* 2005;(436):100-110.

12. Ahmad CS, Kwak SD, Ateshian GA, Warden WH, Steadman JR, Mow VC: Effects of patellar tendon adhesion to the anterior tibia on knee mechanics. *Am J Sports Med* 1998;26(5):715-724.

Chapter 36
Osteotomies About the Knee

Alan M.J. Getgood, MD,
FRCS (Tr&Orth)
J. Robert Giffin, MD,
FRCSC

Key Points

- Patient selection is of paramount importance. Adequate explanation and informed consent helps achieve a satisfactory outcome.
- Use both clinical and radiographic examination to establish the correct diagnosis, define the level of deformity, and plan the osteotomy correction accordingly (tibia or femur).
- Be aware of the potential to alter both the sagittal and coronal axis when performing osteotomies, as this can aid in the treatment of degenerative disease and ligamentous instability.
- When creating an opening wedge, take great care not to fracture the opposite cortex, which could create an unstable construct.
- Understand the intricacies of the fixation system you choose to use, and adjust the rehabilitation protocol as appropriate.
- Make sure patients understand the length of rehabilitation and the goals of treatment.

Dr. Getgood or an immediate family member serves as a paid consultant to or is an employee of Tigenix. Dr. Giffin or an immediate family member has received royalties from Arthrex, serves as a paid consultant to or is an employee of Arthrex, and has received research or institutional support from Arthrex.

Introduction

The baby boomer generation, the first wave of which is now well into their 60s, is known for maintaining an increased activity level into later life. This population may present to health professionals with symptomatic knee osteoarthritis (OA) that interferes with the ability to lead an active lifestyle. Although the cause of OA is known to be multifactorial, the role of abnormal biomechanics and limb malalignment has long been a subject of intense scrutiny. It is generally agreed that in the lower limb, arthrosis is frequently associated with malalignment. The load across the knee joint is a function of alignment, and changes in the axial alignment of the femur or tibia in either the coronal or sagittal plane will influence the distribution of this load. These changes result in abnormal stresses on the articular cartilage.[1] Therefore, assessment and correction of alignment, if indicated, must be at the forefront in the treatment algorithm when considering the management of knee arthrosis in the active baby boomer.

High tibial osteotomy (HTO) was first described by Coventry[2] in 1965. Advances in materials technology, plating systems, and surgical technique, coupled with a greater knowledge of patient selection, has led to improved patient experience and has expanded the indications for the osteotomy technique.

Table 1: Indications for Realignment Osteotomy

Malalignment *and* arthrosis

Malalignment *and* instability

Malalignment *and* arthrosis ± instability

Malalignment *and* articular cartilage procedure ± instability

One primary goal of osteotomy, regardless of anatomic site or technique, is to reposition the weight-bearing line so that the load distribution through the knee is normal or as close to normal as possible, minimizing stresses on the affected compartment.[3,4] Thus, realignment osteotomy has the potential to provide the mature patient with symptom relief, prolonging the life of the native knee joint and delaying the need for total joint arthroplasty until a time when demands have lessened.

HTO was popular in the 1980s and then for a time appeared to fall out of favor. This may have been related to the length of time the patient was left in plaster cast and non–weight bearing. However, the recent interest in combining realignment procedures with ligament reconstruction to address complex instability patterns,[5] the increasing success of concomitant cartilage restoration procedures, and the emergence of new plate technologies have boosted a resurgence of interest in HTO surgery. Consequently, the past 3 years have seen a large increase in published articles on the topic of HTO.

This chapter illustrates how osteotomies about the knee, in particular HTO, can be used to treat abnormal joint mechanics and resultant pathology. The stages of surgery, patient selection, decision making, surgical technique, and rehabilitation are discussed. A short review of current literature provides a summary of HTO results.

Indications

Although knee osteotomy was originally described by Coventry to treat malalignment and arthrosis, its indications are not limited to the patient with medial or lateral arthrosis and corresponding varus or valgus malalignment. The technique is now used in a range of situations, as outlined in **Table 1**. Both coronal and sagittal plane deformities of the tibia and femur can be addressed, allowing surgeons to plan more complex deformity corrections. The latter is particularly applicable in the patient with the malaligned, unstable, ligament-deficient knee.

The treatment of articular cartilage lesions concomitant with osteotomy has been reported.[6] Transferring the load from the articular cartilage in a worn compartment or from cartilage that has undergone a cartilage restoration procedure (microfracture, osteochondral autograft/allograft transplantation, autologous chondrocyte implantation) would appear to protect the maturing regenerate tissue. Load (in particular, shear) has been shown in laboratory experiments to be beneficial for chondrocytes and the development of extracellular matrix; however, as compression can be detrimental, a reduction via realignment surgery is potentially advantageous.[7,8] It is therefore clear that the indications for osteotomy are increasing and the number of relative contraindications are decreasing. Tricompartmental OA is a relative contraindication to knee osteotomy; it may be better addressed with total knee arthroplasty (TKA). However, this decision should be based on the patient's presenting symptoms, age, and activity level. Ultimately, a large deformity may still benefit from a correction to a neutral position rather than the recommended 62.5% "Fujisawa point."[9] Patellofemoral joint arthrosis may be present but does not necessarily exclude patients from an HTO. Again, great attention must be paid to the patient's presenting symptoms and where the patient localizes the pain.

Other relative contraindications include poor bone quality, such as in rheumatoid disease, inflammatory arthritis, or osteoporosis; fixed flexion deformity greater than 20°; morbid obesity; generalized pain; immunosuppression; and impaired bone healing, as may be present in diabetics and smokers.

Patient Assessment

Following a thorough history and physical examination, a radiographic assessment is made of the lower limbs. Attention should be paid to the patient's overall body habitus as well as level of conditioning. Both limbs should be fully examined, including the hip and hindfoot. Particular attention is paid to coronal, sagittal, and rotational plane alignment. Gait should be observed for evidence of thrust in the direction of deformity, indicating the presence of dynamic instability. The knee should be inspected for previous incisions and fully examined to identify any other intra-articular pathology that could be addressed surgically.

Radiographic imaging includes bilateral AP weight-bearing views in full extension, bilateral PA weight-bearing views at 45° of flexion, a Merchant view, and a lateral view of the affected knee to assess the degree of degeneration and compartment involvement. Full-length hip-to-ankle bilateral double-leg–stance radiographs are taken to assess limb alignment; these are taken in a standardized fashion so as to accommodate rotation. Single-leg–stance views potentially exaggerate the degree of soft-tissue laxity and may lead to overcorrection.

Normal Alignment

Before evaluating a patient for malalignment, it is important to understand what normal alignment is. To assess alignment, lines are drawn on the digital film as shown in **Figure 1**. Particular attention is paid to the mechanical axis deviation (MAD; normal = 9.7 ± 6.8 mm), the mechanical tibiofemoral angle (mTFA; normal = 1.3° ± 2°), the anatomic lateral distal femoral angle (aLDFA; normal = 81° ± 2°), the anatomic medial proximal tibial angle (aMPTA; normal = 87° ± 2°), and the proximal posterior tibial articular angle (PPTA; normal = 81° ± 3°).[10] Calculation of these angles allows the anatomic site and plane of deformity to be established. The type of osteotomy can then be decided upon as well as the degree of correction required to establish the desired mechanical axis.

Choosing the Osteotomy Site

In the varus knee, we prefer to use an opening wedge proximal HTO. Although small corrections can be treated with a lateral closing wedge osteotomy, larger corrections can be problematic because proximal tibial bone is removed, often creating tibial translation that can make a later TKA much more technically challenging. Some patients may have symmetric physiologic varus (ie, within population normal limits), with meniscal loss or chondral damage in the medial compartment. In this case, we suggest that this is pathologic varus and an osteotomy is justified to offload the af-

fected compartment, particularly if combined with an articular cartilage or meniscus repair procedure. In the patient with valgus malalignment, the joint must be examined clinically and radiologically to establish whether this is a femoral- or tibial-based deformity. In the event of a femoral-based deformity, where the aLDFA is abnormal, a lateral opening wedge distal femoral osteotomy is preferred, preventing the joint-line obliquity that may result from a tibial-based correction. However, in the setting of normal aLDFA with lateral meniscus or chondral loss, we prefer an opening lateral HTO.

Determining the Degree of Correction Required

Some authors suggest that in varus deformity, the mechanical axis should be shifted to outside the lateral compartment. We believe that this is excessive and prefer to move the mechanical axis to the 62.5% point along the width of the tibial plateau, based on the work of Dugdale et al.[9] Excessive correction can lead to significant angular deformity, which can be cosmetically displeasing, particularly for women. To calculate the degree of correction required, we use the method that Dugdale et al[9] described (**Figure 2**), adjusting it based on the degree of degeneration or injury of the lateral compartment. Lateral arthrosis is a relative contraindication to medial opening wedge HTO. However, in an active person with significant varus and a mild degree of lateral compartment involvement, we believe that benefit can be achieved by realigning the joint to neutral, thereby not overloading the lateral side but providing some mechanical advantage to the more severely affected medial compartment. The advantages and disadvantages of this procedure should be discussed at length with the patient preoperatively so that an understanding is established as to the potential failure of this type of correction. If the patient has reservations about proceeding with surgery, an unloading brace or a lateral heel wedge may be prescribed to see if any symptom relief is achieved before surgery.[11] Although not recommended in the American Academy of Orthopaedic Surgeons (AAOS) guidelines for treatment of primary knee osteoarthritis, we often use these measures to gauge whether patients may potentially respond to realignment surgery. Neither is invasive, and the lateral

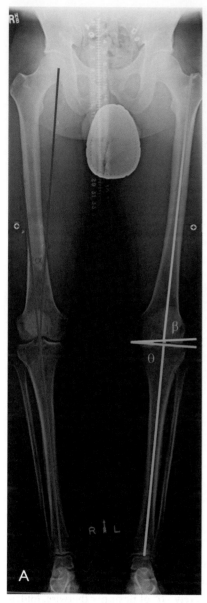

α = mechanical tibiofemoral angle (mTFA)
(normal = 1.3° ± 2°)

β = anatomic lateral distal femoral angle (aLDFA)
(normal = 81° ± 2°)

θ = anatomic medial proximal tibial angle (aMPTA)
(normal = 87° ± 2°)

Δ = proximal posterior tibial articular angle (PPTA)
(normal = 81° ± 3°)

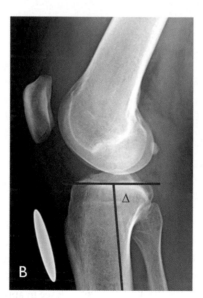

Figure I Long-leg alignment (**A**) and lateral radiographs (**B**) show normal angles in the knee.

heel wedge is often much better tolerated than the unloader brace, although limited efficacy in the former is a potential pitfall.

The clinician should bear in mind that some patients, despite their wish to remain active, may have degenerative disease that is too far advanced to be "rescued" by osteotomy. In some cases, the best option may be activity modification, symptomatic management, or possibly total or partial joint arthroplasty. A unicompartmental knee arthroplasty may be a good option for these patients. However, following HTO, once bone union has been achieved, no restrictions are placed on the patient in terms of recreational sports and activity level. Therefore, we prefer not to be too prescriptive in terms of age regarding which patient gets which treatment. Also, if osteotomy is chosen, the ability to proceed to joint arthroplasty remains a future option.

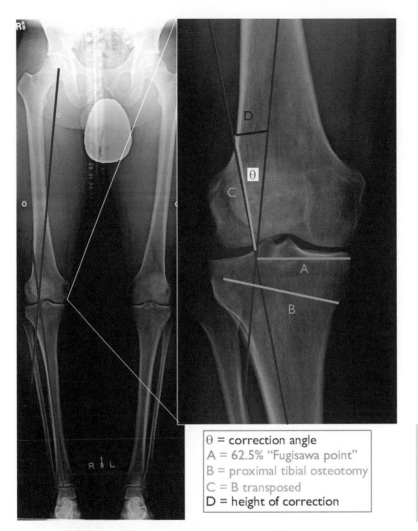

θ = correction angle
A = 62.5% "Fugisawa point"
B = proximal tibial osteotomy
C = B transposed
D = height of correction

Figure 2   The method of calculating the degree of correction to be achieved by high tibial osteotomy is shown on a long-leg alignment radiograph, with the affected area shown in the inset.

In any case, it is of utmost importance to establish the patient's expectations and provide appropriate counsel as to the expected results of surgery. The goals are to achieve pain relief, allow the continuation of an active lifestyle, and delay TKA until the patient's age and activity demand are more appropriate for that operation. It should be stressed, however, that even "good" results tend to deteriorate with time. To help get the point across, we often use the analogy of rotating a worn tire.

Surgical Technique

All patients receive antibiotic prophylaxis before entering the operating room. The procedure is done with the patient supine. A tourniquet is applied and inflated if required. A lateral proximal thigh support is used. If a concomitant anterior cruciate ligament (ACL) reconstruction is planned, a foot post is applied to hold the knee in approximately 70° of flexion; otherwise, folded surgical drapes are used as a bolster under the proximal femur and knee to maintain flexion as indicated. Fluoroscopy is used routinely. Arthroscopy is performed before HTO in all cases to examine the joint surfaces and address any intra-articular pathology. If the degenerative disease is extensive, the HTO may be abandoned. Hemovac drains are routinely used and removed 1 day postoperatively. Patients remain in the

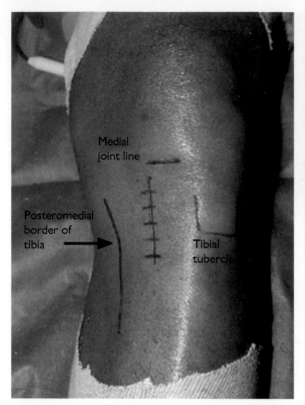

Figure 3   Photograph of a knee with landmarks and the incision for medial opening wedge high tibial osteotomy drawn on the skin.

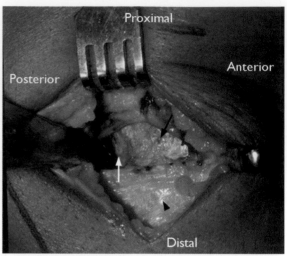

Figure 4   Intraoperative photograph shows the surgical approach for high tibial osteotomy in relation to the pes anserinus (arrowhead), the superficial medial collateral ligament (black arrow), and the posteromedial border of the tibia (white arrow).

hospital overnight for observation and are discharged the following day.

Varus Knee

Medial Opening Wedge HTO

Our preferred technique of medial opening wedge HTO is a modification of the technique described by Amendola et al.[12] This method allows correction of deformity in all planes and, in particular, allows planned alterations to tibial slope in the sagittal plane.

The procedure is performed through a vertical skin incision, which extends 5 cm distally from the medial joint line and is centered between the tibial tubercle and the posteromedial border of the tibia (**Figure 3**). The gracilis and semitendinosus tendons and the superficial medial collateral ligament (MCL) are preserved and retracted medially to expose the posteromedial border

of the proximal tibia (**Figure 4**). The superficial MCL is released distally to allow for large corrections without increasing the medial compartment pressure, as reported by Agneskirchner et al.[13] Great care is taken not to disrupt the deep MCL, to prevent unwanted medial laxity. A guide pin is inserted obliquely along a line proximal to the tibial tubercle from approximately 4 cm below the medial joint line in the region of the transition between metaphyseal and diaphyseal cortical bone on radiographs extending to a point approximately at the tip of the proximal tibiofibular joint, no less than 1 cm distal to the lateral joint line (**Figure 5,** *A*). The starting point for the guide pin should be fairly anterior, to leave room for the placement of the saw and osteotome.

The osteotomy is made below the guide pin using a small oscillating saw to breach the medial, anteromedial, and posteromedial cortices. A retractor is placed posteriorly to protect the neurovascular structures at all times. This is followed by the insertion of narrow, sharp, thin, flexible osteotomes to a point just 1 cm short of the lateral cortex. Frequent imaging helps prevent violation of the lateral cortex and/or misdirection of the osteotome. The osteotomy is opened gradually to the

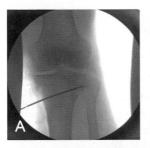 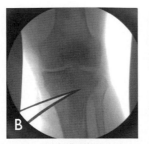 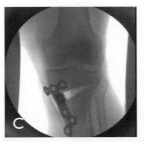 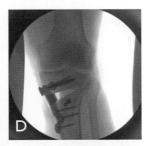

Figure 5   Intraoperative fluoroscopic images show the medial opening wedge high tibial osteotomy technique. **A,** Placement of guide pin. **B,** Opening of osteotomy. **C,** Application of plate along the posteromedial border of the tibia. **D,** Final fixation of osteotomy. Note the screw in the tibial tubercle, from a concomitant tibial tubercle osteotomy.

desired correction angle, first with distracting osteotomes to confirm the mobility of the osteotomy and then a calibrated wedge to the appropriate measured distraction (**Figure 5,** *B*). The wedge is placed posteriorly so as not to open the wedge too much anteriorly, thereby increasing the posterior tibial slope. The proximal tibial metaphysis is triangular in cross section, with the medial tibial cortex being one of the sides of the triangle. When opening the wedge at the posteromedial aspect of the tibia, the anterior part of the wedge in the sagittal plane is more lateral in the coronal plane. If the posterior and anterior gaps are equal, the posterior tibial slope is increased. Thus, as a general rule of thumb, the anterior aspect of the wedge should be opened approximately half as much as the posterior aspect. The distracted osteotomy is then fixed with an appropriate plating system (**Figure 5,** *C* and *D*). The distal screws should be inserted with the knee in extension, which also helps to prevent the tibia being flexed and thereby changing the tibial slope. Bone grafting is recommended in all opening wedge osteotomies greater than 7.5 mm. Allograft cancellous bone chips and/or tricortical blocks may be used unless there is an expressed desire by the patient for autograft bone. In our practice, osteotomies less than 7.5 mm are rarely grafted. In corrections greater than 12.5 mm, a biplane osteotomy to include the tibial tubercle is recommended to prevent patella infera. Great care must be taken to perform the tubercle osteotomy parallel to the posterior cortex, as the tubercle will rotate during the creation of the opening wedge and may fracture or not distract if it engages with the medial cortex of the tibia. The tubercle can

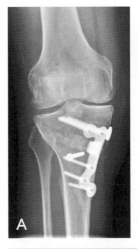 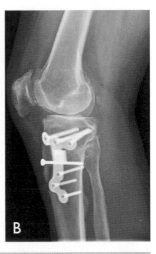

Figure 6   AP (**A**) and lateral (**B**) radiographs of medial opening wedge high tibial osteotomy at 6 months postoperatively. Note the incorporation of the allograft chips and subsequent union of the osteotomy.

then be fixed with a single 4.5-mm cortical lag screw (**Figure 6**).

Lateral Closing Wedge HTO

Currently, our only indication for a lateral closing wedge HTO is a previous lateral closing wedge osteotomy of the contralateral limb. When required, our preferred method for a lateral closing wedge osteotomy is as described by Coventry.[3] The osteotomy is performed through an incision made along a line from the

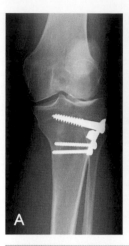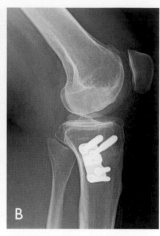

Figure 7   AP (**A**) and lateral (**B**) radiographs of a lateral opening wedge high tibial osteotomy at 6 months postoperatively.

lateral epicondyle over the Gerdy tubercle and extending distally just lateral to the tibial tubercle. The fibular head is not routinely osteotomized, but if this is required to close the osteotomy, the proximal tibiofibular joint is released. The upper limb of the osteotomy is made 2 cm below and parallel to the joint line. The appropriately sized wedge is marked, cut, and removed, and any remaining posterior cortical bone and medial cancellous bone medially is removed using bone rongeurs, small curets, and up-cutting Kerrison rongeurs. Appropriate wedge size is calculated using a modification of the method described by Dugdale et al.[9] The osteotomy is closed with the knee in extension and fixed with one or two stepped staples. Care is taken to ensure that the posterior tibial slope has not been decreased by failure to complete the osteotomy posteriorly, to remove cortical bone from the osteotomy site, and to adequately release the proximal tibiofibular joint when required.

Osteotomy With External Fixation Systems

Various external fixation devices may be used to address large or multiplanar deformities. As described by Adili et al,[14] use of the Ilizarov frame in the treatment of genu varum addresses both the bony and soft-tissue components of the deformity. The authors state that osteotomy distal to the tibial tuberosity allows slight lateral translation of the tibia, which decreases the amount of angular correction required and allows for correction of the tension on the ligamentous and capsular structures. Medial compartment arthritis and posttraumatic deformity are most amenable to acute correction, whereas skeletally mature patients with residual Blount disease deformity and the younger population with idiopathic genu varum may be best treated with gradual correction.

External frames are recommended for deformities greater than 20° to 25° of mechanical varus requiring gradual correction. For the adult population with unicompartmental arthrosis or joint line obliquity and ligament deficiency, we do not routinely use external fixators for correction, as many of the new plating systems can accommodate large corrections.

Valgus Knee

As discussed previously, realignment of the valgus knee may be approached from the femoral or tibial side, depending on where the deformity exists. All techniques—femoral and tibial, opening and closing wedge—have a place in the treatment of the valgus deformity.

Coventry[15] recommended a supracondylar femoral varus osteotomy if the valgus deformity was more than 12° or if the postoperative tilt of the tibiofemoral joint surface exceeded 10°. Bonnin and Chambat,[16] on the other hand, advocated that all valgus deformities be corrected from the tibial side.

With regard to degree of correction, opinions are more uniform than in proximal tibial valgus osteotomy. Several authors recommend correcting the valgus knee to a 0° tibiofemoral angle;[17,18] however, Morrey and Edgerton[19] suggest that the mechanical axis should be repositioned medial to the medial spine.

A proximal tibial varus osteotomy is recommended for smaller valgus deformities or those localized to the tibia, such as can occur after trauma or lateral meniscectomy.[20] A lateral opening wedge osteotomy can be performed, rather than the medial closing wedge osteotomy of Coventry or Bonnin and Chambat. We prefer to use a lateral opening wedge osteotomy in the setting of a primarily tibial deformity because it has the benefit of restoring the anatomy. In our experience, the incidence of delayed union or nonunion of the osteotomy site has not been an issue.

Lateral Opening Wedge Osteotomy

The lateral opening wedge osteotomy (**Figure 7**) is performed through an oblique skin incision similar to that for the lateral closing wedge osteotomy, made with the knee extended (**Figure 8**). The osteotomy also is oblique: it starts 4 cm distal to the lateral joint line just distal to the proximal tibiofibular joint and above the insertion of the patellar tendon and ends 1 to 2 cm distal to the medial articular surface. The fibula is not osteotomized. Residual medial laxity secondary to lengthening of the MCL is less commonly encountered with this technique. This procedure is valuable for corrections of less than 10 mm. The medial structures are not weakened as they are with a medial closing wedge procedure, and dissection around the pes anserinus is avoided.

Medial Closing Wedge Osteotomy

The approach for the medial closing wedge osteotomy is similar to the medial opening wedge osteotomy, with posterior retraction of the pes anserinus tendons and the superficial MCL. The osteotomy is made 2 to 3 cm distal to the joint line, and then a wedge of predetermined size is removed. The superficial MCL is not violated, and reefing or plication of the ligament is not required. Fixation is achieved with one or two osteotomy staples. With respect to alignment, Coventry[15] states that overcorrection is undesirable and that one should aim for a postoperative weight-bearing line that passes through the center of the knee. This approach may be appropriate for small corrections, such as an osteotomy for joint leveling combined with an ACL reconstruction.

Distal Femoral Varus Osteotomy

We prefer to perform a lateral opening wedge distal femoral varus osteotomy in cases of pathologic anatomic lateral distal femoral angle valgus (>81° ± 2° compared with the contralateral side). The degree of correction is calculated as described previously, transposed to the distal femur, with the initial osteotomy from lateral to medial and placed just proximal to the articular cartilage of the lateral trochlea. A standard lateral approach is made, about 2 cm anterior to the posterior border of the iliotibial tract proximally, extending anterior and medial to the Gerdy tubercle. The

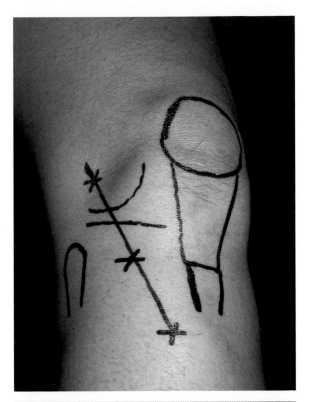

Figure 8 Photograph of a knee with landmarks and the incision for lateral opening wedge high tibial osteotomy drawn on the skin.

iliotibial tract is split anterior to the intermuscular septum, sweeping the fibers of vastus lateralis off it with a Cobb elevator. Perforating vessels should be cauterized. The osteotomy site is identified and subperiosteal dissection is performed while maintaining an intact periosteal sleeve. The starting point for the guide pin is approximately three fingerbreadths above the lateral femoral condyle, and the pin is directed obliquely toward the medial epicondyle. This should be confirmed fluoroscopically. The osteotomy can be performed using the same steps as the proximal tibial opening wedge osteotomy, with a retractor remaining posteriorly at all times to protect the neurovascular structures. A gauze sponge also may be placed posteriorly to sweep away the neurovascular structures from the osteotomy site. Great care must be taken to maintain an intact medial cortical hinge. The osteotomy site can then be distracted to the desired level of correction and fixed with any number of plating systems. Although autograft can be harvested from the proximal tibia, for corrections larger than 7.5 mm, we prefer to use morcellized bone allograft.

Altered Tibial Slope

Altered tibial slope in the sagittal plane, a less clinically prevalent condition, can add to knee instability and create an altered wear pattern and arthrosis. It may be encountered in the primary ligament-deficient knee or, as may be encountered in the active boomer, in the setting of revision of a failed reconstruction or chronic ligament-deficient knee that has developed arthrosis. To maximize the chances of a successful ligament reconstruction in this instance, the tibial slope should be corrected to create a stable joint.

Excessive tibial slope (greater than 13°) results in anterior translation of the tibia, increases chondral wear, and alters joint mechanics and meniscal load sharing. Similarly, decreased tibial slope (less than 7°) as a unilateral deformity is considered pathologic.[21] The degree of recurvatum also should be noted, as this can have an impact on the resultant forces across the joint. These cases of abnormal alignment will stress the cruciate ligaments and could contribute to graft failure in the setting of an ACL or posterior cruciate ligament (PCL) reconstruction.

In patients with a mixture of instability and compartment degeneration with normal tibial slope, a biplane osteotomy can be used to alter the tibial slope to compensate for the ligament deficiency or augment a reconstruction (ie, increase for PCL, decrease for ACL). Simultaneously, it can offload the worn compartment and, in cases such as lateral collateral insufficiency with varus thrust, help correct dynamic instability patterns.

Joint realignment procedures for altered tibial slope are approached anteriorly, with either an anterior closing wedge osteotomy to address increased tibial slope or an opening wedge osteotomy to address decreased tibial slope. Biplane osteotomies are often best approached via an anteromedial opening wedge, as this gives more flexibility. In large complex multiplanar corrections, a circular frame construct with or without navigation may be of benefit. When calculating the amount of correction required, a helpful rule of thumb is that 1 mm equals 2°.

Anterior Closing Wedge Osteotomy

Using an incision similar to that used for the medial opening wedge osteotomy, but slightly more anterior (ie, along the anterior third of the tibia rather than midway), the pes anserinus tendons are retracted and exposure is carried to the posteromedial border of the tibia. Adequate visualization across the anterior tibia must be attained to guide the osteotomy. The osteotomy is completed immediately proximal to the tibial tubercle, and the appropriately sized wedge of bone is removed (1-mm anterior wedge for 1.5 ± to 2° of correction), with the posterior cortex maintained intact initially. The posterior cortex is then fenestrated with a 3.2-mm drill (with careful attention to the adjacent neurovascular structures) to allow a controlled fracture of the posterior cortex while closing the osteotomy, to avoid destabilization. The osteotomy is then fixed with one or two staples.

Anterior Opening Wedge Osteotomy

The skin incision is carried along the medial border of the patellar tendon. The osteotomy is performed at the proximal pole of the tibial tubercle. A tibial tubercle osteotomy can enhance exposure and allow for reattachment such that the position of the patella relative to the femur is preserved. The principal tibial osteotomy is oblique, based on the guide pin position. It runs anterior to posterior from distal to proximal, starting roughly 40 mm distal to the joint line and ending 7 to 10 mm from the joint line posteriorly. This avoids the posterior fibers of the PCL and minimizes disruption of the proximal tibiofibular joint.

The osteotomy is opened to the desired correction with careful maintenance of the posterior cortex, which is fenestrated with a 3.2-mm drill to increase the flexibility of the hinge while avoiding destabilization of the osteotomy. The osteotomy is packed with bone graft when required (ie, when it is greater than 7 mm) and fixed with an anterior plate and screws.

Medial Opening Wedge Biplane Osteotomy

This procedure is performed in the same manner as the standard medial opening wedge technique except that the anterior aspect of the osteotomy is either opened or closed to increase or decrease slope, respectively. To increase slope, we like to use plates with square, rather

Table 2: Rehabilitation Program Following High Tibial Osteotomy

Timeline	Exercise
0 to 3 weeks	Passive ROM using slider board
	Pedal rocking on bicycle
	Isometric quadriceps activation
3 to 6 weeks	Full-circle pedaling on bicycle—spinning or very light resistance only
	Active full range of motion
	Side-lying gluteus medius strengthening
	Hip abduction/adduction, flexion and extension with resistance fixed above knee (ie, pulley or resistance tubing)
	Pool exercises—hip abduction/adduction, flexion and extension, knee flexion and extension
	Gait pattern training with crutches focusing on proper heel strike/toe off.
	Pool: deep-water (chest-level) running or cycling
	Leg press or squat with weight off-loaded to 24-40 lb (important to respect ROM restriction associated with any cartilage/meniscus restoration/repair)
6 to 9 weeks	Pool: shallow-water (waist-level) walking as weight-bearing restrictions allow
	As a general guideline, when 60% of body is submerged, 60% of body weight is off-loaded
	Standing/seated calf raise
	Bilateral wobble-board balancing as weight-bearing status allows
	Knee flexion/extension with very light resistance
Upon full weight bearing	Gait training to restore normal gait
	Step up and step down to work on alignment and eccentric control
	Elliptical trainer and bicycle for cardiovascular conditioning

ROM = range of motion.

than trapezoidal, wedges. These also can be placed more anteriorly as required. To decrease slope, a staple can be used along with the opening wedge plate to gain anterior compression with respect to the posterior opening. Decreasing the posterior tibial slope with opening wedge osteotomies can be technically challenging, however, and should be limited to small corrections.

Rehabilitation

All patients are routinely discharged home on the first postoperative day. Patients are placed in a postoperative brace for 6 weeks with no restriction of movement unless another intra-articular procedure is performed that would require limitation of range of motion. Toe-touch weight bearing with crutches is maintained for at least the first 2 to 4 weeks, with regular radiologic follow-up to guide the length of protected weight bearing, depending on osteotomy stability, choice of fixation, and graft incorporation. We preoperatively warn patients that this may take up to 3 months. With some of the newer fixed-angle devices, patients may be fully weight bearing by 4 to 6 weeks. Our rehabilitation protocol is outlined in **Table 2**. The initial postoperative period (0 to 6 weeks) focuses on the return of range of motion and quadriceps activation. By 6 weeks, patients are started on a stationary bicycle at low resistance and in the swimming pool doing walking and lunges. Once off crutches, further closed-chain quadriceps work is continued, progressing to elliptical training, treadmill, and light jogging by 6 months, depending on

Table 3: Pearls and Pitfalls for Osteotomies About the Knee

Pearls	Pitfalls
All osteotomies	
Thorough patient evaluation, counseling, and goal setting	Violation of opposite cortex—assess stability and stabilize if necessary
Accurate preoperative planning and radiographic evaluation	Making asymmetric bone cuts in sagittal plane
Adequate exposure	Opening the osteotomy before the anterior and posterior cortices are osteotomized
Use of intraoperative fluoroscopy to check guide pin position, and osteotome advancement, prevent lateral cortex violation, and avoid intra-articular screw placement	
Complete exposure of the posterior tibia or femur with protection of the neurovascular structures using a curved, blunt retractor placed directly on bone	
Different types of plate may be indicated for different patients and concomitant ACL reconstruction. We prefer to use a lower-profile nonlocking plate; for individuals heavier than 220 lb, a more rigid construct may be indicated with locking screw technology to allow for early mobilization	
HTO, medial opening	
The osteotomy should always be performed parallel to the joint line in the sagittal plane and below the guide pin to help prevent intra-articular fracture	Poor guide pin positioning
Use oscillating saw to breach cortex only	Neglecting the posterior tibial slope when making the osteotomy (ie, osteotomy performed in nonparallel fashion to the joint line in the sagittal plane)
To avoid altering the posterior tibial slope, the distraction of the osteotomy anteriorly (at the tibial tubercle) should be approximately one-half its distraction posteromedially	Thick, traditional-type osteotomes can apply a greater distraction moment when completing the osteotomy and carry an inherent risk of creating an extra- and/or intra-articular fracture. This is considerably minimized with thin, flexible osteotomes; however, these should be advanced with frequent fluoroscopy checks to avoid misdirection.
Tension of the MCL should be assessed during distraction, and lengthening by fenestration (of the MCL) may assist in achieving larger corrections	
Pay particular attention when securing the osteotomy plate, positioning it on the posteromedial cortex	

Table 3: *(continued)*	
Pearls	**Pitfalls**
HTO, lateral closing	
Make osteotomy 2 cm distal to lateral joint line Complete posterior cortical resection in piecemeal fashion with Kerrison rongeurs	Decreasing tibial slope inadvertently
HTO, lateral opening	

In larger corrections, the anterior capsule of the
  proximal tibiofibular joint may be opened to aid in
  opening the wedge	

ACL = anterior cruciate ligament, HTO = high tibial osteotomy, MCL = medial collateral ligament.	

previous milestones. We emphasize that patients may require up to 1 year before returning to full activity and recreational sport. Although we have several high-level athletes who have returned to competitive sport, particularly skiing, we would agree with most of the published literature that recreational sport is the normal level achieved and return to full competitive sport is less likely.[22,23]

Complications

Several complications have been reported in the literature, many of which are common to any surgery of the lower limb. Specific complications relating to HTO include neurovascular injury, intra-articular fracture, intra-articular screw placement, and violation of the opposite cortex with resultant instability of the osteotomy. The risk of these complications can be greatly diminished with awareness from the surgeon, placement of a retractor posteriorly at all times when working on the posterior cortex, and the use of intraoperative fluoroscopy. **Table 3** lists some pearls and pitfalls of performing osteotomies, which hopefully will help in reducing the frequency of these complications. In the event of an unstable osteotomy, a decision is made as to the degree of instability and whether additional fixation is required. Often with opening wedge HTO a fracture line propagates but the soft-tissue hinge remains intact. Fixed-angle devices often stabilize the osteotomy satisfactorily without additional fixation.[24] If, however, a locking plate construct is not available, a separate lateral

incision is made and fixation is performed with an appropriate device. If this occurs during a closing wedge osteotomy, the opposite side should be fixed. In the event of opposite cortex fracture in a varus distal femoral osteotomy, the fracture should be fixed internally through a separate medial approach.

Early complications such as infection, deep vein thrombosis, and pulmonary embolism can occur with any operation of the lower limb. We routinely use antibiotic prophylaxis but not chemical thromboprophylaxis because the patients are encouraged to mobilize immediately postoperatively. If the patient has underlying risk factors for thromboembolic disease, we use low-molecular-weight heparin.

Results

Interpreting the results of osteotomy about the knee is fraught with difficulty because of the heterogeneity of patient selection, technique, and postoperative rehabilitation reported in the literature. Very few randomized studies exist; therefore, chiefly level IV evidence is available to assess the relative merits of the technique. Due to the resurgence of HTO in the past 5 years, however, a greater amount of literature is appearing on the subject, which helps refine the technique and indications.

Valgus Osteotomy

Valgus tibial osteotomy for medial gonarthrosis has been studied widely, mostly in the form of case series. Early reports were often associated with high complication rates and postoperative rehabilitation, which included a period in plaster cast immobilization. Hernigou et al[25] reported their results in a group of 93 knees that had been treated by proximal tibial opening wedge osteotomy for varus deformity and medial compartment osteoarthritis. At a mean follow-up of 11.5 years, symptomatic relief had deteriorated with time (mean, 7 years after the osteotomy). After 5 years, 90% of the knees had good or excellent results, whereas after 10 years, only 45% (42 knees) were good or excellent. In the 20 knees with a postoperative hip-knee-ankle angle of 183° to 186°, there was no pain and no progression of arthrosis. In those that were undercorrected (an angle of less than 183°), the results were less satisfactory and there was a tendency to a slow deterioration. All five knees that were overcorrected (angle more than 186°) had progressive degenerative changes in the lateral compartment, indicating postoperative alignment to be a significant determinant of long-term survivorship.

Morrey[26] reported on 33 of 34 consecutive lateral closing wedge osteotomies with secondary arthritis and with a mean age of 31.3 years. At a mean follow-up of 7.5 years, 24 were satisfactory, with improved pain and mean activity level, whereas 9 were considered failures, with 5 requiring TKA at a mean of 4.5 years (range, 2 to 8 years) after osteotomy. Coventry et al[27] reported his results on lateral closing wedge proximal tibial osteotomy in knees at a median follow-up of 10 years (range, 3 to 14 years). Using moderate or severe pain or conversion to arthroplasty as a definition of failure, they found an 87% survival rate at 5 years and a 66% survival rate at 10 years. They found relative patient weight and angular correction to be the only risk factors associated with the duration of survival. If valgus angulation at 1 year was less than 8° in a patient whose weight was more than 1.32 times the ideal weight, the rate of survival decreased to 38% at 5 years thereafter and to 19% at 10 years thereafter. These results indicate that patient body mass and angulation correction factor into the survival of the osteotomy; however, the number of patients in each subgroup was not reported.

Although long-term data are not yet available, reports on newer techniques are encouraging. Birmingham et al[28] prospectively evaluated the results of 126 patients who underwent medial opening wedge HTO, in terms of radiographic correction, knee adduction moment on gait analysis, and subjective outcome using the KOOS (Knee injury and Osteoarthritis Outcome Score). At 2 years postoperatively, significant clinical improvements in all parameters were measured, with a reduction in knee adduction moment and subsequent medial compartment loading during the stance phase of the gait cycle. In a similar study with a smaller patient cohort, DeMeo et al[29] prospectively followed 20 patients who underwent medial opening wedge HTO. Evaluation was performed at 2 years postoperatively with objective radiographic and gait analysis, and at a mean of 8 years postoperatively with subjective outcome measurement.[29] At 2 years, 19 of 20 patients rated their knee as good or excellent. Both HSS (Hospital for Special Surgery) and Lysholm scores were improved postoperatively, and gait analysis revealed a 29% increase in adduction moment from preoperatively to that at the 6-month evaluation. Niemeyer et al[30] prospectively evaluated 46 consecutive medial opening wedge HTOs using the TomoFix plate (Synthes, West Chester, PA). Eighty-six percent of patients reported clinical improvement at 24 months compared with baseline as measured by Lysholm and IKDC (International Knee Documentation Committee) scores. An improvement was also seen from 12 to 24 months, with 67% of the study population returning to their preoperative sports activity level.

Return to sports activity following osteotomy has been the subject of several publications. Salzmann et al[23] reviewed a series of 65 patients who underwent HTO for medial compartment knee arthritis. At an average of 36 months after surgery, 90% of patients were engaged in sports and recreational activities compared with 88% before surgery. No patients were involved in competitive sport, but many continued to do high-impact activities such as downhill skiing or mountain biking. On average, a reduction in Tegner activity scale from 4.9 ± 2.3 to 4.3 ± 1.5 was observed. In a review article by Gougoulias et al,[22] 11 level IV studies were evaluated that reported on return to sport following osteotomy of the lower limb. They found that no patients returned to competitive sport; however, most were able to participate in recreational sporting activity, but progression of arthritis was a risk.

The debate regarding closing wedge versus opening wedge osteotomy continues, with more recent studies favoring the opening wedge technique. Cited shortcomings of the lateral closing wedge technique include the need to detach the lateral tibial muscle attachment (anterior compartment musculature), the possible need for fibular osteotomy or proximal tibiofibular joint dissection, the need for dissection of the common peroneal nerve, and potentially a more difficult revision to TKA.[31] Very few comparative studies have been reported, however. In a randomized clinical study by Brouwer et al,[32] no differences in outcome or complication rate were noted at 1 year. Luites et al[33] performed a randomized study assessing the stability of opening wedge versus closing wedge osteotomy using radiostereometry. At 24 months, they found no differences in pain, knee function, or stability. They did, however, conclude that the opening wedge technique was more likely to achieve the intended correction.

Varus Osteotomy

Results of proximal tibial varus osteotomy have previously not equaled those of proximal tibial valgus osteotomy. Shoji and Insall[34] reported "far inferior" results with regard to retention of mobility, relief of pain, and achievement of stability in a group of 49 varus osteotomies that were compared with a previously published series of 63 valgus osteotomies.

Coventry[15] reported that 24 of 31 knees had no pain or only occasional mild pain at a mean follow-up of 9.4 years after a closing wedge varus osteotomy for valgus knees with painful OA of the lateral compartment. The remaining seven still had moderate or severe pain at follow-up.

Recently, Marti et al[20] reported good or excellent results in 30 of 34 patients at a mean follow-up of 11 years using a lateral opening wedge varus osteotomy. These late results are better than those described previously by Harding[35] and certainly seem to reflect more favorably on the lateral opening wedge osteotomy for correction of valgus deformity less than 15°.

Aglietti and Mechetti[36] reported on a series of 18 patients with a mean age of 54 years who underwent distal varus osteotomy for lateral compartment arthritis with a mean tibiofemoral angle of 17.5° preoperatively. At a mean follow-up of 9 years, 13 were rated as having good

or excellent results per the HSS score, and only one knee required a TKA, at 5 years.

In a similar report, Kosashvili et al[37] published results of a consecutive series of 33 distal femoral varus osteotomies with minimum follow-up of 10 years. At a mean follow-up of 15.6 years, 16 had failed, requiring TKA. Of the remaining 17 knees, 10 had good or excellent results.

Amendola and Bonasia[31] published a review of outcomes from HTO, including a summary of survivorship analysis. It is difficult to draw conclusions from these data because of the variability of techniques and fixation systems used, many of which are no longer used in modern clinical practice. That said, 75% to 94% survivorship was observed at 5 years, 51% to 97.6% at 10 years, and 39% to 94.4% at 15 years.

Osteotomy With Ligament Deficiency

Noyes et al[5] showed the benefit of combining HTO with ACL reconstruction to address complex instability patterns. Of the 41 patients who were treated, 16 had intra-articular ACL reconstruction plus HTO, and 14 had an extra-articular tenodesis. At 4.5 years, pain was reduced in 71%, instability was eliminated in 85%, and 66% were able to return to light recreational activities. Thirty-seven percent of patients reported their knees to be normal or very good, and 34% reported them as good. Gait analysis in 17 of the patients showed a significantly increased adduction moment preoperatively compared with controls, with resolution to normal limits postoperatively. In a similar study by Bonin et al,[38] 30 patients were evaluated after combined ACL reconstruction and valgus HTO. At a mean of 12 years, only 5 of 30 knees had progressed by one arthritis grade. In addition, 14 patients were competing in intensive sports and 11 were playing sports at a moderate level.

Giffin et al[39] demonstrated how changing the tibial slope in cadaveric knees affected knee kinematics. They found that an increase in posterior and anterior slope can increase the in situ forces across the ACL and PCL, respectively. Furthermore, increasing posterior slope during HTO can assist with treating the PCL-deficient knee, reducing posterior sag.[21] Since then, a greater emphasis has been placed on the use of combined bony and soft-tissue procedures when treating these patients.

Osteotomy With Cartilage Repair

Although perhaps not indicated as frequently in the baby boomer population as in patients younger than 45 years, cartilage repair techniques may be used in older patients and should be determined on a case-by-case basis. Gomoll et al[40] reported on a series of seven patients who underwent the triad of meniscus transplantation, cartilage repair, and osteotomy, the so-called biologic joint arthroplasty. At 2 years, all reported significant improvement in outcome scores (IKDC, Lysholm, KOOS), with six returning to unrestricted functional activities. It is unclear which of these procedures provided the greatest impact on functional outcome. Sterett et al[6] reported the survivorship of 106 knees in patients with a mean age of 52 years who received medial opening wedge HTO plus microfracture of the medial femoral condyle. At 5 and 7 years, the survivorship was 97% and 91%, respectively, with subjective outcome scores maintained out to 9 years. Interestingly, the authors found that patients who had a medial meniscus injury at the time of surgery were 9.2 times more likely to undergo TKA than patients without. Mahomed et al[41] recommended the use of osteotomy to unload the affected compartment when performing fresh osteochondral allografting for posttraumatic defects of the knee. Results demonstrated an improvement in survivorship and outcome in patients who undergo osteotomy as a combined procedure with the allografting.

Summary

Osteotomy to correct malalignment of the lower limb is a tried and tested procedure. Since the 1960s, surgeons have developed several techniques to off-load diseased compartments in the knee joint in an attempt to prolong the life of the native joints. Although it cannot reverse the degenerative disease pathway, osteotomy can provide a patient with significant pain relief and maintenance of function and activity level, often for at least 10 years. This is very important for mature athletes, as it allows them to maintain a level of activity that a joint arthroplasty cannot offer.

The importance of patient selection and meticulous surgical technique cannot be stressed enough. A patient who understands the goals of the operation and accepts the long rehabilitation will be more likely to gain a satisfactory result. The indications for osteotomy do not lie just with malalignment. It is now indicated in the presence of ligament insufficiency and cartilage repair, and the use of osteotomy will likely grow as techniques and surgical hardware continue to evolve. When coupled with new methods of addressing the biology of the underlying problem, this procedure is sure to be used not only for the current generation of baby boomers but also in the future, to treat generations X and Y.

References

1. Cooke TD: Pathogenetic mechanisms in polyarticular osteoarthritis. *Clin Rheum Dis* 1985;11(2):203-238.

2. Coventry MB: Osteotomy of the upper portion of the tibia for degenerative arthritis of the knee: A preliminary report. *J Bone Joint Surg Am* 1965;47:984-990.

3. Coventry MB: Upper tibial osteotomy for gonarthrosis: The evolution of the operation in the last 18 years and long term results. *Orthop Clin North Am* 1979;10(1):191-210.

4. Maquet P: The biomechanics of the knee and surgical possibilities of healing osteoarthritic knee joints. *Clin Orthop Relat Res* 1980;(146):102-110.

5. Noyes FR, Barber SD, Simon R: High tibial osteotomy and ligament reconstruction in varus angulated, anterior cruciate ligament-deficient knees: A two- to seven-year follow-up study. *Am J Sports Med* 1993;21(1):2-12.

6. Sterett WI, Steadman JR, Huang MJ, Matheny LM, Briggs KK: Chondral resurfacing and high tibial osteotomy in the varus knee: Survivorship analysis. *Am J Sports Med* 2010;38(7):1420-1424.

7. Lane Smith R, Trindade MC, Ikenoue T, et al: Effects of shear stress on articular chondrocyte metabolism. *Biorheology* 2000;37(1-2):95-107.

8. Teramoto M, Kaneko S, Shibata S, Yanagishita M, Soma K: Effect of compressive forces on extracellular matrix in rat mandibular condylar cartilage. *J Bone Miner Metab* 2003;21(5):276-286.

9. Dugdale TW, Noyes FR, Styer D: Preoperative planning for high tibial osteotomy: The effect of lateral tibiofemoral separation and tibiofemoral length. *Clin Orthop Relat Res* 1992;(274):248-264.

10. Paley D, Herzenberg JE, Tetsworth K, McKie J, Bhave A: Deformity planning for frontal and sagittal plane

corrective osteotomies. *Orthop Clin North Am* 1994;25(3):425-465.

11. Cole BJ, Freedman KB, Taksali S, et al: Use of a lateral offset short-leg walking cast before high tibial osteotomy. *Clin Orthop Relat Res* 2003;(408):209-217.

12. Amendola A, Fowler PJ, Litchfield R, Kirkley S, Clatworthy M: Opening wedge high tibial osteotomy using a novel technique: Early results and complications. *J Knee Surg* 2004;17(3):164-169.

13. Agneskirchner JD, Hurschler C, Wrann CD, Lobenhoffer P: The effects of valgus medial opening wedge high tibial osteotomy on articular cartilage pressure of the knee: A biomechanical study. *Arthroscopy* 2007;23(8):852-861.

14. Adili A, Bhandari M, Giffin R, Whately C, Kwok DC: Valgus high tibial osteotomy: Comparison between an Ilizarov and a Coventry wedge technique for the treatment of medial compartment osteoarthritis of the knee. *Knee Surg Sports Traumatol Arthrosc* 2002;10(3):169-176.

15. Coventry MB: Proximal tibial varus osteotomy for osteoarthritis of the lateral compartment of the knee. *J Bone Joint Surg Am* 1987;69(1):32-38.

16. Bonnin M, Chambat P: Current status of valgus angle, tibial head closing wedge osteotomy in media gonarthrosis. *Orthopade* 2004;33(2):135-142.

17. Learmonth ID: A simple technique for varus supracondylar osteotomy in genu valgum. *J Bone Joint Surg Br* 1990;72(2):235-237.

18. McDermott AG, Finklestein JA, Farine I, Boynton EL, MacIntosh DL, Gross A: Distal femoral varus osteotomy for valgus deformity of the knee. *J Bone Joint Surg Am* 1988;70(1):110-116.

19. Morrey BF, Edgerton BC: Distal femoral osteotomy for lateral gonarthrosis. *Instr Course Lect* 1992;41:77-85.

20. Marti RK, Verhagen RA, Kerkhoffs GM, Moojen TM: Proximal tibial varus osteotomy: Indications, technique, and five to twenty-one-year results. *J Bone Joint Surg Am* 2001;83(2):164-170.

21. Giffin JR, Shannon FJ: The role of the high tibial osteotomy in the unstable knee. *Sports Med Arthrosc* 2007;15(1):23-31.

22. Gougoulias N, Khanna A, Maffulli N: Sports activities after lower limb osteotomy. *Br Med Bull* 2009;91:111-121.

23. Salzmann GM, Ahrens P, Naal FD, et al: Sporting activity after high tibial osteotomy for the treatment of medial compartment knee osteoarthritis. *Am J Sports Med* 2009;37(2):312-318.

24. Agneskirchner JD, Freiling D, Hurschler C, Lobenhoffer P: Primary stability of four different implants for opening wedge high tibial osteotomy. *Knee Surg Sports Traumatol Arthrosc* 2006;14(3):291-300.

25. Hernigou P, Medevielle D, Debeyre J, Goutallier D: Proximal tibial osteotomy for osteoarthritis with varus deformity: A ten to thirteen-year follow-up study. *J Bone Joint Surg Am* 1987;69(3):332-354.

26. Morrey BF: Upper tibial osteotomy for secondary osteoarthritis of the knee. *J Bone Joint Surg Br* 1989;71(4):554-559.

27. Coventry MB, Ilstrup DM, Wallrichs SL: Proximal tibial osteotomy: A critical long-term study of eighty-seven cases. *J Bone Joint Surg Am* 1993;75(2):196-201.

28. Birmingham TB, Giffin JR, Chesworth BM, et al: Medial opening wedge high tibial osteotomy: A prospective cohort study of gait, radiographic, and patient-reported outcomes. *Arthritis Rheum* 2009;61(5):648-657.

29. DeMeo PJ, Johnson EM, Chiang PP, Flamm AM, Miller MC: Midterm follow-up of opening-wedge high tibial osteotomy. *Am J Sports Med* 2010;38(10):2077-2084.

30. Niemeyer P, Koestler W, Kaehny C, et al: Two-year results of open-wedge high tibial osteotomy with fixation by medial plate fixator for medial compartment arthritis with varus malalignment of the knee. *Arthroscopy* 2008;24(7):796-804.

31. Amendola A, Bonasia DE: Results of high tibial osteotomy: Review of the literature. *Int Orthop* 2010;34(2):155-160.

32. Brouwer RW, Bierma-Zeinstra SM, van Raaij TM, Verhaar JA: Osteotomy for medial compartment arthritis of the knee using a closing wedge or an opening wedge controlled by a Puddu plate: A one-year randomised, controlled study. *J Bone Joint Surg Br* 2006;88(11):1454-1459.

33. Luites JW, Brinkman JM, Wymenga AB, van Heerwaarden RJ: Fixation stability of opening- versus closing-wedge high tibial osteotomy: A randomised clinical trial using radiostereometry. *J Bone Joint Surg Br* 2009;91(11):1459-1465.

34. Shoji H, Insall J: High tibial osteotomy for osteoarthritis of the knee with valgus deformity. *J Bone Joint Surg Am* 1973;55(5):963-973.

35. Harding ML: A fresh appraisal of tibial osteotomy for osteoarthritis of the knee. *Clin Orthop Relat Res* 1976;(114):223-234.

36. Aglietti P, Menchetti PP: Distal femoral varus osteotomy in the valgus osteoarthritic knee. *Am J Knee Surg* 2000;13(2):89-95.

37. Kosashvili Y, Safir O, Gross A, Morag G, Lakstein D, Backstein D: Distal femoral varus osteotomy for lateral osteoarthritis of the knee: A minimum ten-year follow-up. *Int Orthop* 2010;34(2):249-254.

38. Bonin N, Ait Si Selmi T, Donell ST, Dejour H, Neyret P: Anterior cruciate reconstruction combined with valgus upper tibial osteotomy: 12 years follow-up. *Knee* 2004;11(6):431-437.

39. Giffin JR, Vogrin TM, Zantop T, Woo SL, Harner CD: Effects of increasing tibial slope on the biomechanics of the knee. *Am J Sports Med* 2004;32(2):376-382.

40. Gomoll AH, Kang RW, Chen AL, Cole BJ: Triad of cartilage restoration for unicompartmental arthritis treatment in young patients: Meniscus allograft transplantation, cartilage repair and osteotomy. *J Knee Surg* 2009;22(2):137-141.

41. Mahomed MN, Beaver RJ, Gross AE: The long-term success of fresh, small fragment osteochondral allografts used for intraarticular post-traumatic defects in the knee joint. *Orthopedics* 1992;15(10):1191-1199.

Chapter 37

Foot and Ankle Problems in the Mature Athlete

J.C. Clark, MD
Douglas J. Wyland, MD

Key Points

- Foot and ankle injuries represent a significant portion of the problems encountered by mature athletes.
- Nonsurgical methods of treatment, including oral anti-inflammatory drugs, injections, orthoses, and activity modification, can alleviate most foot and ankle problems in the mature athlete.
- Foot and ankle injuries that occur in youth can lead to chronic conditions in mature athletes that can limit their sports activity.
- Arthritic conditions in the mature athlete include hallux rigidus and ankle osteoarthritis.
- Management of acute foot and ankle injuries in the mature athlete is similar to that used in youth.
- Healing potential and comorbidities need to be taken into consideration when planning a treatment protocol and estimating return to play for the mature athlete.

Introduction

Foot and ankle conditions represent a significant proportion of the ailments that can affect the mature athlete. Because mature athletes are more likely to be endurance-type athletes, chronic overuse injuries predominate in the foot and ankle. For example, in one study of athletes older than 60 years, 20% had Achilles tendon and calf symptoms.[1] This chapter covers many of the more commonly seen tendon disorders, such as peroneal tendinitis, posterior tibial tendinitis, Achilles tendinitis, plantar fasciitis, and flexor hallucis longus tendinitis. It also touches on some of the acute injuries seen in the mature athlete, such as Achilles tendon tears and fractures. Also discussed in this chapter are sections on entrapment neuropathies, stress fractures, and conditions that can be sequelae of previous ankle injuries, such as anterolateral, anterior, and posterior ankle impingement and chronic ankle instability. Last, no chapter on foot and ankle problems in the mature athlete is complete without touching on the arthritides, specifically hallux rigidus and ankle arthritis. Many of these conditions can be managed nonsurgically, with a combination of physical therapy, orthoses, and anti-inflammatory drugs, including corticosteroid injections.

Tendon Disorders

Peroneal Tendons

Dysfunction of the peroneus longus or peroneus brevis tendon is an often-missed cause of acute or chronic lateral ankle pain. Disorders include peroneal tendinitis/tenosynovitis with or without associated tears, tendon subluxation, and frank tendon dislocation.[2-6]

Peroneal Tendinitis/Tenosynovitis

Peroneal tendinitis/tenosynovitis usually occurs as the result of repetitive or prolonged activity and a recent increase in training. In addition to a history and physical examination, the workup often includes MRI to rule out any complete or partial tears of the tendons, particularly peroneal brevis tears, which historically do not do as well with nonsurgical treatment.[7-9] Nonsurgical measures are often successful, so these measures should be exhausted before surgery is considered. Failure of nonsurgical management after 3 to 6 months necessitates peroneal tenosynovectomy, débridement, and/or repair of tears as well as addressing any predisposing factors such as a hypertrophied peroneal tubercle, low-lying peroneus brevis muscle belly, ankle instability, os peroneum, or hindfoot deformity.

If tears of the peroneus longus or brevis tendon are present, several options can be tried, depending on the magnitude of the tear. Simple tears can usually be managed with débridement of up to one half the tendon or with repair or tubularization.[5,6] After appropriate débridement, more complex tears may not be repairable; in these patients, a side-to-side tenodesis of the diseased tendon to the healthier one may be an option. If both tendons are unusable, further options include flexor digitorum longus (FDL), plantaris, or flexor hallucis longus (FHL) tendon transfers, or staged reconstruction with allograft or free hamstring tendon autograft. The decision to perform a tendon transfer or use a tendon graft depends on the excursion and quality of the peroneal muscles.[2,5,6,10] The presence of peroneal tendon tears may reduce the likelihood that patients will return to their preoperative level of play. Steel and DeOrio[11] reported that fewer than 50% of their patients returned to their preoperative level of play after peroneal tendon repair.

Peroneal Tendon Subluxation/Dislocation

Subluxation and dislocation of the peroneal tendons usually occurs after an acute injury wherein the superior peroneal retinaculum (SPR) is avulsed from its fibular insertion, sometimes with a small fleck of bone. In chronic cases, recurrent ankle sprains have been implicated as a cause, as the SPR becomes increasingly attenuated. Although this injury has historically been associated with alpine skiing, more recent studies reveal that it can occur in any sport.[12-16] Symptoms typically include painful snapping or popping over the lateral ankle and reproducible pain with active dorsiflexion and eversion. Radiographs may reveal a small fleck of bone avulsed from the fibula where the SPR usually attaches. MRI can verify any concomitant tendon tears.

Treatment of acute subluxations and dislocations is controversial. Although nonsurgical treatment with immobilization of the foot in neutral to slight inversion and slight plantar flexion to allow the SPR to heal back down to the fibula can be successful, this treatment can be associated with a high rate of recurrence, especially in athletes.[12-14,17-22] Therefore, acute repair may be a better option for the high-demand athlete.[5,6,16,19] For chronic subluxation and dislocations, surgical treatment is recommended.[5,6,13,18]

For either acute or chronic cases of peroneal tendon dislocation, several reconstructive techniques are available; none has been proven to be more effective than the others.[6] Predisposing patient factors such as hindfoot malalignment, shallow retromalleolar groove, congenital absence of the SPR, or lateral ligamentous laxity also should be taken into consideration. First and foremost, direct SPR anatomic repair should be attempted whenever possible. If the retinaculum is severely attenuated, local soft tissues such as a strip of Achilles tendon, periosteum, peroneus brevis, or plantaris can be used for reinforcement.[2,6] Tendon rerouting behind the calcaneofibular ligament also can be used with or without bone blocks.[2,6] Further bony procedures include various osteotomies of the distal fibula to produce bone blocks that can be rotated or transposed to deepen the fibular groove. If an osteotomy is not desired, the retromalleolar groove can be deepened by raising an osteoperiosteal flap from the posterolateral aspect of the fibula, removing underlying cancellous bone with a burr, reducing the flap, and relocating the tendons with a repair of the SPR.[2,6,13-15,23,24] In 2005, Porter et al[13] reported on nine athletes with recurrent peroneal subluxation who underwent a groove-deepening procedure; eight were able to return to their prior level of activity. Timelines for recovery are generally vague, but the athlete can usually get back to sport in 4 to 5 months after a groove-deepening procedure.[25,26]

Posterior Tibial Tendon

Although most orthopaedic surgeons consider posterior tibial tendinitis a condition of women in their fourth to sixth decades of life and associate it with adult-acquired flatfoot deformity, it may affect athletes as well. In fact, 3.6% to 6% of runners presenting to sports medicine physicians may have the condition.[27-30] Prompt recognition and care of the disorder is paramount because as deformity progresses, success with treatment declines. Moreover, some authors agree that progression of this disorder can be rapid.[29,31-33]

Symptoms of posteromedial ankle pain after an increase in training intensity necessitate evaluation of the posterior tibialis tendon. Inability to perform a single-leg toe raise or lack of hindfoot inversion during the test may indicate rupture; failure to perform the maneuver 10 times suggests tendinitis.[3,29] Radiographs can help rule out other possible causes of pain or demonstrate calcification of the posterior tibial tendon, but MRI provides the most information on the integrity of the tendon.

For tenosynovitis, initial nonsurgical care can range from medial arch orthoses, nonsteroidal anti-inflammatory drugs (NSAIDs), physical therapy, and a significant decrease in training to immediate immobilization for 6 to 8 weeks in a short-leg cast. The decision to immediately immobilize the athlete depends on the severity of the inflammation and the disability encountered. Steroid injections are not recommended because of the possibility of tendon rupture. After 3 to 6 months, athletes who have not improved should be considered candidates for a tenosynovectomy. Frayed, hypertrophic, or degenerative areas require débridement, and tears are appropriately repaired. After initial débridement, the surgeon may find that the remaining tendon is elongated or of questionable strength, in which case resection of the diseased portion can be done, followed by a direct end-to-end repair. If this

cannot be done, transfer of the FDL or FHL tendon to the navicular is recommended.[2,3,29] Medial calcaneal displacement osteotomy also may need to be performed if significant hindfoot valgus exists. Depending on the extent of surgery, athletes can return to sport anywhere from 4 to 12 months postoperatively. Athletes who undergo tenosynovectomy alone can expect to return to sport within 4 months.[2,3,29] McCormack et al[34] reported that seven of eight young athletes returned to sport after surgical débridement. Teasdall and Johnson[35] found subjective improvement and return of function in 16 of 18 patients treated with tenosynovectomy alone for tibialis posterior tendinitis.

Rupture of the tibialis posterior tendon is a debilitating situation and return to previous level of athletic activity is guarded. If feasible, advancement and reattachment of the posterior tibial tendon should be performed, but if not, then reconstruction with the FDL should be done.[32,36,37] If a flatfoot deformity exists in these patients at the time of surgery, it will likely remain postoperatively, resulting in some awkwardness with cutting and poor push-off strength.[37] Woods and Leach[37] reported on two mature athletes in their article on tibialis posterior tendon ruptures. One 41-year-old female tennis player who had undergone advancement and reattachment of a ruptured tibialis posterior tendon returned to sport at 9 months, and a 50-year-old female tennis player who underwent an FDL reconstruction of the tibialis posterior tendon was playing without pain by 13 months.

Achilles Tendon

Numerous afflictions of the Achilles tendon occur in athletes and nonathletes alike. The spectrum of disease includes everything from paratenonitis, tendinosis, paratenonitis with tendinosis, retrocalcaneal bursitis, and insertional tendinosis or tendinitis to acute and chronic partial or complete ruptures.[38] This chapter focuses on Achilles tendinitis, insertional tendinitis, and ruptures.

Achilles Tendinitis

Achilles tendinitis is one of the most common overuse syndromes seen by sports medicine physicians. Runners in particular are at an increased risk, with a tenfold increase in Achilles tendon injuries compared with age-matched controls and a lifetime risk in top-level runners of 7% to 9%.[39] For the mature athlete who wants to continue to stay active, immobilization is generally unacceptable treatment. Instead, relative rest by altering the training regimen, performing water-based activities, and decreasing the weekly mileage is recommended.[40] Ice, NSAIDs, a 1/4- to 3/8-in heel lift, orthoses to correct overpronation, eccentric strengthening, and daily gastrocnemius-soleus complex stretching also are included. Injectable corticosteroids are not used because of the risk of rupture. Use of high-energy extracorporeal shock wave therapy also has been reported.[41,42] Rarely, for athletes in whom 3 to 4 months of nonsurgical treatment fails, surgical management with excision of thickened paratenon can be performed. Schepsis et al[40] reported an 87% satisfaction rate for patients with tenosynovectomy. Arthroscopic procedures for débridement of the paratenon and brisement, wherein saline is injected into the paratenon sheath to disrupt adhesions, also have been described.[2,38,40,43,44]

The greatest difficulty in treating Achilles tendinitis arises when degenerative areas of the tendon representing tendinosis are encountered. Removal of these areas at the time of surgery is recommended. Thus, if the surgeon neglects to evaluate for the presence of tendinosis before surgery, a simple tenosynovectomy can turn into a full-blown reconstruction of the Achilles tendon after removal of the diseased portions. If less than 20% of the tendon is involved, a side-to-side repair can generally be performed. Deficiencies of 20% to 50% may require further reinforcement with gastrocnemius fascia turndown flaps or a plantaris weave.[40] When more than 50% of the tendon is involved, authors recommend more robust procedures to augment the repair, such as autologous FHL or FDL transfers, allograft tendon, or semitendinosis and gracilis autografts.[38,40,45] Outcomes after these more extensive procedures have been good to excellent in 88% to 90% of patients in the general population in some reports,[45,46] but critical reviews by Tallon et al[47] and Longo et al[39] show that it is more realistic to expect successful outcomes in approximately 70% of cases.[39,45-47] With this in mind, counseling the mature athlete on realistic expectations regarding return to preoperative level of performance is paramount.

Insertional Achilles Tendinitis

Aside from tendinitis and tendinosis involving the main body of the tendon, the Achilles tendon can develop insertional tendinitis, which is a true inflammatory process often associated with a Haglund deformity (posterior superior calcaneal tuberosity prominence). Aggressive hill-running, running on hard surfaces, and interval training can exacerbate this condition.[38,40] Examination reveals tenderness at the bone-tendon interface and limited passive dorsiflexion due to pain. Radiographs show calcification within the tendon or emanating from the superior part of the calcaneus. MRI helps to delineate any element of intrasubstance tendinosis or change of signal intensity within the tendon, which may eventually help guide treatment.

As with Achilles tendinitis, nonsurgical options for insertional tendinitis are often successful and therefore should be exhausted before surgery is considered.[48] Eccentric exercises are not as effective for this entity as for noninsertional tendinopathies.[49,50] Good to excellent results have been achieved with several surgical techniques, including a central-splitting approach and débridement of the tendon and calcaneus while using the plantaris for reinforcement, débridement and complete detachment of the tendon followed by V-Y lengthening and reattachment with suture anchors, or débridement and FHL transfer.[38,46,48,51] In 1994, Schepsis et al[52] reported on the long-term follow-up of seven patients with insertional tendinitis whose mean age was 44 years. Six of the seven patients had an excellent or good outcome, which correlated with return to preinjury status with only mild or intermittent discomfort.

With any of these procedures, a graduated postoperative regimen is undertaken with emphasis on achievement of range of motion and then strength. Activities such as cycling and swimming are encouraged. For procedures without extensive involvement of the tendon, light jogging may be permitted on softer surfaces at 3 months. For procedures with more extensive tendon involvement, even light jogging should be forbidden until 4 to 5 months and sometimes even 6 months.[40] The surgeon should inform the patient that return of strength comparable to that of the uninjured leg may take 1 year or longer.

Achilles Tendon Rupture

Achilles tendon ruptures are most commonly seen in the 41- to 50-year-old mature athlete.[2] Basketball and racquet sports account for many of these injuries.[3] On histologic examination, degenerative areas of the tendon have been found in the vicinity of the tear, suggesting that a chronic process was present before the overloading incident.[53,54] In fact, most patients report a history of posterior ankle pain as a prodromal symptom prior to frank rupture. On physical examination of the acute rupture, a positive Thompson test, decreased plantar flexion strength, and a palpable gap confirm the diagnosis. In chronic cases, diagnosis by physical examination may be more difficult. The Thompson test is positive in only 80% of chronic cases, and the gap may be filled in with hemorrhage and scar.[3,55] MRI can be ordered if the clinical diagnosis is still in question, but it is not absolutely necessary.

Although debate still exists about nonsurgical versus surgical treatment of acute tendon ruptures for the general population, surgical repair is generally recommended for acute ruptures in the mature athlete.[50,56-60] For simplification, chronic ruptures are considered those that are more than 4 weeks old, although the terms "neglected" or "delayed" ruptures also have been used.[38,61-63] Treatment with surgical repair is recommended for these injuries as well.

Techniques for repair of acute Achilles tendon rupture vary widely, without any one method showing superiority.[40] The ends of the ruptured tendon can usually be reapproximated with plantar flexion of the ankle, allowing the surgeon to use a modified Kessler, Bunnell, or Krackow stitch technique to secure the repair. Interrupted sutures can then be used to reinforce the repair. If the security of the repair is still in question, a pull-out wire, gastrocnemius turndown fascia graft, plantaris tendon weave, or autologous tendon transfer can be used for further reinforcement.[2-4] Chronic Achilles tendon tear reconstructions require additional procedures to fill the gap left in the tendon after scar tissue is resected, which is often greater than 3 cm.[38,64] Options for chronic repairs include direct end-to-end repair, local tissue transfer, tissue augmentation, synthetic biomaterials, and allograft.[38,40] For small gaps of 1 to 2 cm, direct end-to-end repair can usually be accomplished. Defects of 2 to 5 cm will require local

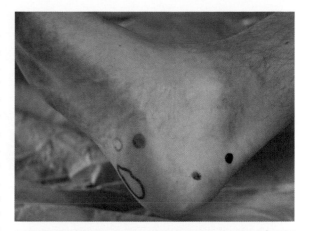

Figure 1   Points of tenderness associated with various etiologies of posterior heel pain are marked on the foot. Note the close proximity of the points of tenderness for the Baxter nerve (pink dot) and plantar fasciitis (green circle). Tenderness deep to the abductor hallucis coincides with irritation of the Baxter nerve, whereas tenderness closer to the medial calcaneal tuberosity is associated with plantar fasciitis. Black dot = retrocalcaneal bursitis; red circle = heel pad syndrome; blue dot = calcaneal stress fracture.

tissue augmentation such as a plantaris weave, V-Y advancement, or a fascial turndown technique. Larger gaps will necessitate local tendon transfers (FHL, FDL, peroneus brevis) or free-tissue transfers with autograft (semitendinosis, gracilis, fascia lata) or allograft.[50,63-67] Synthetic materials are available as well, but often combinations of the above are used.[38,40,68]

Posterior Heel Pain

Inevitably, every surgeon will evaluate a mature athlete with posterior heel pain. Although some of the conditions have overlapping pain patterns, most localize to a certain area, allowing the clinician with a thorough knowledge of the anatomy of the posterior foot and ankle to easily pinpoint the cause on examination (**Figure 1**). Systemic disorders such as the seronegative arthritides, psoriatic arthritis, Reiter disease, diffuse idiopathic skeletal hyperostosis (DISH), rheumatoid arthritis, fibromyalgia, and gout should also be kept in

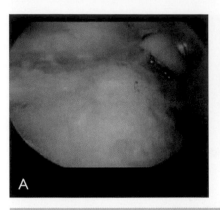
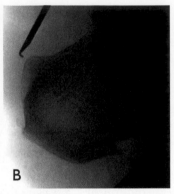
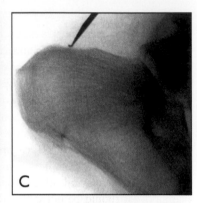

Figure 2 Arthroscopic Haglund deformity resection. **A,** Arthroscopic view of the hindfoot during excision of the retrocalcaneal bursa. Intraoperative fluoroscopic images before (**B**) and after (**C**) Haglund deformity resection.

mind in the workup of posterior heel pain in the mature athlete.

Retrocalcaneal Bursitis

The retrocalcaneal bursa lies in the space between the anterior aspect of the Achilles tendon and the superior tuberosity of the posterior calcaneus. With dorsiflexion of the ankle, pressure is exerted on the bursa, making uphill runners prone to this disorder. Inflammation of the bursa is often associated with Haglund deformity and insertional Achilles tendinitis, but it can exist in isolation own. If concomitant Achilles tendinopathy is suspected or radiographs show calcification of the tendon, MRI may allow better evaluation.

Treatment begins with nonsurgical measures, including decreases in training regimen, avoiding aggravating factors such as hill running, stretching, U-shaped posterior heel pads to relieve pressure from shoe wear, NSAIDs, and possibly immobilization in severe cases. Corticosteroid injections have been described but are generally avoided because of the risk of Achilles tendon rupture. Surgically, partial calcaneal ostectomy and retrocalcaneal bursectomy are performed via either an open or an arthroscopic approach. Studies of the arthroscopic approach have shown shorter surgical time, less morbidity, and fewer complications[69-73] (**Figure 2**). McGarvey et al[48] reported an 82% satisfaction rate in 22 patients of various activity levels; however, only 13 were able to return to sports. Schepsis et al[52] reported 75% satisfactory results in their series of competitive runners treated surgically for retrocalcaneal bursitis,

with 13 of 24 able to get back to their preoperative level of activity without pain.

Plantar Fasciitis

Although most orthopaedic surgeons are familiar with this condition and have treated patients with it, few can agree on the appropriate treatment regimen. Plantar fasciitis is the most common cause of plantar heel pain and is commonly found in runners.[74-76] Acute plantar fasciitis often resolves with little or no treatment, but chronic recurring plantar fasciitis is challenging to treat. Tenderness is located at the origin of the plantar fascia at the medial calcaneal tuberosity. This must be differentiated from the location of pain with entrapment of the nerve to the abductor digiti quinti, the medial calcaneal nerve, and the tarsal tunnel. Nonsurgical treatment involves myriad choices, including training regimen modifications, relative rest, heel cups, night splints, physical therapy, ice, heat, stretching, steroid injections, ultrasound, and extracorporeal shock wave therapy.[2,3,77-79] Typically we prefer to use a combination of gastrocnemius–soleus complex stretching, plantar fascia–specific stretching exercises, ice massage, NSAIDs, heel cups, and a reduction in training regimen. Patient expectations should be that full recovery can take up to 6 to 10 months but is 90% successful.[76] As with other soft-tissue injuries about the foot and ankle, cortisone injections to the plantar fascia origin may increase the risk of plantar fascia rupture and therefore are not recommended. In recalcitrant cases, open partial or complete plantar fasciotomy can be performed with varying results.[76] However, the desire to avoid open procedures and the possible biomechanical consequences of aggressive release of the plantar fascia have led some authors to develop percutaneous plantar fasciotomy and endoscopic plantar fasciotomy with satisfactory results.[80-86] Past studies on return to play after plantar fascia surgery included the study by Snider et al[87] in 1983, in which 8 of 9 patients were able to return to running at an average of 4.5 months, and the 1986 study by Leach et al,[88] in which 14 of 15 athletes returned to full athletic activity, most by 9 weeks.[87,88] It should be noted that these studies used open procedures. In the endoscopic study reported by Ogilvie-Harris and Lobo,[86] a subgroup of 41 patients were athletes. Only 22% were able to participate in sports preoperatively, and all of them had pain during sports. Postoperatively, 76% were able to return to their previous level of play, and 71% had no pain during sports activities.

Heel Pad Syndrome

Sometimes referred to as central heel pain syndrome, fat pad atrophy, or heel pain syndrome, this entity also affects the mature athlete. The location of pain is directly over the central heel without any radiation or aggravation of the pain by extension of the toes as in plantar fasciitis. This fat pad plays a role in resisting torsional and compressive forces during the gait cycle, wherein it is subjected to upwards of 200% of body weight with running.[89] One of the predisposing factors to developing this syndrome is age, as the fat pad gradually loses water, collagen, and adipose tissue after age 40 years. Soft-soled shoes and cushioned heel pads and cups are prescribed for those with atrophy (unpublished data, B. Den Hartog, 2009 American Orthopaedic Foot and Ankle Society [AOFAS], course presentation). Corticosteroid injections should be avoided, as these may exacerbate fat atrophy.

Calcaneal Stress Fracture

Repetitive load to the heel can result in a stress fracture of the calcaneus. In the mature athlete, osteopenia may play an additional role. With regard to the anatomic region of involvement, Sormaala et al[90] used MRI to evaluate military recruits with calcaneal stress fractures and found that most of the fractures occurred in the

posterior and upper half of the calcaneus. Pain is diffuse and nonspecific, but the squeeze test (compression of the medial and lateral walls of the calcaneus) exacerbates the discomfort. Initial radiographs may be negative, as only 15% of MRI-detectable calcaneal stress fractures will be evident on plain radiographs obtained at the initial visit.[90] Further imaging options include MRI and bone scan, especially if swelling is present or the athlete is in season. Initial treatment is nonsurgical, including either immobilization in a non–weight-bearing cast for 4 to 8 weeks or restriction of activities in a walking boot for 4 to 8 weeks, and then gradual resumption of activities. Running should not be started until swelling is absent and radiographs show healing (unpublished data, D. Porter, 2009 AOFAS course presentation). Conversion to an acute fracture is very uncommon, so surgery is rarely needed. In his original series of military recruits, Leabhart[91] reported that most were able to get back to training by 8 weeks. In the study by Sormaala et al,[90] recruits returned to normal training activity within an average of 77 days after first seeking medical attention. Related stress injuries to the navicular, cuboid, and talus should be taken into consideration as well if an athlete has a calcaneal stress fracture.

First Branch of the Lateral Plantar Nerve (Baxter Nerve)

Much attention has been given to the first branch of the lateral plantar nerve, also called the Baxter nerve or the inferior calcaneal branch of the lateral plantar nerve. This branch travels between the abductor hallucis and the quadratus plantae, where it can become entrapped, producing inferior medial heel pain.[2,92] Even though the condition can occur in both athletes and nonathletes, it is predominantly found in middle-aged runners and joggers. Tenderness over the first branch deep to the abductor hallucis with radiation of the pain helps to diagnose this condition. Nonsurgical treatment, involving shock-absorbent heel cups, soft-soled shoes, contrast baths, NSAIDs, and a possible corticosteroid injection, should be exhausted before surgical release of the nerve is performed. Baxter and Pfeffer[92] had excellent or good results in 85% of the athletes they operated on, with 79% obtaining complete relief of pain. More than 80% were able to return to full activity at an average of 2.8 months postoperatively.

FHL Tendinitis

Although FHL tendinitis is more common in ballet dancers, hence the term "dancer's tendinitis," it also can occur in tennis players and runners.[3,93] It is included in this section because pain is referred to the plantar heel or more commonly to the posteromedial aspect of the ankle behind the medial malleolus. Swelling, tenderness, and crepitus can be present. A classic examination finding is pain with resisted great toe flexion. Initial treatment is nonsurgical, including avoidance of the exacerbating activities, NSAIDs, and a walking boot. More severe cases or chronic tendinitis may require a short period of casting. When the tendinitis becomes recalcitrant or triggering develops, surgical release of the tendon sheath with repair of any tears is indicated.

Posterior Ankle Impingement Syndrome

Posterior ankle impingement syndrome (PAIS) refers to pain in the posterior ankle with forced passive plantar flexion.[94] It can occur in up to 18% of runners with impingement-type symptoms.[95] Several different etiologies exist, but this discussion will focus mainly on treatment of os trigonum and chronic impingement of the soft tissues that can lead to calcified inflammatory tissue in the posterolateral corner of the ankle joint.[96] With PAIS, pain is deep and posterolateral, typically behind the peroneal tendons. Discomfort with forced passive plantar flexion of the ankle is the test of choice. Injecting some local anesthetic into the deep posterior ankle behind the peroneal tendons should take away the pain. Ankle radiographs, including a plantar flexion view to evaluate for bony impingement, should be obtained. Calcified ligamentous tissue in the posterolateral corner may be better visualized with an underexposed 25° external rotation radiograph.[94] MRI will help exclude other causes of posterior ankle pain if the diagnosis is in doubt.

Initial treatment of PAIS is always nonsurgical, with successful results achieved approximately 60% of the time.[97] Surgery can involve open or arthroscopic excision of the os trigonum and chronic inflammatory tissues. Arthroscopic approaches may offer a quicker return to activity and less morbidity than open approaches.[71,98-102] Scholten et al[98] reported on 55 ankles treated with endoscopy for posterior ankle impingement; the patients returned to sport at a median time of 8 weeks if the pathology was osseous and 12 weeks if soft-tissue impingement was the predominant pathology. Willits et al[101] reported that 14 of 15 patients were able to return to sporting activities at their preinjury level after endoscopy for posterior ankle impingement. Jerosch and Fadel[100] excised a symptomatic os trigonum in 10 patients; 9 had no symptoms during activities of daily living by 4 weeks. Furthermore, several of the patients who were professional athletes were able to resume sports by 8 weeks.

Hallux Disorders

Hallux Sesamoid Disorders

The medial (tibial) and lateral (fibular) sesamoids lie within the two tendons of the flexor hallucis brevis that are plantar to the first metatarsal head. Mature athletes with pain during the toe-off phase of gait, swelling in the first metatarsophalangeal (MTP) joint, decreased range of motion because of pain, and decreased strength should be evaluated for a hallux sesamoid disorder. The differential is broad, including sesamoidal stress fractures, avulsion fractures, sprain of a bipartite sesamoid, dislocation, osteonecrosis, sesamoid bursitis, neural entrapment, and arthritis of the first metatarsal–sesamoid joint.[2] Runners and golfers are prone to stress fractures. For bony pathology, the axial sesamoid view or CT scans in both the sagittal and coronal planes with 1-mm slices are very useful. If these are negative, soft-tissue etiology must be considered, and a period of nonsurgical treatment can be used before MRI is obtained.[103]

For most sesamoid disorders, including fractures, nonsurgical treatment is undertaken, using modalities that unload the sesamoids, such as metatarsal pads, dorsiflexion-blocking taping techniques, decreased heel height of shoes, and periods of non–weight bearing and immobilization. Steroid injections can be used in cases of bursitis. When nonsurgical treatment is unsuccessful, the symptomatic sesamoid can be removed, keeping in mind that residual weakness of first-ray plantar flexion may result. Saxena reported an average time of return to play of 7.4 weeks in one review and 7.5 weeks in a separate study on professional- and varsity-level athletes.[104] Nonprofessional active patients returned in an average of 12 weeks.[104] For stress fractures, options include partial sesamoidectomy, total sesamoidectomy, and autologous bone grafting with or without internal fixation.[105-107] Techniques for preservation of the hallux sesamoids in elite athletes have been recommended to preserve plantar flexion strength.[105]

Hallux Rigidus

Degenerative arthritis of the first MTP joint is second in prevalence only to bunion deformities in terms of first MTP joint pathology. This can be a debilitating condition for the mature athlete, especially dancers and runners. Pain and limitation of range of motion with radiographic changes establish the diagnosis. The athlete should be counseled that this condition is a form of degenerative joint disease and full symptom relief may not be possible in all instances (unpublished data, R. Anderson, 2009 AOFAS course presentation).

For all grades, initial treatment can involve NSAIDs, cortisone injections, stiff insoles, taping techniques, insoles with Morton extensions, and shoe modifications to make room for dorsal osteophytes. Surgical options will often depend on the initial presenting grade and include cheilectomy with or without a dorsal closing-wedge proximal phalangeal osteotomy, fusion, or resection arthroplasty with soft-tissue interposition (unpublished data, R. Anderson and B. Donley, 2009 AOFAS course presentation). Arthroscopic cheilectomy also has been described with good results.[108,109] In general, greater than 50% involvement of the metatarsal head articular surface warrants fusion or interposition arthroplasty in most cases.[110] For the mature athlete who does not want a fusion, resection arthroplasty with soft-tissue interposition may be an attractive option.[111-113] Plantaris, gracilis autograft, or hamstring allograft can all be used to make the anchovy for interposition. Postoperatively, full activity may be resumed by 8 weeks in most cases (unpublished data, R. Anderson, 2009 AOFAS course presentation). If first MTP joint arthrodesis is planned, the patient must understand the potential functional limitations, restriction on sports participation until the arthrodesis is clinically and radiologically united, and the possible need for a long-term orthosis in their athletic shoes. Although several professional athletes have continued their careers after arthrodesis, too few data on returning to sports after first MTP arthrodesis are available to provide reliable counseling to mature athletes (unpublished data, J.K. DeOrio, 2009 AOFAS course presentation).

Ankle Instability

Chronic Lateral Instability

Although acute lateral ankle sprains are the most ubiquitous injury in sports and are seemingly benign, they can actually lead to residual pain, instability, and sequelae that require surgery.[114,115] If immediate appropriate care is provided and a proper rehabilitation program is followed closely, however, the mature athlete can expect an uneventful recovery. Nonetheless, persistent pain, swelling, and instability after an acute inversion ankle sprain may be related to several causes, including missed hindfoot or metatarsal fractures, osteochondral lesions, peroneal pathology, subtalar instability, nerve entrapment, or anterolateral impingement.[116] Approximately 10% to 20% of athletes with a history of ankle inversion injuries demonstrate chronic instability after nonsurgical treatment.[117] This manifests as repeated instability episodes or a feeling of looseness in the ankle and can be related to mechanical instability of the talocrural joint or a functional instability pattern. Mechanical instability can be objectively defined on examination as 10 mm of anterior translation of the talus on the tibia or a 3-mm difference compared to the contralateral side with the anterior drawer test, or more than 9° of talar tilt on inversion stress radiographs.[116] Either of these methods demonstrates laxity of the lateral ligamentous structures. With functional instability, the ligaments are intact, but the surrounding structures of the ankle are incompetent. With either condition, a program of strengthening of the peroneal muscles, proprioception exercises, coordination training, and functional braces may be successful in up to 90% of cases.[116,118,119]

Failure of nonsurgical options, however, necessitates surgery to restore stability to the lateral ankle. MRI is useful for preoperative evaluation of the lateral ligamentous structures to determine their integrity, help guide the type of reconstruction needed, and rule out simultaneous injuries to the peroneal tendons that may need to be addressed. Hindfoot alignment also needs to be assessed because hindfoot varus can eventually lead to failure of a technically sound lateral ligamentous repair. If hindfoot varus is detected, consideration should be given to performing a valgus-producing calcaneal osteotomy. Both anatomic and nonanatomic reconstructions have been described. Nonanatomic reconstructions such as the Evans, Watson-Jones, and Chrisman-Snook procedures use the peroneus brevis tendon to decrease lateral instability of the ankle. Some long-term follow-up studies have been published, but concerns about these reconstructions have been expressed.[117,120-128] Therefore, we choose to do an anatomic reconstruction with either the Broström procedure, Gould modification of the Broström, or anatomic reconstruction with autograft or allograft. Long-term results of the Broström procedure for chronic lateral ankle instability have been shown to be good or excellent in 91% of patients in a study by Bell et al.[129] Excellent results also have been reported in athletes for the Gould modification of the Broström.[130] Prior to anatomic reconstruction, we routinely perform an arthroscopic examination of the ankle to address any intra-articular pathology.[131,132] Using this approach of arthroscopic examination followed by a modified Broström repair, Ferkel and Chams[132] recently reported excellent outcomes in all 21 patients evaluated. Fourteen patients had postoperative stress radiographs, with all 14 showing a side-to-side difference of less than 3°. With regard to athletes, few studies exist on return to sports after anatomic reconstruction. Recently, Li et al[133] reported on returning 49 of 52 high-demand athletes with chronic ankle instability to their preinjury level by 2 years using the modified Broström repair with suture anchors. Krips et al[134] found better results in athletes with chronic instability who underwent an anatomic reconstruction compared to tenodesis; 36 of 41 patients in the anatomic reconstruction group reported an excellent or good outcome. Postoperatively, return to sports should not be expected before 5 months, as running is generally not allowed until 3 months and sport-specific activities, cutting, and jumping are prohibited until 4 months.

Acute Syndesmosis Injury

Stabilizing the distal tibia and fibula is a set of strong ligamentous structures consisting of the anteroinferior tibiofibular ligament (AITFL), posteroinferior tibiofibular ligament (PITFL), transverse tibiofibular ligament, and the interosseous tibiofibular ligament, which are confluent with the interosseous membrane.[116] Collectively, these ligaments make up the syndesmosis,

which can be injured when an athlete internally rotates the leg and body with the foot planted (unpublished data, B. Den Hartog, 2009 AOFAS course presentation). Physical examination maneuvers such as the squeeze test and external rotation stress test are positive. Radiographs evaluating the tibiofibular clear space, tibiofibular overlap, and medial clear space should be ordered as well as external rotation stress radiographs. An increased tibiofibular clear space (> 6 mm) on either a nonstress AP or mortise view is one of the best indicators of syndesmotic injury.[135] Proximal fibular radiographs to rule out Maisonneuve fracture also are recommended. If the diagnosis is still suspected in the presence of normal radiographs, MRI has been shown to be very sensitive and specific in detecting AITFL and PITFL tears.[136,137]

Treatment can be nonsurgical in the case of an athlete with no associated instability or diastasis on stress radiographs (high ankle sprain) or surgical in the case of frank diastasis, diastasis on stress radiographs, or arthroscopic evidence of syndesmotic instability.[138] Nonsurgical treatment of syndesmosis sprains will reliably have a longer recovery time than similar nonsyndesmotic sprains; this should be communicated to the patient at the start of therapy. If surgery is indicated, anatomic reduction of the fibula to the incisura fibularis of the tibia is imperative for good outcomes.[138-140] The expected time to return after surgical syndesmotic fixation is in the range of 3 to 6 months. The possibility of earlier return was shown by Taylor et al[141] in a 2007 study of six male college athletes; they reported an average time to full activity of 41 days for cortical screw fixation of grade III syndesmosis sprains. Arthroscopy can be added to the procedure for confirmation of syndesmotic injury, assessment of cartilage damage, and verification of anatomic reduction.[138]

Ankle Impingement

Impingement syndromes of the ankle have been increasingly recognized in recent years. Most fall into the category of possible sequelae after ankle inversion injuries. PAIS has already been discussed. Anterolateral and anterior impingement may be encountered in the mature athlete secondary to previous ankle injuries or as part of a degenerative condition.

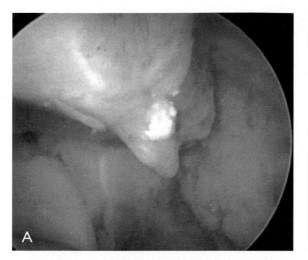
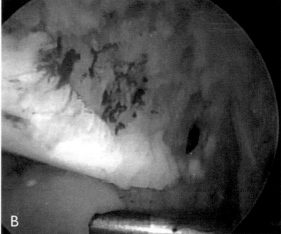

Figure 3   Arthroscopic débridement for anterior ankle impingement. Arthroscopic views of the anterior ankle before (**A**) and after (**B**) resection of a large osteophyte arising from the anterior tibia, which was causing anterior ankle impingement.

Anterolateral Impingement

Consistent pain in the ankle after an inversion sprain may be related to hypertrophic scar tissue or "meniscoid tissue" in the lateral gutter of the ankle.[142,143] On examination, tenderness to palpation over the anterior talofibular ligament is elicited, along with increasing pain in this region as the ankle is dorsiflexed, such as when doing a single-leg squat. Unless some of the scar tissue has calcified, standard and stress ankle radiographs are usually negative. MRI has a diagnostic accuracy of 78.8%.[2] Wolin et al[142] achieved relief of symptoms of anterolateral impingement in all 9 patients they treated with an open technique. Ferkel et al[143] reported good or excellent results in 26 of 31 patients using arthroscopic débridement. The average return to sports in these patients was 6 weeks.[142,143]

Anterior Ankle Impingement

Exostoses on the talus and tibia that cause pain in the anterior tibiotalar sulcus with forced dorsiflexion were described by O'Donoghue in 1957.[144] In this report, several athletes were treated with open débridement with good to excellent results. Now referred to as anterior ankle impingement, this syndrome is common in ballet dancers and soccer players. In fact, these osteo-

phytes have been reported in as many as 60% of professional soccer players.[145] Repeated dorsiflexion or direct microtrauma from kicking a ball can lead to the formation of these tibiotalar spurs.[146] Swelling and tenderness over the anterior ankle as well as painful passive dorsiflexion are present on physical examination. Standard radiographs will typically demonstrate the osseous abnormalities on the lateral view. Nonsurgical management, including using a heel lift to increase the space between the anterior tibia and talus, modification of activities, and steroid injections, can be useful. Surgical management includes open or arthroscopic débridement (**Figure 3**). Arthroscopic resection has found great success in relieving symptoms, identifying concomitant osteochondral lesions, and quicker return to sports.[147-150] With more advanced disease, however, open procedures should be entertained.[150]

Fractures

Stress Fractures

Overall, the vast majority of stress fractures occur in the foot and ankle, with 80% of these involving the tibia, metatarsals, tarsal navicular, and fibula.[2,151] Depending on the age and health of the mature athlete, decreasing bone mass may be a factor in developing a stress fracture. When this is the case, the physician should counsel the patient about bone health and nutrition. Stress fractures can be classified into low risk and high risk, with high-risk stress fractures more likely to recur, go on to nonunion, require surgical treatment, take longer to heal, or progress to complete fracture.[152] Some of these high-risk sites in the foot and ankle are the medial malleolus, talus, navicular, proximal fifth metatarsal, and the sesamoids.[152]

Medial Malleolus Stress Fractures

The incidence of medial malleolus stress fractures ranges from 0.6% to 4.1%, making this a rare injury in the athletic population (unpublished data, J.A. Nunley, 2009 AOFAS course presentation). On examination, tenderness is elicited directly over the medial malleolus and may be accompanied by swelling. Ankle range of motion is not affected. Nonsurgical management, including relative rest for 3 to 8 weeks, protected weight bearing for a limping patient, and cross-training, is always an option for athletes with medial malleolus fractures whether a fracture line is visible on radiographs or not. Shabat et al[153] reported a return to sports at an average of 6.7 months in their review of nonsurgically treated stress fractures. Orava et al[154] reported on eight medial malleolus stress fractures, five of which were treated nonsurgically and healed within 5 months. Surgical fixation should be considered when there is displacement or a visible fracture line on radiographs, when nonsurgical means fail, or in an in-season athlete. In 1988, Shelbourne et al[155] recommended internal fixation and early range of motion for athletes with a medial malleolus stress fracture visible on radiographs who desire to return to sports as soon as possible. Expectations for full return by 6 to 8 weeks were given. Return to play postoperatively has been documented in as little as 24 days, although 4 to 8 weeks is more realistic.[153-156] In the surgical patients reviewed, Shabat et al[153] reported a return to sports at an average of 4.2 months. As these reports indicate, surgically treated patients may return to sports earlier, but the risks of surgical intervention must be taken into consideration given that nonsurgical treatment reliably results in healing.

Lateral Malleolus Stress Fractures

Even though lateral malleolus stress fractures, with an incidence of 4.6% to 21%, are more common than medial malleolus stress fractures, they have not attracted as much attention.[157] This is due in part to the fact that nonsurgical management is the rule for these fractures. In fact, Sherbondy and Sebastianelli[157] commented on the lack of any reports of surgical fixation in the literature. Typically, this stress fracture occurs in the distal 4 to 7 cm of the fibula in runners, leading to its description as the "runner's fracture." Although these stress fractures tend to develop 5 to 6 cm from the tip of the malleolus in younger patients, in middle-aged and older athletes they develop 3 to 4 cm from the tip. Thus, the presence of a lateral malleolus stress fracture should be suspected in the middle-aged female runner with lateral ankle pain. Attention should be paid to any associated hindfoot valgus deformities that can increase stress on the distal fibula. Nonsurgical treatment consisting of symptomatic treatment, cessation of activity, and restriction of weight bearing as necessary can reliably expedite healing.

Navicular Stress Fractures

With increasing recognition by physicians of navicular stress fractures as a possible cause of midfoot pain in the athlete involved in explosive push-off activities, the reported incidence has risen (unpublished data, R. Anderson, 2009 AOFAS course presentation). Nonetheless, diagnosis is still commonly delayed, which is concerning because earlier recognition yields a more favorable outcome. Because of the complex bony anatomy surrounding the midfoot, CT is considered the gold standard for identifying a navicular stress fracture, although MRI is also useful.[2] Typically, the fracture will occur in the central third, a vascular watershed area. Dividing these fractures into complete versus partial and displaced versus nondisplaced will help organize treatment options. For partial and nondisplaced complete fractures, nonsurgical treatment with a non–weight-bearing cast for 6 to 8 weeks is recommended.[2,158,159] If no tenderness is present at the completion of casting, the athlete can start rehabilitation. If the navicular is still tender, a walking boot is recommended until the tenderness resolves. Nonsurgical management in this manner has yielded success in several studies, with Khan et al[160] returning 86% of patients to full activity in an average of 5.6 months, Torg et al[161] returning 100% of patients to activity in 3.8 months, and Saxena et al[162] returning patients to activity at an average of 4.3 months. Although an argument can be made for treating complete and displaced fractures nonsurgically, most authors recommend percutaneous screw fixation of these fractures in athletes.[158,160,161,163] Furthermore, the following have all been proposed as indications for surgery: evidence of sclerotic changes, comminution, cysts, osteonecrosis, failure of nonsurgical methods, delayed union, elite athlete, and nonunion (unpublished data, R. Anderson, 2009 AOFAS course presentation). Bone grafting the fracture site is usually reserved for nonunions or chronic cases.[158] Return to activity after surgical treatment appears to average approximately 4 months. The surgically treated group of Khan et al[160] returned in 3.8 months, and the patients of Saxena et al[162,163] returned in 3.1 months in one study and 4.1 months in another.

Metatarsal Stress Fractures

Commonly known as "march fractures" because they were first described in the military, metatarsal stress fractures also can affect the mature athlete who dances or does long-distance running.[164] The second and third metatarsal shafts account for 80% of these stress fractures.[164] Dorsal pain, tenderness, discomfort with percussion, and swelling can be present. For the second, third, and fourth metatarsals, the pain will be more diaphyseal; in the first and fifth metatarsals, the pain will be more proximal. In the fifth metatarsal, the location is classically in zone III, which is just distal to the fourth and fifth metatarsal articulation (unpublished data, B. G. Donley, 2009 AOFAS course presentation). MRI or bone scan should be obtained if plain radiographs are negative and the diagnosis is still in question. CT is useful for defining the direction and completeness of the fracture line. Stress fractures that are seen on MRI but with no definable fracture line are commonly termed *stress reactions*. For stress reactions, athletes should discontinue activities that cause pain for 3 to 4 weeks, continue aerobic training, and wear stiffer-soled shoes with good arch supports. When a fracture line is present, the limitations should be more aggressive. Protected weight bearing in a boot or cast is recommended along with activity modification for 6 to 8 weeks, except in fifth metatarsal fractures, where non–weight-bearing cast immobilization has been advised. Return to sporting activity is allowed once there is radiographic evidence of a healed fracture and lack of pain on clinical examination. Based on its history of nonunion and extended time to healing, special consideration is given to fifth metatarsal fractures in athletes.[165-170] For competitive athletes who would like to return to play sooner, the risks and benefits of intramedullary screw fixation should be discussed.[170]

Acute Fractures

Lisfranc Fracture-Dislocations

Tarsometatarsal joint injuries can be devastating to the performance of athletes. Maintenance of both the transverse and longitudinal arches of the foot depends on stability in this area. Direct or indirect forces such as twisting on a plantar flexed foot are typical mechanisms of injury. Inability to bear weight, midfoot swelling, tenderness over the base of the second metatarsal, plantar ecchymosis in the first web space, and pain with abduction and pronation of the forefoot can all be present on examination. Initial radiographs include AP, lateral, and oblique views of the forefoot. Proper alignment of the cuneiforms, cuboid, and metatarsals should be assessed. Any indicators of severe injury such as a fleck sign, intermetatarsal widening, or a second metatarsal base fracture should be noted (**Figure 4**). Because 20% of injuries can be missed on standard radiographs, weight-bearing views should be obtained and compared with the contralateral foot if injury is not obvious.[171-173] Widening of the first–second metatarsal space or flattening of the arch compared to the opposite side on weight bearing indicates an unstable injury. Forefoot abduction stress views also can be obtained. At this point, if radiographs are still negative and clinical suspicion is high, MRI or CT can be ordered, with CT being more helpful in identifying this injury.[171]

Treatment depends on the severity of injury, with the goal of all treatment being to maintain the anatomic relationship of the tarsometatarsal joints and provide a painless, plantigrade, stable foot for sports.[171,174-177] For the truly stable Lisfranc or midfoot sprain, nonsurgical measures can be undertaken, including a non–weight-bearing cast for a minimum of 6 weeks

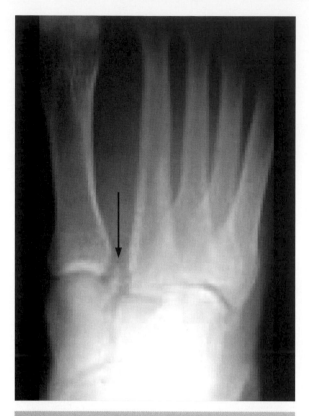

Figure 4 AP radiograph demonstrates widening of the space between the first and second metatarsal bases as well as the associated avulsion fracture, or "fleck sign" (arrow), indicative of a Lisfranc injury. (Reproduced from Thompson MC, Mormino MA: Injury to the tarsometatarsal joint complex. *J Am Acad Orthop Surg* 2003;11(4):260-267.)

followed by repeated clinical and radiographic evaluations to ensure alignment (unpublished data, D.A. Porter, 2009 AOFAS course presentation).[171] Gradual weight bearing in a boot can then begin at 6 weeks. Molded orthotic arch supports are recommended. Return to running depends on the absence of tenderness. Return to play in the patient treated nonsurgically has been reported to be approximately 3 to 4 months.[178-181] Displaced Lisfranc injuries that are obvious on initial radiographs or on stress views should undergo internal screw fixation. For the medial side, ligamentous healing may take upward of 12 to 16 weeks; thus,

Kirschner wires should be avoided. Closed reduction followed by percutaneous screw fixation can be performed in isolated ruptures of the Lisfranc ligament when good-quality intraoperative images show anatomic reduction. If anatomic restoration is not possible, then interposed ligaments, chondral fragments, tibialis anterior tendon, or other debris may need to be removed and open reduction performed before placing screws. Postoperatively, a non–weight-bearing cast is applied for 6 weeks, with protected weight bearing for another 4 to 6 weeks. Return to play is allowed once healing is confirmed with clinical and radiologic examination and the patient has completed a functional rehabilitation program, which may take 5 to 6 months. Controversy exists as to whether or not to remove the screws. A comparison of primary arthrodesis versus open reduction and internal fixation of primarily ligamentous Lisfranc injuries was published in 2006.[182] The primary arthrodesis group had higher AOFAS midfoot scores, higher levels of activity, and a higher percentage of satisfied patients at 2-year follow-up. Thus, primary arthrodesis may be an option in the active mature athlete, but further studies are needed to determine its effect on performance.

Ankle Fractures

In general, ankle fractures in the mature athlete should be managed in the same fashion as ankle fractures in the general population, with focus on stable fixation, anatomic reduction, and preservation of the mortise. Despite attention to anatomic reduction, unsatisfactory results have been seen in as many as 17% to 24% of ankle fractures.[183-185] Postinjury problems include loss of motion, catching, swelling, anterolateral pain, osteonecrosis, and posttraumatic arthritis.[186] Many of these problems are caused by unrecognized traumatic articular surface lesions, which have been documented in up to 79% of ankle fractures.[187-191] Visualization and treatment of these lesions with arthroscopic methods at the time of fracture fixation if possible has been proposed.[190,191] Hopefully, addressing these lesions at the time of injury will result in improved outcomes and allow mature athletes to continue an active lifestyle.

Entrapment Neuropathies

As the superficial peroneal, deep peroneal, and tibial nerves enter the foot and ankle region, they pass through several areas of possible entrapment, including both fibrous and fibro-osseous canals.[2] In these areas, impingement may lead to not only direct axonal compression but also vascular changes that result in abnormal nerve conduction. In general, patients with entrapment neuropathies report dysesthesias and pain in the region that the nerve supplies. Diagnosing these neuropathies is made simpler by knowing the anatomic course these nerves take in the foot and ankle region. Tarsal tunnel syndrome and medial plantar nerve entrapment are discussed briefly here.

Tarsal Tunnel Syndrome

With tarsal tunnel syndrome, typical symptoms are burning, tingling, or numbness throughout the entire plantar foot. A Tinel sign over the tarsal tunnel, localized tenderness, and sensory impairment may be elicited on physical examination.[192] If patients present with the typical history and physical examination findings of tarsal tunnel syndrome, then electrodiagnostic studies are performed to confirm nerve dysfunction. Additionally, MRI to look for potential causes of nerve compression can be ordered if electrodiagnostic studies identify nerve dysfunction.

Identifying the etiology of tarsal tunnel syndrome can be a daunting task, as many cases remain idiopathic. Occasionally, however, a specific etiology such as a synovial cyst, ganglion, venous varicosity, accessory FDL muscle, or hindfoot deformity can be identified as the cause.[3,193-200] Published studies suggest that patients may have a better outcome after decompression when a specific cause is found than patients without a specific identifiable etiology.[201-206] If no specific cause is found in the mature athlete, potential systemic causes such as diabetes, ankylosing spondylitis, rheumatoid arthritis, hypothyroidism, or acromegaly may be sought in the workup.

If no space-occupying lesion is found within the tarsal tunnel, nonsurgical management is typically initiated. Persistent or increasing symptoms despite nonsurgical treatment warrant tarsal tunnel release. After open tarsal tunnel release, the patient undergoes a 2- to 3-week period of non–weight-bearing activity and im-mobilization to allow wound healing. Once the wound is healed, gentle range of motion is encouraged. Weight bearing is initiated at 4 weeks, along with increasing active and passive exercises. If tolerated, a sport-specific return-to-play regimen can be started at 2 months, and the patient can gradually return to sport within 3 to 4 months.

Medial Plantar Nerve Entrapment (Jogger's Foot)

After exiting the tarsal tunnel, the medial plantar nerve runs deep to the abductor hallucis, along the plantar surface of the FDL, and then passes through the knot of Henry. It is at the entrance to the abductor tunnel that the nerve can be compressed, resulting in burning and numbness over the medial plantar aspect of the foot.[192,207,208] Because this classically occurs in joggers, this condition is called "jogger's foot" in most texts. This entrapment can be distinguished from tarsal tunnel syndrome, which predominantly involves the medial plantar nerve, by the location of the Tinel sign. The Tinel sign is positive over the abductor tunnel in medial plantar nerve entrapment; with tarsal tunnel syndrome, it is positive over the tarsal tunnel.[209] This is one entrapment neuropathy in which orthoses may play a role in the etiology through external compression of the nerve; thus, nonsurgical treatment must be carefully selected to avoid placing unwanted pressure over this region with various orthoses. Injections into the area with corticosteroid and anesthetic can help with diagnosis and also offer therapeutic relief. Failure of nonsurgical management warrants release of the medial plantar nerve at the entrance to the abductor tunnel.

Cartilage Problems

Ankle Arthritis

Ankle arthritis is quite common in the mature athlete. Degenerative arthritis may develop secondary to a genetic predisposition, general wear and tear over a lifetime, or as posttraumatic arthritis resulting from chronic sprains or fractures. Degenerative arthritis can involve joints other than the ankle as well, including the subtalar joint, midfoot joints, and the first MTP joint. When a patient presents with nontraumatic joint inflammation and swelling, diagnoses to consider are the systemic arthritides, including rheumatoid and psoriatic arthritis, as well as gouty arthritis, especially if the first MTP joint is involved.

Pain, swelling, stiffness, locking, and catching are often the presenting symptoms of tibiotalar arthritis. In milder cases, the pain and pinching sensation may occur only when the ankle is in certain positions. For example, in an ankle with anterior tibiotalar spurring, the symptoms may occur only when the ankle is maximally dorsiflexed during uphill jogging. In more severe cases, the joint often becomes quite stiff and the discomfort is present with activities of daily living or even at rest.

Mild to moderate ankle arthritis can often be managed by over-the-counter anti-inflammatory medications along with a low- to no-impact exercise program. Joint mobility and proprioceptive strength are the primary goals in this treatment regimen. Inexpensive off-the-shelf inserts can be used for comfort to aid arch and heel support. Heel wedges should be considered if slight varus or valgus heel malalignment is present. It should be noted that this may have effects proximally on the kinetic chain, and may alleviate or exacerbate concomitant knee arthritis. More expensive custom orthoses may be beneficial in some situations and should be carefully considered. Occasionally, the arthritic condition will not respond to these treatments and may require a more aggressive approach such as corticosteroid injections and/or surgery. Corticosteroid injections unfortunately do not result in sustained pain relief, but they can be helpful for acute exacerbations of discomfort. Hyaluronic acid viscosupplementation injections show good promise for use in the ankle as more clinical studies supporting their use for degenerative ankle arthritis have been published, although at the time of writing this chapter, such injections have not been approved by the US Food and Drug Administration and should be considered "off-label" use.[210,211]

Surgical management for ankle arthritis includes arthroscopic débridement, arthrodesis, and total ankle arthroplasty (TAA). Arthroscopy of the ankle can be used for many of the pathologies associated with ankle arthritis, including impingement, loose bodies, and spurs. Moreover, stiffness can be addressed with capsular releases. Results for arthroscopic ankle débridement for these associated pathologies have been very good.[149,150,212-215] For purely osteoarthritic ankles,

however, arthroscopic débridement with limited abrasion arthroplasty and microfracture has had variable results.[212,216-218] In a recent study by Hassouna et al,[219] 28% of patients with osteoarthritic ankles who underwent arthroscopic ankle débridement had a major ankle surgery within 5 years versus none of the patients who had arthroscopic ankle surgery for impingement. Ankle arthrodesis, whether open or arthroscopically assisted, is another option. Although no specific guidelines exist for return to sports after an ankle arthrodesis, most surgeons allow golf and skiing.[220] High-impact sports such as jogging, running, football, and basketball are generally discouraged because of associated periarticular arthroses and stress fractures.[220] TAA is continually evolving and improving the lifestyles, activity levels, and pain scores of many mature athletes.[221] According to studies by Valderrabano et al[222] and Naal et al,[221] the most common sports that patients participate in after TAA are hiking, swimming, cycling, and weight training; significantly fewer patients participate in tennis and jogging. Almost two thirds of the patients of Naal et al[221] participated in sports after TAA, and 56% of the patients of Valderrabano et al[222] were involved in sporting activities after TAA, compared with 36% before surgery. Although these studies have shown that athletic activity after TAA is possible, concern still exists regarding the long-term durability of the replacements. High-impact and stop-and-go sports are generally discouraged in this population.[222]

Osteochondral Lesions of the Talus

A history of prior trauma to the ankle can often be elicited in mature athletes with osteochondral lesions of the talus (OLT). Chronic pain, stiffness, recurrent swelling, or giving way may be present. Although multiple classification systems using radiographs, CT, and MRI have been proposed, imaging should be ordered to primarily determine the location, size, depth, and displacement of the OLT and any associated soft-tissue injuries. Often, CT imaging is better suited to answer these questions, and the injury can be graded based on the Ferkel CT classification of OLT (**Figure 5**).

Treatment of OLT continues to evolve and includes non–weight-bearing cast treatment, primary repair and fixation, arthroscopic débridement with or without microfracture, osteochondral allografts and autografts,

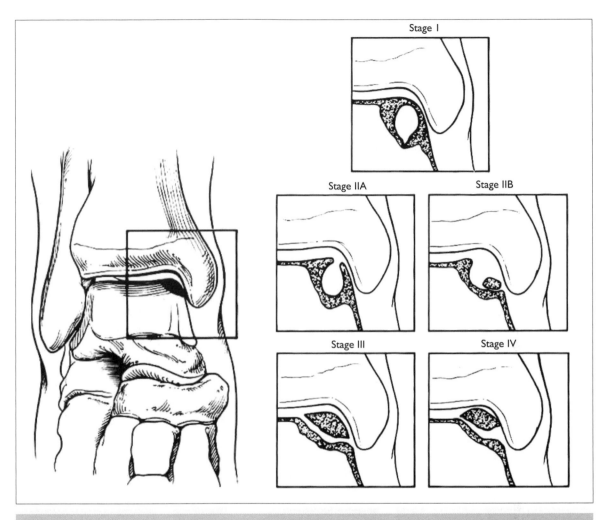

Figure 5 CT staging of osteochondral lesions of the talus. Stage I, cystic lesion within dome of talus, intact roof on all views; stage IIA, cystic lesion with communication to talar dome surface; stage IIB, open articular surface lesion with overlying nondisplaced fragment; stage III, nondisplaced lesion with lucency; stage IV, displaced fragment. (Reproduced with permission from Ferkel RD: Arthroscopic surgery: The foot and ankle, in Whipple TL, ed: *Arthroscopic Surgery Series.* Philadelphia, PA, Lippincott-Raven, 1996, pp 145-170.)

and autologous chondrocyte implantation (ACI). Indications for each technique include the depth and size of the lesion, its chronicity, any previous treatment, and the status of the overlying cartilage. Nonsurgical treatment can initially be tried for most lesions, but success with this method is questionable, even for Berndt and Harty grade I and II lesions, in which there is a small area of subchondral bone compression or the osteo-

chondral fragment is partially detached, respectively.[223]

For many surgeons, failure of nonsurgical means and the presence of a grade III or IV lesion (osteochondral fragment is completely detached) are indications for surgery. If fixation of the cartilage fragment and subchondral bone can be achieved with screws, pins, or bioabsorbable devices, then primary repair should be performed.[224] Otherwise, arthroscopic débridement

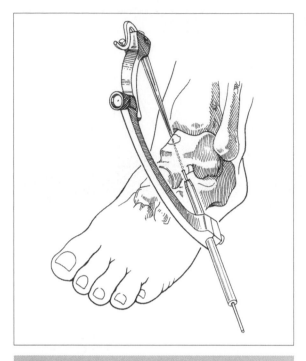

Figure 6 Retrograde drilling of osteochondral lesions of the talus. If the cartilaginous surface is intact, the lesion can be drilled in a retrograde fashion using a drill guide as shown in this drawing. (Reproduced with permission from Taranow WS, Bisignani GA, Towers JD, Conti SF: Retrograde drilling of osteochondral lesions of the medial talar dome. *Foot Ankle Int* 1999;20(8):474-480.)

and excision of the lesion with marrow-stimulation techniques (abrasion arthroplasty, drilling, microfracture) for smaller lesions have been associated with excellent results.[223,225-227] Success in the athletic population with this technique was demonstrated by Saxena and Eakin[228] in 26 microfracture procedures in high-demand athletes, with 96% good to excellent results and return to play in an average of 17 ± 5.3 weeks. If the overlying cartilage is still intact, retrograde drilling of the subchondral bone can be performed[229,230] (**Figure 6**). As with any arthroscopic procedure in the ankle, neurovascular structures should be considered carefully when establishing portal sites. Particular attention should be paid to the branches of the superficial peroneal nerve that run across the anterior ankle. A "nick and spread" maneuver should be used when making portal sites in this region of the ankle.

For larger lesions, such as those larger than 1.5 cm^2 or more than 7 mm deep, lesions associated with subchondral cysts, and lesions that have failed marrow-stimulation techniques, restorative techniques should be used.[231] Few studies exist on osteochondral allografts for talar defects, but their use has been reported.[232] Ostochondral autografts from the lateral trochlear ridge of the ipsilateral femoral condyle, intercondylar notch, medial malleolus, calcaneus, or even ipsilateral talus have all been used with good to excellent results in 90% to 94% of patients[233-240] (**Figure 7**). These procedures are performed arthroscopically or with a mini-open

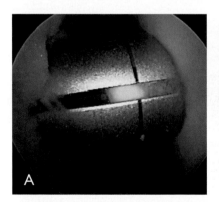
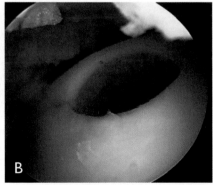
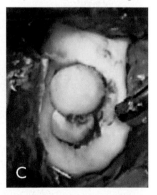

Figure 7 Osteochondral autografts. **A,** Arthroscopic image demonstrates the harvest of an osteochondral autograft from the ipsilateral knee in a patient with a talar osteochondral defect. **B,** Arthroscopic view of the defect after harvesting. **C,** Intraoperative photograph shows osteochondral autograft plugs used to fill in the defect.

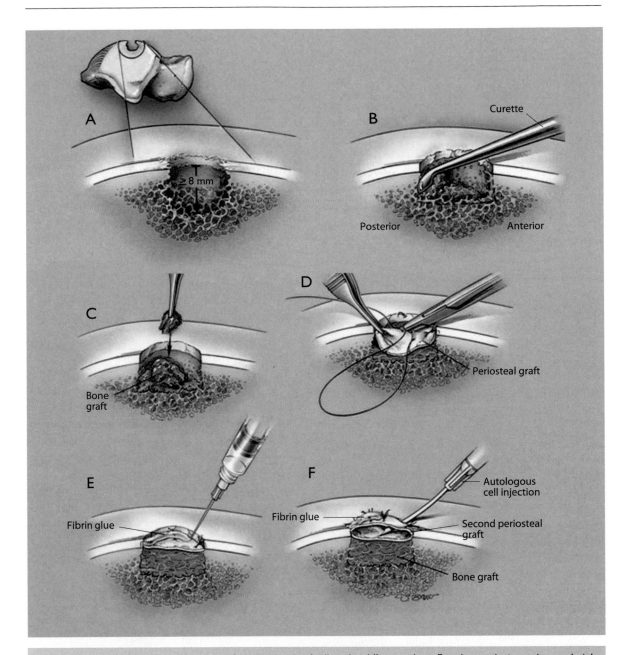

Figure 8 Autologous chondrocyte implantation using the "sandwich" procedure. For deeper lesions, the sandwich procedure involves inspecting and preparing the defect bed (**A** and **B**), impacting enough autologous bone graft to fill the defect up to the subchondral bone plate (**C**), covering the bone graft with a periosteal flap (**D**), and then sealing off the marrow with fibrin glue injected below this deeper periosteal flap (**E**). A second periosteal flap is sutured to the cartilage edges, creating a space between the periosteal flaps where the chondrocytes are injected (**F**). (Reproduced with permission from Nam EK, Ferkel RD, Applegate GR: Autologous chondrocyte implantation of the ankle: A 2- to 5-year follow-up. *Am J Sports Med* 2009;37(2);274-284.)

approach. However, in some cases, an open approach with tibial or fibular osteotomies may be necessary to gain adequate (perpendicular) access to the lesion. Return to sporting activities has been recommended after 6 months, with several authors reporting patients who have returned to marathon running after the procedure.[237,241]

Another option for treatment of larger OLTs is ACI. Although it has been associated with success in the knee, this procedure has only recently been applied to the ankle.[242] ACI requires two operations: one to harvest chondrocytes from the ipsilateral knee, and a second to implant them into the talar lesion several weeks to months later. Joint malalignment must be addressed if present and the procedure is contraindicated in cases of an abutting cartilage lesion on the distal tibial plafond. Good to excellent early results of ACI in the treatment of talar lesions with a mean area of 1.95 cm^2 were found by Whittaker et al[243] in 2005. Recently, Nam et al[242] demonstrated good to excellent results in 9 of 11 patients with an average talar lesion size of 273 mm^2 treated by standard ACI or the "sandwich" procedure (described in **Figure 8**) at a mean follow-up of 38 months. These patients had significant improvements in the Finsen and AOFAS ankle hindfoot scores, with coinciding increases in the postoperative Tegner activity level scores.[242] Patients returned to nonimpact sports by 6 months and to impact sports by 9 months. Furthermore, at a mean follow-up of 63 months, Baums et al[244] reported good or excellent results in 11 of 12 patients who underwent ACI for an average talar lesion size of 2.3 cm^2. All patients involved in competitive sports were able to return to full activity. Although a recent randomized controlled study comparing chondroplasty, microfracture, and osteochondral autograft for OLT demonstrated no difference in outcome ratings,[245] there have been no randomized studies to date comparing ACI with these other techniques.

Summary

Many foot and ankle injuries can occur in the mature athlete. Most of these injuries are chronic in nature and represent overuse syndromes from repetitive trauma to tissues and joints that are unable to withstand the repeated loads that they could once handle. These conditions can be treated with various combinations of therapy, anti-inflammatory drugs, relative rest, orthoses, injections, and activity modification. For foot and ankle injuries that are acute in onset, principles of management are similar to treating the same injuries in any aging athlete, keeping in mind the healing potential and baseline condition of the mature athlete's musculoskeletal tissues.

References

1. Kannus P, Niittymäki S, Järvinen M, Lehto M: Sports injuries in elderly athletes: A three-year prospective, controlled study. *Age Ageing* 1989;18(4):263-270.

2. Coughlin MJ, Mann RA, Saltzmann CL, eds: *Surgery of the Foot and Ankle*, ed 8. Philadelphia, PA, Mosby, 2007.

3. DeLee JC, Drez D, Miller M, eds: *Delee & Drez's Orthopaedic Sports Medicine: Principles and Practice*, ed 2. Philadelphia, PA, Saunders, 2003.

4. Zivot ML, Pearl SH, Pupp GR, Pupp JB: Stenosing peroneal tenosynovitis. *J Foot Surg* 1989;28(3):220-224.

5. Philbin TM, Landis GS, Smith B: Peroneal tendon injuries. *J Am Acad Orthop Surg* 2009;17(5):306-317.

6. Heckman DS, Reddy S, Pedowitz D, Wapner KL, Parekh SG: Operative treatment for peroneal tendon disorders. *J Bone Joint Surg Am* 2008;90(2):404-418.

7. Krause JO, Brodsky JW: Peroneus brevis tendon tears: Pathophysiology, surgical reconstruction, and clinical results. *Foot Ankle Int* 1998;19(5):271-279.

8. Saxena A, Cassidy A: Peroneal tendon injuries: An evaluation of 49 tears in 41 patients. *J Foot Ankle Surg* 2003;42(4):215-220.

9. Dombek MF, Lamm BM, Saltrick K, Mendicino RW, Catanzariti AR: Peroneal tendon tears: A retrospective review. *J Foot Ankle Surg* 2003;42(5):250-258.

10. Redfern D, Myerson M: The management of concomitant tears of the peroneus longus and brevis tendons. *Foot Ankle Int* 2004;25(10):695-707.

11. Steel MW, DeOrio JK: Peroneal tendon tears: Return to sports after operative treatment. *Foot Ankle Int* 2007;28(1):49-54.

12. Sarmiento A, Wolf M: Subluxation of peroneal tendons: Case treated by rerouting tendons under

calcaneofibular ligament. *J Bone Joint Surg Am* 1975;57(1):115-116.

13. Porter D, McCarroll J, Knapp E, Torma J: Peroneal tendon subluxation in athletes: Fibular groove deepening and retinacular reconstruction. *Foot Ankle Int* 2005;26(6):436-441.

14. McGarvey WC, Clanton TO: Peroneal tendon dislocations. *Foot Ankle Clin* 1996;1(2):325-342.

15. Kollias SL, Ferkel RD: Fibular grooving for recurrent peroneal tendon subluxation. *Am J Sports Med* 1997;25(3):329-335.

16. Arrowsmith SR, Fleming LL, Allman FL: Traumatic dislocations of the peroneal tendons. *Am J Sports Med* 1983;11(3):142-146.

17. Adachi N, Fukuhara K, Tanaka H, Nakasa T, Ochi M: Superior retinaculoplasty for recurrent dislocation of peroneal tendons. *Foot Ankle Int* 2006;27(12): 1074-1078.

18. Selmani E, Gjata V, Gjika E: Current concepts review: Peroneal tendon disorders. *Foot Ankle Int* 2006;27(3): 221-228.

19. Eckert WR, Davis EA Jr: Acute rupture of the peroneal retinaculum. *J Bone Joint Surg Am* 1976;58(5):670-672.

20. Stover CN, Bryan DR: Traumatic dislocation of the peroneal tendons. *Am J Surg* 1962;103:180-186.

21. McLennan JG: Treatment of acute and chronic luxations of the peroneal tendons. *Am J Sports Med* 1980;8(6):432-436.

22. Escalas F, Figueras JM, Merino JA: Dislocation of the peroneal tendons: Long-term results of surgical treatment. *J Bone Joint Surg Am* 1980;62(3):451-453.

23. Zoellner G, Clancy W Jr: Recurrent dislocation of the peroneal tendon. *J Bone Joint Surg Am* 1979;61(2): 292-294.

24. Maffulli N, Ferran NA, Oliva F, Testa V: Recurrent subluxation of the peroneal tendons. *Am J Sports Med* 2006;34(6):986-992.

25. Ferran NA, Oliva F, Maffulli N: Recurrent subluxation of the peroneal tendons. *Sports Med* 2006;36(10): 839-846.

26. Raikin SM: Intrasheath subluxation of the peroneal tendons: Surgical technique. *J Bone Joint Surg Am* 2009;91(suppl 2 Pt 1):146-155.

27. Lysholm J, Wiklander J: Injuries in runners. *Am J Sports Med* 1987;15(2):168-171.

28. Macintyre JG, Taunton JE, Clement DB, Lloyd-Smith DR, McKenzie DC, Morrell RW: Running injuries: A

clinical study of 4,173 cases. *Clin J Sport Med* 1991;1(2):81-87.

29. Fink BR, Mizel MS: Management of posterior tibial tendinitis in the athlete. *Oper Tech Sports Med* 1999;7(1):28-31.

30. Cavanagh PR: *The Running Shoe Book*. Mountain View, CA, Anderson World, 1980, p 270.

31. Conti SF: Posterior tibial tendon problems in athletes. *Orthop Clin North Am* 1994;25(1):109-121.

32. Mann RA, Thompson FM: Rupture of the posterior tibial tendon causing flat foot: Surgical treatment. *J Bone Joint Surg Am* 1985;67(4):556-561.

33. Jahss MH: Spontaneous rupture of the tibialis posterior tendon: Clinical findings, tenographic studies, and a new technique of repair. *Foot Ankle* 1982;3(3):158-166.

34. McCormack AP, Varner KE, Marymont JV: Surgical treatment for posterior tibial tendonitis in young competitive athletes. *Foot Ankle Int* 2003;24(7): 535-538.

35. Teasdall RD, Johnson KA: Surgical treatment of stage I posterior tibial tendon dysfunction. *Foot Ankle Int* 1994;15(12):646-648.

36. Johnson KA: Tibialis posterior tendon rupture. *Clin Orthop Relat Res* 1983;(177):140-147.

37. Woods L, Leach RE: Posterior tibial tendon rupture in athletic people. *Am J Sports Med* 1991;19(5):495-498.

38. Reddy SS, Pedowitz DI, Parekh SG, Omar IM, Wapner KL: Surgical treatment for chronic disease and disorders of the Achilles tendon. *J Am Acad Orthop Surg* 2009;17(1):3-14.

39. Longo UG, Ronga M, Maffulli N: Achilles tendinopathy. *Sports Med Arthrosc* 2009;17(2):112-126.

40. Schepsis AA, Jones H, Haas AL: Achilles tendon disorders in athletes. *Am J Sports Med* 2002;30(2): 287-305.

41. Furia JP: High-energy extracorporeal shock wave therapy as a treatment for chronic noninsertional Achilles tendinopathy. *Am J Sports Med* 2008;36(3):502-508.

42. Chung B, Wiley JP: Extracorporeal shockwave therapy: A review. *Sports Med* 2002;32(13):851-865.

43. Saltzman CL, Tearse DS: Achilles tendon injuries. *J Am Acad Orthop Surg* 1998;6(5):316-325.

44. Maquirriain J, Ayerza M, Costa-Paz M, Muscolo DL: Endoscopic surgery in chronic achilles tendinopathies: A preliminary report. *Arthroscopy* 2002;18(3):298-303.

45. Wilcox DK, Bohay DR, Anderson JG: Treatment of chronic achilles tendon disorders with flexor hallucis longus tendon transfer/augmentation. *Foot Ankle Int* 2000;21(12):1004-1010.

46. Den Hartog BD: Flexor hallucis longus transfer for chronic Achilles tendonosis. *Foot Ankle Int* 2003;24(3):233-237.

47. Tallon C, Coleman BD, Khan KM, Maffulli N: Outcome of surgery for chronic Achilles tendinopathy: A critical review. *Am J Sports Med* 2001;29(3):315-320.

48. McGarvey WC, Palumbo RC, Baxter DE, Leibman BD: Insertional Achilles tendinosis: Surgical treatment through a central tendon splitting approach. *Foot Ankle Int* 2002;23(1):19-25.

49. Fahlström M, Jonsson P, Lorentzon R, Alfredson H: Chronic Achilles tendon pain treated with eccentric calf-muscle training. *Knee Surg Sports Traumatol Arthrosc* 2003;11(5):327-333.

50. Heckman DS, Gluck GS, Parekh SG: Tendon disorders of the foot and ankle, part 2: Achilles tendon disorders. *Am J Sports Med* 2009;37(6):1223-1234.

51. Wagner E, Gould JS, Kneidel M, Fleisig GS, Fowler R: Technique and results of Achilles tendon detachment and reconstruction for insertional Achilles tendinosis. *Foot Ankle Int* 2006;27(9):677-684.

52. Schepsis AA, Wagner C, Leach RE: Surgical management of Achilles tendon overuse injuries: A long-term follow-up study. *Am J Sports Med* 1994;22(5):611-619.

53. Kannus P, Józsa L: Histopathological changes preceding spontaneous rupture of a tendon: A controlled study of 891 patients. *J Bone Joint Surg Am* 1991;73(10):1507-1525.

54. Arner O, Lindholm A: Subcutaneous rupture of the Achilles tendon: A study of 92 cases. *Acta Chir Scand Suppl* 1959;116(suppl 239):1-51.

55. Beskin JL, Sanders RA, Hunter SC, Hughston JC: Surgical repair of Achilles tendon ruptures. *Am J Sports Med* 1987;15(1):1-8.

56. Cetti R, Christensen SE, Ejsted R, Jensen NM, Jorgensen U: Operative versus nonoperative treatment of Achilles tendon rupture: A prospective randomized study and review of the literature. *Am J Sports Med* 1993;21(6):791-799.

57. Häggmark T, Liedberg H, Eriksson E, Wredmark T: Calf muscle atrophy and muscle function after non-operative vs operative treatment of achilles tendon ruptures. *Orthopedics* 1986;9(2):160-164.

58. Khan RJ, Fick D, Keogh A, Crawford J, Brammar T, Parker M: Treatment of acute Achilles tendon ruptures: A meta-analysis of randomized, controlled trials. *J Bone Joint Surg Am* 2005;87(10):2202-2210.

59. Möller M, Movin T, Granhed H, Lind K, Faxén E, Karlsson J: Acute rupture of tendon Achillis: A prospective randomised study of comparison between surgical and non-surgical treatment. *J Bone Joint Surg Br* 2001;83(6):843-848.

60. Bhandari M, Guyatt G, Siddiqui F, et al: Treatment of acute Achilles tendon ruptures: A systematic overview and metaanalysis. *Clin Orthop Relat Res* 2002;400 :190-200.

61. Ibrahim SA: Surgical treatment of chronic Achilles tendon rupture. *J Foot Ankle Surg* 2009;48(3):340-346.

62. Porter DA, Mannarino FP, Snead D, Gabel SJ, Ostrowski M: Primary repair without augmentation for early neglected Achilles tendon ruptures in the recreational athlete. *Foot Ankle Int* 1997;18(9):557-564.

63. Wapner KL: Delayed repair of the Achilles tendon, in Kitaoka HB, ed: *Masters Techniques in Orthopaedic Surgery: The Foot and Ankle*. Philadelphia, PA, Lippincott Williams & Wilkins, 2002, pp 323-335.

64. Wapner KL, Pavlock GS, Hecht PJ, Naselli F, Walther R: Repair of chronic Achilles tendon rupture with flexor hallucis longus tendon transfer. *Foot Ankle* 1993;14(8):443-449.

65. Turco V, Spinella AJ: Team physician #2: Peroneus brevis transfer for Achilles tendon rupture in athletes. *Orthop Rev* 1988;17(8):822-824, 827-828.

66. Mann RA, Holmes GB Jr, Seale KS, Collins DN: Chronic rupture of the Achilles tendon: A new technique of repair. *J Bone Joint Surg Am* 1991;73(2):214-219.

67. Pérez Teuffer A: Traumatic rupture of the Achilles tendon: Reconstruction by transplant and graft using the lateral peroneus brevis. *Orthop Clin North Am* 1974;5(1):89-93.

68. Dalton G: Achilles tendon rupture. *Foot Ankle Clin* 1996;1:225-236.

69. Leitze Z, Sella EJ, Aversa JM: Endoscopic decompression of the retrocalcaneal space. *J Bone Joint Surg Am* 2003;85(8):1488-1496.

70. Ortmann FW, McBryde AM: Endoscopic bony and soft-tissue decompression of the retrocalcaneal space for the treatment of Haglund deformity and retrocalcaneal bursitis. *Foot Ankle Int* 2007;28(2):149-153.

71. van Dijk CN, Scholten PE, Krips R: A 2-portal endoscopic approach for diagnosis and treatment of posterior ankle pathology. *Arthroscopy* 2000;16(8): 871-876.

72. van Dijk CN, van Dyk GE, Scholten PE, Kort NP: Endoscopic calcaneoplasty. *Am J Sports Med* 2001;29(2):185-189.

73. Schunck J, Jerosch J: Operative treatment of Haglund's syndrome: Basics, indications, procedures, surgical techniques, results and problems. *Foot Ankle Surg* 2005;11(3):123-130.

74. Lutter LD: Surgical decisions in athletes' subcalcaneal pain. *Am J Sports Med* 1986;14(6):481-485.

75. McBryde AM Jr: Plantar fasciitis. *Instr Course Lect* 1984;33:278-282.

76. Neufeld SK, Cerrato R: Plantar fasciitis: Evaluation and treatment. *J Am Acad Orthop Surg* 2008;16(6):338-346.

77. Digiovanni BF, Nawoczenski DA, Malay DP, et al: Plantar fascia-specific stretching exercise improves outcomes in patients with chronic plantar fasciitis: A prospective clinical trial with two-year follow-up. *J Bone Joint Surg Am* 2006;88(8):1775-1781.

78. Barry LD, Barry AN, Chen Y: A retrospective study of standing gastrocnemius-soleus stretching versus night splinting in the treatment of plantar fasciitis. *J Foot Ankle Surg* 2002;41(4):221-227.

79. Malay DS, Pressman MM, Assili A, et al: Extracorporeal shockwave therapy versus placebo for the treatment of chronic proximal plantar fasciitis: Results of a randomized, placebo-controlled, double-blinded, multicenter intervention trial. *J Foot Ankle Surg* 2006;45(4):196-210.

80. Barrett SL, Day SV, Pignetti TT, Robinson LB: Endoscopic plantar fasciotomy: A multi-surgeon prospective analysis of 652 cases. *J Foot Ankle Surg* 1995;34(4):400-406.

81. Lundeen RO, Aziz S, Burks JB, Rose JM: Endoscopic plantar fasciotomy: A retrospective analysis of results in 53 patients. *J Foot Ankle Surg* 2000;39(4):208-217.

82. Berlin MJ: Percutaneous plantar fasciotomy. *Curr Podiatr Med* 1985;2:32.

83. Benton-Weil W, Borrelli AH, Weil LS Jr, Weil LS Sr: Percutaneous plantar fasciotomy: A minimally invasive procedure for recalcitrant plantar fasciitis. *J Foot Ankle Surg* 1998;37(4):269-272.

84. Boyle RA, Slater GL: Endoscopic plantar fascia release: A case series. *Foot Ankle Int* 2003;24(2):176-179.

85. Kinley S, Frascone S, Calderone D, Wertheimer SJ, Squire MA, Wiseman FA: Endoscopic plantar fasciotomy versus traditional heel spur surgery: A prospective study. *J Foot Ankle Surg* 1993;32(6): 595-603.

86. Ogilvie-Harris DJ, Lobo J: Endoscopic plantar fascia release. *Arthroscopy* 2000;16(3):290-298.

87. Snider MP, Clancy WG, McBeath AA: Plantar fascia release for chronic plantar fasciitis in runners. *Am J Sports Med* 1983;11(4):215-219.

88. Leach RE, Seavey MS, Salter DK: Results of surgery in athletes with plantar fasciitis. *Foot Ankle* 1986;7(3):156-161.

89. Perry J: Anatomy and biomechanics of the hindfoot. *Clin Orthop Relat Res* 1983;(177):9-15.

90. Sormaala MJ, Niva MH, Kiuru MJ, Mattila VM, Pihlajamäki HK: Stress injuries of the calcaneus detected with magnetic resonance imaging in military recruits. *J Bone Joint Surg Am* 2006;88(10):2237-2242.

91. Leabhart JW: Stress fractures of the calcaneus. *J Bone Joint Surg Am* 1959;41:1285-1290.

92. Baxter DE, Pfeffer GB: Treatment of chronic heel pain by surgical release of the first branch of the lateral plantar nerve. *Clin Orthop Relat Res* 1992;(279):229-236.

93. Hamilton WG: Tendonitis about the ankle joint in classical ballet dancers. *Am J Sports Med* 1977;5(2): 84-88.

94. Maquirriain J: Posterior ankle impingement syndrome. *J Am Acad Orthop Surg* 2005;13(6):365-371.

95. McBryde A: Disorders of the ankle and foot, in Brana WA, Kalenak A, eds: *Clinical Sports Medicine.* Philadelphia, PA, WB Saunders, 1991, pp 466-489.

96. Jaivin JS, Ferkel RD: Arthroscopy of the foot and ankle. *Clin Sports Med* 1994;13(4):761-783.

97. Hedrick MR, McBryde AM: Posterior ankle impingement. *Foot Ankle Int* 1994;15(1):2-8.

98. Scholten PE, Sierevelt IN, van Dijk CN: Hindfoot endoscopy for posterior ankle impingement. *J Bone Joint Surg Am* 2008;90(12):2665-2672.

99. van Dijk CN: Hindfoot endoscopy. *Sports Med Arthrosc Rev* 2000;8(4):365-371.

100. Jerosch J, Fadel M: Endoscopic resection of a symptomatic os trigonum. *Knee Surg Sports Traumatol Arthrosc* 2006;14(11):1188-1193.

101. Willits K, Sonneveld H, Amendola A, Giffin JR, Griffin S, Fowler PJ: Outcome of posterior ankle arthroscopy for hindfoot impingement. *Arthroscopy* 2008;24(2):196-202.

102. Marumoto JM, Ferkel RD: Arthroscopic excision of the os trigonum: A new technique with preliminary clinical results. *Foot Ankle Int* 1997;18(12):777-784.

103. Vanore JV, Christensen JC, Kravitz SR, et al: Diagnosis and treatment of first metatarsophalangeal joint disorders: Section 4. Sesamoid disorders. *J Foot Ankle Surg* 2003;42(3):143-147.

104. Saxena A, Krisdakumtorn T: Return to activity after sesamoidectomy in athletically active individuals. *Foot Ankle Int* 2003;24(5):415-419.

105. Anderson RB, McBryde AM Jr : Autogenous bone grafting of hallux sesamoid nonunions. *Foot Ankle Int* 1997;18(5):293-296.

106. Biedert R, Hintermann B: Stress fractures of the medial great toe sesamoids in athletes. *Foot Ankle Int* 2003;24(2):137-141.

107. Blundell CM, Nicholson P, Blackney MW: Percutaneous screw fixation for fractures of the sesamoid bones of the hallux. *J Bone Joint Surg Br* 2002;84(8):1138-1141.

108. Iqbal MJ, Chana GS: Arthroscopic cheilectomy for hallux rigidus. *Arthroscopy* 1998;14(3):307-310.

109. Frey C, van Dijk CN: Arthroscopy of the great toe. *Instr Course Lect* 1999;48:343-346.

110. Coughlin MJ, Shurnas PS: Hallux rigidus: Grading and long-term results of operative treatment. *J Bone Joint Surg Am* 2003;85(11):2072-2088.

111. Barca F: Tendon arthroplasty of the first metatarsophalangeal joint in hallux rigidus: Preliminary communication. *Foot Ankle Int* 1997;18(4):222-228.

112. Coughlin MJ, Shurnas PJ: Soft-tissue arthroplasty for hallux rigidus. *Foot Ankle Int* 2003;24(9):661-672.

113. Hamilton WG, O'Malley MJ, Thompson FM, Kovatis PE: Roger Mann Award 1995: Capsular interposition arthroplasty for severe hallux rigidus. *Foot Ankle Int* 1997;18(2):68-70.

114. Gerber JP, Williams GN, Scoville CR, Arciero RA, Taylor DC: Persistent disability associated with ankle sprains: A prospective examination of an athletic population. *Foot Ankle Int* 1998;19(10):653-660.

115. Konradsen L, Bech L, Ehrenbjerg M, Nickelsen T: Seven years follow-up after ankle inversion trauma. *Scand J Med Sci Sports* 2002;12(3):129-135.

116. Reed ME, Fiebel JB, Donley BG, Giza E: Athletic ankle injuries, in Kibler WB, ed: *Orthopaedic Knowledge Update: Sports Medicine*, ed 4. Rosemont, IL, American Academy of Orthopaedic Surgeons, 2009, pp 199-203.

117. Krips R, van Dijk CN, Halasi PT, et al: Long-term outcome of anatomical reconstruction versus tenodesis for the treatment of chronic anterolateral instability of the ankle joint: A multicenter study. *Foot Ankle Int* 2001;22(5):415-421.

118. Broström L: Sprained ankles: VI. Surgical treatment of "chronic" ligament ruptures. *Acta Chir Scand* 1966;132(5):551-565.

119. Stewart MJ, Hutchins WC: Repair of thelateral ligaments of the ankle. *Am J Sports Med* 1978;6(5):272-275.

120. Barnum MJ, Ehrlich MG, Zaleske DJ: Long-term patient-oriented outcome study of a modified Evans procedure. *J Pediatr Orthop* 1998;18(6):783-788.

121. Becker HP, Ebner S, Ebner D, et al: 12-year outcome after modified Watson-Jones tenodesis for ankle instability. *Clin Orthop Relat Res* 1999;358(358): 194-204.

122. Korkala O, Tanskanen P, Mäkijärvi J, Sorvali T, Ylikoski M, Haapala J: Long-term results of the Evans procedure for lateral instability of the ankle. *J Bone Joint Surg Br* 1991;73(1):96-99.

123. Rosenbaum D, Becker HP, Sterk J, Gerngross H, Claes L: Functional evaluation of the 10-year outcome after modified Evans repair for chronic ankle instability. *Foot Ankle Int* 1997;18(12):765-771.

124. Snook GA, Chrisman OD, Wilson TC: Long-term results of the Chrisman-Snook operation for reconstruction of the lateral ligaments of the ankle. *J Bone Joint Surg Am* 1985;67(1):1-7.

125. Younes C, Fowles JV, Fallaha M, Antoun R: Long-term results of surgical reconstruction for chronic lateral instability of the ankle: Comparison of Watson-Jones and Evans techniques. *J Trauma* 1988;28(9): 1330-1334.

126. Sugimoto K, Takakura Y, Akiyama K, Kamei S, Kitada C, Kumai T: Long-term results of Watson-Jones tenodesis of the ankle: Clinical and radiographic findings after ten to eighteen years of follow-up. *J Bone Joint Surg Am* 1998;80(11):1587-1596.

127. Karlsson J, Bergsten T, Lansinger O, Peterson L: Lateral instability of the ankle treated by the Evans procedure: A long-term clinical and radiological follow-up. *J Bone Joint Surg Br* 1988;70(3):476-480.

128. Krips R, Brandsson S, Swensson C, van Dijk CN, Karlsson J: Anatomical reconstruction and Evans tenodesis of the lateral ligaments of the ankle: Clinical and radiological findings after follow-up for 15 to 30 years. *J Bone Joint Surg Br* 2002;84(2):232-236.

129. Bell SJ, Mologne TS, Sitler DF, Cox JS: Twenty-six-year results after Broström procedure for chronic lateral ankle instability. *Am J Sports Med* 2006;34(6):975-978.

130. Hamilton WG, Thompson FM, Snow SW: The modified Brostrom procedure for lateral ankle instability. *Foot Ankle* 1993;14(1):1-7.

131. Komenda GA, Ferkel RD: Arthroscopic findings associated with the unstable ankle. *Foot Ankle Int* 1999;20(11):708-713.

132. Ferkel RD, Chams RN: Chronic lateral instability: Arthroscopic findings and long-term results. *Foot Ankle Int* 2007;28(1):24-31.

133. Li X, Killie H, Guerrero P, Busconi BD: Anatomical reconstruction for chronic lateral ankle instability in the high-demand athlete: Functional outcomes after the modified Broström repair using suture anchors. *Am J Sports Med* 2009;37(3):488-494.

134. Krips R, van Dijk CN, Lehtonen H, Halasi T, Moyen B, Karlsson J: Sports activity level after surgical treatment for chronic anterolateral ankle instability: A multicenter study. *Am J Sports Med* 2002;30(1):13-19.

135. Harper MC, Keller TS: A radiographic evaluation of the tibiofibular syndesmosis. *Foot Ankle* 1989;10(3):156-160.

136. Takao M, Ochi M, Oae K, Naito K, Uchio Y: Diagnosis of a tear of the tibiofibular syndesmosis: The role of arthroscopy of the ankle. *J Bone Joint Surg Br* 2003;85(3):324-329.

137. Oae K, Takao M, Naito K, et al: Injury of the tibiofibular syndesmosis: Value of MR imaging for diagnosis. *Radiology* 2003;227(1):155-161.

138. Williams GN, Jones MH, Amendola A: Syndesmotic ankle sprains in athletes. *Am J Sports Med* 2007;35(7):1197-1207.

139. Zalavras C, Thordarson D: Ankle syndesmotic injury. *J Am Acad Orthop Surg* 2007;15(6):330-339.

140. van den Bekerom MP, Lamme B, Hogervorst M, Bolhuis HW: Which ankle fractures require syndesmotic stabilization? *J Foot Ankle Surg* 2007;46(6):456-463.

141. Taylor DC, Tenuta JJ, Uhorchak JM, Arciero RA: Aggressive surgical treatment and early return to sports in athletes with grade III syndesmosis sprains. *Am J Sports Med* 2007;35(11):1833-1838.

142. Wolin I, Glassman F, Sideman S, Levinthal DH: Internal derangement of the talofibular component of the ankle. *Surg Gynecol Obstet* 1950;91(2):193-200.

143. Ferkel RD, Karzel RP, Del Pizzo W, Friedman MJ, Fischer SP: Arthroscopic treatment of anterolateral impingement of the ankle. *Am J Sports Med* 1991;19(5):440-446.

144. O'Donoghue DH: Impingement exostoses of the talus and tibia. *J Bone Joint Surg Am* 1957;39(4):835-852.

145. Massada JL: Ankle overuse injuries in soccer players: Morphological adaptation of the talus in the anterior impingement. *J Sports Med Phys Fitness* 1991;31(3):447-451.

146. Tol JL, Slim E, van Soest AJ, van Dijk CN: The relationship of the kicking action in soccer and anterior ankle impingement syndrome: A biomechanical analysis. *Am J Sports Med* 2002;30(1):45-50.

147. Branca A, Di Palma L, Bucca C, Visconti CS, Di Mille M: Arthroscopic treatment of anterior ankle impingement. *Foot Ankle Int* 1997;18(7):418-423.

148. Tol JL, Verheyen CP, van Dijk CN: Arthroscopic treatment of anterior impingement in the ankle. *J Bone Joint Surg Br* 2001;83(1):9-13.

149. Ogilvie-Harris DJ, Mahomed N, Demazière A: Anterior impingement of the ankle treated by arthroscopic removal of bony spurs. *J Bone Joint Surg Br* 1993;75(3):437-440.

150. Scranton PE Jr, McDermott JI: Anterior tibiotalar spurs: A comparison of open versus arthroscopic debridement. *Foot Ankle* 1992;13(3):125-128.

151. Wall J, Feller JF: Imaging of stress fractures in runners. *Clin Sports Med* 2006;25(4):781-8002.

152. Diehl JJ, Best TM, Kaeding CC: Classification and return-to-play considerations for stress fractures. *Clin Sports Med* 2006;25(1):17-28, vii.

153. Shabat S, Sampson KB, Mann G, et al: Stress fractures of the medial malleolus: Review of the literature and report of a 15-year-old elite gymnast. *Foot Ankle Int* 2002;23(7):647-650.

154. Orava S, Karpakka J, Taimela S, Hulkko A, Permi J, Kujala U: Stress fracture of the medial malleolus. *J Bone Joint Surg Am* 1995;77(3):362-365.

155. Shelbourne KD, Fisher DA, Rettig AC, McCarroll JR: Stress fractures of the medial malleolus. *Am J Sports Med* 1988;16(1):60-63.

156. Kor A, Saltzman AT, Wempe PD: Medial malleolar stress fractures: Literature review, diagnosis, and treatment. *J Am Podiatr Med Assoc* 2003;93(4): 292-297.

157. Sherbondy PS, Sebastianelli WJ: Stress fractures of the medial malleolus and distal fibula. *Clin Sports Med* 2006;25(1):129-137.

158. Jones MH, Amendola AS: Navicular stress fractures. *Clin Sports Med* 2006;25(1):151-158.

159. Lee S, Anderson RB: Stress fractures of the tarsal navicular. *Foot Ankle Clin* 2004;9(1):85-104.

160. Khan KM, Fuller PJ, Brukner PD, Kearney C, Burry HC: Outcome of conservative and surgical management of navicular stress fracture in athletes: Eighty-six cases proven with computerized tomography. *Am J Sports Med* 1992;20(6):657-666.

161. Torg JS, Pavlov H, Cooley LH, et al: Stress fractures of the tarsal navicular: A retrospective review of twenty-one cases. *J Bone Joint Surg Am* 1982;64(5):700-712.

162. Saxena A, Fullem B, Hannaford D: Results of treatment of 22 navicular stress fractures and a new proposed radiographic classification system. *J Foot Ankle Surg* 2000;39(2):96-103.

163. Saxena A, Fullem B: Navicular stress fractures: A prospective study on athletes. *Foot Ankle Int* 2006;27(11):917-921.

164. Fetzer GB, Wright RW: Metatarsal shaft fractures and fractures of the proximal fifth metatarsal. *Clin Sports Med* 2006;25(1):139-150.

165. Dameron TB Jr: Fractures and anatomical variations of the proximal portion of the fifth metatarsal. *J Bone Joint Surg Am* 1975;57(6):788-792.

166. DeLee JC, Evans JP, Julian J: Stress fracture of the fifth metatarsal. *Am J Sports Med* 1983;11(5):349-353.

167. Kavanaugh JH, Brower TD, Mann RV: The Jones fracture revisited. *J Bone Joint Surg Am* 1978;60(6):776-782.

168. Stewart IM: Jones's fracture: Fracture at the base of the fifth metatarsal. *Clin Orthop* 1960;16:190-198.

169. Torg JS, Balduini FC, Zelko RR, Pavlov H, Peff TC, Das M: Fractures of the base of the fifth metatarsal distal to the tuberosity: Classification and guidelines for non-surgical and surgical management. *J Bone Joint Surg Am* 1984;66(2):209-214.

170. Weinfeld SB, Haddad SL, Myerson MS: Metatarsal stress fractures. *Clin Sports Med* 1997;16(2):319-338.

171. Thompson MC, Mormino MA: Injury to the tarsometatarsal joint complex. *J Am Acad Orthop Surg* 2003;11(4):260-267.

172. Coss HS, Manos RE, Buoncristiani A, Mills WJ: Abduction stress and AP weightbearing radiography of purely ligamentous injury in the tarsometatarsal joint. *Foot Ankle Int* 1998;19(8):537-541.

173. Kaar S, Femino J, Morag Y: Lisfranc joint displacement following sequential ligament sectioning. *J Bone Joint Surg Am* 2007;89(10):2225-2232.

174. Calder JD, Whitehouse SL, Saxby TS: Results of isolated Lisfranc injuries and the effect of compensation claims. *J Bone Joint Surg Br* 2004;86(4):527-530.

175. Myerson MS, Fisher RT, Burgess AR, Kenzora JE: Fracture dislocations of the tarsometatarsal joints: End results correlated with pathology and treatment. *Foot Ankle* 1986;6(5):225-242.

176. Richter M, Thermann H, Huefner T, Schmidt U, Goesling T, Krettek C: Chopart joint fracture-dislocation: Initial open reduction provides better outcome than closed reduction. *Foot Ankle Int* 2004;25(5):340-348.

177. Kuo RS, Tejwani NC, Digiovanni CW, et al: Outcome after open reduction and internal fixation of Lisfranc joint injuries. *J Bone Joint Surg Am* 2000;82(11):1609-1618.

178. Meyer SA, Callaghan JJ, Albright JP, Crowley ET, Powell JW: Midfoot sprains in collegiate football players. *Am J Sports Med* 1994;22(3):392-401.

179. Shapiro MS, Wascher DC, Finerman GA: Rupture of Lisfranc's ligament in athletes. *Am J Sports Med* 1994;22(5):687-691.

180. Curtis MJ, Myerson M, Szura B: Tarsometatarsal joint injuries in the athlete. *Am J Sports Med* 1993;21(4):497-502.

181. Nunley JA, Vertullo CJ: Classification, investigation,

and management of midfoot sprains: Lisfranc injuries in the athlete. *Am J Sports Med* 2002;30(6):871-878.

182. Ly TV, Coetzee JC: Treatment of primarily ligamentous Lisfranc joint injuries: Primary arthrodesis compared with open reduction and internal fixation. A prospective, randomized study. *J Bone Joint Surg Am* 2006;88(3):514-520.

183. Brown OL, Dirschl DR, Obremskey WT: Incidence of hardware-related pain and its effect on functional outcomes after open reduction and internal fixation of ankle fractures. *J Orthop Trauma* 2001;15(4):271-274.

184. Beris AE, Kabbani KT, Xenakis TA, Mitsionis G, Soucacos PK, Soucacos PN: Surgical treatment of malleolar fractures: A review of 144 patients. *Clin Orthop Relat Res* 1997;341(341):90-98.

185. Day GA, Swanson CE, Hulcombe BG: Operative treatment of ankle fractures: A minimum ten-year follow-up. *Foot Ankle Int* 2001;22(2):102-106.

186. Utsugi K, Sakai H, Hiraoka H, Yashiki M, Mogi H: Intra-articular fibrous tissue formation following ankle fracture: The significance of arthroscopic debridement of fibrous tissue. *Arthroscopy* 2007;23(1):89-93.

187. Hintermann B, Regazzoni P, Lampert C, Stutz G, Gächter A: Arthroscopic findings in acute fractures of the ankle. *J Bone Joint Surg Br* 2000;82(3):345-351.

188. Loren GJ, Ferkel RD: Arthroscopic assessment of occult intra-articular injury in acute ankle fractures. *Arthroscopy* 2002;18(4):412-421.

189. Leontaritis N, Hinojosa L, Panchbhavi VK: Arthroscopically detected intra-articular lesions associated with acute ankle fractures. *J Bone Joint Surg Am* 2009;91(2):333-339.

190. Aktas S, Kocaoglu B, Gereli A, Nalbantodlu U, Güven O: Incidence of chondral lesions of talar dome in ankle fracture types. *Foot Ankle Int* 2008;29(3): 287-292.

191. Ono A, Nishikawa S, Nagao A, Irie T, Sasaki M, Kouno T: Arthroscopically assisted treatment of ankle fractures: Arthroscopic findings and surgical outcomes. *Arthroscopy* 2004;20(6):627-631.

192. Oh SJ, Meyer RD: Entrapment neuropathies of the tibial (posterior tibial) nerve. *Neurol Clin* 1999;17(3): 593-615, vii.

193. Burks JB, DeHeer PA: Tarsal tunnel syndrome secondary to an accessory muscle: A case report. *J Foot Ankle Surg* 2001;40(6):401-403.

194. Kinoshita M, Okuda R, Morikawa J, Abe M: Tarsal tunnel syndrome associated with an accessory muscle. *Foot Ankle Int* 2003;24(2):132-136.

195. Sammarco GJ, Stephens MM: Tarsal tunnel syndrome caused by the flexor digitorum accessorius longus: A case report. *J Bone Joint Surg Am* 1990;72(3):453-454.

196. Sammarco GJ, Conti SF: Tarsal tunnel syndrome caused by an anomalous muscle. *J Bone Joint Surg Am* 1994;76(9):1308-1314.

197. Canter DE, Siesel KJ: Flexor digitorum accessorius longus muscle: An etiology of tarsal tunnel syndrome? *J Foot Ankle Surg* 1997;36(3):226-229.

198. Wittmayer BC, Freed L: Diagnosis and surgical management of flexor digitorum accessorius longus-induced tarsal tunnel syndrome. *J Foot Ankle Surg* 2007;46(6):484-487.

199. Cimino WR: Tarsal tunnel syndrome: Review of the literature. *Foot Ankle* 1990;11(1):47-52.

200. Frey C, Kerr R: Magnetic resonance imaging and the evaluation of tarsal tunnel syndrome. *Foot Ankle* 1993;14(3):159-164.

201. Lau JT, Daniels TR: Tarsal tunnel syndrome: A review of the literature. *Foot Ankle Int* 1999;20(3):201-209.

202. Pfeiffer WH, Cracchiolo A III: Clinical results after tarsal tunnel decompression. *J Bone Joint Surg Am* 1994;76(8):1222-1230.

203. Takakura Y, Kitada C, Sugimoto K, Tanaka Y, Tamai S: Tarsal tunnel syndrome: Causes and results of operative treatment. *J Bone Joint Surg Br* 1991;73(1):125-128.

204. Stern DS, Joyce MT: Tarsal tunnel syndrome: A review of 15 surgical procedures. *J Foot Surg* 1989;28(4):290-294.

205. Linscheid RL, Burton RC, Fredericks EJ: Tarsal-tunnel syndrome. *South Med J* 1970;63(11): 1313-1323.

206. Radin EL: Tarsal tunnel syndrome. *Clin Orthop Relat Res* 1983;(181):167-170.

207. Oh SJ, Lee KW: Medial plantar neuropathy. *Neurology* 1987;37(8):1408-1410.

208. Rask MR: Medial plantar neurapraxia (jogger's foot): Report of 3 cases. *Clin Orthop Relat Res* 1978;(134):193-195.

209. Mann RA: Tarsal tunnel syndrome. *Orthop Clin North Am* 1974;5(1):109-115.

210. Cohen MM, Altman RD, Hollstrom R, Hollstrom C,

Sun C, Gipson B: Safety and efficacy of intra-articular sodium hyaluronate (Hyalgan) in a randomized, double-blind study for osteoarthritis of the ankle. *Foot Ankle Int* 2008;29(7):657-663.

211. Salk RS, Chang TJ, D'Costa WF, Soomekh DJ, Grogan KA: Sodium hyaluronate in the treatment of osteoarthritis of the ankle: a controlled, randomized, double-blind pilot study. *J Bone Joint Surg Am* 2006;88(2):295-302.

212. Cheng JC, Ferkel RD: The role of arthroscopy in ankle and subtalar degenerative joint disease. *Clin Orthop Relat Res* 1998;(349):65-72.

213. Hawkins RB: Arthroscopic treatment of sports-related anterior osteophytes in the ankle. *Foot Ankle* 1988;9(2):87-90.

214. Feder KS, Schonholtz GJ: Ankle arthroscopy: Review and long-term results. *Foot Ankle* 1992;13(7): 382-385.

215. van Dijk CN, Scholte D: Arthroscopy of the ankle joint. *Arthroscopy* 1997;13(1):90-96.

216. Amendola A, Petrik J, Webster-Bogart S: Ankle arthroscopy: Outcome in 79 consecutive patients. *Arthroscopy* 1996;12(5):565-573.

217. Ogilvie-Harris DJ, Sekyi-Otu A: Arthroscopic debridement for the osteoarthritic ankle. *Arthroscopy* 1995;11(4):433-436.

218. Martin DF, Baker CL, Curl WW, Andrews JR, Robie DB, Haas AF: Operative ankle arthroscopy: Long term follow-up. *Am J Sports Med* 1989;17(1):16-23.

219. Hassouna H, Kumar S, Bendall S: Arthroscopic ankle debridement: 5-year survival analysis. *Acta Orthop Belg* 2007;73(6):737-740.

220. Vertullo CJ, Nunley JA: Participation in sports after arthrodesis of the foot or ankle. *Foot Ankle Int* 2002;23(7):625-628.

221. Naal FD, Impellizzeri FM, Loibl M, Huber M, Rippstein PF: Habitual physical activity and sports participation after total ankle arthroplasty. *Am J Sports Med* 2009;37(1):95-102.

222. Valderrabano V, Pagenstert G, Horisberger M, Knupp M, Hintermann B: Sports and recreation activity of ankle arthritis patients before and after total ankle replacement. *Am J Sports Med* 2006;34(6):993-999.

223. Tol JL, Struijs PA, Bossuyt PM, Verhagen RA, van Dijk CN: Treatment strategies in osteochondral defects of the talar dome: A systematic review. *Foot Ankle Int* 2000;21(2):119-126.

224. Schachter AK, Chen AL, Reddy PD, Tejwani NC: Osteochondral lesions of the talus. *J Am Acad Orthop Surg* 2005;13(3):152-158.

225. Ferkel RD, Zanotti RM, Komenda GA, et al: Arthroscopic treatment of chronic osteochondral lesions of the talus: Long-term results. *Am J Sports Med* 2008;36(9):1750-1762.

226. Thermann H, Becher C: Microfracture technique for treatment of osteochondral and degenerative chondral lesions of the talus: 2-year results of a prospective study. *Unfallchirurg* 2004;107(1):27-32.

227. Becher C, Thermann H: Results of microfracture in the treatment of articular cartilage defects of the talus. *Foot Ankle Int* 2005;26(8):583-589.

228. Saxena A, Eakin C: Articular talar injuries in athletes: Results of microfracture and autogenous bone graft. *Am J Sports Med* 2007;35(10):1680-1687.

229. Taranow WS, Bisignani GA, Towers JD, Conti SF: Retrograde drilling of osteochondral lesions of the medial talar dome. *Foot Ankle Int* 1999;20(8): 474-480.

230. Kono M, Takao M, Naito K, Uchio Y, Ochi M: Retrograde drilling for osteochondral lesions of the talar dome. *Am J Sports Med* 2006;34(9):1450-1456.

231. Giannini S, Vannini F: Operative treatment of osteochondral lesions of the talar dome: Current concepts review. *Foot Ankle Int* 2004;25(3):168-175.

232. Gross AE, Agnidis Z, Hutchison CR: Osteochondral defects of the talus treated with fresh osteochondral allograft transplantation. *Foot Ankle Int* 2001;22(5):385-391.

233. Mendicino RW, Hallivis RM, Cirlincione AS, Catanzariti AR, Krause N: Osteochondral autogenous transplantation for osteochondritis dissecans of the ankle joint. *J Foot Ankle Surg* 2000;39(5):343-348.

234. Assenmacher JA, Kelikian AS, Gottlob C, Kodros S: Arthroscopically assisted autologous osteochondral transplantation for osteochondral lesions of the talar dome: An MRI and clinical follow-up study. *Foot Ankle Int* 2001;22(7):544-551.

235. Scranton PE Jr, McDermott JE: Treatment of type V osteochondral lesions of the talus with ipsilateral knee osteochondral autografts. *Foot Ankle Int* 2001;22(5):380-384.

236. Al-Shaikh RA, Chou LB, Mann JA, Dreeben SM, Prieskorn D: Autologous osteochondral grafting for talar cartilage defects. *Foot Ankle Int* 2002;23(5):

381-389.

237. Baltzer AW, Arnold JP: Bone-cartilage transplantation from the ipsilateral knee for chondral lesions of the talus. *Arthroscopy* 2005;21(2):159-166.

238. Sammarco GJ, Makwana NK: Treatment of talar osteochondral lesions using local osteochondral graft. *Foot Ankle Int* 2002;23(8):693-698.

239. Hangody L: The mosaicplasty technique for osteochondral lesions of the talus. *Foot Ankle Clin* 2003;8(2):259-273.

240. Hangody L, Füles P: Autologous osteochondral mosaicplasty for the treatment of full-thickness defects of weight-bearing joints: Ten years of experimental and clinical experience. *J Bone Joint Surg Am* 2003;85(suppl 2):25-32.

241. Kreuz PC, Steinwachs M, Erggelet C, Lahm A, Henle P, Niemeyer P: Mosaicplasty with autogenous talar autograft for osteochondral lesions of the talus after failed primary arthroscopic management: A

prospective study with a 4-year follow-up. *Am J Sports Med* 2006;34(1):55-63.

242. Nam EK, Ferkel RD, Applegate GR: Autologous chondrocyte implantation of the ankle: A 2- to 5-year follow-up. *Am J Sports Med* 2009;37(2):274-284.

243. Whittaker JP, Smith G, Makwana N, et al: Early results of autologous chondrocyte implantation in the talus. *J Bone Joint Surg Br* 2005;87(2):179-183.

244. Baums MH, Heidrich G, Schultz W, Steckel H, Kahl E, Klinger HM: Autologous chondrocyte transplantation for treating cartilage defects of the talus. *J Bone Joint Surg Am* 2006;88(2):303-308.

245. Gobbi A, Francisco RA, Lubowitz JH, Allegra F, Canata G: Osteochondral lesions of the talus: Randomized controlled trial comparing chondroplasty, microfracture, and osteochondral autograft transplantation. *Arthroscopy* 2006;22(10):1085-1092.

Chapter 38

Spine Problems in the Mature Athlete

Eeric Truumees, MD

Key Points

- Because the population is aging and more individuals are participating in sports later in life, clinicians are seeing more mature athletes with spine problems.
- Although nonspecific diagnoses are commonly rendered for neck and back pain, the evaluation of the older athlete is complicated by higher rates of coexisting or previously undetected disease.
- Degenerative changes are nearly universal in imaging studies obtained in mature athletes, but early testing may be needed if red flags are detected during the history or physical examination.
- For typical sports-induced injuries, management begins with reversing precipitating factors: core strength and flexibility should be increased, bone density should be improved, and sport-specific technique should be optimized (eg, the patient should work on the golf swing).
- Temporary bracing may be required for acute bone injuries, such as vertebral compression fractures.
- Rarely, surgical intervention is indicated for myelopathy or recalcitrant radiculopathy.
- Return to play must be decided individually, based on the patient's neurologic and skeletal stability.

Introduction

Because older adults today remain athletically more active than previous generations, athletic injuries to the spine are more common as well. In the literature, the term *mature athlete* is used to refer to individuals from 30 to 90 years of age. In this chapter, *mature athlete* refers to an individual born in 1964 or earlier. Similarly, *athlete* refers to an individual who participates at any of varying levels, from a weekend warrior to an elite athlete on the senior tour.

Mature athletes can present with injuries on a spectrum ranging from simple myofascial strains to exacerbation of underlying spondylosis. In addition, sports injuries may confer other, specific risks in mature athletes. For example, acquired cervical stenosis confers a small but real risk of central cord syndrome with hyperextension. Similarly, older individuals are more likely to have had previous surgery, peripheral arterial disease, Paget disease, or osteoporosis. Sacral insufficiency, vertebral compression, and other spinal fractures occur with lower energy mechanisms of injury in patients with diminished bone mass.

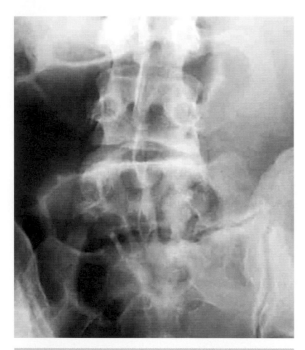

Figure 1   AP radiograph demonstrates a lumbar transitional vertebra in a patient with sports-related low back pain. The patient has mechanical abnormalities that may impact his prognosis and likelihood of improvement with observation alone.

As with the population at large, low back pain in older athletes usually arises from benign and self-limited mechanical dysfunction (**Figure 1**). Unlike younger athletes, however, mature athletes return to sports more slowly and often at a lower participation level. Red flag conditions, such as posterior penetrating ulcers, pancreatitis, renal calculi, or abdominal aortic aneurysm, manifest as back pain and may be falsely attributed to sports. Older athletes more often exhibit "mimic" conditions, such as overlapping shoulder or hip disease.

As a result, management of spine problems in the mature athlete necessitates careful evaluation and decision making. To assist the clinician with these patients, this chapter reviews the epidemiology, pathophysiology, evaluation, treatment, and return-to-play issues for the older athlete with spine injury. When mature athletes present with spinal symptoms, their injuries can be stratified by sport and mechanism of loading, patient age and sex, anatomic region, or presence of radicular symptoms.

Epidemiology

The pervasiveness of neck and low back pain, coupled with the near universality of degenerative changes on imaging, complicates the assessment of older athletes. More than 80% of adults report low back pain episodes, and up to 5% have major pain episodes yearly.[1,2] These incidents often occur without a precipitating event but are subsequently attributed to a sports injury. Although back pain is common in athletes, it is more common in those less physically active. In one study of low back pain in athletes, an incidence of up to 30% was reported.[3]

Only a minute percentage of these episodes of back pain reflect true, radiographically evident trauma. In cross-sectional studies, only 15% of low back pain patients are given a specific diagnosis. Because the vast majority of low back pain episodes are benign and self-limited, a "wait and see" attitude is reasonable in many cases. Within the wide swath of the population that could be considered mature athletes, the risk profile for different injuries varies from group to group.[4,5] For example, pars interarticularis fractures are more frequently encountered in teenage athletes, and vertebral compression fractures are more common in older athletes. In most mature athletes, only degenerative changes are seen. Because virtually all mature athletes exhibit age-appropriate degeneration, the clinical relevance of these radiographic findings is unclear. For example, MRI studies revealed disk degeneration in 93% of patients 60 to 80 years of age.[6] Most of these radiographically "abnormal" structures do not cause symptoms.[2]

Although radiographic spinal degeneration worsens with age, reports of pain peak at 60 years of age and then wane. In a cross-sectional survey of 34,902 Danish twins, subjects were asked to self-report pain by area.[4] In this cohort, aged 20 to 71, pain in the low back, neck, and thoracic area for at least 30 days in the past year was reported by 12%, 10%, and 4%, respectively. Although most (20%) had pain limited to one region, 13% reported pain in two areas. Diffuse spinal pain (all three areas) was reported by 8%. A smaller subset reported radicular or radiating pain. In that group, leg pain was the most common (22%), followed by arm (16%) and trunk (5%) symptoms.

Risk Factors

Given the prevalence of back and neck pain in the mature population at large, understanding which sports and activities confer additional risk assists the clinician in assessing and advising patients. These risk factors are important for two reasons. First, back and neck pain are often falsely attributed to the sport, and the temporal connection between the activity and the symptoms is tenuous. Second, at-risk subgroups may require more aggressive investigation for subtle injuries or even counseling to avoid certain loading mechanisms.

It is known that older athletes are much more likely to injure themselves than are younger athletes in the same sport.[7] When older athletes are injured, the pain tends to last longer. On the other hand, even accounting for an increased likelihood of injury, older athletes are still physically better off than inactive, age-matched peers.

Regional pain around the spine is more common in mature female athletes. Women not only report more pain episodes than do men, but the episodes last longer and affect more areas (eg, neck and back). Neck and back pain in women tends to be more functionally incapacitating than in men. In one study of patients with severe back pain, women were three to four times more likely to report difficulty with light housework, shopping, mobility tasks, and basic activities of daily living.[5,8] A study examining the correlation between lifting, repetitive activity, and the incidence of back pain reported that women were at higher risk for low back pain even though they were less often exposed to lifting and other "heavy" work.[9]

Other predictors for neck and back pain that are more common in older athletes include prior surgeries, lifelong heavy work, lower functional levels, and higher body mass index.[10-12] For example, surgical menopause or inadequate rehabilitation after pelvic or abdominal surgery puts patients at higher risk for later low back pain.[13]

Although the relative risk conferred by age, sex, and past history is important, the relationship between symptom onset and athletic activity also must be ex-plored. Twisting injuries, for example, are more likely than falls to cause pain.[14]

Back pain sufferers have decreased range of motion and less lumbar extension strength. One study showed that increasing lumbar extension strength through 20 sessions with a MedX lumbar extension machine (MedX, Ocala, FL) significantly decreased back pain.[15]

In adults, a vicious cycle often arises. Lower fitness levels increase the likelihood of back pain, which further decreases activity levels, increasing pain. Studies demonstrate decreased core muscle fatigue strength and co-contraction, diminished cross-sectional area, and increased fatty infiltration in patients with persistent or recurrent pain.[16-19] Unfortunately, aging alone also leads to loss of core muscle strength.[20] Pain further limits activity and fitness and adds mental stress, dissatisfaction with life, and sleep problems.[21] Depression in turn increases the incidence of pain episodes and the associated disability, perhaps through fear avoidance behavior.[12,22] Pain, or even the fear of pain, affects electromyographic (EMG) firing patterns,[23] but interestingly, older patients demonstrate less fear avoidance behavior than their younger counterparts.[24] Understanding this interplay between lower fitness levels and pain may assist diagnosis as well as subsequent rehabilitation and return to sport. For example, EMG studies demonstrate a training effect in patients using a bike ergonometer.[25]

Impact of Sports in Youth

Older athletes who report neck and back pain often blame the sports they played in their youth. Understanding the long-term impact of sports can assist clinical evaluation and recommendations for return to activity.

In 1977, Murray-Leslie et al[26] analyzed the spines of 109 ex-military and 112 sport parachutists aged 50 years or older.[26] The ex-military parachutists demonstrated an 84.7% rate of lumbar disk degeneration on radiographic examination. Of that group, 17.4% had "moderate" changes and 10.8% had "severe" changes. Several occult spine fractures were identified. Of note, the study did not implicate parachuting as a cause of lumbar pain. In this group, the only significant association with back pain was body weight ($P < 0.01$); no correlation was found with age or the number of descents. Despite the frequency of the spinal trauma, the authors concluded that parachute descents rarely led to long-term disability.

Since then, a variety of studies have reported increased degenerative change in athletes when compared with age-matched norms. Athletes cited include Olympians, gymnasts, wrestlers, and water-ski jumpers.[27-30] Even "excessive" competitive swimming was found to increase radiographic degeneration, especially at L5-S1.[31] In most of these studies, radiographic changes did not correlate with increased back pain. In one study, participation in multiple sports as an adolescent predicted less pain later.[32] In later adulthood, former elite athletes report *less* back pain than control groups.[33]

Nicholas et al[34] refuted the perception that retired professional football players have poor health. Thirty-five years after the event, the authors studied 36 of 41 members of the 1969 Super Bowl winning team through Short Form 36 (SF-36), medical history, and football-specific questionnaires. The SF-36 scores for physical and mental health were not different from age-matched norms. The most prevalent health problems were arthritis (24 of 36 players), hypertension (13 players), and chronic low back pain (13 players). Both arthritis and low back pain decreased SF-36 physical health scores approximately 20%. The authors concluded that, despite a high prevalence of arthritis, these professional football players had long and fulfilling careers with no apparent long-term detrimental effects.

Pathophysiology

Age, sex, and sport affect not only the rate but also the types of injuries seen.[35] As with spine symptoms in general, neck and back pain after sports is often treated without a specific diagnosis. Most short-term, acute low back pain stems from myofascial inflammation or injury.

The unrelenting changes aging confers render the entire spinal motion segment more vulnerable to injury.[36] From an early age, motor control over the spine steadily decreases.[8,37] In older patients, muscle bulk, primarily comprised of type IIA (fast-twitch) fibers, also declines (so-called "senile sarcopenia").[38] Decreased muscular activation in mature adults leads to loss of coordination and strength. Together, these factors impair self-protection ability and increase injury rates.[39]

Testosterone has been studied as a means of reversing this trend, but its use remains controversial (see chapter 6).[40]

Interestingly, muscular pain is *less* common in older adults, despite the diminutions in their function.[38] On the other hand, when muscle pain occurs in older athletes, they take longer to recover. In patients with persistent and more diffuse symptoms, myofascial pain syndromes such as fibromyalgia should be considered. Although nonspecific back and neck pain syndromes are common overall, they affect active adults less frequently than the population at large.[41]

Even when the primary injury is nonmuscular, back and neck function impacts the types of injuries to which patients are subject and their recovery profile. Thus, an understanding of the static and dynamic spinal stabilizers is critical in both the assessment and treatment phases of mature athletes with spine injury. For example, although any direction of loading can affect the disk, the spine is most vulnerable to rotational and combined force vectors (such as rotation with axial loading).[11]

Spinal stabilizers are divided into the static stabilizers (the longitudinal ligaments, intervertebral disks, and facet joint capsules) and the dynamic stabilizers (the core and superficial muscles). The lumbar extensors are critical, but so are the abdominal and pelvic muscles, including the hip flexors, extensors, and abductors. Well-balanced dynamic stabilizers act synergistically to reduce the shear forces.

Nonmuscular disruptions are seen in the disks, bones, ligaments, and articular processes.[42,43] The specific injury depends on the position of the spine at the time of impact and the force vector imparted. The increased stiffness and decreased bone mineral content of the older spine further impacts the relative frequency of injuries seen. For example, in the cervical spine, stingers and burners are less likely. Exacerbation of spondylosis with radicular or myelopathic symptoms (eg, central cord syndrome) is more common.

Spinal alignment determines the ability of the stabilizers to function together and the loading vectors to which the injured segment is subjected.[44] Increased lordosis, typically from anterior pelvic tilt, weak abdominals, or tight hip flexors, increases shear loading to the posterior elements (eg, the facets). Decreased lordosis resulting from posterior pelvic tilt due to weak extensors or tight hamstrings increases shear loading to the disk.

At the disk level, degenerative processes start during the first decade of life. Biochemical changes in the disk are followed by macroscopic alterations, including annular tears and fissures. As the disk collapses anteriorly, facet loading is compromised, precipitating facet degeneration, subluxation, and osteophytosis. The facet capsules hypertrophy and become lax with associated ligamentum flavum enlargement. Together, these changes narrow the spinal canal and are the most common causes of myelopathy, neurogenic claudication, and radiculopathy in older athletes.

The disk is the motion segment structure most vulnerable to athletic injury.[45,46] With annular disruption, intervertebral disk injuries can be seen in mature athletes. Traumatic disk herniations are rare but are probably more common with torsional loading.[47] The degenerative disk itself may be a source of pain in that the outer third of the anulus receives branches of the sinuvertebral nerve.[48]

Bone injury may occur more readily in older patients because of the combination of bone loss and decreased shock absorption.[49] Thus, older athletes are predisposed to both stress and acute fractures. Avulsion fractures can include the spinous or transverse processes or disk-level osteophytes. With increasing axial loads, vertebral body failure occurs. Most frequently, these injuries affect the thoracolumbar junction.

Vertebral compression fractures cause anterior vertebral body height loss but preserve the posterior vertebral cortex and the spinal canal. More severe axial loading, with or without hyperflexion forces, causes burst fractures. Clinically, the term burst fracture encompasses a spectrum of injuries, from minimal canal intrusion to devastating injuries with marked vertebral body comminution and severe neurologic injury.

Sacral injuries are frequently missed because the affected anatomy is hard to visualize. Acute sacral ala fractures may irritate the L5 root as it passes over the ala anteriorly. In mature athletes, sacral injuries can stem from either acute trauma or chronic, repetitive overloading (ie, stress fracture).

Major, destabilizing sports-related spine injuries most often result from high-velocity collisions between players or sudden acceleration or deceleration mechanics.[43] Most often, such catastrophic spine injuries occur in contact sports such as football, hockey, rugby, and wrestling. Although some mature athletes continue to participate in hockey and other contact sports, they are more likely to participate in and sustain major spinal column injury from noncontact sports such as skiing, diving, surfing, power lifting, and equestrian sports.

A variety of other factors seen in older athletes, such as declines in proprioceptive function and reaction times, impact injury patterns.[8] These neurophysiologic changes modulate how much back pain a given amount of degenerative disk disease causes and how much functional limitation is associated with a given amount of pain.[50] Further, increased spinal stiffness occurs in tandem with increased appendicular skeleton stiffness. Decreased flexibility forces the joints to bear stresses rather than dissipating them to the surrounding muscles. Older adults with chronic low back pain are increasingly likely to exhibit hip and knee degeneration.[8]

In addition to acute spinal column trauma and exacerbation of degenerative conditions, older athletes are vulnerable to a wide array of problems that are far less common in their younger counterparts.[14,42] The conditions, all seen almost exclusively in persons older than 50 years, include malignancy, aortic aneurysm, Paget disease, and polymyalgia rheumatica. To identify these conditions, red flags should be sought in the history and physical examination (**Table 1**).

Evaluation of the Mature Athlete's Spine

In an ocean of benign, self-limited axial neck and low back pain, the clinician's first challenge lies in early detection of the rare but dangerous lesions, as these lesions are more common in older athletes. Nonspinal pain generators such as vascular or intra-abdominal pathology should be excluded (**Table 2**). Next, nonmechanical spine problems such as neoplasm or infection should be ruled out. For mechanical spinal column compromise, root and cord compression from axial problems should be differentiated. In mature athletes, early establishment of neurologic and mechanical stability expedites return to play.

Table 1: Clinical Red Flags

- By patient group
  - Age >50 years
  - History of cancer or recent infection
  - Recent history of major trauma
  - Prior spine surgery
  - Immunocompromise
  - Use of blood thinners
  - History of intravenous drug abuse
  - History of metabolic bone disease (osteoporosis, osteomalacia)
  - History of inflammatory conditions (rheumatoid arthritis, lupus, inflammatory bowel disease)

- Symptoms concerning for major spine pathology
  - Progressive neurologic deficit
  - Gait disturbance, history of falls
  - Bowel or bladder difficulties
  - Constitutional symptoms: malaise, fever, chills, weight loss
  - Nonmechanical pain pattern (worse when supine or at night)

- Symptoms concerning for intra-abdominal, intrapelvic, and other nonspine pathology
  - Colicky pain
  - Pain that radiates to testes or groin
  - Vaginal or penile discharge
  - Gastrointestinal or genitourinary blood
  - Nausea, constipation, change in appetite
  - Pain from front to back

- Other indications that special attention may be needed
  - Peripheral vascular disease
  - Risk for osteoporosis (eg, steroid use)
  - Diabetes
  - Psychosocial overlay: depression, active legal proceedings, etc

History

Clinical assessment begins with a thorough history. Where does it hurt? What kind of pain is it (sharp, aching, burning, etc)? How long has it hurt? Mature athletes often attribute the onset of their pain to a sports injury, but further questioning may uncover little true correlation. When patients describe unremitting or night pain, tumor or infection should be suspected. In older athletes in particular, a history of previous spine problems should be elicited.[51] Previous occurrences imply a higher risk of recurrence.

Next, the patient should be questioned about radiating radicular, funicular, or sclerotomal symptoms. In older patients, herpes zoster (shingles) is more common, and radiating pain may precede the rash. Precipitating and palliating factors allow partial differentiation of potential pain generators. For example, disk pain usually worsens when sitting. Symptoms that worsen with Valsalva maneuvers such as coughing, sneezing, and straining imply space-occupying lesions in the canal. Vascular claudication should be distinguished from neurogenic claudication. The patient should be asked about weakness, ataxia, and difficulty manipulating fine objects. More subtle functional decline, such as trouble getting out of a chair or ascending the stairs, may imply early weakness or cord compression. Painless weakness warrants an aggressive workup and may represent myelopathy, paraneoplastic syndrome, or other neurologic diseases such as multiple sclerosis or amyotrophic lateral sclerosis.

In older athletes, especially women, previous activity level and bone health assessments are critical. In patients who have recently increased their activity level, new-onset back pain generates a differential diagnosis unlike that in patients with a long history of high-level sports participation. Although lifelong training improves lean body mass and bone health, women whose history includes long amenorrheic episodes, on the other hand, are at increased risk for osteoporosis.

Past medical history and review of systems are more relevant in the mature athlete than in younger patients. Specifically, patients should be asked about inflammatory spondyloarthropathies such as rheumatoid arthritis and ankylosing spondylitis, cancer, immunocompromise, trauma, neurologic problems, and major infections. In the review of systems, the patient should

Table 2: Differential Diagnosis of Low Back Pain in the Athlete

Diagnosis	Presentation
Low back strain	Beltline or paravertebral pain with motion
Degenerative disk disease	Midline pain with sitting or loading
Lumbar transitional vertebra	Midline low back pain
Facet-mediated pain	Midline and paramedian pain with extension
Spondylolisthesis	Mechanical midline and paramedian pain
Traumatic fracture	Midline pain at the level of injury
Disk herniation	Pain, numbness, and weakness radiating into the leg
Lumbar spinal stenosis	Low back, buttock, and leg pain, improved with flexion
Cauda equina syndrome	Radicular symptoms with bowel and bladder dysfunction and saddle anesthesia
Spinal infection	Constant low back pain with fevers, chills, night sweats, recent infection, or dental procedure
Tumor	Night pain, fever, older age (>60 years), weight loss
Intra-abdominal or intrapelvic processes	Boring nonmechanical pain, GI disturbance
Renal disease/stones	Colicky pain, GI disturbance
Hip pathology	Groin pain, pain with rotation or weight bearing
Sacroiliac pathology	Buttock and PSIS area pain, pain with loading
Abdominal aortic aneurysm	Constant, boring front-to-back pain

GI = gastrointestinal, PSIS = posterior superior iliac spine.

be questioned about fevers, chills, night sweats, and unanticipated weight loss.

Examination

Physical examination of the mature athlete's spine should begin with observation. The patient's gait, pain, and distress level should be observed. Difficulties with single-toe rise, sitting to standing, or Romberg testing should be noted. Effective heel-toe walking excludes a wide number of pathologies. Ambulatory aids, a wide-based gait, ataxia, or a Trendelenburg gait should be documented. Spinal alignment should be assessed, as well as iliac crest heights, to screen for functional limb-length discrepancy or listing. Paraspinal spasms, scoliosis, muscle atrophies, or asymmetries should be identified and recorded. Mature athletes are more likely to have thoracic hyperkyphosis that may lead to malalignment above and below.

The spine and the paravertebral musculature should be palpated. The presence of tenderness, fluctuance, or skin changes should be documented. Muscular pain syndromes often include tenderness at the insertion on bone. In the cervical spine, this includes the spinous processes at C7 and T1, the medial scapular border, and the occiput. In the low back, the gluteals and extensors attach at the posterior superior iliac spine. Pain in this area is often mistaken for sacroiliac joint inflammation. The Patrick test can test for sacroiliac pathology or sacral stress fracture.[52]

The active and passive arc of motion of the neck, back, and extremities should be assessed. Extensor muscle strength should be tested through the arc of motion. Patients with true or functional core weakness often demonstrate an "instability catch"—that is, they push off from their thighs with their arms when they extend back to neutral. Older patients are more likely to have extremity joint problems; thus shoulder, hip, and knee motion, stability, and pain should be assessed. An abdominal examination is useful to check for aortic aneurysm or visceral problems.

Any potential spine pathology requires a thorough neurovascular examination. When testing strength, functional tests are more sensitive than resistance against the examiner's arm. Reflexes and other cord-mediated signs should be tested. Provocative testing includes nerve tension signs (straight-leg raise and femoral nerve stretch) and re-creation of arm symptoms with neck range of motion or sustained extension.

In addition to providing information for the initial assessment and diagnosis, the physical examination improves decisions regarding return to play. Increasingly, authors recommend a battery of sport-specific tests.[53,54] For example, given the popularity of golf among mature athletes and the frequency with which low back pain is reported among golfers, golf-specific testing is becoming more common. One third of the Professional Golfers Association (PGA) touring membership reported playing with low back pain.[55] Amateurs, who play less frequently, have an even higher rate of symptoms. Sport-specific tests evaluate functional spinal stability such as postural control, proprioception, and muscle activation.

The golf swing is often the major cause of injury. The lumbar spine rotates at the top of the backswing. The subsequent uncoiling, through the downswing and follow-through, generates rotational, sagittal plane shear, axial compression, and lateral bending forces. Amateur golfers generate higher forces than professionals.[55] Quantitatively, these loads are similar to those found to disrupt the lumbar disk in cadaver studies. Before mature athletes return to golf, they must learn proper mechanics and undertake lumbar strengthening. If the physician is unsure of proper sports mechanics, the patient should be referred to a professional teacher, such as a golf professional or athletic trainer.

Cycling, which also is popular among mature athletes, can be associated with neck and back problems. The clinician must be aware of the complex interplay of the individual's seated posture on the bike, riding style, and seat height. Lowering the seat often improves low back pain but can increase neck extension. Saddle problems can also lead to radicular irritation.

Radiographic Evaluation

Radiographic evaluation of the mature athlete begins with plain radiographs, which are necessary only after a trial of symptomatic management.[56] For both cervical and lumbar symptoms, weight-bearing AP and lateral views should be obtained (**Figure 2**). In patients with suspected instability, flexion-extension views also should be ordered. In patients with lumbar symptoms, oblique views, a lateral L5-S1 coned-down view, and an AP pelvic view to check the hip and sacroiliac joints should be considered. Similarly, in patients with neck pain, radiographs of the shoulder on the symptomatic side should be obtained to evaluate possible shoulder problems as a cause of neck pain.

Most mature athletes have at least some of the cardinal findings of spondylosis, including end-plate sclerosis and disk-space loss. Other findings include loss of lordosis, subluxations, vacuum phenomenon, and osteophytes. Disk height loss with end-plate disruption, or in the absence of other spondylotic change, should alert the clinician to the possibility of infection.

Because spondylosis is frequently painless, its usefulness as a diagnostic entity in mature athletes with spinal symptoms is limited. In one study, disk degeneration was present in 90% of the adults examined, half of whom had no pain. In Murray-Leslie et al's[26] study of parachutists, on the other hand, spondylolysis was found in 2 of 46 ex-military parachutists and spondylolisthesis unassociated with spondylolysis in 4. Although most degenerative changes were asymptomatic, spondylolisthesis was always associated with low back pain. In other series, spondylolisthesis accounts for up to 5% of chronic low back pain.

In older patients or those with medical risk factors, bone integrity of the vertebrae should be scrutinized. Danger signs include cortical erosion or expansion, vertebral collapse, or the "winking owl sign" on the AP view, which represents unilateral pedicle destruction that may suggest the presence of neoplasm. The paraspinal soft-tissue contours, such as the psoas shadows on a lumbar AP view, should be assessed. It is important to

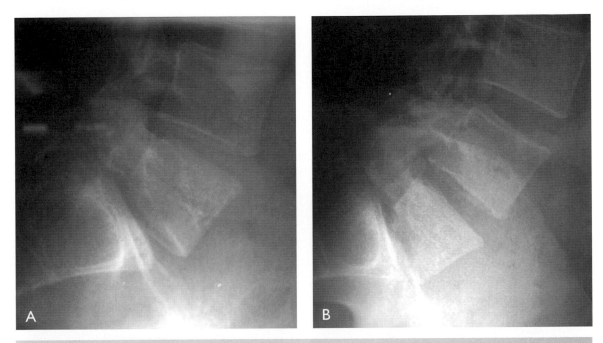

Figure 2   Lateral radiographs obtained in April (**A**) and September (**B**) of the same year demonstrate gradual disk height loss and end plate erosion in a patient with constant back pain. Recommendations to obtain MRI had been made, but unfortunately this individual's diskitis was not diagnosed until an abscess formed with lower extremity weakness in the ensuing month.

note that evidence of osteopenia is not evident on plain radiographs until 30% of bone mineral density has been lost.

In patients with purely axial, mechanical symptoms, imaging and other testing is not required unless the symptoms fail to respond to first-line, symptomatic management. In patients with red flags, earlier imaging is recommended. For example, higher energy injuries prompt early plain radiographs. In patients with suspected osteoporosis, the fracture risk is higher. In that group, dual-energy x-ray absorptiometry (DEXA) scanning and plain radiographs should be obtained.

MRI should be obtained in patients with systemic illness, night or rest pain, or weakness (**Figures 3** and **4**). In mature athletes with higher energy injuries, short tau inversion recovery (STIR) sequences should be obtained to assess for dens fracture, ligament integrity, and end-plate injuries. Gadolinium contrast may be helpful in patients with previous spine surgery or those in whom infection or tumor is suspected. Typically, tu-

mors demonstrate decreased signal intensity on T1-weighted images and increased signal intensity on T2-weighted images.

As with plain radiographs, the nearly universal presence of degenerative changes on MRI in the mature athlete may prompt overreferral or overtreatment. For example, Savage et al[57] studied MRIs of 149 working men in five occupational groups and found L5-S1 degeneration to be significantly more prevalent ($P < 0.01$) in older individuals (31 to 58 years; 52% prevalence) than in younger individuals (20 to 30 years; 27% prevalence). Although low back pain was more prevalent in the older subjects in this study, appearance of degeneration on MRI was not related to reports of low back pain. No differences among occupational groups were noted, suggesting that activity has, at most, a limited impact on the development of spondylosis. At 1-year follow-up, 13 of the subjects reported first-time low back pain, but no MRI change could account for the new symptoms.

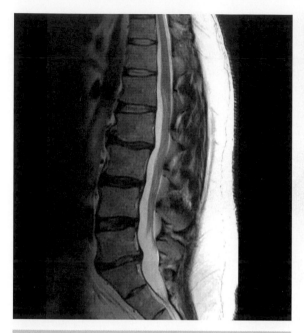

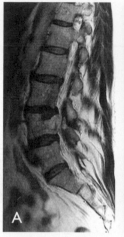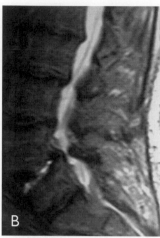

Figure 3   Sagittal T2-weighted MRI scan demonstrates multilevel disk degeneration in a patient with recurrent low back pain. Note the end plate anomalies at L2-L3 and the disk height loss at L5-S1. These changes, although common in asymptomatic individuals, may affect normal loading mechanics.

Figure 4   Sagittal MRIs demonstrate other red flag conditions to be considered in mature athletes presenting with low back pain. In both cases, a history of minor trauma was reported. **A,** This patient's constant, unrelenting pain was associated with increased radicular symptomatology. **B,** In another patient, focal tenderness was noted in the midline over the palpable slip at L4-L5. Back and leg pain symptoms were noted. Subsequent evaluation demonstrated significant, but previously undiagnosed, osteoporosis.

Other tests that can be considered include technetium Tc-99m bone scans, which are sensitive to many tumors, infection, stress fracture, or rib injuries. In mature athletes, CT is useful to look for subtle pars or end-plate disruptions (**Figure 5**). Extensor muscle thinning on CT, as on MRI, has been correlated with increased low back pain.[58]

Treatment and Return to Play

In one cross-sectional study of low back pain in athletes, more than 90% improved without formal medical attention.[3] Of those formally treated, the most common myofascial neck and back injuries improved within 1 week. More than 90% of the treated cohort had recovered fully at 3 months.

At the other end of the injury spectrum, high-energy fractures and dislocations require intensive, multidisciplinary care, often in a level 1 trauma center. In any high-energy trauma situation, an early transfer is optimal. Event physicians must first attend to the ABCs of resuscitation: airway, breathing, and circulation. Regardless of pain level, the patient should be immobilized on a backboard and placed in a cervical collar. Levels of consciousness and a neurologic examination should be documented and repeated at regular intervals until the trauma transfer is complete. The injury mechanism, early symptoms, and early neurologic status should be communicated to the spine specialist assuming care.

Although the benefits of early surgery remain controversial, recent retrospective studies support reduction, decompression, and stabilization within 8 hours when possible.[59,60] A randomized trial is currently underway. Therapeutic cooling for acute spinal cord injury received much media attention after the rapid recovery of Buffalo Bills tight end Kevin Everett in 2007. At this

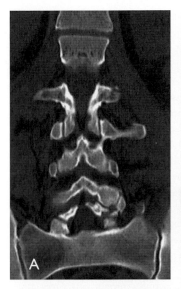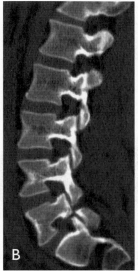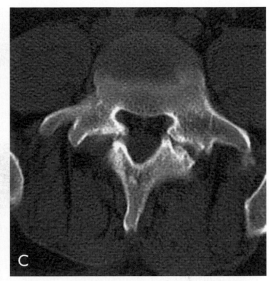

Figure 5 CT images demonstrate a chronic pars fracture in the coronal (**A**), sagittal (**B**), and axial (**C**) planes. The loss of the pars affects the spine's resistance to shear loading. In the absence of spondylolisthesis, it is not clear whether the pars defect places the patient at significantly increased risk during sports.

time, the benefits of that approach have been convincingly demonstrated only in animal models and small series.[61,62] Immobilization, maintenance of blood pressure, and oxygenation are far more likely to optimize neurologic outcome.

In the office, the orthopaedic surgeon most typically encounters the mature athlete with ongoing mechanical back pain. In this setting, treatment varies as a function of symptom duration and severity. It can be divided into three phases—acute, rehabilitation, and maintenance.[14,63]

Acute Phase

In mature athletes with acute low back pain, pain control should be initiated. Traditionally, pain medications include nonsteroidal anti-inflammatory drugs, narcotics, and muscle relaxers. Narcotics should be used sparingly, because in patients with more chronic low back pain, the side effects of opioids are more prevalent than in the general population and outcomes are no better than for patients on nonnarcotic agents.[64] Muscle relaxers are also controversial, but probably less so. In patients with acute, radicular pain, a steroid dose pack may be considered. A wide variety of other agents, such as gabapentin, may have utility for radicular symptoms. Intravenous pamidronate has been shown to decrease neurogenic claudication symptoms.[65]

Some authors recommend ice for tenderness. Heat may be helpful for those with muscular symptoms, but it should be avoided after acute injury, especially in the presence of soft-tissue injury or bruising. Heat is useful in the rehabilitative phase to improve muscular blood flow and to reduce stiffness.

Physical therapy remains the mainstay of mechanical pain treatment. In the acute phase, physical therapy focuses on reducing pain, using modalities such as massage, ultrasound, and transcutaneous electrical nerve stimulation (TENS).[44,63] Pool therapy can be helpful, but no more so than other treatments.[66] Pool therapy seems most useful to allow an earlier return to activity in the most functionally limited patients. In more affected athletes, especially those who are unsteady or weak, ambulatory aids such as a cane, walker, or wheelchair should be considered.

In the acute phase, activity limitations, but *not* bed rest, should be recommended. Low-impact aerobic activity, such as walking, is encouraged. Typical restrictions include avoidance of the following: bending, lifting more than 5 lb, twisting, and overhead activities. Other activity recommendations are injury-specific and are designed to avoid loading injured structures. For disk-mediated pain, excessive sitting, bending, and lifting should be avoided. Patients with radicular symptoms should avoid postures that increase pain radiation. Osteoporotic patients probably benefit from similar restrictions. Physical therapy can also be very helpful in instructing the patient in proper posture and body mechanics to protect injured structures, reduce symptoms, and prevent further injury during activities of daily living.

Rigid bracing, such as a thoracolumbosacral orthosis or Philadelphia collar, is reserved for patients with acute spinal fractures or an active infection. Semirigid bracing, such as a corset or soft collar, is occasionally helpful in mature athletes as a proprioceptive reminder. Intermittent bracing, such as a rucksack-type orthosis, may relieve pain and fatigue during prolonged standing and walking.[67]

Rehabilitation Phase

Several rehabilitation phase protocols have been described. Many strategies seek to centralize referred or radicular pain, often through identification of postures that minimize symptom radiation. Once accomplished, active stabilization is sought.[63] The therapist teaches the patient how to find a neutral spinal alignment and maintain it during everyday activities. This position, specific to the individual, is determined by the pelvic and spinal postures that place the least stress on the spine and its supporting structures.

For mature athletes in particular, the physician and physical therapist both must assess the entire kinetic chain.[68] Lower extremity and core strength are intricately linked.[69,70] Restricted motion or weakness in one area precipitates problems in other parts of the chain. For example, decreased hip range of motion increases stress on the lumbar spine. Conversely, by altering gait and ground reaction forces, low back pain increases the risk for other lower extremity problems.[71] Core strengthening programs improve rotational control of the leg and thus decrease the risk of anterior cruciate ligament injury. For sports requiring arm movement and strength, any rehabilitation program must include both upper and lower extremity closed-kinetic-chain exercises.

Active stabilization affords spinal control and protection through synergistic activation of the trunk and spinal musculature. Abdominal and gluteal muscle strengthening is stressed.[58] After rehabilitation, the maintenance phase focuses on eccentric strengthening exercises.[58] Dynamic conditioning (eg, exercise ball) and endurance exercises are added. Several programs have been described. In a bicycle endurance program studied specifically for older adults with chronic low back pain, a set level of energy expenditure was achieved three times a week for 12 weeks. For the 18 patients who completed the trial, exercise effectively decreased low back pain and improved function.[72]

Outcomes of these rehabilitation efforts are generally positive, but they vary considerably. Preinjury fitness level has been shown to impact outcomes both positively and negatively. Winters-Stone and Snow[73] found that the patients with the lowest initial functional level exhibited the greatest gains. Hartvigsen and Christensen[41] reported that individuals participating in strenuous exercise at least once a week had the best outcomes. No one type or frequency of exercise could be recommended. In all likelihood, individuals with the lowest preinjury functional levels have the greatest room for improvement, but fitter individuals recover faster and attain higher postrehabilitation function. Some programs may be better suited to different patients' needs, but clear recommendations cannot currently be supported by the literature.

When mature athletes recover—and often sooner—they ask about return to activity in general, and their sport in particular. Unfortunately, the literature is noteworthy for a "striking lack of objective data" and a complete absence of level I evidence to guide these recommendations.[74,75] Even lower level evidence, such as expert opinion, is confounded by a "marked lack of consensus among treating physicians."[76,77] In a survey of practice patterns regarding return to play after a cervical spine injury,[77] half of the respondents reported using published guidelines. But in the accompanying case review, only one in ten consistently followed those guidelines. The authors noted that spine specialists tended to allow earlier return to play and physicians with longer practice histories took a more conservative approach.

The grading system of Watkins et al, which attempts to quantify risk of return to sport, is often quoted (**Table 3**).[78] However, the specific head and neck issues addressed are not broadly relevant in mature athletes. Many authors' guidelines for return to sport in older athletes vary little from those for younger athletes, such as full resolution of symptoms and a return to full range of motion.[7,42-44] At the least, resolution of neurologic signs and symptoms should occur. Complete resolution of other symptoms, such as low back pain, may not be achievable. Similarly, older athletes may return to their previous arc of motion, but not, perhaps, full range of motion.

The mature athlete is more likely than younger counterparts to have had previous spinal surgery. The surgeon must decide which sports remain appropriate in the postoperative period and when the patient can return. Generally, a well-healed single-level cervical or lumbar fusion does not bar return to sports, although when polled, most spine surgeons will never allow healed athletes to return to contact sports, like rugby, and fall-prone sports, like skiing. Some mature athletes have irremediable issues such as poor bone quality, spondylolisthesis, and spinal canal stenosis that preclude some, but not all, athletic pursuits. Other specific issues seen mainly in older patients include ankylosing spondylitis, diffuse idiopathic skeletal hyperostosis, Klippel-Feil syndrome, and degenerative autofusion. These conditions alter the spine's mechanics and its response to sudden loading. The clinician should be very cautious about allowing a return to high-impact sports in patients with multilevel fusions, abnormal sagittal alignment, or poor bone quality.[79]

Unlike younger athletes, who often quickly resume their previous sports at full participation, mature athletes are best returned to their sports gradually.[14] On the other hand, older athletes are more compliant with rehabilitation and are less likely to be involved in high-impact sports and engage in overly risky behavior. Medical comorbidities, which are uncommon in younger athletes, often have to be considered in mature athletes. Cardiopulmonary changes that are a part of normal aging include a decrease in maximum heart rate and maximum cardiac output.[80,81] In older athletes, the cardiac muscle is less able to increase wall muscle size than in younger athletes. To increase cardiac output

---

Table 3: Risk Categories for Return to Sports in Mature Athletes[a]

- Low-risk conditions
    Asymptomatic bone spurs
    Healed, nondisplaced fractures
    Stingers/burners
    Healed disk herniations or asymptomatic
      foraminal stenosis
    Low-grade slips
- Moderate-risk conditions
    Facet and lateral mass fractures
    Nondisplaced, healed odontoid and C1 ring
      fractures
    High-grade, kyphotic, or mobile slips
- High-risk conditions
    Os odontoideum, odontoid fractures
    Ruptured transverse atlantal ligament
    Occipitocervical or cervical
      fracture-dislocations
    Cord anomalies
    Central disk herniations with high-grade
      stenosis

[a]Information adapted from reference 78.

---

with exertion, an increased heart rate is required.[69] Older patients also have decreased lung capacity and decreased temperature regulation. They are also vulnerable to delirium from dehydration. Major health problems such as hypertension, heart disease, lung disease, and hearing and sight loss should be addressed with the patient's primary physician before returning these patients to active participation.

Maintenance Phase

Seasonal athletes should be encouraged to cross-train year round or precondition before returning to their sport. To prevent reinjury, patient education and preseason, sport-specific training should be emphasized.[44] Sport-specific training improves body mechanics and minimizes forces on the spine. These forces are additionally counteracted by strengthening the spine's dynamic stabilizers. Proper flexibility should be maintained to avoid stress concentration. Improvements in aerobic fitness increase tissue blood flow and oxygenation.[27] In older athletes, deteriorating balance should be addressed by the addition of balance exercises to the workout regimen.

Good sport-specific mechanics are critical in the prevention of recurrent injury.[44] In golfers, low back pain often recurs with return to sport. Much of this risk stems from the significant stress imparted on the lumbar spine by the golf swing.[82] To assess the impact of skill on spinal force generation, Cole and Grimshaw[83] compared surface EMG measurements of erector spinae and external oblique activity during 20 golf drives in a cohort of 12 symptomatic and 18 asymptomatic golfers.[83] These cohorts were further divided by handicap. Low-handicap golfers with low back pain tended to demonstrate reduced erector spinae activity both at the top of the backswing and at impact, whereas greater external oblique activity was seen throughout the swing.

Using a triaxial electrogoniometer, Lindsay and Horton[84] compared spinal motion in three planes during swings in professional golfers with and without low back pain.[84] Golfers with low back pain demonstrated more spinal flexion and significantly more side bending on the backswing. In the downswing of golfers with no history of low back pain, more than twice as much trunk flexion velocity was demonstrated. The authors believed this difference was related to increased abdominal muscle activity.

In the high-handicap group, golfers with low back pain demonstrated more erector spinae activity. Reduced erector spinae activity was associated with a reduced capacity to protect the spine and its surrounding structures at the top of the backswing and at impact, where the torsional loads are high. The authors concluded that the distinct differences in swing mechanics between the symptomatic and asymptomatic golfers could guide recovery from golf-related low back pain.[83]

The mature athlete should have proper equipment, whether sport-specific, such as a bicycle seat at the correct height or golf clubs of proper length, or more general, such as proper shoe wear. Older patients are more sensitive to shoe wear. Runners, in particular, need good midsole cushioning and should change shoes every 250 to 500 miles.[85] Grass, dirt, wooden, and rubber tracks are less stressful to the body than concrete

and are particularly recommended for older runners. Various insoles have been shown to reduce low back pain.[86,87] In one study, a viscoelastic heel decreased vertical strain transients in the lumbar spine.[86]

Whether beginning a new season or returning an injured mature athlete to sports, the following four elements[88] should be incorporated into the protocol: (1) injury rehabilitation coordinated by a physical therapist; (2) preactivity warm-up routines; (3) coaching on proper, sport-specific technique; and (4) preseason conditioning programs. Mature athletes also should adopt the routine of postactivity cooldown exercises and stretches.

For the subgroup of patients with multiply recurrent or more severe symptoms, more definitive intervention may be available through a spine specialist. These treatments can range from injection therapies to surgical stabilization. Patients with weakness, myelopathy, or other red flags should be referred early. Patients with recalcitrant, moderate radiculopathy may benefit from referral at the 6- to 8-week mark. In patients with severe axial symptoms, invasive treatment may be considered if 4 to 6 months of intensive nonsurgical management fails to relieve symptoms. Clearly, professional athletes are more economically invested in their physical performance. For example, the professional masters golfer will likely be referred sooner, and more aggressive treatment may be justified. In the medically frail or osteoporotic patient, a more deliberate approach is recommended.

Conclusions

The mature athlete could be 30 or 90, and may engage in sports ranging from walking to professional tennis. When these individuals have neck or back pain, potential etiologies range from transient myofascial irritation to fractures from vertebral metastasis. Typically, activity-mediated symptoms are reported in patients with evidence of spondylosis on imaging studies. Given that both low back pain and asymptomatic radiographic degeneration are extremely common, establishing the true "pain generator" remains challenging in most patients without focal injury.

Older athletes carry higher risks of injury than their younger peers, but the benefits of sports participation outweigh the risks. Overall, active adults have lower pain and higher functional levels than their less active peers. Despite having relatively more free time, older adults are typically reluctant to take up new activities. Injuries and fear avoidance behaviors most typically lead to a gradual disengagement from previous activities.

Understanding this population's risk factors for spinal pain guides their evaluation. Although most pain is transient, recurrent or recalcitrant symptoms should be explored aggressively, both to allow earlier return to activity and to catch potentially serious conditions. Mature athletes are not only at greater risk for mechanical problems but also are more likely to have bone loss, cancer, and major infection. These conditions require a different evaluation and management algorithm than most mechanical pain generators.

For most patients with mechanical symptoms, return to activity requires rehabilitation of both the core muscles and associated "downstream" joint and muscle groups (eg, the hip and the knee). Endurance exercise and preseason conditioning, appropriate warm-up, and sport-specific technique instruction all convey additional benefits.

References

1. Dwyer AP: Backache and its prevention. *Clin Orthop Relat Res* 1987;(222):35-43.

2. Svensson HO, Andersson GB, Johansson S, Wilhelmsson C, Vedin A: A retrospective study of low-back pain in 38- to 64-year-old women: Frequency of occurrence and impact on medical services. *Spine (Phila Pa 1976)* 1988;13(5):548-552.

3. Graw BP, Wiesel SW: Low back pain in the aging athlete. *Sports Med Arthrosc* 2008;16(1):39-46.

4. Leboeuf-Yde C, Nielsen J, Kyvik KO, Fejer R, Hartvigsen J: Pain in the lumbar, thoracic or cervical regions: Do age and gender matter? A population-based study of 34,902 Danish twins 20-71 years of age. *BMC Musculoskelet Disord* 2009;10:39.

5. Leveille SG, Guralnik JM, Hochberg M, et al: Low back pain and disability in older women: Independent association with difficulty but not inability to perform daily activities. *J Gerontol A Biol Sci Med Sci* 1999; 54(10):M487-M493.

6. Boden SD, Davis DO, Dina TS, Patronas NJ, Wiesel SW: Abnormal magnetic-resonance scans of the lumbar spine in asymptomatic subjects: A prospective investigation. *J Bone Joint Surg Am* 1990;72(3): 403-408.

7. Hubert HB, Fries JF: Predictors of physical disability after age 50: Six-year longitudinal study in a runners club and a university population. *Ann Epidemiol* 1994;4(4):285-294.

8. Yagci N, Cavlak U, Aslan UB, Akdag B: Relationship between balance performance and musculoskeletal pain in lower body comparison healthy middle aged and older adults. *Arch Gerontol Geriatr* 2007;45(1): 109-119.

9. Alcouffe J, Manillier P, Brehier M, Fabin C, Faupin F: Analysis by sex of low back pain among workers from small companies in the Paris area: Severity and occupational consequences. *Occup Environ Med* 1999; 56(10):696-701.

10. Gnudi S, Sitta E, Gnudi F, Pignotti E: Relationship of a lifelong physical workload with physical function and low back pain in retired women. *Aging Clin Exp Res* 2009;21(1):55-61.

11. Hangai M, Kaneoka K, Kuno S, et al: Factors associated with lumbar intervertebral disc degeneration in the elderly. *Spine J* 2008;8(5):732-740.

12. Hartvigsen J, Frederiksen H, Christensen K: Physical and mental function and incident low back pain in seniors: A population-based two-year prospective study of 1387 Danish Twins aged 70 to 100 years. *Spine (Phila Pa 1976)* 2006;31(14):1628-1632.

13. Ericksen JJ, Bean JF, Kiely DK, Hicks GE, Leveille SG: Does gynecologic surgery contribute to low back problems in later life? An analysis of the women's health and aging study. *Arch Phys Med Rehabil* 2006;87(2): 172-176.

14. Buschbacher R: The aging athlete's spine. *J Back Musculoskel Rehabil* 1995;5:55-74.

15. Holmes B, Leggett S, Mooney V, Nichols J, Negri S, Hoeyberghs A: Comparison of female geriatric lumbar-extension strength: asymptotic versus chronic low back pain patients and their response to active rehabilitation. *J Spinal Disord* 1996;9(1):17-22.

16. Burnett AF, Cornelius MW, Dankaerts W, O'sullivan PB: Spinal kinematics and trunk muscle activity in cyclists: A comparison between healthy controls and non-specific chronic low back pain subjects-a pilot investigation. *Man Ther* 2004;9(4):211-219.

17. Hicks GE, Simonsick EM, Harris TB, et al: Cross-sectional associations between trunk muscle composition, back pain, and physical function in the

health, aging and body composition study. *J Gerontol A Biol Sci Med Sci* 2005;60(7):882-887.

18. Ranson CA, Burnett AF, Kerslake R, Batt ME, O'Sullivan PB: An investigation into the use of MR imaging to determine the functional cross sectional area of lumbar paraspinal muscles. *Eur Spine J* 2006;15(6): 764-773.

19. Takahashi I, Kikuchi S, Sato K, Iwabuchi M: Effects of the mechanical load on forward bending motion of the trunk: Comparison between patients with motion-induced intermittent low back pain and healthy subjects. *Spine (Phila Pa 1976)* 2007;32(2):E73-E78.

20. Mannion AF, Käser L, Weber E, Rhyner A, Dvorak J, Müntener M: Influence of age and duration of symptoms on fibre type distribution and size of the back muscles in chronic low back pain patients. *Eur Spine J* 2000;9(4):273-281.

21. Miranda H, Viikari-Juntura E, Punnett L, Riihimäki H: Occupational loading, health behavior and sleep disturbance as predictors of low-back pain. *Scand J Work Environ Health* 2008;34(6):411-419.

22. Vlaeyen JW, Kole-Snijders AM, Boeren RG, van Eek H: Fear of movement/(re)injury in chronic low back pain and its relation to behavioral performance. *Pain* 1995;62(3):363-372.

23. Lamoth CJ, Daffertshofer A, Meijer OG, Lorimer Moseley G, Wuisman PI, Beek PJ: Effects of experimentally induced pain and fear of pain on trunk coordination and back muscle activity during walking. *Clin Biomech (Bristol, Avon)* 2004;19(6):551-563.

24. Cook AJ, Brawer PA, Vowles KE: The fear-avoidance model of chronic pain: Validation and age analysis using structural equation modeling. *Pain* 2006; 121(3):195-206.

25. Watanabe S, Eguchi A, Kobara K, Ishida H, Otsuki K: Electromyographic activity of selected trunk muscles during bicycle ergometer exercise and walking. *Electromyogr Clin Neurophysiol* 2006;46(5):311-315.

26. Murray-Leslie CF, Lintott DJ, Wright V: The spine in sport and veteran military parachutists. *Ann Rheum Dis* 1977;36(4):332-342.

27. Durall CJ, Udermann BE, Johansen DR, Gibson B, Reineke DM, Reuteman P: The effects of preseason trunk muscle training on low-back pain occurrence in women collegiate gymnasts. *J Strength Cond Res* 2009; 23(1):86-92.

28. Hellström M, Jacobsson B, Swärd L, Peterson L: Radiologic abnormalities of the thoraco-lumbar spine in athletes. *Acta Radiol* 1990;31(2):127-132.

29. Horne J, Cockshott WP, Shannon HS: Spinal column damage from water ski jumping. *Skeletal Radiol* 1987; 16(8):612-616.

30. Ong A, Anderson J, Roche J: A pilot study of the prevalence of lumbar disc degeneration in elite athletes with lower back pain at the Sydney 2000 Olympic Games. *Br J Sports Med* 2003;37(3):263-266.

31. Kaneoka K, Shimizu K, Hangai M, et al: Lumbar intervertebral disk degeneration in elite competitive swimmers: A case control study. *Am J Sports Med* 2007;35(8):1341-1345.

32. Auvinen JP, Tammelin TH, Taimela SP, Zitting PJ, Mutanen PO, Karppinen JI: Musculoskeletal pains in relation to different sport and exercise activities in youth. *Med Sci Sports Exerc* 2008;40(11):1890-1900.

33. Videman T, Sarna S, Battié MC, et al: The long-term effects of physical loading and exercise lifestyles on back-related symptoms, disability, and spinal pathology among men. *Spine (Phila Pa 1976)* 1995;20(6): 699-709.

34. Nicholas SJ, Nicholas JA, Nicholas C, Diecchio JR, McHugh MP: The health status of retired American football players: Super Bowl III revisited. *Am J Sports Med* 2007;35(10):1674-1679.

35. Iwamoto J, Takeda T, Sato Y, Matsumoto H: Retrospective case evaluation of gender differences in sports injuries in a Japanese sports medicine clinic. *Gend Med* 2008;5(4):405-414.

36. Benoist M: Natural history of the aging spine. *Eur Spine J* 2003;12(Suppl 2):S86-S89.

37. Brumagne S, Cordo P, Verschueren S: Proprioceptive weighting changes in persons with low back pain and elderly persons during upright standing. *Neurosci Lett* 2004;366(1):63-66.

38. Seto JL, Brewster CE: Musculoskeletal conditioning of the older athlete. *Clin Sports Med* 1991;10(2):401-429.

39. Hwang JH, Lee YT, Park DS, Kwon TK: Age affects the latency of the erector spinae response to sudden loading. *Clin Biomech (Bristol, Avon)* 2008;23(1):23-29.

40. Morley JE, Kaiser FE, Sih R, Hajjar R, Perry HM III: Testosterone and frailty. *Clin Geriatr Med* 1997; 13(4):685-695.

41. Hartvigsen J, Christensen K: Active lifestyle protects against incident low back pain in seniors: A population-based 2-year prospective study of 1387 Danish twins

aged 70-100 years. *Spine (Phila Pa 1976)* 2007;
32(1):76-81.

42. Hackley DR, Wiesel SW: The lumbar spine in the aging athlete. *Clin Sports Med* 1993;12(3):465-468.

43. Tall RL, DeVault W: Spinal injury in sport: Epidemiologic considerations. *Clin Sports Med* 1993;12(3):441-448.

44. Dreisinger TE, Nelson BW: Management of back pain in athletes. *Sports Med* 1996;21(4):313-320.

45. Kosaka H, Sairyo K, Biyani A, et al: Pathomechanism of loss of elasticity and hypertrophy of lumbar ligamentum flavum in elderly patients with lumbar spinal canal stenosis. *Spine (Phila Pa 1976)* 2007; 32(25):2805-2811.

46. Vernon-Roberts B, Moore RJ, Fraser RD: The natural history of age-related disc degeneration: the pathology and sequelae of tears. *Spine (Phila Pa 1976)* 2007; 32(25):2797-2804.

47. Kahler DM: Low back pain in athletes. *J Sport Rehabil* 1993;2(1):63-78.

48. Grignon B, Grignon Y, Mainard D, Braun M, Netter P, Roland J: The structure of the cartilaginous end-plates in elder people. *Surg Radiol Anat* 2000;22(1): 13-19.

49. Stucki G, Ewert T: How to assess the impact of arthritis on the individual patient: The WHO ICF. *Ann Rheum Dis* 2005;64(5):664-668.

50. Weiner DK, Rudy TE, Morrow L, Slaboda J, Lieber S: The relationship between pain, neuropsychological performance, and physical function in community-dwelling older adults with chronic low back pain. *Pain Med* 2006;7(1):60-70.

51. Tong HC, Haig AJ, Geisser ME, Yamakawa KS, Miner JA: Comparing pain severity and functional status of older adults without spinal symptoms, with lumbar spinal stenosis, and with axial low back pain. *Gerontology* 2007;53(2):111-115.

52. Blake SP, Connors AM: Sacral insufficiency fracture. *Br J Radiol* 2004;77(922):891-896.

53. Malliou P, Gioftsidou A, Beneka A, Godolias G: Measurements and evaluations in low back pain patients. *Scand J Med Sci Sports* 2006;16(4):219-230.

54. Stevens VK, Bouche KG, Mahieu NN, Cambier DC, Vanderstraeten GG, Danneels LA: Reliability of a functional clinical test battery evaluating postural control, proprioception and trunk muscle activity. *Am J Phys Med Rehabil* 2006;85(9):727-736.

55. Hosea TM, Gatt CJ Jr: Back pain in golf. *Clin Sports Med* 1996;15(1):37-53.

56. Greenan TJ: Diagnostic imaging of sports-related spinal disorders. *Clin Sports Med* 1993;12(3):487-505.

57. Savage RA, Whitehouse GH, Roberts N: The relationship between the magnetic resonance imaging appearance of the lumbar spine and low back pain, age and occupation in males. *Eur Spine J* 1997;6(2): 106-114.

58. Keller A, Gunderson R, Reikerås O, Brox JI: Reliability of computed tomography measurements of paraspinal muscle cross-sectional area and density in patients with chronic low back pain. *Spine (Phila Pa 1976)* 2003; 28(13):1455-1460.

59. Bagnall AM, Jones L, Duffy S, Riemsma RP: Spinal fixation surgery for acute traumatic spinal cord injury. *Cochrane Database Syst Rev* 2008;1:CD004725.

60. Cengiz SL, Kalkan E, Bayir A, Ilik K, Basefer A: Timing of thoracolombar spine stabilization in trauma patients; impact on neurological outcome and clinical course. A real prospective (RCT) randomized controlled study. *Arch Orthop Trauma Surg* 2008; 128(9):959-966.

61. Kwon BK, Curt A, Belanger LM, et al: Intrathecal pressure monitoring and cerebrospinal fluid drainage in acute spinal cord injury: A prospective randomized trial. *J Neurosurg Spine* 2009;10(3):181-193.

62. Levi AD, Green BA, Wang MY, et al: Clinical application of modest hypothermia after spinal cord injury. *J Neurotrauma* 2009;26(3):407-415.

63. Kaul MP, Herring SA: Rehabilitation of lumbar spine injuries in sports. *Phys Med Rehabil Clin N Am* 1994; 5(1):133-156.

64. Kalso E, Simpson KH, Slappendel R, Dejonckheere J, Richarz U: Predicting long-term response to strong opioids in patients with low back pain: Findings from a randomized, controlled trial of transdermal fentanyl and morphine. *BMC Med* 2007;5:39.

65. Feld J, Rosner I, Avshovich N, Boulman N, Slobodin G, Rozenbaum M: An open study of pamidronate in the treatment of refractory degenerative lumbar spinal stenosis. *Clin Rheumatol* 2009;28(6):715-717.

66. Waller B, Lambeck J, Daly D: Therapeutic aquatic exercise in the treatment of low back pain: A systematic review. *Clin Rehabil* 2009;23(1):3-14.

67. Ishida H, Watanabe S, Yanagawa H, Kawasaki M, Kobayashi Y, Amano Y: Immediate effects of a rucksack type orthosis on the elderly with decreased lumbar

lordosis during standing and walking. *Electromyogr Clin Neurophysiol* 2008;48(1):53-61.

68. Nadler SF, Wu KD, Galski T, Feinberg JH: Low back pain in college athletes: A prospective study correlating lower extremity overuse or acquired ligamentous laxity with low back pain. *Spine (Phila Pa 1976)* 1998;23(7): 828-833.

69. Arendt EA: Core strengthening. *Instr Course Lect* 2007;56:379-384.

70. Zazulak BT, Hewett TE, Reeves NP, Goldberg B, Cholewicki J: Deficits in neuromuscular control of the trunk predict knee injury risk: A prospective biomechanical-epidemiologic study. *Am J Sports Med* 2007;35(7):1123-1130.

71. Lee CE, Simmonds MJ, Etnyre BR, Morris GS: Influence of pain distribution on gait characteristics in patients with low back pain: Part 1. Vertical ground reaction force. *Spine (Phila Pa 1976)* 2007;32(12): 1329-1336.

72. Iversen MD, Fossel AH, Katz JN: Enhancing function in older adults with chronic low back pain: A pilot study of endurance training. *Arch Phys Med Rehabil* 2003;84(9):1324-1331.

73. Winters-Stone KM, Snow CM: Musculoskeletal response to exercise is greatest in women with low initial values. *Med Sci Sports Exerc* 2003;35(10): 1691-1696.

74. Bono CM: Low-back pain in athletes. *J Bone Joint Surg Am* 2004;86-A(2):382-396.

75. Eck JC, Riley LH III: Return to play after lumbar spine conditions and surgeries. *Clin Sports Med* 2004;23(3): 367-379.

76. Morganti C: Recommendations for return to sports following cervical spine injuries. *Sports Med* 2003; 33(8):563-573.

77. Morganti C, Sweeney CA, Albanese SA, Burak C, Hosea T, Connolly PJ: Return to play after cervical spine injury. *Spine (Phila Pa 1976)* 2001;26(10): 1131-1136.

78. Vaccaro AR, Klein GR, Ciccoti M, et al: Return to play criteria for the athlete with cervical spine injuries resulting in stinger and transient quadriplegia/paresis. *Spine J* 2002;2(5):351-356.

79. Kohrt WM, Bloomfield SA, Little KD, Nelson ME, Yingling VR, American College of Sports Medicine: American College of Sports Medicine Position Stand: Physical activity and bone health. *Med Sci Sports Exerc* 2004;36(11):1985-1996.

80. Hood S, Northcote RJ: Cardiac assessment of veteran endurance athletes: A 12 year follow up study. *Br J Sports Med* 1999;33(4):239-243.

81. Morley JE, Reese SS: Clinical implications of the aging heart. *Am J Med* 1989;86(1):77-86.

82. Gluck GS, Bendo JA, Spivak JM: The lumbar spine and low back pain in golf: A literature review of swing biomechanics and injury prevention. *Spine J* 2008;8(5): 778-788.

83. Cole MH, Grimshaw PN: Trunk muscle onset and cessation in golfers with and without low back pain. *J Biomech* 2008;41(13):2829-2833.

84. Lindsay D, Horton J: Comparison of spine motion in elite golfers with and without low back pain. *J Sports Sci* 2002;20(8):599-605.

85. Ting AJ: Running and the older athlete. *Clin Sports Med* 1991;10(2):319-325.

86. Folman Y, Wosk J, Shabat S, Gepstein R: Attenuation of spinal transients at heel strike using viscoelastic heel insoles: An in vivo study. *Prev Med* 2004;39(2): 351-354.

87. Shabat S, Gefen T, Nyska M, Folman Y, Gepstein R: The effect of insoles on the incidence and severity of low back pain among workers whose job involves long-distance walking. *Eur Spine J* 2005;14(6):546-550.

88. Cann AP, Vandervoort AA, Lindsay DM: Optimizing the benefits versus risks of golf participation by older people. *J Geriatr Phys Ther* 2005;28(3):85-92.

Index

Page numbers with *f* indicate figures.
Page numbers with *t* indicate tables.
